Telemedicine and E–Health Services, Policies, and Applications:

Advancements and Developments

Joel J. P. C. Rodrigues
Instituto de Telecomunicações, University of Beira Interior, Portugal

Isabel de la Torre Diez
University of Valladolid, Spain

Beatriz Sainz de Abajo
University of Valladolid, Spain

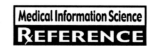

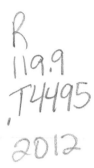

Managing Director: Lindsay Johnston
Senior Editorial Director: Heather A. Probst
Book Production Manager: Sean Woznicki
Development Manager: Joel Gamon
Development Editor: Hannah Abelbeck
Acquisitions Editor: Erika Gallagher
Typesetter: Russell A. Spangler
Cover Design: Nick Newcomer, Lisandro Gonzalez

Published in the United States of America by
    Medical Information Science Reference (an imprint of IGI Global)
    701 E. Chocolate Avenue
    Hershey PA 17033
    Tel: 717-533-8845
    Fax: 717-533-8661
    E-mail: cust@igi-global.com
    Web site: http://www.igi-global.com

Library of Congress Cataloging-in-Publication Data

Telemedicine and E-health services, policies, and applications: advancements and developments / Joel J.P.C. Rodrigues, Isabel de la Torre Diez and Beatriz Sainz de Abajo, Editors.
       p. cm.
  Summary: "This book offers a comprehensive and integrated approach to telemedicine by collecting E-health experiences and applications from around the world and by exploring new developments and trends in medical informatics"-- Provided by publisher.
  Includes bibliographical references and index.
  ISBN 978-1-4666-0888-7 (hardcover) -- ISBN 978-1-4666-0889-4 (ebook) -- ISBN 978-1-4666-0890-0 (print & perpetual access) 1. Telecommunication in medicine. 2. Medical informatics. I. Rodrigues, Joel, 1972- II. De la Torre Diez, Isabel, 1979- III. Sainz de Abajo, Beatriz, 1974-
  R119.9.T4495 2012
  362.10285'4678--dc23
                        2011050943

British Cataloguing in Publication Data
A Cataloguing in Publication record for this book is available from the British Library.

All work contributed to this book is new, previously-unpublished material. The views expressed in this book are those of the authors, but not necessarily of the publisher.

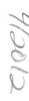

Editorial Advisory Board

List of Reviewers

Table of Contents

Kai Lin, Dalian University of Technology, China
Min Chen, Huazhong University of Science and Technology, China
Joel J. P. C. Rodrigues, Instituto de Telecomunicações, University of Beira Interior, Portugal
Hongwei Ge, Dalian University of Technology, China

Begonya Otal, Institute of Biomedical Research August Pi Sunyer (IDIBAPS), Spain
Luis Alonso, Technical University of Catalonia (UPC), Spain
Christos Verikoukis, Telecommunications Technological Centre of Catalonia (CTTC), Spain

Nuno M. Garcia, Instituto de Telecomunicações, Portugal & University of Beira Interior, Portugal
*   & Lusophone University of Humanities and Technologies, Portugal*
Paula Sofia Sousa, Instituto de Telecomunicações, Portugal & University of Beira Interior, Portugal
Isabel G. Trindade, University of Beira Interior, Portugal
Rui Miguel, University of Beira Interior, Portugal
José Lucas, University of Beira Interior, Portugal

Diana Bri, Universitat Politècnica de Valencia, Spain
Jaime Lloret, Universitat Politècnica de Valencia, Spain
Carlos Turro, Universitat Politècnica de Valencia, Spain
Miguel Garcia, Universitat Politècnica de Valencia, Spain

Detailed Table of Contents

    Kai Lin, Dalian University of Technology, China
    Min Chen, Huazhong University of Science and Technology, China
    Joel J. P. C. Rodrigues, Instituto de Telecomunicações, University of Beira Interior, Portugal
    Hongwei Ge, Dalian University of Technology, China

Body Sensor Networks (BSNs) are formed by the equipped or transplanted sensors in the human body, which can sense the physiology and environment parameters. As a novel e-health technology, BSNs promote the deployment of innovative healthcare monitoring applications. In the past few years, most of the related research works have focused on sensor design, signal processing, and communication protocol. This chapter addresses the problem of system design and data fusion technology over a bandwidth and energy constrained body sensor network. Compared with the traditional sensor network, miniaturization and low-power are more important to meet the requirements to facilitate wearing and long-running operation. As there are strong correlations between sensory data collected from different sensors, data fusion is employed to reduce the redundant data and the load in body sensor networks. To accomplish the complex task, more than one kind of node must be equipped or transplanted to monitor multi-targets, which makes the fusion process become sophisticated. In this chapter, a new BSNs system is designed to complete online diagnosis function. Based on the principle of data fusion in BSNs, we measure and investigate its performance in the efficiency of saving energy. Furthermore, the authors discuss the detection and rectification of errors in sensory data. Then a data evaluation method based on Bayesian estimation is proposed. Finally, the authors verify the performance of the designed system and the validity of the proposed data evaluation method. The chapter is concluded by identifying some open research issues on this topic.

    Begonya Otal, Institute of Biomedical Research August Pi Sunyer (IDIBAPS), Spain
    Luis Alonso, Technical University of Catalonia (UPC), Spain
    Christos Verikoukis, Telecommunications Technological Centre of Catalonia (CTTC), Spain

The aging population and the high expectations towards quality of life in our society lead to the need of more efficient and affordable medical systems and monitoring solutions. The development of wireless

Body Sensor Networks (BSNs) offers a platform to establish such a healthcare monitoring systems. However, BSNs in the healthcare domain operate under conflicting requirements. These are the maintenance of the desired reliability and message latency of data transmissions (i.e. quality of service), while simultaneously maximizing battery lifetime of individual body sensors. In doing so, the characteristics of the entire system, especially the Medium Access Control (MAC) layer, have to be considered. For this reason, this chapter aims for the optimization of the MAC layer by using energy-saving techniques for BSNs. The fact that the IEEE 802.15.4 MAC does not fully satisfy BSNs requirements highlights the need for the design of new scalable MAC solutions, which guarantee low-power consumption to the maximum number of body sensors in high density areas (i.e., in saturation conditions). In order to emphasize IEEE 802.15.4 MAC limitations, this chapter presents a detailed overview of this de facto standard for Wireless Sensor Networks (WSNs), which serves as a link for the introduction and description of the here proposed Distributed Queuing (DQ) MAC protocol for BSN scenarios. Within this framework, an extensive DQ MAC energy-consumption analysis in saturation conditions is presented to be able to evaluate its performance in relation to IEEE 802.5.4 MAC in highly dense BSNs. The obtained results show that the proposed scheme outperforms IEEE 802.15.4 MAC in average energy consumption per information bit, thus providing a better overall performance that scales appropriately to BSNs under high traffic conditions. These benefits are obtained by eliminating back-off periods and collisions in data packet transmissions, while minimizing the control overhead.

Chapter 3

Nuno M. Garcia, Instituto de Telecomunicações, Portugal & University of Beira Interior, Portugal
    & Lusophone University of Humanities and Technologies, Portugal
Paula Sofia Sousa, Instituto de Telecomunicações, Portugal & University of Beira Interior, Portugal
Isabel G. Trindade, University of Beira Interior, Portugal
Rui Miguel, University of Beira Interior, Portugal
José Lucas, University of Beira Interior, Portugal

The use of wearable technologies in medicine and health care has become of important in order to considerably improve benefits for patients and health service providers. Within telemedicine, biomedical clothing plays a crucial role. The main technology advances and the research of the Textile and Paper Materials Research Unit (UMTP) and of the Assisted Living Computing and Telecommunications Laboratory (ALLab) teams, in the area, will be addressed. Issues that remain unsolved will be presented. The chapter presents an overview of the key concepts for telemedicine and the role of textile electrodes and their integration in smart clothing. The development of software algorithms that specifically handle signals that are collected using biomedical clothing, integrating resiliency and a proper set of alarms, is presented and discussed in the context of classical biomedical signal processing. Finally, biomedical clothing design will be discussed in social, psychological, and esthetical contexts.

Chapter 4

Diana Bri, Universitat Politècnica de Valencia, Spain
Jaime Lloret, Universitat Politècnica de Valencia, Spain
Carlos Turro, Universitat Politècnica de Valencia, Spain
Miguel Garcia, Universitat Politècnica de Valencia, Spain

Specific Absorption Rate (SAR) is used to measure the body tissue exposure to electromagnetic fields. This chapter describes how SAR values can be estimated from a deployed Wireless Local Area Network (WLAN). We carried out this work using the Received Signal Strength (RSS) obtained from the access points. This parameter is easily obtained by an ordinary wireless network scanner. RSS variations are measured for a different number of people in the same room and without people. It will allow us to estimate how much energy is absorbed by a group of people and by a single person on average. Moreover, we have included the weight of the people in order to know the RSS lost by kilogram. These measurements were taken at the Higher Polytechnic School of Gandia, Universitat Politècnica de València, Spain, in two placements: the library and inside an anechoic camera.

Chapter 5

Ahmad Taher Azar, Modern Science and Arts University (MSA), Egypt

Biomedical Engineering is a branch that unites engineering methods with biological and medical sciences in order to enhance the quality of our lives. It focuses on understanding intricate systems of living organisms, and on technology development, algorithms, methods, and advanced medical knowledge, while enhancing the conveyance and success of clinical medicine. With engineering principles, biomedical engineering improves the procedures and devices to overcome health care and medical problems by combining both biology and medicine with engineering principals. In the field of Biomedical Engineering, engineers usually need to have background knowledge from such different fields of engineering as electronics, mechanical, and chemical engineering. Specialties in this field like bioinstrumentation, biomechanics, biomaterials, medical imagining, clinical engineering, bioinformatics, telemedicine and rehabilitation engineering, which will be introduced in this chapter together with an overview of the field of biomedical engineering.

Chapter 6

Henrique M. G. Martins, University of Beira Interior, Portugal

This chapter is a theoretical in-depth review of three conceptual groups that serve as the fundamental basis for m-health technology development—both at hardware and software levels—as well as for technology adaptation to work/life practices, and for adoption and usage studies. Objectively the review will focus on the concepts of Time (clock, event, practice-based, and timeless time), experiences of time (subjective construction of the "past," "present," and "future," time aggregation/"episodification" frequency, rhythm, cycles, "spiraling," and mono-polichronicity), space, and mobility (namely physical mobility, remote versus local, modalities of travelling/visiting/ wandering, micro-mobility).

Chapter 7

Mowafa Househ, King Saud Bin Abdul Aziz University for Health Sciences, Saudi Arabia
Elizabeth Borycki, University of Victoria, Canada
Andre Kushniruk, University of Victoria, Canada
Sarah Alofaysan, King Saud Bin Abdul Aziz University for Health Sciences, Saudi Arabia

The mHealth field focuses on the use of mobile technologies to support hospital care, healthy behavior, patient monitoring, and educational awareness. It is a new field that is developing rapidly, with thousands of mHealth applications developed within the last two years alone. In this chapter, the authors discuss the current state of, and the opportunities and challenges within, the mHealth field. They also introduce the term Mobile Social Networking Healthcare (MSN-Healthcare), which they define as follows: "The use of mobile health applications that incorporate social networking tools to promote healthy behaviors and awareness among patient groups and communities." This concept has not been introduced in previous literature. This chapter is organized as follows: 1) introduction and background of mHealth; 2) opportunities for the implementation of mHealth in relation to chronic disease management, the education of health professionals, the needs of health professionals, and the decision-making process for patients and clinicians; 3) challenges concerning implementation and usability, information needs, and interactions with clinical work; 4) current application uses; and 5) future trends and conclusion.

Chapter 8

Ubiquitous Health (U-Health) smart homes are intelligent spaces capable of observing and correctly recognizing the activities and health statuses of their inhabitants (context) to provide the appropriate support to achieve an overall sense of health and well-being in their inhabitants' daily lives. With the intrinsic heterogeneity and large number of sources of context information, aggregating and reasoning on low-quality raw sensed data may result in conflicting and erroneous evaluations of situations, affecting directly the reliability of the U-Health systems. In this environment, the evaluation and verification of Quality of Context (QoC) information plays a central role in improving the consistency and correctness of context-aware U-Health applications. Therefore, the objective of this chapter is to highlight the impact of QoC on the correct behavior of U-Health systems, and introduce and analyze the existing approaches of modeling, evaluating, and using QoC to improve its context-aware decision-making support.

Chapter 9

The tremendous growth in the use of Web 2.0 technologies, interactive computer technologies, electronic records, and mobile devices for delivery of e-health necessitates attention to design. Designing e-health requires consideration of research, including best practices embodied in design principles. This chapter reviews key background information, including central definitions, concepts, and research, followed by a presentation of 9 key considerations that are recommended for guiding the design of e-health messages. An illustrative case example demonstrates how a typology that codifies design principles gave rise to a research tool that permits the evaluation of health care websites. The case example underscores the important role of findings from research evaluations in creating a feedback loop for designers, permitting research to inform refinements in design. Overall, the 9 key considerations suggest a new paradigm for design, while also giving rise to corresponding recommendations for future research to support evolution in the field of e-health.

Health surveillance practices date back to decades ago. Traditionally, such practices to gather health data have been manual; more recently, however, computerized health information systems have been applied to enhance and facilitate health information acquisition for surveillance. The so-called *health surveillance systems* put in practice the systematic acquisition of health data, which is stored and processed for expert analysis. This chapter makes a survey of health surveillance systems dedicated to syndromic and epidemiological surveillance, identifying the different design and technological strategies adopted in the development of such systems. The aims of such a survey are: (1) to provide practitioners with some information about the collective expertise of health information system architects in the design and implementation of syndromic and epidemiological surveillance systems; and (2) to pave the way for the establishment of software product lines dedicated to such systems.

Chapter 11

The system presented in this chapter is mainly destined to offer support and to monitor chronic and elderly patients. In accordance with the new tendencies in the field, it integrates innovative components for data acquisition systems, Web-based virtual instrumentation, personalized user interfaces, and relational data in a complex, modular, flexible, and opened structure. Compared with other similar integrated communication systems, which are based on Wi-Fi technology, the presented one has as distinctive features: small dimensions, low power consumption, and a considerable autonomy. A large set of experiments and the corresponding results illustrates the functionality of the configurable virtual web instrument principle materialized in the E-Health Monitoring and Supervising System (EMSS) that has many possible applications. As an example, a cheap, easy to use, and personalized support destined to improve the quality of life for subjects suffering from chronic diseases or elderly patients was chosen. The implementation of the complete application included a model for gesture recognition, which allows the classification and assessment of the characteristics of the subject's movement, highlighting even small progresses of the monitored patients.

Chapter 12

In this chapter, the authors review software that enables the proper management of EHR. The different types of software share the feature of being open source and offer the best opportunity in health care to developing countries—an overall integrated approach. The authors analyze the main free software programs (technical features, programming languages, places for introduction, etc.). Then they focus on the description and the comparison of the three most important open source software programs EHR (OpenMRS, OpenVistA, and OpenEMR) that are installed on two operating systems (Linux Ubuntu and Windows). Finally, the authors show the results of the various parameters measured in these systems after using different Web browsers. The results show us how the three main EHR applications work depending on which operating system is installed and which web browser is used.

Peter J. Hawrylak, The University of Tulsa, USA

Nakeisha Schimke, The University of Tulsa, USA

John Hale, The University of Tulsa, USA

Mauricio Papa, The University of Tulsa, USA

Electronic healthcare or E-Health promises to offer better care at lower cost. This is critical as the cost of healthcare continues to increase and as the population ages. Radio Frequency Identification (RFID) technology is one form of wireless technology that will be part of the E-Health environment. RFID provides the ability to identify, track, and monitor patients and staff members. This enables better resource allocation, reduction of medical errors, and increased independence for patients. One part of E-Health is the Electronic Medical Record (EMR). New developments in RFID technology now enable the storage of all or part of the EMR on an RFID tag that remains with the patient. This chapter investigates the use of RFID in E-Health, how RFID can be used to store the EMR, and the security and privacy risks associated with using RFID to store the EMR.

Josipa Kern, University of Zagreb, Croatia & Andrija Štampar School of Public Health, Croatia

Marijan Erceg, Croatian National Institute of Public Health, Croatia

Tamara Poljičanin, Merkur Clinical Hospital, Croatia

Slavica Sović, University of Zagreb, Croatia & Andrija Štampar School of Public Health, Croatia

Kristina Fišter, University of Zagreb, Croatia & Andrija Štampar School of Public Health, Croatia

Davor Ivanković, University of Zagreb, Croatia & Andrija Štampar School of Public Health, Croatia

Silvije Vuletić, University of Zagreb, Croatia & Andrija Štampar School of Public Health, Croatia

The *Public Health Surveillance System* (PHSS) is defined as the ongoing, systematic collection, analysis, interpretation and dissemination of health-related data essential to the planning, implementation, and evaluation of public health practice. It serves as an early warning system, guides public health policy and strategies, documents the impact of an intervention or progress towards specified public health targets/ goals, and understands and monitors the epidemiology of a condition to set priorities and guide public health policy and strategies. For this purpose, the PHSS should: be ICT-based and comprehensive with clearly defined sources, volumes, and standards of data; include all the stakeholders with information they produce, with enough flexibility in the dynamic of constructing indicators; be safe and able to produce information on demand and on time; and be able to act as a risk management system by providing warnings/reminders/alerts to prevent unwanted events.

Riccardo Spinelli, Università degli Studi di Genova, Italy

Clara Benevolo, Università degli Studi di Genova, Italy

In this chapter, the authors analyze the impact of the new ICT-driven economic paradigm—the digital economy—on healthcare services. The increasing adoption of ICT in healthcare has been very fruitful and has led to the innovative approach to healthcare practice commonly known as e-health. Here the authors first propose a framework, consisting of six elements, whose mutual interaction outlines the structure and the dynamics of the digital economy. Then, a classification scheme of services is presented, which considers their characteristics and their delivery modes; this scheme supports understanding the way in which the adoption of ICT impacts healthcare services. Finally, an overall explanatory outline is constructed that allows one to analyze and understand the origins, implications, and future perspectives of the changes that ICT has brought to healthcare services. Examples of e-health applications are traced back to the building blocks of the framework, isolating the impact of each driver on their structure, configuration, and delivery modes.

Chapter 16

Maria J. Treurnicht, Stellenbosch University, South Africa
Liezl van Dyk, Stellenbosch University, South Africa

Telemedicine could effectively aid hospital referral systems in bringing specialized care to rural communities. South Africa has identified telemedicine as part of its primary health care strategic plan, but similar to many other developing countries, the successful implementation of telemedicine programs is a daunting challenge. One of the contributing factors is the insufficient evidence that telemedicine is a cost-effective alternative. Furthermore, many telemedicine services are implemented without a thorough needs assessment. Throughout this chapter, the authors investigate the use of medical informatics in quantitative telemedicine needs assessments. A framework is introduced to direct implementation policies towards a proven clinical need rather than pushing technology into practise. This clinical-pull strategy aims to reduce the amount of failed projects, by providing decision support to implement appropriate technologies that have the potential to contribute towards better quality healthcare.

Chapter 17

Xiaohong W. Gao, Middlesex University, UK
Martin Loomes, Middlesex University, UK
Richard Comley, Middlesex University, UK

In this chapter, a comprehensive review of the development of telemedicine in China, with the focus on the establishment of PACS (Picture Archiving and Communications Systems) and image-guided tele-surgery, will be accounted for together with a comparative study in reference to the counterparts in Europe, leading to a framework of a sustainable, scalable, and flexible e-health infrastructure for the future global digital (paper-less) hospital. The study is drawn from the first-hand knowledge gained through the conduction of a 3-year networking project on *Telemedicine: Tele-Imaging in Medicine* (TIME, 2005-2007) funded by the European Commission under the Asia-link programme. It is the authors' hope that this chapter resonates with the future prospect of telemedicine by providing the right contents, at the right time and to the right extent, especially when the implementations taking place are in countries with disparate economic development.

Preface

E-health field has a great potential. According to the World Health Organisation (WHO), e-health is the combined use of electronic communication and information technology in the health sector. Moreover, it enables a safer, higher quality, more equitable and sustainable health system. The book seeks to show interesting e-health experiences and applications around the world. It wants to take account of developments and trends that are taking place in the area of Medical Informatics and it offers s a comprehensive and integrated approach to healthcare. The mission of the book is to be a fundamental source for the advancement of knowledge, application, and practice in the interdisciplinary areas of healthcare, e-health, m-health, u-health, sensors, biomedical engineering, and telemedicine.

Due to its grounding in research and theory evidence, this book is designed for use in graduate courses in health management, medicine, nursing, health professionals and medical informatics. The book can help to e-health contents, applications and interesting experiences. It is an important way to communicate e-health concepts.

The book will address innovative concepts and critical issues in the emerging field of e-health and it treats a range of services that are at the edge of medicine/healthcare and information technology. It is formed by 17 chapters. Chapter 1 addresses the problem of system design and data fusion technology over a bandwidth and energy constrained body sensor network. Compare with the traditional sensor network, miniaturization and low-power are more important to meet the requirements of facilitate wearing and long-running operation. Chapter 2 aims for the optimization of the MAC layer by using energy-saving techniques for BSNs and presents a detailed overview of this de facto standard for WSNs, which serves as a link for the introduction and description of our here proposed Distributed Queuing (DQ) MAC protocol for BSN scenarios. Chapter 3 presents an overview of the key concepts for Telemedicine, the role of textile electrodes and its integration in smart clothing. Moreover, biomedical clothing design will be discussed in social, psychological and esthetical contexts. Chapter 4 analyzes the Specific Absorption Rate (SAR) of the human body when it is exposed to WLANs devices working at the 2.4GHz radio frequency ISM band. In order to make these measurements we will use a controlled indoor place and an uncontrolled environment where no variable can be fixed.

In the field of Biomedical Engineering, engineers usually need to have background knowledge from different fields of engineering as electronics, mechanical and chemical engineering. Specialties in this field like bioinstrumentation, biomechanics, biomaterials, medical imagining, clinical engineering, bioinformatics, telemedicine and rehabilitation engineering, which will be introduced in Chapter 5 together with an overview of the field of biomedical engineering. Chapter 6 provides a theoretical review of three conceptual groups that serve as fundamental basis for m-health technology development as well as for technology adaptation to work/life practices, and for adoption and usage studies. Chapter 7 focuses on the current state, opportunities, and challenges of the mHealth field. The evaluation and verification of

Quality of Context (QoC) information play a central role to improve the consistency and correctness of context-aware U-Health applications. Therefore, the objective of Chapter 8 is to highlight the impact of QoC on the correct behavior of U-Health systems, and introduce and analyze the existing approaches of modeling, evaluating, and using QoC to improve its context-aware decision-making support. Chapter 9 reviews key background information, including central definitions, concepts, and research, followed by a presentation of 9 key considerations that are recommended for guiding the design of e-health messages.

Chapter 10 makes a survey of HISes dedicated to syndromic and epidemiological surveillance, identifying the different design and technological strategies adopted in the development of such systems. The adopted methodology for structuring this survey comprises the definition of a set of criteria for comparative analysis of the discussed HISes as well as the presentation and comparison of such HISes in the light of the defined criteria. Chapter 11 presents a system destined to offer support and to monitor the chronic and elderly patients. Compared with other similar integrated communication systems which are based on the Wi-Fi technology, the presented one has as distinctive features small dimensions, low power consumption and a considerable autonomy. Chapter 12 reviews a set of software that enables the proper management of EHRs. The authors analyze the main free software programs (technical features, programming languages, places for introduction, etc.) and they focus on the description and the comparison of the three most important open source software programs EHR (OpenMRS, OpenVistA, and OpenEMR) that are installed on different operating sytems. Chapter 13 investigates the use of RFID in E-Health, how RFID can be used to store the EMR, and the security and privacy risks associated with using RFID to store the EMR.

Chapter 14 presents different aspects about Public Health Surveillance System. This system is defined as the ongoing, systematic collection, analysis and interpretation of health-related data essential to the planning, implementation, and evaluation of public health practice. Chapter 15 analyzes the impact of the new ICT-driven economic paradigm—the digital economy—on healthcare services. The authors present a classification scheme of services which considers their characteristics and their delivery modes; this scheme supports understanding the way in which the adoption of ICT impacts on healthcare services. Chapter 16 argues the case for using medical informatics in needs assessments, towards evidence-based telemedicine management and clinical-pull approaches for implementation. The aim is to reduce telemedicine projects that employ unnecessary systems and equipment, by providing them with an alternative for better planning, prior to implementation. Chapter 17 gives a detailed account on the latest development of telemedicine and PACS systems with a focus on China. In comparison with their counterparts in Europe, the results are drawn from the completed TIME project funded by EU and the initial work conducted from the newly funded FP7 project WIDTH on *Infrastructure for the Digital Hospital*.

Acknowledgment

The editors of the book *Telemedicine and E-Health Services, Policies and Applications: Advancements and Developments* would like to thank to all the authors for their ideas and excellent work. We appreciate the originality of their works. Moreover, we would like to express our deep appreciation to our colleagues for their excellent review of the book chapters. The editors acknowledge the remarkable collaboration and the effort of all the reviewers to ensure the technical quality of this book.

Finally, but not least, this book is the result of great teamwork. For this we would like to thank all the efforts of the editorial staff at IGI Global.

Joel J. P. C. Rodrigues
Instituto de Telecomunicações, University of Beira Interior, Portugal

Isabel de la Torre Díez
University of Valladolid, Spain

Beatriz Sainz de Abajo
University of Valladolid, Spain

Chapter 1
System Design and Data Fusion in Body Sensor Networks

Kai Lin
Dalian University of Technology, China

Min Chen
Huazhong University of Science and Technology, China

Joel J. P. C. Rodrigues
Instituto de Telecomunicações, University of Beira Interior, Portugal

Hongwei Ge
Dalian University of Technology, China

ABSTRACT

Body Sensor Networks (BSNs) are formed by the equipped or transplanted sensors in the human body, which can sense the physiology and environment parameters. As a novel e-health technology, BSNs promote the deployment of innovative healthcare monitoring applications. In the past few years, most of the related research works have focused on sensor design, signal processing, and communication protocol. This chapter addresses the problem of system design and data fusion technology over a bandwidth and energy constrained body sensor network. Compared with the traditional sensor network, miniaturization and low-power are more important to meet the requirements to facilitate wearing and long-running operation. As there are strong correlations between sensory data collected from different sensors, data fusion is employed to reduce the redundant data and the load in body sensor networks. To accomplish the complex task, more than one kind of node must be equipped or transplanted to monitor multi-targets, which makes the fusion process become sophisticated. In this chapter, a new BSNs system is designed to complete online diagnosis function. Based on the principle of data fusion in BSNs, we measure and investigate its performance in the efficiency of saving energy. Furthermore, the authors discuss the detection and rectification of errors in sensory data. Then a data evaluation method based on Bayesian estimation is proposed. Finally, the authors verify the performance of the designed system and the validity of the proposed data evaluation method. The chapter is concluded by identifying some open research issues on this topic.

DOI: 10.4018/978-1-4666-0888-7.ch001

INTRODUCTION

In these years, many technologies have experienced great development, including biomedicine, wireless sensor network, multi-media process, intelligent information process, and so on. As a dominant application framework for the evolving body sensor network technology, human health monitoring is increasingly emerging by using both in-body and out-of-body sensors. Body Sensor Networks (BSNs) are formed by the equipped or transplanted sensors in the human body. These sensors need to collect the important physiology signals (temperature, blood sugar, blood pressure), human activity or action signals, and the environment; then process this information and transmit it to the base station. Being a new solution for universal medical care, disease monitoring, and prevention, the purpose of BSNs is to provide a public computational platform integrated with hardware, software, and wireless communication technology. It becomes ubiquitous and the marketing opportunities for advanced consumer electronics and services will be expanded extensively (Tan & Wang, 2008; Pantelopoulos & Bourbakis, 2010). More and more interests in the design and development of BSN systems for applications of improving people's daily life are growing, which also leads to the introduction of other technologies into BSNs, such as RFID technology, Zigbee, Bluetooth, video surveillance system, WPAN, WLAN, Internet, and cellular network.

According to the inquiry results of World Health Organization (WHO), aging population is becoming a significant problem, which causes millions of people to suffer from obesity or chronic diseases. This trend results in the decline of service quality and the healthcare system overloaded (Venkatasubramanian, Gupta, 2010). BSNs can be used to solve this problem by being applied to medical care, health regeneration, aiding the aged and disabled. Additionally, BSNs can be extended to entertainment like cartoon industry, dance design and training; physical culture like the simulation and analysis of fencing education; other industry like automobile engine, state monitoring and failure detection of machine equipment; even the military area like monitoring and health of soldiers; or in the public area of society like large scale incident and psychological relief. In summary, the following typical applications will benefit from the advanced integration of BSNs and emerging wireless technologies:

- Remote health/fitness monitoring: Health and motion information are monitored in real-time, and delivered to nearby diagnosis or storage devices, through which data can be forwarded to health service center and diagnosed by doctors for further processing.
- Military and sports training: For example, motion sensors can be worn at both hands and elbows, for accurate feature extraction of soldiers and sports players' movements.
- Interactive gaming: BSNs enable game players to perform actual body movements, such as boxing and shooting, that can be feedback to the corresponding gaming console, thereby enhancing their entertainment experiences.
- Personal information sharing: Private or business information can be stored in body sensors for many applications in daily life such as shopping and information exchange.
- Secure authentication: This application involves resorting to both physiological and behavioral biometrics schemes, such as facial patterns, fingerprints, and iris recognition. The potential problems, e.g., proneness to forgery and duplicability, have motivated the investigations into new physical/behavioral characteristics of the human body, e.g., Electroencephalography (EEG) and gait, and multimodal biometric systems.

Figure 1. Application of BSNs

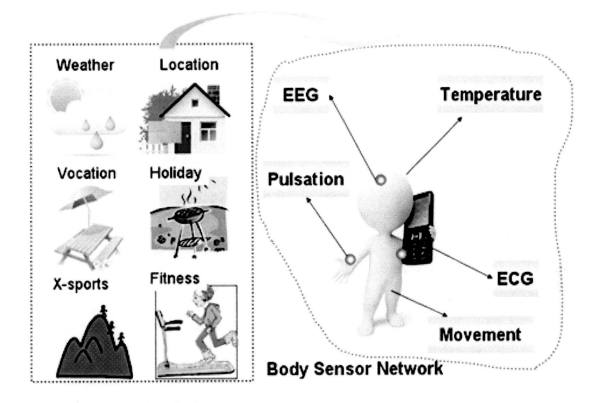

Figure 1 shows some applications of BSNs, which changes the communication method among people by connecting the logical and physical worlds together. People can get their health situations directly from exchanging physiological information, location information, entertainment information, movement information, weather information, and environment information.

There are several special advantages introduced by using BSNs as followings:

- **Flexibility:** Non-invasive sensors can be used to automatically monitor physiological readings, which being forwarded to nearby devices, such as a cell phone, a wrist watch, a headset, a PDA, a laptop, or a robot based on the application needs
- **Effectiveness and efficiency:** the signals that body sensors provide can be effectively processed to obtain reliable and accurate physiological estimations. In addition, their ultra-low power consumption makes their batteries long-lasting
- **Cost-effective:** With the increasing demand of body sensors in the consumer electronics market, more sensors will be mass-produced at a relatively low cost

Currently, many BSN systems have already been developed for different applications, especially for using body sensors to collect patient information and by deploying diverse wireless networking systems for enhanced diagnosis assistance and action handling. The Duofertility Project (DuoFertility, 2009) was already developed as a trail commercial system for monitoring and analyzing female body temperatures. This system can detect and calculate both ovulation and fertile periods. It measures a female's body skin temperature by placing a sensor reader under her arm. The sensor device under the arm only collects the skin temperature measurements. Aiming to establish a correlation between core body temperature and skin temperature, ANOM project integrated their system with a skin temperature sensor (Anliker, et al., 2004). Unfortunately, this attempt was unsuccessful because the correlation between core body temperature and skin temperature could not be established as the skin temperature could vary with change in environmental conditions. The above-mentioned projects based their temperature studies on measurement and analysis of skin temperature. However, the skin temperature could be influenced by environmental conditions as reported in Campbell (2008) and Brengelmann (2000).

These existing systems are not adaptable to special environments, particularly the cold region. Hence, new strategies of application systems need to be developed. In this chapter, we explore how to use BSNs for healthcare monitoring in cold region, which refers to those areas with temperatures below zero degrees. BSNs ought to simultaneously collect the accurate surrounding environment information and human characteristics of the monitoring targets, like heartbeat and blood pressure. The incorrect judgment of the surrounding environment will result in the wrong evaluation to human healthcare. Therefore, the monitoring and process in cold regions are facing the following challenges:

- The environment condition changes in uncertain ways and must be observed by more than one single parameter.
- Human being as a complex creature system, it is also the comprehensive reflection of multi-characteristic. These multi-characteristics have complicated association and subordinating relations.
- The parameters of environment and human characteristic change randomly in a certain range.

Considering the deployment of sensor nodes in high density, some redundant sensory data will generate, which results in the waste of energy and bandwidth. For the sake of improving the resource utilization, data fusion is employed in BSNs with some benefits: Firstly, as the monitoring area is overlapped, energy consumption can be saved by deleting abundant data and reducing transmission energy. Secondly, as the accuracy of one sensor node is low, more accurate data can be obtained after fusing several sensory data. Thirdly, the data fusion is beneficial for improving efficiency of data collection. The reduction of data transmission can decrease the transmission conflict and delay. Due to these functions, data fusion becomes an indispensable technology for BSNs and can be combined with other technologies.

In this chapter, the state-of-the-art of the related schemes are summarized and compared. We analyze the requirement of BSNs for monitoring healthcare and design the available system model. Then we discuss the data fusion process in BSNs, and analyze the effect of saving energy by a fusion process. To eliminate the inaccuracy of sensory information during data collecting, we adopt Bayesian estimation where the time and spatial distribution are considered. This method can achieve the reliable evaluation of the information in uncertain, multi-source, and inhomogeneous. Furthermore, we analyze the effect of detection and rectification of errors in sensory data. Finally, we verify the performance of designed system and the validity of the proposed data evaluation method based on Bayesian estimation. Some of these works have been published on ICC 2011(Lin, et al., 2011).

The remainder of this chapter is organized as follows. Section 2 presents some related works, Section 3 introduces BSN architecture and system design. Section 4 describes data fusion in BSN. Section 5 presents the simulation and numerical results. We summarize our work and conclude the chapter in Section 7 after mentioning the future research directions in Section 6.

RELATED WORK

Our work is closely related to the system design in BSNs, data fusion in BSNs, the context-aware mechanism in BSNs, detection and rectification of errors in sensory data. We will give a brief review of the works in these four aspects.

Related Work in System Design in BSNs

The wearable factor is an important problem in body sensor network design. Currently, many researchers have developed many valuable application systems. Chen et al. designed a four level health condition monitoring system consisting of communication system and control system (Chen, et al., 2007). Vehkaojal et al. designed sport-monitoring system with portable sensors to complete the synergy process of physical movement, where the environment sensors are simultaneously used to simplify the data process. Liang et al. designed a real-time monitoring system of human activities with data fusion in body sensor networks, by distinguishing and tracing of the embedded mathematical module and estimating the ordinary movement of the targets (Liang, et al., 2007). Tatbul et al. capsulated the embedded sensors in a unit, measuring the physical parameters to monitor the health condition of soliders (Tatbul, et al., 2004), physical environment, low band, and personal area based on forwarding which result in the uncertainty and accuracy of this module. Javanov et al. traced the body sensor network by the health recovery with computer-aided design (Jovanov, et al., 2005). This system can analyze the real-time data, supply direction, and send feedback. All the recorded information can be sent back to medical service and be seamlessly aggregated to the medical information card for the following database study. As the surface temperature changes with the environment, the relationship is hard to establish, ANOM finally withdraws from the medical system. Jones et al.

developed a monitoring system aimed at American football sportsmen (Jones, 2006), including "wireless pill" and wireless data readings. According to the surface temperature shown in the readings, the coach and team can arrange the proper rest. Rodrigues et al. compared the node feature feedback in body sensor networks and proposed an interface classification method based on characteristic parameters, which have been applied in sensor equipments (Rodrigues, et al., 2011). Chen et al. investigated the lock system to prevent the trailer and truck by MRAC control technology, where MARAC simulated how to deal with the lock in case of different loading (Chen & Shieh, 2011).

Related Work in Data Fusion in BSNs

In the real application, BSN will generate a large amount of physiological parameters for processing, transmitting, and visiting. The basic problem is how to operate this data. The significance of BSN is not only to improve the reaction speed but also reduce the data amount to increase the lifetime of node and BSN. Additionally, data fusion can filter the noise component and make the prediction and reasoning. Data fusion can be classified from different viewpoints. There are three types of typical data: (1) information content, (2) the relationship between data fusion, and (3) application data semantic meaning.

Judging from the information content before and after fusion process, the data fusion can be divided into lossless fusion and loss fusion. In lossless fusion, all the detailed data information is saved. The usual process is to eliminate the abundant data. According to information theory, the total information and entropy is limited by lossless data fusion while some information detail might be ignored and data quality is reduced, which can reduce storage and transmission amount to save more energy. The upper bound of information loss is maintaining the necessary data of total information. Many loss fusions aim at the data requirement of intra-network.

Depending on the operation level, the data fusion can be divided into pixel level fusion, feature level fusion, decision-making level fusion. Here, the pixel level fusion is the bottom level facing to data. The operation target includes pixel data classification, combination, and reduction of the abundant data. The feature-level fusion abstracts some data characterization and decision-making level fusion can complete the judgment and classification. By some simple logical operation, the final decision can be obtained. As the calculating power and energy are limited for sensor node, there is less decision-making level fusion process in the current applications of WSNs.

In terms of the semantics of data, the data fusion can be divided into application dependent fusion and independent fusion. The application dependent fusion should understand the semantic of data from the application layer and obtain the maximum compression. However, this may result in a large information loss. Additionally, the semantic problem of multi-layer causes more difficulty to protocol stack. For the independent fusion, it is not necessary to understand the data semantic of application layer but fuse the data from data link layer directly. This technology realizes the data fusion as an independent level and simple relationships between different layers. As the data fusion is preceded by the data from different layers, these methods will not lose any information. However, the data fusion efficiency is lower than that of the application dependent fusion.

Either in research or application, BSNs are a sub-branch or sub-group of WSN. Many data fusion technologies in WSN are also suitable for BSN. In the data fusion of BSN, relative technologies include suspection method, estimation method, and characteristic mapping method. In general, the suspections are applied in the strategy fusion based on the perception of environment, such as Bayesian prediction, fuzzy logic, neural network, adductive reasoning, and semantic data fusion. From the viewpoint of estimation, the data fusion technology includes maximum likelihood estimation, maximum a posteriori estimation, the least squares estimation, moving average filtering, Kalman filtering, and particle filtering. To some BSN applications, it is impossible to directly use the original sensory data. In this case, the characteristic data of different environments can be abstracted to generate a special reflection. The data fusions in BSN have made great achievements, aggregate attachment, average value integration, and principal component analysis. Other technologies includes Gauss mix module, Bayesian network, and Markov module. The existing data fusion in the sensor network depends on the suspection of classification. Most data fusion is adopted to fuse or preprocess the generated data, and then a Bayesian network is used to classify the precepted data, or use the Kalman filtering and Markov model to identify a series of actions and activities.

Krishnamachari et al. investigated the impact of data aggregation on various networking metrics by surveying the existing data aggregation protocols in WSNs (Krishnamachari, 2002). Intanagonwiwat et al. proposed a novel approach that adjusts aggregation points in order to increase the amount of path sharing and reduced energy consumption (Intanagonwiwat, et al., 2002). The results suggested that greedy aggregation could achieve up to 45% energy savings over opportunistic aggregation in high-density networks, without adversely impacting latency or robustness. Pattem et al. proposed several data aggregation techniques to study the performance of various data aggregation schemes across the range of spatial correlations (Pattem, Krishnamachari, & Govindan, 2004). The analysis and simulations revealed that the characteristics of optimal routing with compression did depend on the level of correlation. Specially, there existed a practical static clustering scheme, which could provide near-optimal performance for a wide range of spatial correlations. Yu et al. employed the data aggregation tree to extract the packet flow (Yu, Krishnamachari, & Prasanna, 2004). Goel et al. proposed a hierarchical matching algorithm, which resulted in an aggregation tree with simultaneous logarithmic approximation for all concave aggregation functions (Goel & Estrin, 2003). In this model, each node can theoretically obtain the joint entropy of its subtree to achieve the maximal aggregation ratio. Anandkumar et al. (2009) presented a novel formulation for optimal sensor selection and in-network fusion for distributed inference known as the Prize-Collecting Data Fusion (PCDF) in terms of the optimal trade-off between the costs of aggregating the selected set of sensor measurements and the resulting inference performance at the fusion center (Xing, et al., 2009). PCDF is then analyzed under a correlation model specified by a Markov Random Field (MRF) with a given dependency graph. For a special class of dependency graphs, a constrained version of PCDF reduces to the prize-collecting Steiner tree on an augmented graph. In this case, an approximation algorithm is given with an approximation ratio that depends only on the number of profitable cliques in the dependency graph. Zhang and Shen (2009) formulate the energy consumption balancing problem as an optimal transmitting data distribution problem by combining the ideas of corona-based network division and mixed-routing strategy together with data aggregation. Luo, Liu, and Das (2006) proposed a routing algorithm called Minimum Fusion Steiner Tree (MFST) for data gathering with aggregation in wireless sensor networks. MFST not only optimizes data transmission cost, but also incorporates the cost for data fusion, which could be significant for emerging sensor networks with vectorial data and security requirements. They further found that fusion costs were comparable to those of communications for certain applications (Luo, et al., 2006). Motivated by the limitations of MFST, they designed a novel routing algorithm, called Adaptive Fusion Steiner Tree (AFST) for energy efficient data gathering in sensor networks.

Related Work in Context-Aware Mechanism in BSNs

Context-aware calculation can explain the physical and biochemical signals, providing the necessary movement condition and environment information for on-line disease diagnosis. The typical research is: the context-aware BSN system with new proposed algorithm, like that Li et al. presented a QRS BSN system based on context-aware (Chaczko, et al., 2008) and Chaczko et al. presented home aware and health monitoring system (Lenzini, 2009). Lenzini et al. introduced a software structure used for context-aware, the specialty is the authentication dependent on trust and context-aware. Context-aware is responsible for combining the different data scenarios to solve the potential conflicts and decide the activity of human activity (Patel & Schmidt, 2011). Patel et al. discussed how to manage the download in the Web robot interface (Arroyo-Valles, et al., 2011). Arroyo et al. use the forwarding structure established by random tool to solve the different context-aware. The structure parameters include the power efficiency, energy consumption of retransmission, and information importance (Atallah, et al., 2007). The second type is the context-aware technology for identifying human activities, like Atallah et al. proposed the behavior model based on hidden Markov which can effectively monitor the ordinary activities of the patients at home (Pansiot, et al., 2007). Pansion et al. combined the environment sensor based on Blob with ear wearable sports sensor to identify the accuracy of activity (Stauffer & Grimson, 2000). Stauffer et al. proposed the real-time tracing learning algorithm (Rinderle-Ma, Reichert, & Jurisch, 2011), Rinderle et al. introduced the composition of life cycle in network service and the corresponding characteristics, and gave the definition of design, run, and development (Van & Gellersen, 2004). The third is the direct or indirect SOM technology to realize the application of context-aware. Bao et al. proposed the classification method for the complicated diseases to measure the heart rate (Thiemjarus, Lo, & Yang, 2006). Thiemjarus et al. established the SOM configuration to solve the categories separation, and nodes extension, and proposed a distributed suspection model based on STSOM (Heimbigner, 2011). Now, the context-aware technology in BSNs is still facing challenges from the disorder movement and environment instantaneous.

Related Work in Detection and Rectification of Errors in Sensory Data in BSNs

Limited by price, the accuracy of data collection from sensor nodes in BSN is low and easily disrupted. For example, disordered respiration and sudden movement can generate the abnormal signal with low signal-to-noise, which can influence the accuracy of gathered data from physiology and movement. Additionally, the instantaneous changing of the monitoring environment can also affect the gathered data. Hence, the feature is uncertain and fuzzy. It is important to measure and rectify the gathered data. Palpanas et al. designed a model method for abnormal detection and predicted the behavior of normal models, and the measured error is the abnormal data (Palpanas, et al., 2003). The method is highly dependent on the management of sensors, other sensors in the group, detection ability of abnormal models. Branch et al. proposed an intra-network structure for detecting the abnormal behaviors among neighbor nodes (Branch, et al., 2006), where the setting and cost of ordinary parameters are expensive. Subramaniam et al. proposed the on-line anomaly detection structure, each sensor equipped with one slider window can predict the data distribution. This method with high miss rate needs extra storage space (Subramaniam, et al., 2006). Hida et al. proposed an anomaly detection method for inquiry process to improve the reliability of the measured results. All the above mentioned methods aim to the single data without the consideration of space similarity. Pessi et al. analyzed the lightning detection and lightning sensor image data from TRMM and compared with latent heat and vapor data from TRMM. This research is helpful to replace the sparse data of lightning rate in ocean area to vapor data supported NWP models (Pessi & Businger, 2009). The movement of nodes will bring the error to the system detection, when the node is in some region, the system might misjudge the position of the node. Kim et al. proposed a method by detecting the connection state and power lifetime of mobile nodes to monitor the input and output state (Kim & Chung, 2010). Grubb introduced the prediction equation of glomerulus filtration rate, combined with other body parameters to measure the loss of renal function (Grubb, 2010). The insufficient is that the instantaneous abnormal is the absolute abnormal, while the BSN needs to comprehensively consider the gathered data in the target area.

ARCHITECTURE AND SYSTEM DESIGN OF BSN

Architecture of BSNs

BSNs supply a kind of service platform integrated with hardware, software, and wireless communication technology, which can achieve the ubiquitous monitoring of healthcare. Sensors are made to easily wear and transplant, and operate with low energy consumption. Different sensors are used to collect important physiology signals. Here, all the monitoring physiology signals are divided into: continuous physiology signals that the waves are generally the most, like electromyography and pulse wave, corresponding to EEG scanning, vision sensor, electrocardiogram, and so on; discrete periodical physiological signals that include temperature, blood pressure, oxygen saturation, and other physiological parameters, corresponding to temperature sensor, blood pressure monitoring, and pulse detection sensors. Additionally, human activities, action signals, and environment information also need to be collected and processed, and then transmitted to the base station.

Sensors can be classified to three types according to their position in BSNs, named as implantable sensors like implantable biosensors and inhalable sensor (e.g. camera pill); wearable sensors like glucose sensor, noninvasive blood pressure sensor, oxygen saturation sensor, and temperature sensor; surrounded sensor that is distributed near the targets and used to identify human activity and environment. Based on the above classification, BSNs can be divided into three types: (1) The implanted BSNs, (2) The wearable BSNs, (3) The hybrid BSNs.

The architecture of BSNs is the logical organization of the equipment in the system, which generally includes star, mesh, ring, and bus topology. The selection of topology can affect the system performance, like energy consumption, flow load, robustness of failure node, and so on. In general, the star topology and the mesh topology are corresponding to one hop and multi-hop wireless communication method, respectively. In large scale BSNs, the selection of topology should consider many factors with the real application. Mesh and hybrid topologies are suitable for this situation and have great research value. Additionally, the mesh and hybrid topology can improve the reliability of a network, then intelligently identify and monitor by the distributed interference method or strategy.

Combined with different BSNs topologies, Figure 2 shows a comprehensive architecture of BSNs. The architecture consists of three layers. The first layer consists of a group of monitoring sensors. These nodes can measure and proceed the physiological and the surrounded environment information of human targets, then transmit this data to the BSN head/master node in the second level. The second layer includes mobile personal server, or BSN head/mater nodes, or sink node/base station. They are responsible for the communication with the outside network, analyzing the local data, detecting the abnormal physiological situation, executing safety tasks, sending warnings, collecting the generated data from the first layer, and managing each sensor node and equipment. They can be hosted by portable PDA or cell phone with enough power supply. Moreover, it can be used as a router between node and server, connect the short distance network (Bluetooth/ZigBee/WiFi) or long distance network (GSM/GPRS/3G). The third layer includes the outside network, which can supply many kinds of applications in long-distance, like the electro-medical records of registered users.

Requirement for System Design

In this world, many regions are in severe environments, such as cold regions, with the properties of low temperatures, long periods of cold time, many cold waves, and huge temperature shifts between day and night (the South Pole and Arctic). Under this environment, the materials are easy to distort and fault ratio of equipment will be increased so that the system is difficult to deploy and more likely to break down. The movement of human targets, weather, and geographic mutation make the environment indexes change an uncertainty. Hence, the system design should consider the following factors:

Computing ability: Sensors in BSNs are required to have the ability to successfully complete the tasks in the different environments even when the monitoring targets are various and fuzzy, which means the sensors should have excellent computing and process ability. Take the cold-resistance test as an example; the monitoring data includes the surrounding environment, shell temperature, terminal temperature, central temperature, heart rhythm, blood pressure, and so on. All these parameters are vague and uncertain. Simple logical judgment

Figure 2. Comprehensive architecture of BSNs

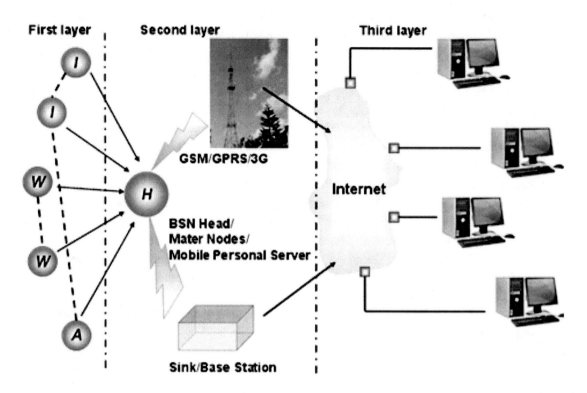

and the monitoring on each parameter cannot efficiently estimate the real state of monitoring objective. Hence, the system must have enough computing ability.

Low energy consumption: Although sensors of BSNs are carried on human targets, they still cannot be charged or replace the battery conveniently in severe environments, such as snow mountain, polar region, and other cold region. Hence, it is necessary to assure the low energy consumption in BSNs, which can keep the network operating in the long term.

Robustness: Ratio of device failure will be high under severe environment. It is important to guarantee the sensitivity of the global performance to individual device failures. The failure of one device should not cause the collapse of the entire network. Furthermore, the performance of the system degrade is often desirable as gracefully as possible with respect to component failures.

Besides of the above properties, BSNs should meet the dynamic data requirement with the following characteristics: 1) Sensors are connected by a wireless self-organized method, which is easier to be extended and maintained with lower cost. 2) Network can support online programming, which can dynamically update the program of sensors so that it can achieve the different functions of network. 3) Sensors are module designed, where the separate modules have different functions. The design of process, communication, and gathering make the sensors flexible according to the applications. 4) Sensors in compact size are easier to carry. 5) Sensors have independent processing and storage ability, which can process the gathered information in distributed method and make the data gathering and information process simultaneously. 6) Single sensor in low price can achieve the deployment in high density, which can improve the gathering security of environment and physiological characteristic.

Figure 3. The designed BSNs system structure

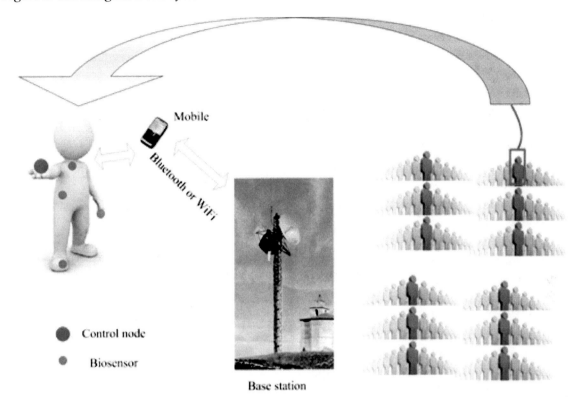

Base station

System Design of BSNs

Our system is illustrated in Figure 3, which consists of four kinds of components, named as biosensor, control node, mobile agent, and base station. The biosensor and control nodes are equipped on human body, which form one local network. A biosensor consists of a processor, memory, transceiver, sensors, and a power unit. These biosensors will perform the tasks like sensing and processing sensory data of the human body and transmit them to the control node, and also receive external signals to adjust their action. The control nodes also equipped with some kinds of sensors to monitor the environment. They periodically receive the sensory data generated by biosensors, and then transmit the data received and generated by themselves to the mobile agent. The mobile agents connected to a movable base station through wireless communication (Bluetooth or WiFi), where all sensory data are stored for further processing. As compared to the biosensors and the control nodes, the mobile agent and base station have significantly higher transmission and processing capabilities. The following is the detailed introduction of the components.

Biosensors: Various types of biosensors are employed to constantly measure related information and perform multiple sensing functions simultaneously, such as temperature, heartbeat, blood pressure, blood oxygen content, and so on. Biosensors participate in three types of wireless communication links, which is between the biosensors, between the biosensor and control node, and between the biosensors and the mobile agent. Biosensors have limited power supply and cannot afford heavy tasks of computation and communication. For the biosensor nodes implanted in human body, it must be in small size. Additionally, we choose accelerator to complete information gathering combined with the requirement of the real application environment of BSN and diversity of human activities. These accelerators can be embedded in common items like watches, mobile phones, belts, and shoes. Human targets can wear them a long time without any discomfort. The moving characteristic can be extracted from the 3D accelerated signal, which can conquer the weakness that the vision characteristic abstraction is easily influenced by environment and the high cost.

Control node: These nodes are responsible for receiving and forwarding the sensory data sent from biosensors, and then monitoring the movement information of human beings and the surrounding environmental condition. We have referred MicaZ to design the processing unit and sensor board of control node, ATMega128L adopted as the CPU and CC2420 adopted as wireless communication chip. In the sensor board, it includes one sensor detector PT25, and the temperature range is from −80 to 200°C. The accuracy is ±0.03°C with the resolution of 0.01°C, which can meet the requirement of environment measurement. The humidity sensor is Rh36 with the accuracy of ±2% under the working temperature of −40°C to 85°C. The wind sensor is GW2423550 under the working temperature of −40°C to 55°C. Additionally, each control node adopts the cellular insulate material.

Mobile agent: These devices serve for data collection from biosensors and control nodes to complete the local data processing, then transmitting the data to base station. As cell phones are widely used and can support high data rate transmission, they are suitable for medical care as mobile agents due to the inherited characteristics.

Base station: These devices are also movable and responsible for the final data collecting and process. Their work model can be changed according to the different applications, like different transmittal rates and package formats. The base station is different from the usual control node, which is only responsible for data collection not

data gathering. Therefore, there are no sensors equipped in the base station but it consists of two communication modules. One is a wireless module communicating with usual sensor nodes, and the other one is used to connect with the outside network for further diagnose and telemedicine.

DATA FUSION IN BSNs

System Models

Network Model

We assume that all the nodes are uniformly distributed in a circular area of radius. Only one base station is located at the center of the area. All the nodes have the same initial energy budget. During data collection, the maximum communication distance is also the same for all nodes. Each node has a unique ID number and knowledge of its geographical location. Without loss of generality, we make the following assumptions in this paper:

Except for the base station and mobile node, all the biosensors and control nodes are isomorphic with the same initial energy, computation capacity, and data fusion capacity. The mobile node and base station have no limitations of energy and computation capacity.

Based on the distance to the receiver, the biosensors and control nodes can adjust the transmission power to save energy consumption.

When the biosensors and control nodes have no tasks, they can switch to the sleeping state to save energy consumption.

Fusion Model

Similar to Luo, Liu, and Das (2006), a data fusion model is employed in our research, where the sensor nodes are required to send their data constantly. In this model, if a node v needs to receive the data sent from node u, which is marked as

Figure 4. Data fusion in heterogeneous network

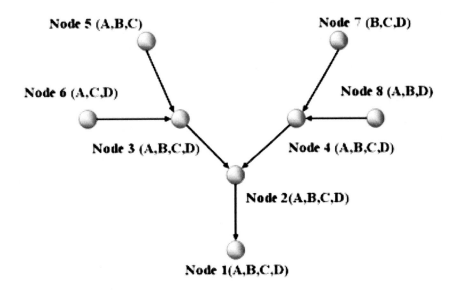

$w(u)$. The total data amount after fusion process at node v is expressed as:

$$w(v) = \max(\tilde{w}(v), w(u)) + \min(\tilde{w}(v), w(u))(1 - \rho) \tag{1}$$

Where $\tilde{w}(v)$ represents the data amount generated by node v. ρ represents the data correlation between node u and v, which is affected by data attribute.

In heterogeneous BSNs, the attributes of the packets generated by different biosensors and control nodes are not the same, which increases the difficulty of the fusion process. As shown in Figure 4, there are four kinds of sensors in the network, which can separately generate four kinds of attributive data represented by types A, B, C, and D. Each control node is equipped with three kinds of sensors. Figure 4 shows the data gathering and fusion process for nodes 5, 6, 7, and 8. The attributive data in packets generated by them are types A, B, and C; types A, C, and D; types B, C, and D; and types A, B, and D. For easy illustration, the packets generated by nodes 1, 2, 3, and 4 are not shown in this figure.

Although the data attributes of these nodes are not identical, there is still some redundancy if some of the same attributes exist. For example, node 3 can fuse the components of type A and C, which coexist in packets generated by node 5 and 6. This shows that data fusion can still be used to reduce redundancy in heterogeneous BSNs if the same attributes exist in different packets.

Energy Model

We assume that all the control nodes have the same initial energy E_0, while the mobile nodes and base station are without energy limitation. Similar to Heinzelman, Chandrakasan, and Balakrishnan (2002), the energy consumption of transmitting one bit data over distance d is $W(v,u) > W(z,u)$, where $W(v,u) = W(z,u)$ and (ID_u, ID_v) are the energy spent by transmitter electronics and transmitting amplifier, respectively. $ID_v(k \geq 2)$ is the propagation loss exponent. Consequently, the energy dissipation in receiving one bit data is $T(e)$. Data fusion process can introduce the extra energy consumption, which is represented by d_s. Specially, the fusion cost will be increased with the using of encryption and other security mechanisms.

Saving Energy Efficiency of Data Fusion in BSN

In addition to a comprehensive understanding of various data, the fusion process also can reduce unnecessary data transmission for the sake of reducing energy consumption. The efficiency is mainly dependent on the correlation among fused data. When various data are fused, the length of the generated new data will be decreased with increasing the correlation. Here, the correlation coefficient is denoted by ρ.

Additionally, it is also affected by the energy consumption of the fusion process. Data fusion cannot save the energy of network anymore when the energy consumption reaches a certain degree. To measure the efficiency of saving energy, both the cost of transmission and fusion should be considered, denoted by $C_t(S_i)$ and $C_f(S_i)$, respectively. $C_t(S_i)$ is the energy consumption of data transmission of node S_i and can be calculated as:

$$C_t(S_i) = \sum D_t(S_i, g) \cdot e_t \tag{2}$$

Where $\sum D_t(S_i, g)$ represents the amount of transmitted data and g represents the data attribute, e_t represents the energy consumption of transmitting one bit data. The value of e_t is given by the earlier model.

The energy consumption of fusion process of node S_i is given by:

$$C_f(S_i) = \sum D_f(S_i, g) \cdot e_f \tag{3}$$

Where $\sum D_f(S_i, g)$ represents the total data amount of data fusion, and e_f represents the

energy consumption of fusing one bit data. The value of e_f is affected by the adopted fusion algorithm.

For easier analysis, we make the following hypothesis: When node S_i transmits data to node S_j, the node S_j is responsible for fusing the data. $\sum D(S_i, g)$ and $\sum D(S_j, h)$ represents data amount of node S_i and S_j before fusion, respectively. $\hat{D}(S_j)$ represents the generated data amount after fusion. According to the data fusion model, if the sensory data generate from node S_i and S_j including same attributive and the correlation coefficient is $\rho(S_i, S_j)$, we have:

$$\hat{D}(S_j) = \sum_{g \neq h} \left[D(S_i, g) + D(S_j, h) \right]$$
$$+ \sum_{g = h} \left[\begin{array}{l} \max\left(D(S_i, g), D(S_j, h) \right) \\ + \min\left(D(S_i, g), D(S_j, h) \right) \\ \cdot \left(1 - \rho(S_i, S_j) \right) \end{array} \right] \tag{4}$$

According to whether node S_j fusing data or not, there are two different cases. One is node S_j does not fuse data but transmits the received and generated data directly, thus the total data amount transmitted by node S_j can be calculated as:

$$D'(S_j) = \sum \left[D(S_i, g) + D(S_j, h) \right] \tag{5}$$

The energy consumption of node v in this case is expressed as:

$$E_1(S_j) = D'(S_j) \cdot e_t$$
$$= \sum \left[D(S_i, g) + D(S_j, h) \right] \cdot e_t \tag{6}$$

In the other case, the node S_j fuses the data and the total energy consumption is written as:

$$E_2\left(S_j\right) = D'\left(S_j\right) \cdot e_f + \hat{D}\left(S_j\right) \cdot e_t$$
$$= \sum \left[D\left(S_i, g\right) + D\left(S_j, h\right)\right] \cdot e_f$$
$$+ \sum_{g \neq h} \left[D\left(S_i, g\right) + D\left(S_j, h\right)\right] \cdot e_t$$
$$+ \sum_{g = h} \left[\begin{array}{l} \max\left(D\left(S_i, g\right), D\left(S_j, h\right)\right) \\ + \min\left(D\left(S_i, g\right), D\left(S_j, h\right)\right) \\ \cdot \left(1 - \rho\left(S_i, S_j\right)\right) \end{array}\right] \cdot e_t$$

$$(7)$$

It can be deduced that the efficiency of saving energy by fusion process at node S_j is:

$$P\left(S_j\right) = E_2\left(S_j\right) - E_1\left(S_j\right)$$
$$= \sum \left[D\left(S_i, g\right) + D\left(S_j, h\right)\right] \cdot e_f$$
$$- \min\left(D\left(S_i, g\right), D\left(S_j, h\right)\right) \cdot \rho\left(S_i, S_j\right) \cdot e_t$$

$$(8)$$

Above all, both the correlation among nodes and the energy consumption of fusion process can determine the energy-conservation efficiency of data fusion. If the energy consumption of fusion is high or the correlation among the fused data is low, the data fusion may not save energy for BSNs. The energy-conservation efficiency of data fusion can be used to optimize the establishment of routing and determine how to proceed with the data fusion.

Data Detection and Fusion Rectification

The purpose of BSNs application is to supply the warning in time when human beings are sick. However, limited by price, the accuracy of biosensors is low and easily interrupted, which may result in the wrong diagnosis. From the work module of BSNs, it can be known that the global information is lack and the design of distributed strategy is necessary.

In ordinary sensor networks, many significant studies on detecting the abnormal data by wavelet transform have been developed. As targets, movement, environment variation, and sudden sickness will cause the risk of misjudgment by the BSNs; a new method to be applied in this technology still needs to be found. The estimation of abnormal data cannot be detected by a single sensor appearing outlier behavior or an individual sensor with abnormal data. The cooperation strategy and fusion process needs to be applied to improve the accuracy and rectification to abnormal data.

The generated data of a single sensor has relativity in time domain and frequency domain; moreover, sensory data from different nodes have relativity in spatial domain. The relativities among time, frequency, and spatial domains should be connected to rectify the abnormal data. Firstly, wavelet transform can judge the data generated from each sensor node from time and frequency domain and complete filtration, delete those noise interruptions. Then, a new transmission strategy is set combined with link information, which can improve the quality of data transmission and reduce the occurrence of abnormal data. Additionally, it is important to design the QoS insurance, fault-tolerant, and load equilibrium routing, and make the error rate of transmission as factor of the routing standard. The efficiency of fusion is fully enlarged during digging multi-source data during transmission, and data with the same target are fused. Non-linear errors of sensor nodes are reduced and eliminated.

Data Evaluation Based on Bayesian Estimation

As we mentioned above, although the human healthcare is main target when BSNs are applied in different regions, it is of great importance to accurately monitor the surround environment of the target human. Similar to the physiological parameters of human target, the indexes of environment monitoring also have complex subjection relationship, which includes temperature, relative humidity, wind speed, light, and other comprehensive factors. As biosensor and control nodes are deployed in the low density and the single biosensor or control nodes can only obtain the local and unilateral information, they cannot obtain accurate condition of human targets and natural environment due to the limited information. Moreover, the data collecting is affected by sensor property and outside noise. There is an obvious unavoidable difference between the gathered information and real condition, even mistake. It is necessary to find an efficient method to collect the information of the environment and human characteristics.

Combined with system design, we collect data of the same monitoring target by multi biosensors, which exhibit the multi-source information collecting property. Compared to using a single sensor, the advantage of multi-source collecting is able to collect overall information. The essence of this method is taking advantage of redundancy and complementation. Hence, the uncertain multi-source collecting and fusion process can be completed by biosensor and control nodes to obtain the reliable evaluation result. This kind of distributed and multi-dimensional process can be used to filter and merge the worthless information, wrong information, repeat information, and other invalid information. It can be regarded as a collection of many groups of single monitoring targets. Each group focused on a single monitoring target composes one local region. The data from nodes in each region only reflect the target condition in this area. The relativity among the data in one region is strong while it is weak in different regions. Therefore, the multi-group data collecting can be analyzed to single target collecting of multi-node in local region.

In severe environments, the single monitoring result of biosensor or control node is more likely to generate an error and become unreliable. To obtain the accurate evaluation result, it is needed to

judge whether the monitoring value is in the reliable range. The direct judgment can only describe the data information of one node at one time, but cannot fuse the multi-source data and describe the overall monitoring information. As the time and spatial distribution of a node can meet the deficiency of uncertain single data, we introduce the distributed Bayesian estimation to solve this problem. In BSNs, it is not difficult to obtain the three kinds of information needed in Bayesian estimation, including the general information, sample information, and prior information. Since the collected data is in accordance with the property of Bayesian estimation, the overall or local monitoring information is able to be evaluated. Considering the data relativity between the single node and multi-node, two steps are designed to complete the Bayesian evaluation based on time and spatial distribution.

Time distribution evaluation: Each biosensor or control node is an evaluable system and the information collecting process is operating on a series of discrete-time. We hypothesize that there are n discrete time of data collecting in $T = \{t_1, t_2, t_3, ..., t_n\}$. S_i represents sample in time T, which is the actual sample value on T, then it can be represented by $S_i = \{S_i(t_1), S_i(t_2), S_i(t_3), ..., S_i(t_n)\}$. The measured value is uncertainty and S_i needs to be processed by Bayesian estimation. Corresponding to S_i, there are a group of evaluating values matched with $\bar{S}_i = \{\bar{S}_i(t_1), \bar{S}_i(t_2), \bar{S}_i(t_3), ..., \bar{S}_i(t_n)\}$. For $\forall m \in [0, n]$, $\bar{S}_i(t_m)$ is calculated by the prior $\pi_i(\theta_m)$ on time t_m and the measured value $S_i(t_m)$. As prior value of t_m from time t_1 to t_m is calculated step by step. Hence, the $S_i(t_m)$ reflects not only the single measured value in t_m but also the fusion of all the measured values before t_m. To obtain the prior information in Bayesian estimation, the first key step is to determine the prior distribution.

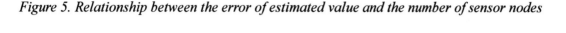

Figure 5. Relationship between the error of estimated value and the number of sensor nodes

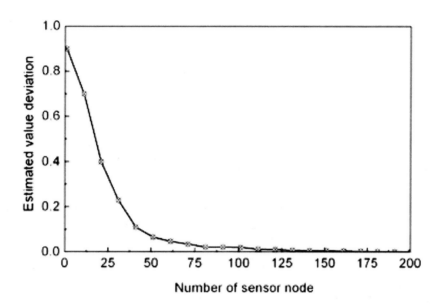

Although the sensory data is obtained by discrete time sampling, the overall data distribution is still continuous. To find the information distribution of biosensor and control node, we need to find the proper prior distribution by histogram and then evaluate the hyper parameters. A large amount of sensory data needs to be collected to draw the column diagram. Figure 5 is a diagram drawn on 200 samples collected at -10 cent degree per minute, which exhibits the gathered sensory data following normal distribution. We make the likelihood function $L(\theta) = p(x|\theta)$ as prior distribution, which means the prior distribution is also normal distribution. Each monitoring value of biosensor and control node should meet the normal distribution $N(\theta, \gamma^2)$ of the expected value as center. The next step is to find the prior distribution $\pi(\theta|x)$. We use normal distribution $N(\vartheta, \gamma^2)$ as the prior distribution of θ, which can be described as:

$$\pi(\theta) = \frac{1}{\gamma\sqrt{2\pi}} \exp- \frac{(\theta - \vartheta)^2}{2\gamma^2} \tag{9}$$

Based on Bayesian estimation, the likelihood function of original value of node j is:

$$p(S_j|\theta) = \prod_{i=1}^{n}(S_j|\theta)$$

$$= \left(\frac{1}{\sigma\sqrt{2\pi}}\right)^n \exp\left\{-\frac{1}{2\pi\sigma^2}\sum_{i=1}^{n}[S_j(t_i - \theta)]^2\right\} \tag{10}$$

The joint distribution of sample S and parameter θ is:

$$h(S,\theta) = p(S|\theta)\pi(\theta)$$

$$= \frac{1}{\gamma\delta^n}(2\pi)^{-\frac{n+1}{2}} \exp\left\{-\frac{1}{2}\left[\frac{n\theta^2 - 2n\theta\sum_{i=1}^{n}\frac{S_j(t_i)}{n}}{\sigma^2} + \frac{1}{\sigma^2}\sum_{i=1}^{n}S_j(t_i)^2 + \frac{\theta^2 - 2\theta\vartheta + \vartheta^2}{\gamma^2}\right]\right\} \tag{11}$$

If we set $\delta_0 = \sqrt{\dfrac{\delta^2}{n}}$, $\alpha = \dfrac{n}{\delta^2} + \dfrac{1}{\gamma^2}$,

$$\beta = \frac{1}{\delta^2}\sum_{i=1}^{n} S_j(t_i) + \frac{\vartheta}{\gamma^2},$$

$$\lambda = \frac{1}{\delta^2}\sum_{i=1}^{n} S_j(t_i) + \frac{\vartheta^2}{\gamma^2}.$$

Then:

$$\pi(\theta|S_j) = \frac{h(S_j,\theta)}{m(S_j)}$$

$$= \sqrt{\frac{2\pi}{\alpha}}\exp\left\{-\frac{1}{2}\alpha\left(\theta - \frac{\beta}{2}\right)^2\right\} \tag{12}$$

The evaluation of single node measured value is:

$$\overline{S}_j(t_i) = \overline{\theta}$$

$$= \frac{\delta^2\vartheta + \gamma^2\sum_{i=1}^{n} S_j(t_i)}{\delta^2 + n\gamma^2} \tag{13}$$

Evaluation of Spatial distribution: When the evaluation of time distribution is obtained, fusion is needed to proceed based on spatial distribution. We hypothesize there are k nodes in the monitoring region, each node is independent in macro but has indivisibility relationship in micro. For the measuring targets with the spatial distribution property, the abundant measured valued from many nodes can eliminate the uncertainty from single node. The prior evaluation of $\overline{S}_j(t_i)$ in t_i can be obtained after k nodes posterior evaluation:

$$\overline{S}(t_i) = \sum_{j=1}^{k} \alpha_j \overline{S}_j(t_i) \tag{14}$$

Here, α_j represents the weight of each node after prior evaluation to the overall evaluation,

the value is distributed by mobile agent according to the following equation:

$$\begin{cases} \alpha_j\left|\overline{S}_j(t_i) - S_j(t_i)\right| = \alpha_k\left|\overline{S}_k(t_i) - S_k(t_i)\right| \\ \sum_{j=1}^{K} \alpha_j = 1 \end{cases} \tag{15}$$

It can be seen that the higher weight of posterior evaluation can be obtained for the node with smaller difference between the evaluation and measured value.

Identification of Human Movement

Identification of human movement includes data gathering, characteristic parameter abstraction, movement model, and statistic study. Moreover, how to acquire the movement information and use the energy of portable equipment in high efficiency is another important challenge.

To solve the problem of high dimensionality, nonlinearity, and quantity analysis, classification needs to complete simultaneous and continuous movement identification during the fusion process. The most useful identification is to train the identified movement data with relative learning algorithm. More identified data is helpful by the high probability of physical identification. In the current running environment of BSNs, it is impossible for the monitoring target to acquire a large amount of training data. Utilizing the semi-supervised learning method and non-supervised clustering method can automatically select the key characterization, which can identify with less training data. Additionally, smooth restrain characterization can be introduced to improve the accuracy of identification.

Hidden Markov model can be used to achieve the continuous identification over a sustained period of time. Here, the active type of human targets is determined by the biggest output probability. At the same time, the complexity of Markov model can be reduced by clustering method. The configuration of movement identification of human beings can be achieved. First, the simulation signal of the accelerator sensor is transformed to data signals by modulus transformation. Then, window detection, smooth filtrate, and signal normalization are handled. The signal after terminate sport node processing can complete the relative calculation of characterization and select the characterization for training by cluster algorithm.

SIMULATION AND NUMERICAL RESULTS

In this section, we evaluate the performance of the proposed system and fusion process method. Our simulation experiments are organized as follows: Firstly, we describe the experimental environment. Secondly, we demonstrate how to obtain the enough information for Bayesian estimation. Thirdly, we investigate the performance of the design data evaluation method during the fusion process with the proposed system.

Experimental Environment

Experiment data gathering includes two parts: environment characterization, like room temperature, air humidity, and wind speed; and experimental entity like physiological and movement state. None of each part of the experiment data, which compose the description of experiment process, is unnecessary. The floor space, structure property, and airflow in the test environment are different, it is important to guarantee the accuracy and smooth monitoring results whether the tests are in the reliable range or the experiment reaches the inquired level. From the viewpoint of target state and environment monitoring, it needs the following conditions:

When the test targets enter the experiment environment, the gathering and analysis are completed under safety safe and controllable station.

During the experiment, the environment state can also be efficiently monitored, besides of the physiological and movement monitoring.

Proper safety monitoring is necessary for the participants and equipment.

To make the monitoring result achieve the requirement of minimum local environment, each local environment of participant must be under control to make the deployment density.

The experiment area is 200 m², and each space for the participant is only 2 m³. We set 25 participants in 100 m² and each one carries 4 control nodes and 20 biosensors. The real difference of each environment can well be reflected. Temperature, relative humidity, and wind speed needs measurement, hence each control node is equipped with three sensor devices. To obtain the intermediate data for detecting the reasonability of fusion algorithm, we add more data gathering sensor nodes to record the sensory value during monitoring. The data gathering sensor nodes are general MicaZ nodes without data gathering function. Each sensor gathering node will set N distributed node as the real-time detection to the base station. Technically, all the tasks of data gathering nodes are responsible for data transmission. The real existence of data gathering is unnecessary; here it is only for the use of verification of the algorithm. Each experiment only tests one group of data. The experiment environment is shown as Table 1.

Temperature, humidity, and wind speed are separately recorded as environment parameters. Table 1 lists values of measurement characterization for Bayesian estimation. All the parameters

Table 1. The range of environment test measurement

Environment index	μ_0	σ_0	α_0
Wind speed	Set value	0.4	0.5
Humidity	Set value	1	0.5
Temperature	Set value	0.2	0.25

have close relationship with sensor accuracy, measurement accuracy, and confidence.

Experimental Result and Analysis

To obtain enough information for Bayesian estimation, the node deployment density should be considered firstly. A series of experiments are carried out under the environment of minus 5 degrees.

Figure 5 gives the changing trend of estimated value with increasing the node density. The estimated error decreases when more nodes are deployed. When the number of nodes is 100, the changing becomes slower and slower. The estimated value becomes stable and very close to the sample value. The optimal result can be used to determine the proper deployment density of nodes. According to Figure 5, more than one node deployed per square meter can reflect the real condition of the environment.

Figure 6 gives the estimated value of each node after Bayesian estimation for monitoring the environmental temperature. It can be seen that the estimated value is close to the sample value and fluctuates in a small range.

Figure 7 shows the comprehensive evaluation of 20 experiments to single node. It can be seen that the error between the sample value and estimated value from Bayesian is smaller than that of the sample value. The distributed Bayesian estimation can meet the accurate requirement of data collecting.

The body is most sensitive to cold environments; the fingers and toes are easily frozen. As a result, it is important to measure these parts. The fingers of each person are equipped with temperature sensors. These sensors can calculate one evaluation value as the mean temperature of all fingers by Bayesian distribution. Figure 8 shows the estimated value and distribution evaluation with time changing based on Bayesian distribution. It can be seen that the stable estimated value can be obtained after a certain period, although there is high error between the estimated value and the sample value at the beginning.

FUTURE RESEARCH DIRECTIONS

As a future work, we are interested in considering the data fusion efficiency in BSNs. We need to

Figure 6. Estimated temperature value of each node

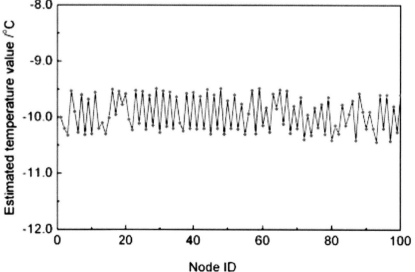

Figure 7. Comparison of sample and estimated value

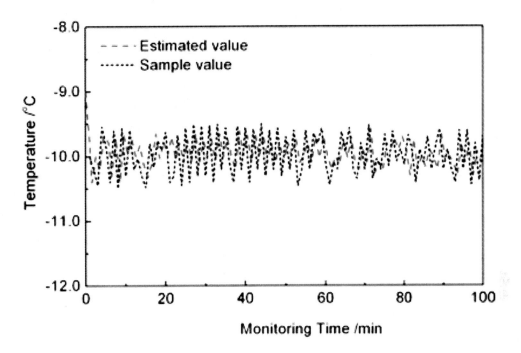

Figure 8. Trends of finger and estimated temperature

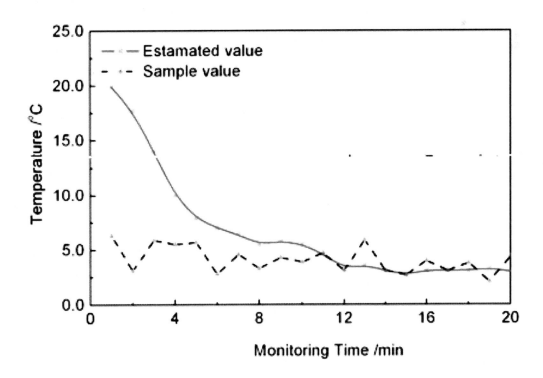

analyze the interaction among various fusion methods on relation coefficient in depth. Especially for the fusion process method in context-aware environments; the data types of human being are different under various circumstances. It is necessary to find an efficient method to quickly obtain the decision result. Hence, this could be a very attractive research issue for further investigation.

CONCLUSION

In this chapter, we studied the system design and data fusion in BSNs. Then, we designed a new BSN system, which can be used in different environments, such as cold regions. As there are strong correlations between data gathered from sensor nodes in close physical proximity, the effective in-network fusion schemes involve minimizing such redundancy and hence reducing the load in BSNs. Under various applications of BSNs, the data collection must be multiple attribute for each sensor node equipped with more than one kind of sensor. An increase in complexity for the fusion process is unavoidable due to the existence of various physical attributes. In this chapter, for the property of uncertainty, multi-source, and the huge amount and complex subjection, systematical and deep research is carried out. The evaluation of Bayesian estimation based on distribution is adopted to solve the accuracy problem facing environmental and human characteristics. The experiment result shows that the accuracy of monitoring can be efficiently guaranteed.

REFERENCES

Amft, O., Troster, G., Lukowicz, P., & Schuster, C. (2006). Sensing muscle activities with body-worn sensors. In *Proceedings of the International Workshop on Wearable and Implantable Body Sensor Networks (BSN 2006)*, (pp. 138-141). Washington, DC: IEEE Computer Society.

Anandkumar, A., Meng, W., Lang, T., & Swami, A. (2009). Prize-collecting data fusion for cost-performance tradeoff in distributed inference. In *Proceedings of IEEE INFOCOM* (pp. 2150–2158). Rio de Janeiro, Brazil: IEEE Press. doi:10.1109/INFCOM.2009.5062139

Anliker, U., Ward, J. A., Lukowicz, P., Troster, G., Dolveck, F., & Baer, M. (2004). AMON: A wearable multiparameter medical monitoring and alert system. *IEEE Transactions on Information Technology in Biomedicine, 8*, 415–427. doi:10.1109/TITB.2004.837888

Arroyo-Valles, R., Marques, A. G., & Cid-Sueiro, J. (2011). Optimal selective forwarding for energy saving in wireless sensor networks. *IEEE Transactions on Wireless Communications, 10*(1), 164–175. doi:10.1109/TWC.2010.102810.100014

Atallah, L., Elhelw, M., Pansiot, J., et al. (2007). Behavior profiling with ambient and wearable sensing. In *Proceedings of the 4th International Workshop on Wearable and Implantable Body Sensor Networks,* (pp. 133-138). Berlin, Germany: Springer.

Branch, J., Szymanski, B., Giannella, C., Wolff, R., & Kargupta, H. (2006). In-network outlier detection in wireless sensor networks. In *Proceedings of ICDCS 2006*. Lisboa, Portugal: ICDCS.

Brengelmann, G. L. (2000). Body surface temperature: Manifestation of complex anatomy and physiology of the cutaneous vasculature. In *Proceedings of the 22nd Annual International Conference of the IEEE,* (pp. 1927-1930). IEEE Press.

Campbell, I. (2008). Body temperature and its regulation. *Anaesthesia and Intensive Care Medicine, 9*, 259–263. doi:10.1016/j.mpaic.2008.04.009

Chaczko, Z., Klempous, R., Nikodem, J., et al. (2008). Applications of cooperative WSN in homecare systems. In *Proceedings of the 3rd International Conference on Broadband Communications, Information Technology & Biomedical Applications*, (pp. 215-220). Washington, DC: IEEE Press.

Chen, L. K., & Shieh, Y. A. (2011). Jackknife prevention for articulated vehicles using model reference adaptive control. *Journal of Automobile Engineering, 225*(1), 28–42. doi:10.1243/09544070JAUTO1513

Chen, S., Lee, H., Chen, C., et al. (2007). A wireless body sensor network system for healthcare monitoring application. In *Proceedings of IEEE Biomedical Circuits and Systems Conference (BIOCAS)*, (pp. 243-246). Washington, DC: IEEE Press.

DuoFertility. (2009). *Website.* Retrieved from http://www.duofertility.com.

Goel, A., & Estrin, D. (2003). Simultaneous optimization for concave costs: Single sink aggregation or single source buy-at-bulk. In *Proceedings of ACM-SIAM Symposium on Discrete Algorithms*, (pp. 499-505). Baltimore, MD: ACM Press.

Grubb, A. (2010). Non-invasive estimation of glomerular filtration rate (GFR): The Lund model: Simultaneous use of cystatin C- and creatinine-based GFR-prediction equations, clinical data and an internal quality check. *Scandinavian Journal of Clinical and Laboratory Investigation, 70*(2), 65–70. doi:10.3109/00365511003642535

Heimbigner, D. (2011). A tamper-resistant programming language system. *IEEE Transactions on Dependable and Secure Computing, 8*(2), 194–206. doi:10.1109/TDSC.2010.51

Heinzelman, W. B., Chandrakasan, A. P., & Balakrishnan, H. (2002). An application-specific protocol architecture for wireless microsensor networks. *IEEE Transactions on Wireless Communications, 1*(4), 660–670. doi:10.1109/TWC.2002.804190

Intanagonwiwat, C., Estrin, D., Govindan, R., & Heidemann, J. (2002). Impact of network density on data aggregation in wireless sensor networks. In *Proceedings of the 22nd International Conference on Distributed Systems*, (pp. 457-458). Vienna, Austria: IEEE.

Jones, W. D. (2006). Taking body temperature, inside out. *IEEE Spectrum, 43*, 13–15. doi:10.1109/MSPEC.2006.1572338

Jovanov, E., Milenkovic, A., & Otto, C. (2005). A wireless body area network of intelligent motion sensors for computer assisted physical rehabilitation. *Journal of Neurological Engineering and Rehabilitation, 2*(1), 1–10.

Kim, K., & Chung, C. W. (2010). In/out status monitoring in mobile asset tracking with wireless sensor networks. *Sensors (Basel, Switzerland), 10*(4), 2709–2730. doi:10.3390/s100402709

Krishnamachari, B. (2002). The impact of data aggregation in wireless sensor networks. In *Proceedings of International Workshop on Distributed Event-Based Systems*, (pp. 575-578). IEEE.

Lenzini, G. (2009). Trust-based and context-aware authentication in a software architecture for context and proximity-aware services. *Architecting Dependable Systems, 6*, 284–307.

Liang, D., Wu, J., & Chen, X. (2007). Real-time physical activity monitoring by data fusion in body sensor networks. In *Proceedings of the 10th Internaional Conference on Information Fusion*, (pp. 1-7). Washington, DC: IEEE.

Lin, K., Lai, C., & Chen, M. (2011). Research on body sensor networks in cold region. In *Proceedings of IEEE ICC*. Kyoto, Japan: IEEE Press.

Luo, H., Liu, Y., & Das, S. K. (2006). Routing correlated data with fusion cost in wireless sensor networks. *IEEE Transactions on Mobile Computing, 5*(11), 1620–1632. doi:10.1109/TMC.2006.171

Luo, H., Luo, J., Liu, Y., & Das, S. K. (2006). Adaptive data fusion for energy efficient routing in wireless sensor networks. *IEEE Transactions on Computers, 55*(10), 1286–1299. doi:10.1109/TC.2006.157

Ouchi, K., Suzuki, T., & Doi, M. (2002). Lifeminder: A wearable healthcare support system using user's context. In *Proceedings of ICDCSW,* (pp. 791-792). ICDCSW.

Palpanas, T., Papadopoulos, D., Kalogeraki, V., & Gunopulos, D. (2003). Distributed deviation detection in sensor networks. *SIGMOD Record, 32*(4). doi:10.1145/959060.959074

Pansiot, J., Stoyanov, D., Mcilwraith, D., et al. (2007). Ambient and wearable sensor fusion for activity recognition in healthcare monitoring systems. In *Proceedings of the Internatinal Workshop on Wearable and Implantable Body Sensor Networks,* (pp. 208-212). Berlin, Germany: Springer.

Pantelopoulos, A., & Bourbakis, N. G. (2010). A survey on wearable sensor-based systems for health monitoring and prognosis. *IEEE Transactions on Systems, Man and Cybernetics. Part C, Applications and Reviews, 40*(1), 1–12. doi:10.1109/TSMCC.2009.2032660

Patel, A., & Schmidt, N. (2011). Application of structured document parsing to focused web crawling. *Computer Standards & Interfaces, 33*(3), 325–331. doi:10.1016/j.csi.2010.08.002

Pattem, S., Krishnamachari, B., & Govindan, R. (2004). The impact of spatial correlation on routing with compression in wireless sensor networks. In *Proceedings of the Third International Symposium on Information Processing in Sensor Networks,* (pp. 28-35). Berkeley, CA: ACM.

Pessi, A. T., & Businger, S. (2009). Relationships among lightning, precipitation, and hydrometeor characteristics over the north Pacific ocean. *Journal of Applied Meteorology and Climatology, 48*(4), 833–848. doi:10.1175/2008JAMC1817.1

Pollard, J. K., Santarelli, C., Rohman, S., & Fry, M. E. (2002). Wireless and web-based medical monitoring in the home. *Medical Informatics and the Internet in Medicine, 27*(3), 219–227. doi:10.1080/1463923021000014130

Rinderle-Ma, S., Reichert, M., & Jurisch, M. (2011). On utilizing web service equivalence for supporting the composition life cycle. *International Journal of Web Services Research, 8*(1), 41–67. doi:10.4018/jwsr.2011010103

Rodrigues, J. J. P. C., Pereira, O. R. E., & Neves, P. A. C. S. (2011). Biofeedback data visualization for body sensor networks. *Journal of Network and Computer Applications, 34*(1), 151–158. doi:10.1016/j.jnca.2010.08.005

Stauffer, C., & Grimson, W. E. (2000). Learning patterns of activity using real time tracking. *IEEE Transactions on Pattern Analysis and Machine Intelligence, 22*(8), 747–757. doi:10.1109/34.868677

Subramaniam, S., Palpanas, T., Papadopoulos, D., Kalogeraki, V., & Gunopulos, D. (2006). Online outlier detection in sensor data using non-parametric models. In *Proceedings of VLDB 2006*. VLDB.

Tan, C., & Wang, H. (2008). Body sensor network security: An identity-based cryptography approach. In *Proceedings of WiSec 2008*. WiSec.

Tatbul, N., Buller, M., Hoyt, R., et al. (2004). Confidence based data management for personal area sensor networks. In *Proceeedings of the 1st International Workshop on Data Management for Sensor Networks*. VLDB.

Thiemjarus, S., Lo, B., & Yang, G. (2006). A spatio temporal architecture for context aware sensing. In *Proceedings of the International Workshop on Wearable and Implantable Body Sensor Networks (BSN)*, (pp. 1-4). Washington, DC: IEEE Press.

Van, L. K., & Gellersen, H. W. (2004). A study in distributed wearable activity recognition. In *Proceedings of the 8th IEEE International Symposium on Wearable Computers (ISWC)*, (pp. 142-149). Washington, DC: IEEE Press.

Venkatasubramanian, K. K., & Gupta, S. K. S. (2010). Physiological value-based efficient usable security solutions for body sensor networks. *ACM Transactions on Sensor Networks*, 6(4), 1–36. doi:10.1145/1777406.1777410

Xing, G., Tan, R., Liu, B., Wang, J., Jia, X., & Yi, C. (2009). Data fusion improves the coverage of wireless sensor networks. In *Proceedings of the International Conference on Mobile Computing and Networking*, (pp. 157-168). Beijing, China: IEEE.

Yu, Y., Krishnamachari, B., & Prasanna, V. K. (2004). Energy-latency tradeoffs for data gathering in wireless sensor networks. In *Proceedings of IEEE INFOCOM 2004 - Conference on Computer Communications - Twenty-Third Annual Joint Conference of the IEEE Computer and Communications Societies*, (pp. 244-255). Hong Kong, China: IEEE Press.

Zhang, H., & Shen, H. (2009). Balancing energy consumption to maximize network lifetime in data-gathering sensor networks. *IEEE Transactions on Parallel and Distributed Systems*, 20(10), 1526–1539. doi:10.1109/TPDS.2008.252

Chapter 2
Body Sensors and Healthcare Monitoring:
Design and Optimization of a Wireless Communication Protocol

Begonya Otal
Institute of Biomedical Research August Pi Sunyer (IDIBAPS), Spain

Luis Alonso
Technical University of Catalonia (UPC), Spain

Christos Verikoukis
Telecommunications Technological Centre of Catalonia (CTTC), Spain

ABSTRACT

The aging population and the high expectations towards quality of life in our society lead to the need of more efficient and affordable medical systems and monitoring solutions. The development of wireless Body Sensor Networks (BSNs) offers a platform to establish such a healthcare monitoring systems. However, BSNs in the healthcare domain operate under conflicting requirements. These are the maintenance of the desired reliability and message latency of data transmissions (i.e. quality of service), while simultaneously maximizing battery lifetime of individual body sensors. In doing so, the characteristics of the entire system, especially the Medium Access Control (MAC) layer, have to be considered. For this reason, this chapter aims for the optimization of the MAC layer by using energy-saving techniques for BSNs. The fact that the IEEE 802.15.4 MAC does not fully satisfy BSNs requirements highlights the need for the design of new scalable MAC solutions, which guarantee low-power consumption to the maximum number of body sensors in high density areas (i.e., in saturation conditions). In order to emphasize IEEE 802.15.4 MAC limitations, this chapter presents a detailed overview of this de facto standard for Wireless Sensor Networks (WSNs), which serves as a link for the introduction and description of the

DOI: 10.4018/978-1-4666-0888-7.ch002

here proposed Distributed Queuing (DQ) MAC protocol for BSN scenarios. Within this framework, an extensive DQ MAC energy-consumption analysis in saturation conditions is presented to be able to evaluate its performance in relation to IEEE 802.5.4 MAC in highly dense BSNs. The obtained results show that the proposed scheme outperforms IEEE 802.15.4 MAC in average energy consumption per information bit, thus providing a better overall performance that scales appropriately to BSNs under high traffic conditions. These benefits are obtained by eliminating back-off periods and collisions in data packet transmissions, while minimizing the control overhead.

INTRODUCTION

Wireless Sensor Networks (WSNs) and Body Sensor Networks (BSNs) are enabling technologies for the application domain of unobtrusive medical monitoring. This field includes continuous cable-free monitoring of vital signs in intensive care units (Ragil, 2005), remote monitoring of chronically ill patients (BASUMA Project, 2006; MobiHealth Project, 2004; HealthService24 Project, 2009; Lo & Yang, 2005), monitoring of patients in mass casualty situations (Anliker, Ward, Lukowicz, Tröster, Dolveck, & Baer, 2004), monitoring people in their everyday lives to provide early detection and intervention for various types of disease (Malan, Fulford-Jones, Welsh, & Moulton, 2004), computer-assisted physical rehabilitation in ambulatory settings (MyHeart Project, 2006), and assisted living of elderly at home (Jovanov, Milenkovic, Otto, & de Groen, 2005; Eklund, Hansen, Sprinkle, & Sastry, 2005). In these scenarios, the sensors range from on-body sensors, to ambient sensors like positioning devices, to mobile devices such as cellular phones or PDAs. Depending on the application scenario BSNs are employed stand-alone or in combination with mobile phones or ambient WSNs. In order to have a better overview of potential new medical and personal healthcare applications, we will analyse and further study this field.

Like other wireless data networks, BSNs are formed by nodes (body sensors), which dynamically establish and break radio links among them in order to deliver an effective and trustworthy communication. The radio channel is common and shared by all body sensors that belong to the BSN. The Medium Access Control (MAC) layer is responsible for coordinating channel accesses, by avoiding collisions and scheduling data transmissions, to maximize throughput efficiency at an acceptable packet delay and minimal energy consumption. Therefore, it is required to define proper MAC protocols with a number of rules that guarantee the efficient use of the radio channel, and take stringent medical requirements into account (IEEE, 2003).

Bear in mind that considerable research efforts have been put into improving the efficiency of individual layers. For example, at the Physical layer (PHY), advanced signal processing techniques have been devised to face problems such as noise, interference and unwanted signal replicas caused by the random and time-varying nature of radio channels. Besides, a great variety of MAC schemes have been developed for wireless systems. However, advances attained in the different layers had barely taken into account those achieved in other layers. Actually, since a few years ago, each layer research has widely ignored the other layers. It seems clear that system performance improvements could arise from some communications between different layers, having in mind in the system design certain smart interaction among them. This foresight has led to a new paradigm: cross-layer optimization, where for instance, different layers will actuate accordingly to adapt to the actual channel conditions, performing the cross-layer interaction. Some research has been developed for general unspecific wireless systems, focusing specially on MAC issues (Maharshi, Tong, & Swami, 2003; Tong, Zhao, & Mergen, 2001), while others study in depth the optimal bandwidth allocation (Shyu, Chen, & Luo, 2002), or the optimal power assignment for this kind of systems (Wang, 2004). Regarding specific types of networks or applications, for instance, ad hoc wireless networks have been an extensive field of cross-layer research (Yuen, Lee, & Andersen, 2002) due to the totally wireless nature of the communications system. Also, wireless sensor networks have been a target for some cross-layer optimization developments (Woo, Madden, & Govindan, 2004), where mostly energy-saving techniques are applied. Energy in sensor nodes is consumed by multiple functions such as processing, radio communications, and power supplies among others. Shutdown and scaling are the main techniques used to minimize energy consumption for radios. The idea behind shutdown is that the node operates at a fixed transmission rate and power level, and shuts down the radio after transmitting, thus avoiding any superfluous energy consumption. Scaling is based on the relation between performance and energy requirements. The node varies properties such as modulation and error coding, trading off energy consumption for transmission time.

The medical domain generally implies more rigorous requirements on reliability and obviously on energy consumption. Since vital signals are measured for real-time monitoring and diagnostic purposes, BSNs must have a guaranteed maximum latency and a low packet loss (i.e. Quality of Service [QoS]). Moreover, in order to avoid frequent battery-replacement and to keep the size of body sensors small, reducing the energy-consumption for data communication is of dramatic importance. Hence, these stringent medical requirements and the unreliability of wireless communication create a specific need for further improving MAC protocols in future demanding BSNs (Bourgard, Catthoor, Daly, Chandrakasam, & Dehaene, 2005; Yang, 2006).

This chapter aims for the analysis of BSNs under saturation conditions and the optimization of properly adapted MAC protocol solutions with the proposal of cross-layer energy-saving techniques. Energy-saving mechanisms to prolong body sensors' battery lifetime and smart scheduling mechanisms to enable the efficient use of the radio channel will allow the future development of novel healthcare monitoring, diagnostic and therapeutic applications, and additionally widen a brand new personal healthcare market. Additionally, novel cross-layer scheduling algorithms to increase QoS in the medical domain based on the here proposed design are depicted by the same authors in (Otal, Alonso, & Verikoukis, 2009).

BACKGROUND

As previously mentioned, the MAC layer is responsible for coordinating channel access, by avoiding collisions and scheduling data transmissions, to maximize throughput at an acceptable end-to-end packet delay and minimal energy consumption. Despite being the de facto standard for most current research studies in BSNs, the IEEE 802.15.4 MAC (IEEE, 2003) is not actually intended to serve any set of applications with stringent QoS and varying data rate demands, like the ones existing in healthcare and medical environments. In the literature, it is already possible to find some publications in relation to BSNs in healthcare systems, such as (Chevrollier & Golmie, 2005; Golmie, Cypher, & Rebala, 2005), where the authors performed an evaluation analysis of IEEE 802.15.4 MAC under specific medical settings. It was pointed out that the scalability of IEEE 802.15.4 is not a given feature, since the current IEEE 802.15.4 MAC design does not support a high sensor density area and its use is extremely restricted under interference scenarios. Simulation results in (Cavalcanti, Schmitt, & Soomro, 2007) confirm that the IEEE 802.15.4 MAC may be energy efficient in controlled environments, (i.e.

without interference), but it fails in supporting QoS in co-existing scenarios, which is a serious issue for medical applications. Human monitoring BSNs must support high degrees of reliability under specific message latency requirements, without endangering sensor power consumption to avoid frequent battery replacements. The fact that the IEEE 802.15.4 MAC does not fully satisfy BSN requirements highlights the need for the design of new scalable MAC solutions. These guarantee low-power consumption to all different sorts of body sensors, while ensuring rigorous QoS, and data rate requirements for future BSNs under co-existent scenarios in healthcare systems.

The release of IEEE 802.15.4 for Low Rate Wireless Personal Area Networks (LR-WPAN) (IEEE, 2003) represented a milestone in Wireless Sensor Networks (WSNs), and is, as aforementioned, the current standard of choice for most BSNs studied scenarios with its limitations, though. It targets low data rate, low power consumption, and low cost wireless networking and offers device level wireless connectivity. It is expected to be used in a wide variety of embedded applications, including home automation, industrial sensing, environmental control, and medical monitoring. In these applications, numerous embedded devices running on batteries are distributed in an area communicating via wireless radios. The key concern is thereby that of extremely low power consumption, since it is often infeasible to replace or recharge batteries for the devices on a regular basis.

Similar to all IEEE 802 wireless standards, the IEEE 802.15.4 standard standardizes only the Physical (PHY) and Medium Access Control (MAC) layers (IEEE, 2003). Here we concentrate however on MAC layer protocols, which play a significant role in determining the efficiency of wireless channel bandwidth sharing an energy cost of communication. In the IEEE 802.15.4 MAC layer, a central controller in a LR-WPAN, called the Personal Area Network (PAN) coordinator, builds the network in its personal operating space.

The standard supports three topologies: star, peer-to-peer, and cluster-tree. The star topology communication is established between devices and the PAN coordinator; in the peer-to-peer topology any device can communicate with each other device within its range; and in the cluster-tree topology, most devices can communicate with each other within the cluster, but only some of them may connect to the infrastructure. The standard identifies two channel access mechanisms:

1. Beacon-enabled networks use a slotted Carrier Sense Multiple Access Mechanism with Collision Avoidance (CSMA/CA), and the slot boundaries of each device are aligned with the slot boundaries of the PAN coordinator. The communication is then controlled by the PAN coordinator, which transmits regular beacons for device synchronization and network association control. The PAN coordinator defines the start and the end of the superframe by transmitting a periodic beacon. The length of the beacon period and hence the duty cycle of the system can be defined by the user between certain limits as specified in the standard (IEEE, 2003). There are 16 time slots in a superframe. Among them, there are at most 7 Guaranteed Time Slots (GTS) that form the Contention Free Period (CFP), and the others are Contention Access Period (CAP). The advantage of this mode is that the coordinator can communicate at will with all nodes. The disadvantage is that nodes must wake up to receive the beacon.

2. In non-beacon mode, a network node can send data to the coordinator at will, using a simpler unslotted CSMA/CA, if required. If the channel is idle, following a random back-off, the transmission is performed. If a busy channel is detected, the device shall wait for another random period before trying to access the channel again. To receive data from the coordinator the node must power up and poll the coordinator. To achieve the required node lifetime the polling frequency must be predetermined by power reserves and expected data quantity. The advantage of the non-beacon

Figure 1. A star-based BSN in a potential medical scenario

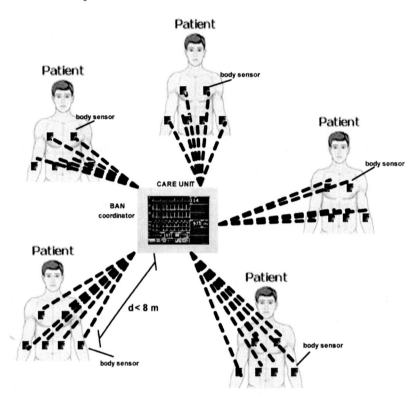

mode is that the node's receiver does not have to regularly power-up to receive the beacon. The disadvantage is that the coordinator cannot communicate at will with the node but must wait to be invited by the node to communicate.

PROBLEM STATEMENT

We focus here on single-hop beacon-enabled star-based BSNs, where a Body Area Network (BAN) coordinator is elected. That is, from now on we refer to a BAN instead of a PAN, while using either the IEEE 802.15.4 MAC or our newly proposed Distributed Queuing (DQ) MAC. In a ward BSN as portrayed in Figure 1, the BAN coordinator can be for example a bedside monitoring system, with several ward-patients wearing body sensors. Single-hop communication from body sensors to BAN coordinator (uplink), from BAN coordinator

to body sensors (downlink), or even from body sensor to body sensor (ad hoc) is possible. In the following, we model the uplink communication, which occurs more often than downlink or ad hoc communication for regular patient monitoring BSNs in hospital environments (see Figure 1). That is, we consider hereby that a single-hop star-based (uplink) setting is more directly suitable than an ad hoc or multi-hop setting for current BSNs, since we think of healthcare scenarios in which most wearable medical body sensors report to a single medical care unit in the nearby with more energy-resources (see next *section*). Further, it might be pointed out that a multi-hop scenario may be too energy-hungry for some specific body sensors (e.g. the ones close to the care unit) and thus jeopardize their own medical data transmissions. It is therefore assumed that the single-hop star-based topology is the most energy-efficient, because this does not put body

Figure 2. IEEE 802.15.4 MAC superframe structure in beacon-enabled mode (active)

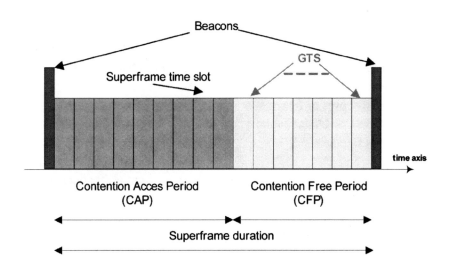

sensor's own medical data transmission at risk, avoiding unnecessary battery replacements.

In an IEEE 802.15.4 star-based BSN, the beacon-enabled mode appears to allow for the greatest energy efficiency. Indeed, it allows the transceiver to be completely switched off up to 15/16 of the time when nothing is transmitted/received, while still allowing the transceiver to be associated to the network and able to transmit or receive a packet at any time (Bourgard, Catthoor, Daly, Chandrakasam, & Dehaene, 2005). The beacon mode introduces the so-called superframe structure (Figure 2).

As previously mentioned, the superframe structure starts with the beacon, which is a small synchronization packet sent by the BAN coordinator, carrying service information for the BSN maintenance and notifying body sensors about pending data in the downlink. The inter-beacon period is partially or entirely occupied by the superframe, divided into 16 slots. The number of slots at the tail of the superframe may be used as GTS, *i.e.*, they can be dedicated to specific body sensors with no contention (see Figure 2, CFP). This functionality targets very low latency applications, but does not scale properly to highly dense BSNs (*i.e.*, saturation conditions), since the

number of dedicated slots would not be sufficient to accommodate more than seven body sensors at a time. In such conditions, it is better to use the contention access mode, where the sparse data is statistically multiplexed. In the contention access period, distributed channel accesses in the uplink are coordinated by a slotted CSMA/CA mechanism, while indirect transmission is used in the downlink. As we will see later, the CSMA/CA mechanism has a significant impact on the overall energy and performance of the uplink. According to the slotted CSMA/CA algorithm in (Bourgard, Catthoor, Daly, Chandrakasam, & Dehaene, 2005), a node must sense the channel free at least twice before being able to transmit, this corresponds to the decrement of the so-called contention windows. The first sense must be delayed by a random delay chosen between 0 and 2^{BE-1}, where BE is the back-off exponent. This randomness serves to reduce the probability of collision when two nodes simultaneously sense the channel, assess it free and decide to transmit at the same time. When the channel is sensed busy, transmission may not occur and the next channel sense is scheduled after a new random delay computed with an incremented back-off exponent. If the latter has been incremented twice and the channel is not sensed to be free, a transmission failure is notified and the procedure is aborted. When a packet collides or is corrupted, it can be retransmitted after a new contention procedure. The contention procedure starts immediately after the end of the beacon transmission (see Figure 2, CAP). All channel senses or transmissions must be aligned with the CSMA slot boundaries that are separated by a fixed period.

IEEE 802.15.4 Suitability for BSNs in Medical Applications

From the traffic point of view, we can broadly group the BSN medical applications into three categories: real time low data rate, best-effort low data rate, and real time high data rate. The first category includes EEG (Electroencephalography), ECG (Electrocardiogram), blood analysis, *etc.* The second category consists of supervisors, control and alarms, *etc.* The third category covers EMG (Electromyography) and endoscope. All of these medical signals have very strict requirements in terms of accuracy, reliability and latency, since some of them are life critical. ECG is an electrical recording of voltage in the heart in the form of continuous strip graph, which has a prime function in screening and diagnosis of cardiovascular diseases (Yang, 2006).

In healthcare scenarios, where different patients are treated simultaneously, the traffic generated by the body sensors deployed in a hospital room can also be classified in two different types: periodic and aperiodic. Periodic traffic contains the routine check-up values for the patients and physical status of the room. Usually, these values do not have strict timeliness requirements. Therefore, normal contention access method (CSMA/CA) may be used for such traffic. However, the aperiodic traffic, which is generated on the basis of some unexpected event, occurred with the patients or within the room, is very critical and needs guaranteed access to the channel and bandwidth as they must report before a worse case situation happens (*i.e.*, strict latency requirements). Examples for such traffic are; (1) a dramatically increase/decrease in the blood pressure; or, (2) a heart-attack to the patient; or, (3) an unexpected temperature change in the room. GTS services can be used for such traffic.

It looks straightforward to implement IEEE 802.15.4 in such scenarios, but following limitations of the protocol must be figured out before attempting this. The first and foremost problem with the current GTS allocation is the bandwidth under utilization. Most of the time, a device uses only a small portion of the allocated GTS slots, the major portion remains unused resulting in an empty hole in the CFP, which represents a waste of the already scarce radio resources. As shown in Figure 2, the protocol explicitly supports only seven GTS allocations. In the medical field, where one illness usually boost-ups other illnesses, many devices should be able to reach the coordinator via such guaranteed services. Besides, the current protocol only supports first come first serve based GTS allocation and does not take into account the traffic specification, delay requirements, and the energy resources. In medical scenarios, many critical events may occur at a time, and some of them are more critical and need most urgent response. With the current protocol, the device can request for all seven GTS slots, even if it is not really needed. Such unbalanced slot distribution can block other needful devices to take such timeliness advantages. Moreover, the protocol uses GTS expiration on the basis of some constant factors and the assigned GTS slots are broadcasted for the constant number of times in the superframes. Such restrictions also cause unnecessary energy consumption and CFP slots blockage for longer time. Even if CFP is not present in the superframe, the beacons transmitted by the coordinator always use unnecessarily one byte of the CFP, resulting in certain energy inefficiency. Last but not least, the current IEEE 802.15.4 superframe structure contains a constant size CAP. For most urgent scenarios, we may need flexible size CAP rather than the fixed one.

IEEE 802.15.4 Limitations on Energy Consumption

The performance evaluation study in (Gang, Krishnamachari, & Raghavendra, 2004) reveals some of the key throughput-energy-delay tradeoffs in the IEEE 802.15.4 MAC. The authors provide an analysis comparing the energy costs of beacon and non-beacon modes for synchronization, showing that the optimum choice depends upon the combination of duty cycles and data rates. In (Mišic, Shafi, & Mišic, 2006), a Markov chain model of the IEEE 802.15.4 MAC is proposed, where each state is based on the counter values as the 802.11 model in Bianchi (2000). Both models describe the behavior of the protocols using the probability that the device is in the channel accessing states. However, in the IEEE 802.15.4 MAC, this probability is not suitable for describing the behaviors because the channel sensing should be performed twice before entering accessing states. Park *et al.* (2005) propose a new Markov chain model of IEEE 802.15.4 and analyze the throughput and energy consumption in saturation conditions. The proposed model utilizes the probability of a device in the channel sensing states instead of in the channel accessing states. A similar approach for evaluating the performance of slotted IEEE 802.15.4 was followed by Pollin *et al.* (2008). The model and analysis are similar in form to Bianchi's (2000), but here the key approximation in their model is the independence of the carrier sensing probability, which determines when nodes become active to listen to the channel.

Both analytical models in Park, Kim, Choi, Choi, and Kwon (2005) and Pollin *et al.* (2008) show how the gross saturation throughput, expressed as the number of occupied slots for successful packet transmissions of size L (ignoring protocol over-head), drastically decreases as the number of sensors in the network increases. Energy consumption per information bit is also obtained through both of these models, presenting their worst results for a high number of nodes (e.g.,

20–40 nodes). Information bit is here defined as the payload bit in the data packet, *i.e.*, non-control bit.

It is therefore deduced that the IEEE 802.15.4 MAC may jeopardize the deployment and scalability of BSNs, not only in terms of throughput, but also especially in terms of energy consumption. Thus, the IEEE 802.15.4 MAC performance should be improved, targeting at low power consumption MAC protocols that scale up within BSN scenarios, while fulfilling medical application requirements. We observe that Distributed Queuing (DQ) MAC protocols (Alonso, Ferrús, & Agustí, 2005; Xu & Campbell, 1992) present a large number of advantages with respect to CSMA-based wireless communications systems. Therefore, we further analyze and optimize this DQ MAC scheme in order to prove its performance within BSN scenarios, and to improve the radio channel utilization taking the 802.14.5 MAC standard as a reference.

Please note that the introduction of energy-aware radio activation polices into a DQ MAC mechanism, as also an energy-consumption analysis in non-saturation conditions was already introduced in (Otal, Alonso, & Verikoukis, 2010). There, the authors further compare the here proposed DQ MAC to the BSN-MAC in non-saturation conditions. The Body Sensor Network MAC (BSN-MAC) is based on IEEE 802.15.4 which supports both star and peer-to-peer network topologies. The authors in Li and Tan (2005) concentrate also on the star topology because in their analyzed BSN the number of sensors is limited and an external mobile device such as a cell phone, is usually available. In Otal, Alonso, and Verikoukis (2010), the authors use the BSN-MAC as a reference benchmark and compare the energy consumption results with respect to IEEE 802.15.4 MAC in non-saturation conditions.

An optimization design and evaluation of the here characterized DQ MAC protocol in terms of quality-of-service was presented in Otal, Alonso, and Verikoukis (2009) under different healthcare scenarios. The aim of Otal, Alonso, and Verikoukis

(2009) was to study a novel cross-layer fuzzy-rule based scheduling algorithm, which allowed packet transmissions to be scheduled taking into account the channel quality among body sensors, each sensor specific medical constraints and their residual battery lifetime.

In the next sections, we further analyze the potential benefits of DQ MAC in terms of energy efficiency per information bit in BSNs under saturation conditions. That is, analytical results of average energy consumption per information bit are presented in order to get a measure of the obtainable benefits of using this DQ MAC proposal compared to IEEE 802.15.4 MAC in extensive healthcare scenarios with a raising number of body sensors in the same area (*i.e.,* high-density area).

AN ENERGY-SAVING DQ MAC PROTOCOL FOR BSNs

The Distributed Queuing Random Access Protocol (DQRAP) is a random access protocol based on a queuing system shared among nodes. It was proposed for the first time by Xu and Campbell (1992), starting from a previous protocol called DQDB (Distributed Queuing Dual Bus), they developed the DQRAP protocol for a TDMA environment proposing an analytical model and showing, by means of computer simulations, how the protocol approaches the performance of the theoretical optimum system M/M/1. DQRAP divides the TDMA slot into a "reservation subslot" or "control subslot," that is further divided into access minislots and a data subslot. The basic idea of DQRAP is to concentrate user accesses in the control subslot, while the data subslot is devoted to collision free data transmission. The DQRAP provides a collision resolution tree algorithm that results stable for every traffic load even over the system transmission capacity. One of the most interesting features of the DQRAP protocol is its capacity to behave like an ALOHA-type protocol for light traffic load and to smoothly switch to a

reservation system as the traffic load increases, reducing automatically collisions. Moreover, it must be taken into account that the protocol is fair as all nodes get, on average, the same service from the system. An interesting property of the DQRAP comes from the distributed queue adoption. Nodes can estimate the system load simply considering the number of busy positions in each queue. The load estimation is important information in a network environment.

Based on their previous research works, Alonso et al. (2005) presented the Distributed Queuing Collision Avoidance (DQCA), which is a distributed high-performance medium access protocol designed for WLAN environments. The protocol behaves as a random access mechanism under low traffic conditions and switches smoothly and automatically to a reservation scheme when traffic load grows. DQCA has the following main features:

- It eliminates back-off periods and collisions in data packet transmissions.
- It performs independently of the number of stations transmitting in the system.
- It does not suffer from instability under all traffic conditions like slotted Aloha and keeps maximum achieved transmission rate if arrival rate keeps growing.

Crucial success of BSNs is the availability of small, lightweight, low-cost body sensors. Even more important for medical applications, the body sensors must consume low power to eliminate frequent battery replacement, at the same time that high reliability is guaranteed (Otal, Alonso, & Verikoukis, 2009). The preceding IEEE 802.15.4 MAC has all the aforementioned weaknesses when employed in BSNs for medical applications. However, the DQ MAC family introduces a range of advantages that we would like to further analyze from the energy-consumption perspective under BSNs in saturation conditions (*i.e.,* highly dense area).

Figure 3. General superframe structure of a DQ MAC scheme

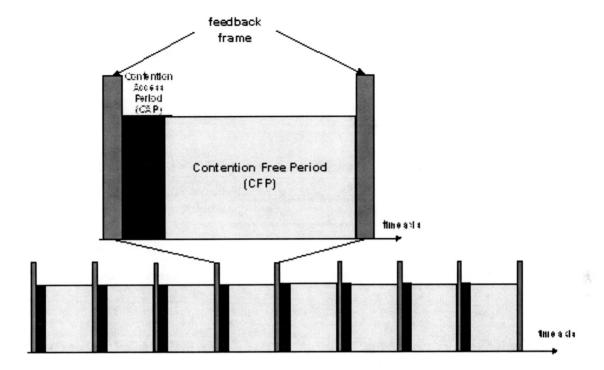

Energy-Saving DQ MAC Superframe

The proposed DQ MAC mechanism is a distributed always-stable high performance protocol, which behaves as a random access mechanism for low traffic load and switches smoothly and automatically to a reservation scheme when traffic load grows. The key feature of the proposed protocol is that it eliminates collisions and backoff periods in data packet transmissions. Figure 3 portrays the general superframe format of a DQ MAC mechanism. In our proposal for a star-based wireless BSN, the complete DQ MAC superframe structure comprises two differential parts:

1. From body sensors to BAN coordinator (uplink). This is through a CAP, specifically for body sensors' access requests, and a CFP, exclusively for collision-free data transmissions;
2. From BAN coordinator to body sensors (downlink). The BAN coordinator uses the

feedback frame in order to acknowledge the previous data transmission and to broadcast control information to all body sensors in the BSN, so that they can follow independently the protocol rules (see Alonso, Ferrús, & Agustí, 2005; Xu & Campbell, 1992).

Figure 4 depicts in more detail the superframe format of our adapted energy-saving DQ MAC first proposal for BSNs in healthcare environments.

DQ MAC Contention Access Period (CAP)

The CAP is further divided into m access minislots. Within these access minislots, Access Requests Sequences (ARS) of duration t_{ARS} are sent to gather a position within the CFP. ARS are the minimum signal required for the BAN coordinator to detect channel access. That means, the PHY level only needs to detect three different states (empty, success, collision), but in principle no information

Figure 4. Energy-saving DQ MAC superframe for BSNs

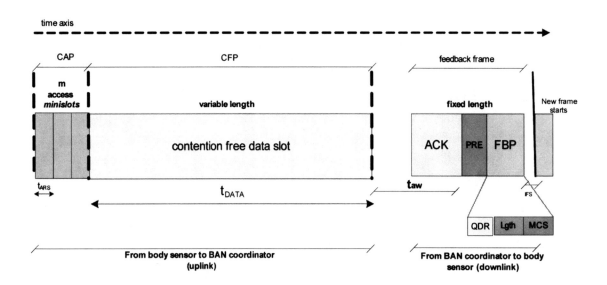

bits are required (Alonso, Ferrús, & Agustí, 2005; Xu & Campbell, 1992), though it is implementation dependant.

DQ MAC Contention Free Period (CFP)

Immediately after the CAP, the CFP allows contention free data transmissions within the contention free data slot of variable duration t_{DATA} or variable length (*i.e.*, payload length) (see Figure 4).

DQ MAC Feedback Frame

Following the contention free data slot, we define here t_{aw} as the maximum time to wait for an Acknowledgement (ACK) of duration t_{ACK}, as in IEEE 802.15.4 (IEEE, 2003). Bear in mind that the DQ MAC superframe is bounded by the hereby named Feedback Packet (FBP), of fixed duration t_{FBP}, contained in the depicted feedback frame (see Figure 3). Similar to IEEE 802.15.4 MAC superframe format, one of the main uses of the FBP is to synchronize the attached body sensors to the BAN coordinator. The FBP always contains relevant MAC control information, which

is essential for the right functioning of all the attached body sensors to the BSN using the DQ MAC protocol. In our energy-saving DQ MAC superframe proposal, the FBP is preceded by a novel synchronization Preamble (PRE), which follows immediately after t_{aw} elapses. The functionality of PRE is to enable power management solutions and energy-aware radio activation policies among the different time intervals in order to prolong body sensors' battery lifetime. At the end of the DQ MAC superframe, an Inter Frame Space (IFS) is added to allow the MAC layer to process the data received from the PHY layer.

All in all, the main differences of this new energy-saving DQ MAC superframe format with respect to the previous DQ MAC ones are the following:

1. A Preamble (PRE) is newly introduced within the broadcasted feedback frame, concretely between the ACK and the FPB, to enable synchronization after power-sleep modus (*i.e.*, either idle or shutdown, see Bourgard, Catthoor, Daly, Chandrakasam, & Dehaene, 2005). The intuitive reasoning is the following: (1) The feedback frame is an aggregation of an ACK and the

FBP in order to save PHY header overhead and therefore energy-consumption at reception. That is, the ACK is essential only to the body sensor, who transmitted in the previous contention free data slot. Hence, body sensors can prolong their power-sleep modus until the immediate reception of the FBP. (2) The precise position of the PRE between the ACK and the FBP is mainly due to scalability in terms of energy-efficiency. This means that in a future system design or downlink multicast applications, several ACKs or any other type of info, may be aggregated just before the preamble—PRE. Body sensors within the DQ MAC system not being addressed in this multicast/aggregated communication shall only receive the FBP. That is the reason why a preamble is suitable in this explicit position.

2. FBP is here of fixed length (*i.e.*, independent of the number of sensors in the BSN) and contains two brand new fields for specific energy-saving purposes; the Modulation and Coding Scheme (MCS) and Length of the packet transmitting in the next contention free data slot. This facilitates independent energy-aware radio activation policies; so that body sensors can calculate the time, they can remain in power-sleep modus. Further, the MCS field is also thought for future multi-rate medical applications in BSNs (*i.e.*, scalability).

Note that the FBP always contains a specific field named QDR (Queuing Discipline Rules), which contains the updating information regarding the aforementioned ARS. That is, the QDR field contains the state of each of the access minislots, which can be empty, success, or collision. Two bits are necessary to encode the state of each access minislot, so $2 \cdot m$ is the total number of bits devoted to the QDR field, see (Alonso, Ferrús, & Agustí, 2005; Xu & Campbell, 1992). Additionally, there is the possibility to transmit data packets of variable length (t_{DATA}), using the same frame structure, at the same time that energy-saving benefits are maintained.

DQ MAC Data Transaction in a Star-Based BSN

Three types of direct data transfer transactions may exist in a stand-alone BSN. The first one is the data transfer from any body sensor to the BAN coordinator. The second type of transaction is the data transfer from the BAN coordinator to body sensors. The third transaction is the data transfer between two peer body sensors. In a star-based topology, only two of these transactions are used, because data may be exchanged only between the BAN coordinator and a body sensor. Hereby we choose to model and further study the single-hop star-based topology, because:

1. it is the most feasible topology in current BSN medical applications scenarios (see Yang, 2006).
2. it is the most suitable topology using DQ MAC. That is to say that a DQ MAC scheme already requires a centralized architecture (Xu & Campbell, 1992), in spite of the distributed and independent behavior of all body sensors in the BSN.
3. it is the most energy-efficient topology within direct short-range communication between body sensors and the BAN coordinator, taking single body sensor battery life-time into account.

Body sensors in medical applications are especially stringent in terms of power consumption. The replacement of batteries may cost more than the devices themselves, like for example in implantable devices. It is not only very cumbersome, but also practically impossible to replace the batteries in some applications at once. In a single-hop star-based BSN, body sensors save energy resources, because all data transmissions are directly to the BAN coordinator (within low-power range), which is elected considering its superiority in terms of power resources. That is, since no multi-hop data transmission is allowed, body sensors can manage their power consumption considering their own residual battery lifetime. That is the reason why a well-designed single-hop star-based BSN is more reasonable for short-range medical applications.

Data Transfer from a Body Sensor to a BAN Coordinator in a BSN

Our here referred DQ MAC protocol is based on two distributed queues. Note that for clarity reasons; only a brief explanation is included here. A more detailed description can be found in Alonso, Ferrús, and Agustí (2005) and Xu and Campbell (1992):

1. the Collision Resolution Queue (CRQ); and
2. the Data Transmission Queue (DTQ).

The CRQ is devoted to the collision resolution algorithm (for resolving ARS collisions) and the DTQ to collision-free data packet transmission scheduling. Both queues are simply represented by four integer numbers, recorded at every body sensor (*i.e.*, distributed queues), which correspond to the specific sensor position and the total number of sensors in each queue. Every body sensor updates these four numbers upon synchronization through the PRE and reception of the FBP. The information contained in the QDR field carries this specific information, see Figure 4 (Xu & Campbell, 1992). Thereafter, every body sensor applies a set of rules to actualize its position in the CRQ and DTQ queues accordingly. At the appropriate time, a body sensor transmits whether an ARS within the CAP or its data packet within the CFP to the BAN coordinator. The BAN coordinator acknowledges the successful reception of the data packet by transmitting ACK. This sequence is summarized in more detail in the illustration of Figure 5.

Further, Figure 6 specifically depicts a state-of-the-art DQ MAC data transfer from a body sensor to a BAN coordinator in a BSN, following

DQ MAC protocol rules regarding CRQ and DTQ, after updating the state of the queues thanks to the information in the QDR field in FBP.

As aforementioned, a body sensor willing to transmit a packet must first synchronize with the BSN through the FBP broadcasted by the BAN coordinator to update the state of the system queues (CRQ & DTQ). Note that when both queues are empty, the protocol uses an exception of slotted-Aloha (see Xu & Campbell, 1992). However, if CRQ is empty—but DTQ is not—, the body sensor sends an ARS—randomly selecting one of the access minislots—to grant its access into DTQ. If its ARS collides with any of another body sensor in the selected access minislot, these body sensors involved therein occupy the same position in CRQ (following the order of the selected minislot position), and wait for a future frame to compete for a free access minislot again to grant its access into a DTQ exclusive position. New body sensors, with a packet to send, are not allowed to enter the system until CRQ is empty (*i.e.*, all current collisions are resolved). When a

Figure 5. Communication between a body sensor and the BAN coordinator

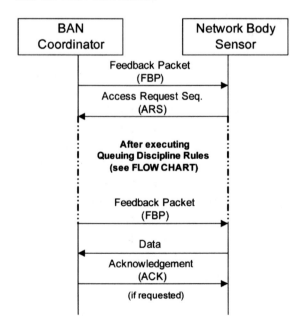

Figure 6. DQ MAC flow chart for energy-saving BSNs based on original DQRAP algorithm

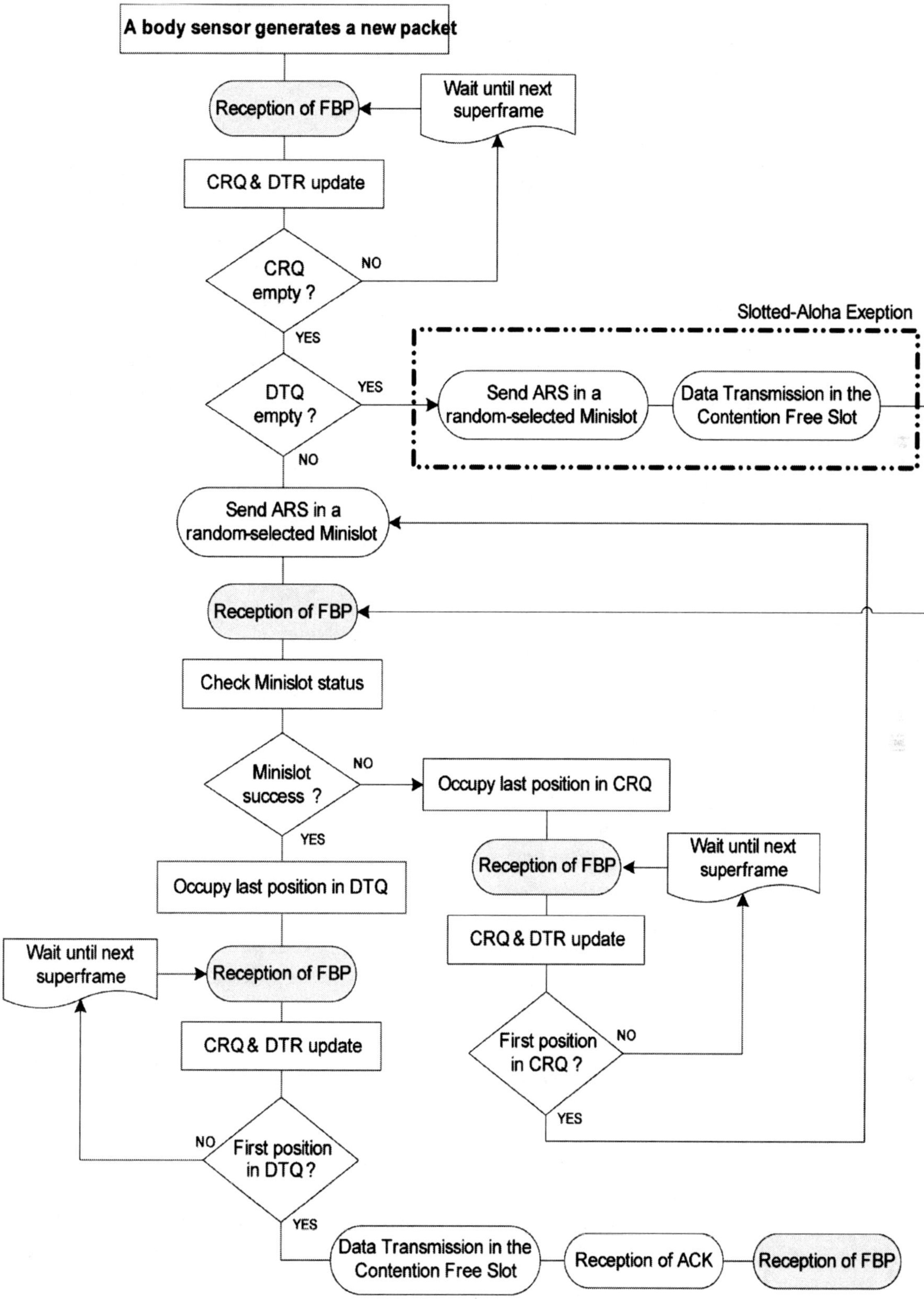

body sensor selects successfully a free access minislot (known at the reception of the FBP), it takes immediately a place in DTQ up. If DTQ is now empty, it may be in the first position of DTQ, thus transmitting directly in the next DQ MAC superframe data slot.

Note that a body sensor is just allowed to send an ARS in a random-selected minislot if and only if CRQ is empty. If CRQ is not empty, this body sensor has to wait until the next superframe and recheck again CRQ condition via the FBP. Therefore, the inherent behaviour of the protocol avoids new ARSs entering the system, if there are still old ARS to be resolved. That is, CRQ only has new entries, whenever it becomes empty.

ENERGY CONSUMPTION ANALYSIS IN SATURATION CONDITIONS

Like other different types of sensors, body sensors are limited in stored energy, computational capacity and memory. New MAC protocols and algorithms must be designed with special attention to these aspects and above all to their limited and sometimes non-renewable power storage. Significant power is consumed at a body sensor when it either transmits or receives a packet. Here we proceed to evaluate body sensors' energy consumption in a star-based BSN using DQ MAC with respect to IEEE 802.15.4 MAC in saturation conditions (*i.e.,* highly dense BSNs), in which we suppose there are always sensors transmitting, and CRQ and DTQ are never empty (see Figure 6). That is, we assume a specific window size at a time for evaluating CRQ inner ARS resolution.

The DQ MAC energy consumption per information bit in saturation conditions ε_{bit} (*i.e.,* efficiency) is here calculated as the average energy consumption to transmit one DQ MAC superframe $E_{Superframe}$ over the payload packet length in bits L_{bit} of a superframe, considering all body sensors always have packets to send. Thus, the total energy consumption per information bit ε_{bit} in saturation

conditions for the whole superframe transmission can be expressed as follows:

$$\varepsilon_{bit} = \frac{E_{Superframe}}{L_{bit}}, \tag{1}$$

where L_{bit} corresponds to the payload length in bits of the data packet transmitted in the collision-free data slot and $E_{Superframe}$ is defined as the energy consumption of the whole DQ MAC superframe from a body sensor perspective, taking uplink and downlink into consideration (see Figure 4).

To calculate the body sensor energy consumption for the whole DQ MAC superframe duration $E_{Superframe}$ (see Figure 4), let us first define the following:

1. E_{ARS}, and E_{DATA}, as the energy consumption for ARS and data frame transmissions; and,
2. E_{ACK}, and E_{FBP}, as the energy consumption for ACK and FBP frame receptions, respectively.

These energies can be obtained as:

$$\begin{aligned}
E_{ARS} &= m t_{ARS} P_{tx\_ARS}, \\
E_{DATA} &= t_{DATA} P_{tx\_DATA}, \\
E_{ACK} &= t_{ACK} P_{rx}, \\
E_{FBP} &= (t_{PRE} + t_{FBP}) P_{rx}.
\end{aligned} \tag{2}$$

where P_{tx_DATA} is the power consumption in transmission mode for a data frame, which according to Chipcon specifications (Chipcon, 2004) could differ from the power consumption of transmitting ARS (P_{tx_ARS}), since in IEEE 802.15.4 MAC different transmission modes are allowed. Additionally, P_{rx} is the power consumption in receiving mode. Further, (2) also contains the average time the transceiver is in each of these four energy-consumption states corresponding to the DQ MAC superframe duration (see Figure 4), t_{ARS} for ARS transmissions, t_{DATA} for data transmission, t_{ACK} for

ACK reception, and, t_{PRE}, t_{FBP} for PRE synchronization and FBP reception, as aforementioned. Thus, here $E_{Superframe}$ is computed as:

$$
\begin{aligned}
E_{Superframe} = {} & E_{ARS} + E_{DATA} + E_{ACK} + E_{FBP} \\
& + (t_{aw} - t_{ACK} + t_{IFS})P_{idle}.
\end{aligned}
\tag{3}
$$

Therefore, DQ MAC energy consumption efficiency ε_{bit} is expressed in Joules per information bit (J/bit). Note that P_{idle} corresponds to the state when a body sensor is neither transmitting nor receiving bits. That is to say, that a body sensor is not active or it is in idle mode. Typically, in general WSNs, the power consumed during receiving mode is larger than in transmitting mode (Bourgard, Catthoor, Daly, Chandrakasam, & Dehaene, 2005). The figures of the power consumptions utilized here in our case study are listed in Table 1 and based on Chipcon specifications (Chipcon, 2004). For the sake of simplicity, in our calculations, we consider that both power consumptions in transmission mode (*i.e.*, P_{tx_DATA} and P_{tx_ARS}) have the same value, although they could differ from each other based on hardware specifications (Chipcon, 2004).

The reference scenario is defined by a set of parameters provided in Table 2, whose fields correspond to IEEE 802.15.4 MAC default values (IEEE, 2003).

Notice that the maximum Packet Service Data Unit (PSDU) the PHY layer shall be able to receive a packet in the IEEE 802.15.4 MAC standard is 127 bytes (IEEE, 2003). That is the reason why we study several lengths up to 118 bytes (approx. 120 bytes), assuming the minimum MAC overhead

length of 9 bytes as indicated in Table 2. Further, in our DQ MAC protocol, the number of access minislots m is also 3, as in (Alonso, Ferrús, & Agustí, 2005; Xu & Campbell, 1992). As previously said, the duration of the ARS (t_{ARS}) could be reduced to a very small value (*i.e.*, between 2 μs and 10 μs), since no data information is needed to be carried through (Alonso, Ferrús, & Agustí, 2005; Xu & Campbell, 1992). For our calculations though, we use 128 μs as ARS duration value in order to consider the worst-case scenario. This is equivalent to the duration of the Preamble sequence in IEEE 802.15.4 MAC and might be fare with a feasible hardware prototype implementation. Figure 7 characterizes the energy consumption per information bit of DQ MAC mechanism for BSNs derived from Equation (1) and the parameter values of Table 1 and Table 2. As expected, DQ MAC energy consumption per information bit decreases rapidly at increasing the payload length, due to the smaller relative overhead. DQ MAC mechanism maximum energy consumption is obtained for small-sized packets and reaches its maximum of 3.5×10^{-7} J/bit of the overall normalized energy consumption.

Following DQ MAC protocol specific rules, a body sensor is just allowed to send an ARS in a random-selected minislot, if and only if CRQ is empty. Unless CRQ is empty, this body sensor has to wait until the next superframe and recheck again CRQ condition via FBP (see Figure 6). Therefore, the inherent behavior of the protocol avoids new ARSs entering the system, if there are still old ARS to be resolved. That is, CRQ only

Table 1. IEEE 802.15.4 transceiver power consumption (–25 dBm)

$P_{tx\ ARS}$	P_{tx_DATA}	P_{rx}	P_{idle}
15 mW	15 mW	35.23 mW	712 μW

Table 2. IEEE 802.15.4 MAC & DQ MAC parameter values

Parameter	Value	Parameter	1Value
PHY header	6 bytes	ACK	11 bytes
MAC header	9 bytes	Beacon	11 bytes
Data payload	8 to 120 bytes	t_{aw}	864 μs
Data rate	250 Kb/s	t_{IFS}	192 μs

Figure 7. Energy consumption per information bit of DQ MAC protocol for BSNs

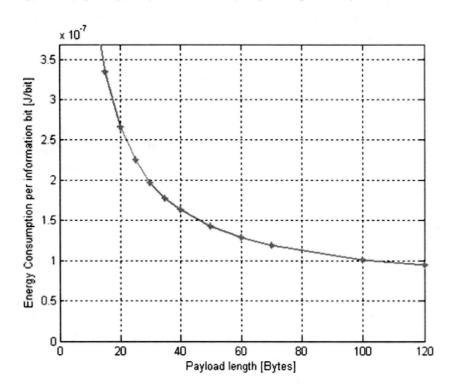

has new entries, whenever it becomes empty. In this particular scenario, we modeled a non-empty CRQ per window size, assuming on average *m* ARSs transmissions at a time in the process of CRQ becoming empty. That is in practice independently of which access minislot has been used, but in theory, we assume that there is no empty access minislot within that transmission. This assumption is valid in this specific conditions and scenario, since in (Xu & Campbell, 1992), there is an example (for highly dense networks) where it can be seen that in stable conditions, with *m*=3, after the third round trip, most devices have already entered DTQ. There, it is also proved the small difference between using *m*=3 or *m*=16 (a bigger number of minislots), showing that the delay to resolve collisions is minimal independently of the number of minislots. The specific rules of DQRAP (original DQ MAC) are explained in more detail in Alonso, Ferrús, and Agustí (2005) and Xu and Campbell (1992).

It is assumed that all blocked stations are supposed to transmit immediately whenever CRQ becomes empty, here synchronized via the FBP, and thereafter the protocol follows with the same behavior. DQ MAC assures that the speed of contention resolution in the CRQ subsystem is faster than the speed of data transmission, thus guaranteeing that the CRQ subsystem will not block input traffic to the whole system (Alonso, Ferrús, & Agustí, 2005; Xu & Campbell, 1992).

DQ MAC Energy Consumption Performance Evaluation

To get example figures, a scenario with an increasing number of always-active body sensors in a star-based BSN in saturation has been selected. The next Figure 8 depicts the achievable estimated energy consumption improvement per information bit of DQ MAC mechanism versus IEEE 802.15.4 MAC protocol, derived from expressions (1) and from Park, Kim, Choi, Choi, and Kwon (2005), respectively. All IEEE 802.15.4 MAC curves are as a function of the payload length (in bytes) and the number of body sensors in the BSN. In saturation conditions, the IEEE 802.15.4 MAC shall deal with a certain level of data collisions, which steadily increases with the number of body sensors in the network. This results in a progressive reduction of the energy efficiency of the IEEE 802.15.4 MAC. In contrast, when evaluating DQ MAC protocol energy consumption per information bit in the same saturation conditions, we observed that DQ MAC energy efficiency is independent of the number of body sensors in the BSN, similar to the previous throughput analysis (see Alonso, Ferrús, & Agustí, 2005; Xu & Campbell, 1992). That is, because of the inherent behavior of DQ MAC of eliminating back-off periods and collisions in data transmissions by means of the distributed queuing system. This means, that in saturation conditions, DTQ is always non-empty, and collisions are gradually being resolved in the CRQ. As a result, no collisions are produced in the information data part of DQ MAC superframe (see Figure 4), and therefore no energy per information bit is wasted due to unwilling collisions. Like in the previous studied case, the reference scenario is defined by a set of parameters provided in Table 1 and Table 2, whose fields correspond to IEEE 802.15.4 MAC default values (IEEE, 2003).

All data transmissions are supposed to be successful, except from the ones that fail anyway due to channel conditions, such as fading or Doppler Effect. Thus, although the collision resolution mechanism requires some energy consumption, the complete elimination of data collisions represents a remarkable enhancement in the overall network. That is:

- up to 98% improvement with respect to IEEE 802.15.4 MAC for a 40 body-sensor network size.
- up to 92% improvement with respect to IEEE 802.15.4 MAC for a 20 body-sensor network size.

- up to 77% improvement with respect to IEEE 802.15.4 MAC for a 10 body-sensor network size.
- up to 52% improvement with respect to IEEE 802.15.4 MAC for a 5 body-sensor network size.

OVERALL MAC OVERHEAD COMPARISON IN SATURATION CONDITIONS

Previously, we have compared the energy consumption per information bit of IEEE 802.15.4 MAC analytical model in Park, Kim, Choi, Choi, and Kwon (2005) versus our proposed DQ MAC analytical scheme in saturation conditions. Next, we evaluate the overall MAC superframe overhead in terms of energy consumption based on the analysis in Bourgard, Catthoor, Daly, Chandrakasam, and Dehaene (2005). As sketched in both superframe structures of IEEE 802.15.4 MAC and DQ MAC in Figure 9, the IEEE 802.15.4 MAC introduces significant overhead, which has consequential impact on the overall energy consumption in saturation conditions. Please be aware that all depicted MAC fields follow IEEE 802.15.4 MAC values specified in Table 2 (IEEE, 2003). As aforementioned, to be fair in the comparison both IEEE 802.15.4 MAC and DQ MAC data packet lengths are the same, and the beacon and FBP fields have the same value respectively in their MAC superframes, *i.e.*, 11 bytes. In the following, we assume that body sensors attempt to transmit a single packet per superframe. Let us here assess the overall MAC overhead of the whole superframe structure in saturation conditions (*i.e.*, there is always a packet to be transmitted). To do so, in Figure 9 we clearly distinguished among the different power consumption states: transmit, receive and idle, like aforementioned in the previous studied scenario. In the IEEE 802.15.4 MAC superframe, a body sensor first listens to the beacon, after having preemptively turned on

Figure 8. Achievable estimated energy consumption improvement per information bit of DQ MAC vs. IEEE 802.15.4 MAC

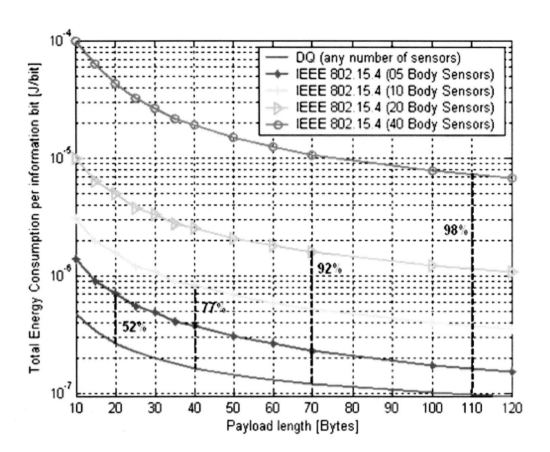

its radio in receive mode. After the beacon is received, the body sensor can enter in idle mode. The contention procedure requires at least two channel senses for Clear Channel Assessment (CCA) (IEEE, 2003), which requires turning the receiver on. Within the CCAs, the receiver can return to the idle state. Once the channel is assessed clear twice, the transmission can start. If the packet is well received, a short ACK is fed back to the body sensor (in receiving mode) after a minimum time t_{aw} when it is in idle state.

Figure 9 also shows our here proposed DQ MAC procedure, whose relative overhead compared to that of IEEE 802.15.4 is remarkably lower in saturation conditions. To compute the whole MAC overhead in DQ MAC in saturation

conditions, we assume a body sensor is transmitting in the collision-free data slot, while its ARS has already been transmitted in a previous DQ MAC superframe. That is, in saturation conditions we compute the DQ MAC superframe energy-consumption per information bit.

To lower power consumption in future designs, it is valuable to know the power breakdown of both DQ MAC and IEEE 802.15.4 MAC superframe structures, taking previous. Figure 10 presents the power breakdown between the different phases of the DQ MAC and IEEE 802.15.4 MAC considering their illustrations in Figure 9 and specified values in Table 2. We notice that the effective transmission in DQ MAC uses already more than 50% of the total energy consumption,

Figure 9. Energy consumption per information bit of DQ MAC protocol for BSNs

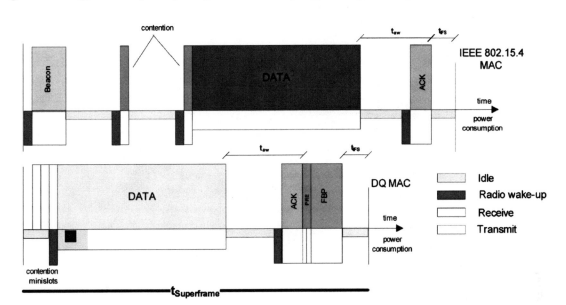

which is an improvement with respect to IEEE 802.15.4, as analyzed in Bourgard, Catthoor, Daly, Chandrakasam, & Dehaene (2005). Less than 15% is spent during DQ MAC contention taking radio wake up polices into account. The ACK mechanism uses more than 15% of the energy, mainly because of the necessity of activating the receiver during the acknowledgement waiting-time t_{aw}. For listening to the FBP, around 10% of the energy is used, compared to the 20% of energy spent in IEEE 802.15.4 in beacon mode. The rest is used for Inter-Frame Space (IFS) purposes (*i.e.*, processing). Please note that all our analysis take radio wake up policies into account, for both DQ MAC and IEEE 802.15.4 MAC protocols.

DISCUSSION: TOWARDS A SMART SCHEDULING ALGORITHM FOR QoS IN BSNs

As already explained, in medical environments, a centralized architecture is appropriate, since the BAN coordinator (e.g. the Care Unit in Figure 1) is superior to the rest of the body sensors in terms of processing memory, storage and power resources. Thus, releasing body sensors of un-necessary energy-consumption, and other scarcely resources. Note that if the traffic load (or rather, the number of ambient or body sensors) in the BSN notably increases be-yond saturation limits, a cluster-tree architecture with several BAN coordinators can be adopted, as also allowed in IEEE 802.15.4 (IEEE, 2003).

Based on our here presented DQ MAC protocol and our work presented in Otal, Alonso, and Verikoukis (2010), we further develop the Distributed Queuing Body Area Network (DQBAN) protocol (Otal, Alonso, & Verikoukis, 2009), to introduce an overall system characterization specially modified for energy-efficient wireless BSNs with special QoS demands in healthcare environments. This article mainly studies the DQBAN behavioural bounds in a star-based BSN with a single BAN coordinator close to saturation limits under two specific hospital scenarios. The main goal is to evaluate DQBAN scalability, in terms of QoS and energy-consumption, in highly dense scenarios, i.e. with a sudden increase of traffic load, which turns to be the most difficult in

Figure 10. Breakdown of energy consumption

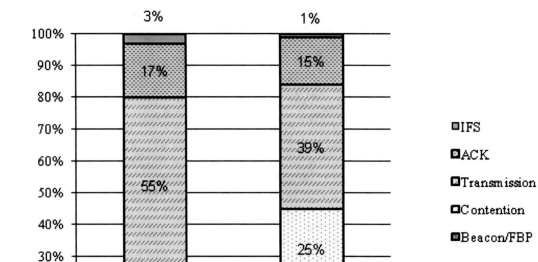

current MAC protocol designs. These two specific medical scenarios are the following:

Medical Homogenous Scenario

One possible scenario is a ward with several hospitalized patients that are real-time monitored by several ECG body sensors sending their data to a central-room care unit, as portrayed in Figure 1. This scenario is defined as homogenous, because all body sensors belong to the same type of application, i.e. ECG. That is, we first study DQBAN in a homogenous setting with an increasing number of ECG body sensors until reaching saturation traffic conditions, in order to validate its performance within a high density area (i.e. many patients wearing body sensors at once). Nowadays, realistic

healthcare settings of these characteristics may range from a hospital waiting room to a geriatric clinic rest room (i.e. within 6–8 m distance from the BAN coordinator). In those situations, several patients are being monitored for a period of time in order to achieve a specific diagnosis, verify a given treatment, or simply as a preventive monitoring measure to avoid any acute episode. Note that we use here ECGs, but a similar scenario can be portrayed using EEGs (encephalograms) or any other sort of body sensors. The focus is to evaluate DQBAN overall performance and its QoS benefits in front of a plain DQ MAC protocol.

Medical Heterogeneous Scenario

In practice, most archetypal healthcare scenarios conform to a centralized infrastructure with heterogeneous sets of applications and data traffic. An example may be a star-based BSN, where the vital signs data of several hospitalized real-time monitoring patients (wearing different on-body sensors on bed or walking, such as ECG, respiratory rate, blood pressure, oxygen saturation [SpO2]) and doctors' notes (working on a PDAs or Laptops) are transmitted to a central-floor care unit for controlling within a short distance. Simple realistic scenarios can also be either a wide corridor of a hospital floor or a clinic rest room. Note that a star-based BSN with DQBAN is also appropriate inside the operating theatre, where different sorts of applications are utilised. Nonetheless, in order to evaluate DQBAN scalability, its study is most required in large-scale scenarios with an increasing number of patients, or rather, an increasing number of active body sensors.

New System Modelling

DQBAN corresponds to an overall improvement of the previous designed energy-saving DQ MAC model. Specifically, DQBAN is modified by means of a novel cross-layer fuzzy-logic scheduling mechanism apart from the energy-aware radio activation policies to satisfy both energy-efficient and stringent QoS demands in healthcare scenarios. Like in the original DQ MAC protocols, back-off periods and collisions in data packets are eliminated, thereby increasing also goodput efficiency with respect to IEEE 802.15.4 MAC (IEEE, 2003). Hence, DQBAN supports high application-dependant performance requirements in terms of reliability, message latency, and power consumption, while being adaptable to changing conditions, such as heterogeneous traffic load, interferences, and the number of sensors in a hospital BSN. DQBAN also utilizes the two common logical distributed queues CRQ and DTQ, for serving access requests (via the "access minislots") and data packets (via the "data slot"), respectively. In the new logic system model though, instead of keeping a first-come-first-served discipline in DTQ, a cross-layer fuzzy-rule based scheduler is introduced (Otal, Alonso, & Verikoukis, 2009). The use of the scheduler permits a body sensor, though not occupying the first position in DTQ, to transmit its data in the next collision-free "data slot" in order to achieve a far more reliable system performance for medical applications. Practically speaking, this is obtained by integrating a fuzzy-logic system in each body sensor in the BSN. A fuzzy-logic approach allows each particular body sensor to individually deal with multiple cross-layer inputs of diverse nature. The basic idea is that body sensors consider their own QoS criteria, current channel quality and battery constraints, and make use of fuzzy-logic theory, as a control mechanism, to demand or refuse the next frame "data slot," according to their particular needs.

Note that the cross-layer Fuzzy-Logic System (FLS) is implemented in each body sensor. That means that the own FLS could learn about the body sensor behaviour taken the current channel conditions into account. However, there are still a lot more different types of existing services that may be offered for ambient and BSNs in the clinical field. Thus, apart from our analysis and performance evaluation in terms of QoS, delay efficiency, and power consumption, there are many other parameters, depending on the medical application scenario, that still require some special emphasis. In particular, we would like to find out if our designed DQBAN protocol model is especially suitable for other specific kind of medical or personal healthcare settings. For that, we will further adapt and optimize the DQBAN protocol for different sorts of medical applications following their specific requirements in future trends.

FUTURE TRENDS

This chapter aims at contributing to the evolution of BSNs, not only with the main given inputs summarized in the previous sections, but also with the fundamental analysis to many open topics that have been identified through the course of this work, though have not been covered in this chapter. Some of these recognised open lines of research are the following:

Selection of a New IEEE 802.15 as a Standard-the-Facto of Reference for BSNs

The selection of IEEE 802.15.4 (IEEE, 2003) as a standard-the-facto of reference for BSNs is going to change in the immediate future, since wireless BSN systems will be standardized in the brand-new IEEE 802.15.6 task group. This new group may include specific characteristic and features of IEEE 802.15.4 PHY/MAC. We could follow the new lines within the standardisation world in order to foresee new upcoming medical and personal healthcare application scenarios and detect their potential new requirements for BSNs. For instance, one of the goals of the standardisation group IEEE 802.15.4b (IEEE, 2005) is to enhance the current IEEE 802.15.4 868/915 MHz PHY with a higher data rate in the future. The current IEEE 802.15.4b draft introduces two new PHY that enable 100 to 250 kb/s for the 868 MHz band and 250 kb/s for the 915 MHz band. However, due to the current draft status of IEEE 802.15.4b and eventual changes in radio regulations, the future evolution of the IEEE 802.15.4 868/915 MHz band with respect to the achievable data rate remains uncertain. At the current time, the relation and final status with the new IEEE 802.15.6 is still unclear, though it may be compliant to IEEE 802.15.4.

For the time being, owing to the data rate requirements of BSNs, the 2.450 MHz PHY seems appropriate to enable the envisaged medical use cases. However, two drawbacks of the utiliza-

tion of the 2.4 GHz ISM frequency band are still considerable:

1. body attenuation, and;
2. the potentially high interference levels.

These topics could be further discussed in future work.

Evaluation of the Proposed DQ MAC Protocol in a Stand-Alone Mesh-Based BSN

In this chapter, we aimed at evaluating the DQ MAC protocol constraints in a star-based topology, considering most current medical applications. However, there might be future medical applications requiring one or even both sorts of topologies, i.e. star-based and mesh-based BSN. The star-based topology implies a centralized architecture, which has been straightforward from our proposed DQ MAC protocol perspective. The mesh topology, on the other hand, is a new challenge to evaluate, since every body sensor could send packets peer-to-peer to its neighbouring sensors. This means that our proposed DQ MAC protocol approach, ideal for a star-based topology BSN, will obviously have to be extended to the mesh topology. For a mesh-topology without any BAN coordinator, we can intuitively suggest a table-based solution, through which every body sensor should be able to actualise the inherent information of the DQ MAC protocol in a decentralised way, via its first-hop neighbouring sensors. However, we should also study this solution in terms of scalability. Nevertheless, there is already in the literature, in Alonso-Zárate, Kartsakli, Alonso, and Verikoukis (2010), a similar approach for the 802.11 family in using cluster-tree architecture with several BAN coordinators though with peer-to-peer communication. We could also analyse and compare this possibility, and if it results in a better performance, we will adapt it to our protocol definition.

Wireless Ambient Sensor Network Discovery and Association

From now on, we are not just dealing with stand-alone BSNs, but with the combination of WSNs and BSNs (i.e. Ambient and Body Sensor Networks) that cooperate in conjunction for performing the same type of medical or personal healthcare application e.g. a telecare monitoring system used to monitor elderly individuals living alone in their own home. We will therefore study and adapt discovery schemes for a BSN neighbouring ambient sensor network that could match our DQ MAC approach. Once the discovery went through, the following step is the association establishment via a candidate sensor from the BSN that will link both networks, ambient-body network (see Otal, 2010). In order to do so, a candidate sensor of the BSN should be selected for this type of linking-forwarding role. In a star-based topology, it could be the BAN coordinator, the one also in charge of this new function, since this new role should just be a small fraction to add on its coordination tasks. However, in a mesh-based topology, the selection of the candidate sensor is not that straightforward. We should apply prior to the association establishment, a self-configuration algorithm, so as to select the appropriate candidate sensor that will act as a linking and afterwards forwarding node with the new discovered wireless ambient network. In this case, the candidate node could be interchangeable within the sensors configuring the BSN.

Integration of Self-Configuration Setup Algorithms Based on Cross-Layer Information

We will deal with a rule-based self-configuration set-up, based on smart algorithms, such as fuzzy-logic algorithms, that may take the sensor functionality and power consumption into account in order to establish the most appropriate and stateless configuration. Therefore, depending on the medi-

cal application the BSN is attached to, the selected central sensor could be either the one with higher power capacity, or the one being closer to e.g. a PC/PDA that collects all information (i.e. minimising therefore power transmission by reducing distance attenuation), or the sensor performing a concrete function, which is not of vital importance, and can devote time and power capacity to acting as a coordinator. Having said that, we will analyse whether this initial self-configuration setup may be possible via a PHY-MAC cross-layer dialogue. The new idea herewith is that the initial minislots for petition requests inherent of the DQ MAC protocol (Otal, Alonso, & Verikoukis, 2009) are used to initiate the self-configuration set-up, in terms of power capacity of the sensor.

Another totally different possibility we would like to study is the fact of using a MAC-APP cross-layer dialog, where the coordinator of the star-based topology BSN is chosen application-wise. That is, depending on what the function of the sensor is, it will be decided, if it is feasible that it becomes a coordinator. The next straight forward approach is to try to combine both concepts and develop a PHY-MAC-APP tri-cross-layer dialog, which will be a hybrid of the aforementioned mechanisms, and matches completely DQBAN strategy. In order to do so we can use smart algorithms that should take a decision from a balanced perspective, i.e. DQBAN cross-layer fuzzy-logic algorithm.

Study of Interference Mitigation Solutions and Adaptation to the Medical Domain

In medical applications running on stand-alone BSNs, the propagation conditions are likely to vary mainly due to interferences in the neighbourhood of the BAN. The IEEE 802.15.4 PHY (IEEE, 2003) uses Direct Sequence Spread Spectrum (DSSS) to fight against the potentially high interference levels from other standards (e.g. 802.11 families) in the unlicensed frequency bands (i.e. 2.450

MHz PHY). We would like to further analyze this approach to introduce an adaptive multi-code algorithm based on Alonso, Agusti, and Sallent (2000). Unlike Alonso, Agusti, and Sallent (2000), where multicode is used as a way to increase the overall throughput performance for UMTS (i.e. CDMA) oriented applications, herewith we would like to use adaptive codes as a way to mitigate interferences and as a signal protection. That is, the data from a sensor which requires a special treatment in terms of QoS (i.e depending on the functionality of the sensor) may use an additional code derived from the proposed MAC protocol in order to mitigate the interferences in the neighbourhood and achieve a better protection.

Efficiency Analysis of Multi-Rate and Receiver Aggregation Algorithms as Energy-Saving Measurements for Future Medical Applications

In the current IEEE 802.15.4 release the data rate of the 2.450 MHz PHY shall be 250 kb/s, being for the moment the maximum and unique data rate for medical applications using this frequency band. However, the IEEE 802.15.4b draft introduces already two new PHY that enable 100 to 250 kb/s for the 868 MHz band and 250 kb/s for the 915 MHz band, being in the current IEEE 802.15.4, only 20 kb/s and 40 kb/s respectively. We envisage that in future medical and personal healthcare sensing networking applications, ambient and body sensors may need to support higher data throughput demands with variable rates, at expenses of reducing their power capacity. Therefore, we would like to study some means to allow sensors to send data to several receivers (i.e. multicasting) using different multiple rates. Based on our new energy-saving DQ MAC superframe structure and the new smart scheduling approach (see Otal, Alonso, & Verikoukis, 2009), we aim at solutions at the MAC layer that may increase sensors data throughput without putting their battery life at risk. Thus, we are considering potential brand new medical use

case scenarios for BSNs requiring variable application rates and multiple sensor receivers with power management constraints.

Traditional aggregation schemes link MAC Protocol Data Units (MPDUs) between the same source and destination device together (IEEE, 2003). The main purpose of aggregation is to reduce the number of access attempts to the medium and thereby significantly increase the protocol efficiency and data throughput. An improvement to the traditional type of aggregation is to aggregate packets that are intended for more than one receiver. This feature will be especially useful for a BAN coordinator (star-based topology or equivalent configuration), whenever it may have to sent packets to many different receivers. For delay-critical applications traditional aggregation poses problems, because of the delay that is introduced by waiting for subsequent data packets for the same destination and buffering older packets in the meantime. If MPDUs for different receivers are aggregated, a reasonable aggregate size can be reached much faster and thereby the buffering delay is reduced. In the case of multiple receiver aggregation, the distance and propagation conditions between the sender and the different receivers can differ significantly.

For example, if MPDUs of the three sensor nodes with different Modulating and Coding Schemes (MCSs) (i.e. different rates) are aggregated and transmitted at the same MCS, the lowest MCS of all links requires to be chosen, which limits the throughput of all other sensors. In this case, either the whole aggregate has to be transmitted at the lowest rate or another option is not to aggregate and access the medium three times at different MCSs. Choosing the first option, aggregation at a single MCS, may result in a major decrease in efficiency in such a scenario. Therefore, under these circumstances, transmitting the MPDUs separately at different MCS and not aggregating gives rise to better performance. It is up to the sender, rsp. BAN coordinator (star-based topology) to decide in which situations linking of

MPDUs for different receivers together, makes sense and in which not. We would like to avoid this sort of time-consuming decisions at the BAN coordinator and make multiple receiver aggregation feasible in future multi-rate BSNs.

Therefore, we will propose a new multi-rate and receiver aggregation schemes based on our studies in Otal and Habetha (2005) and apply the introduced scheme good performance results to multi-rate BSNs. The presented multiple aggregation scheme, thereby named Multiple MCS and Receiver Aggregation (MMRA) (Otal & Habetha, 2005), allows the aggregation of MPDUs for several receivers to be transmitted at different MCSs. For this purpose MMRA information (i.e. MCS, MAC Addresses, Length, etc.) is transmitted in the PHY Header (although it could be also in the MAC Header), and sub-aggregates of different MCS are separated by preambles to allow PHY layer synchronisation. An evaluation methodology of our new multi-rate and receiver aggregation scheme adapted from our work in Otal and Habetha (2005) and a performance analysis will also be described.

Aggregation on MAC level requires that a receiving sensor stays awake during the whole aggregate (at least until its own MPDUs have been received) in order to keep PHY layer synchronization. With long aggregates, remaining awake during the entire aggregate can lead to very inefficient power saving at the receiving sensor. We will see that MMRA scheme solves this problem by introducing preambles inside the aggregate (as we did at designing DQ MAC energy-saving superframe). Preambles allow the receiving sensors to go into sleep-mode and re-synchronize after waking-up acting as an efficient power saving method. Analytical computations in Otal and Habetha (2005) show that MMRA performs better not only in time efficiency compared to other single-rate aggregation schemes, where MPDUs aggregates belonging to different receivers are limited to the lowest MCS, but above all MMRA outperforms single-rate aggregation schemes in terms of power efficiency. MMRA

provides a power saving frame format structure, which will allow receiving sensors to reduce power consumption and save battery life, crucial for body sensors in BSNs.

Please be aware, that the use of the preamble field PRE in DQ MAC is strategic, since in a downlink MMRA using the DQ MAC superframe, there might be several ACKs corresponding to different body sensors. Thus, the DQ MAC downlink feedback frame structure ACKs/PRE/FBP shall be maintained in order to save battery lifetime to all active body sensors in the BSN. That has already been previously commented.

Evaluation of Key Management Schemes in Order to Guarantee Secure Multicast Transmissions in BSNs

Our previous foreseen solution for allowing multiple sensor receivers gives rise mainly to one drawback; there is an issue of security resulting from the fact that encryption could be potentially more difficult when data for different receivers is combined. In order to handle this additional difficulty, we will study key management schemes to guarantee secure multicast (i.e. multiple receivers) transmissions.

In medical applications, broadcast encryption will address the problem of the allocation of secret keys to sensors in order to enable a BAN coordinator to securely broadcast data to a selected subset of sensor nodes. This has already been an important problem in the larger area of network security, so we would like to tackle this issue as an optimization of our previously studied multi-rate and receiver aggregation mechanism using the DQ MAC protocol in BSNs. Each time the BAN coordinator needs to establish a new broadcast key (i.e. to encrypt the data for a subset of sensors) it enacts an establishment protocol. This protocol consists of a sequence of transmissions; each transmission is encrypted using a different establishment key. A transmission can only be decrypted by the sensors that have the corresponding establishment key in their personalized set. The broadcast encryption system should be designed so that only privileged sensors in the subset are able to compute the new broadcast key when the protocol ends. Subsequent transmissions by the BAN coordinator are encrypted using the newly establishment broadcast key.

As an example, consider the simple broadcast encryption system in which each sensor has a unique establishment key. To establish a new broadcast key, select a random key B and send one transmission for each of the privileged sensors, encrypting B with the establishment key of the sensor. This protocol only requires a small amount of storage as each sensor holds just one establishment key. However, it requires a large amount of communication because the number of transmissions is equal to the number of sensors in the privileged set. At the opposite end of the spectrum, consider the broadcast encryption system that assigns to each set of sensors a unique establishment key and each sensor holds the keys for all sets in which it is a member. To establish a new broadcast key, select a random key B and send one transmission encrypting B using the establishment key associated with the set of privileged sensors. This system only requires one transmission (low communication). However, it requires each sensor to hold as many establishment keys as there are privileged sets in which it is a member (high storage). These two examples suggest there is a trade-off between the number of transmissions needed to establish a new broadcast key and the number of establishment keys held by each sensor. Thus, we would like to find some means to better handle this trade-off between the number of establishment keys held by each sensor (storage) and the number of transmissions required to establish a new broadcast key (communication and battery life).

CONCLUSION

This chapter aims at contributing to the incessant growth of Wireless Sensor Networks and particularly Body Sensor Networks (BSNs) considering essential medical equipments. The focus has been set on the optimization design, analysis, and performance evaluation of energy-saving MAC protocol solutions for BSNs in healthcare scenarios. Firstly, we analyzed the requirements and most convenient topology scenarios of new evolving BSNs for specific medical and healthcare settings. Following the new lines within the standardization world, we foresee new upcoming medical and personal healthcare application scenarios and detect the depicted potential new requirements for BSNs.

The core of this chapter is the proposal of a better conditioned energy-saving frame format of an enhanced Distributed Queuing Medium Access Protocol (DQ MAC) for Body Sensor Networks (BSN) in healthcare scenarios. Further, we presented an analytical evaluation of this enhanced DQ MAC protocol for a star-based BSN until reaching saturation conditions (*i.e.*, high-density area). It has been shown that our here proposed DQ MAC mechanism outperforms IEEE 802.15.4 MAC in terms of overall energy-consumption per information bit. All in all, we have shown that our proposed DQ MAC protocol represents a remarkable improvement of the overall network energy efficiency, which scales well for very dense BSNs and it is particularly suitable in medical scenarios. In fact, the work presented in the future trends of this chapter still leaves many open challenges to be solved and it does not conclude our studies on the field of optimization of BSNs in healthcare and medical scenarios, but it is a milestone in our way. The authors mentioned their work in relation to smart scheduling algorithms to increase QoS in the medical domain based on the here proposed DQ MAC protocol design. In previous work, we evaluated the performance of our complete proposed protocol structure for several sorts of medical and personal healthcare working scenarios.

ACKNOWLEDGMENT

This work was partially funded by the WSN4QoL (286047-PEOPLE-2011-IAPP) and CO2GREEN (TEC2010-20823).

REFERENCES

Alonso, L., Agusti, R., & Sallent, O. (2000). A near-optimum MAC protocol based on the distributed queuing random access protocol (DQRAP) for a CDMA mobile communication system. *IEEE Journal on Selected Areas in Communications, 18*, 1701–1718. doi:10.1109/49.872957

Alonso, L., Ferrús, R., & Agustí, R. (2005). WLAN throughput improvement via distributed queuing MAC. *IEEE Communications Letters, 9*(4), 310–312. doi:10.1109/LCOMM.2005.1413617

Alonso-Zárate, J., Kartsakli, E., Alonso, L., & Verikoukis, C. (2010). Performance analysis of a cluster-based MAC protocol for wireless ad hoc networks. *EURASIP Journal on Wireless Communications and Networking, n.d.*, 16.

Anliker, U., Ward, J. A., Lukowicz, P., Tröster, G., Dolveck, F., & Baer, M. (2004). AMON: A wearable multi-parameter medical monitoring ans alert system. *IEEE Transactions on Information Technology in Biomedicine, 8*(4), 415–427. doi:10.1109/TITB.2004.837888

BASUMA Project. (2006). *Webpage*. Retrieved from http://www.basuma.de/.

Bianchi, G. (2000). Performance analysis of the IEEE 802.11 distributed coordination function. *IEEE Journal on Selected Areas in Communications, 18*(3), 535–547. doi:10.1109/49.840210

Bourgard, B., Catthoor, F., Daly, D. C., Chandrakasam, A., & Dehaene, W. (2005). Energy efficiency of the IEEE 802.15.4 standard in dense wireless microsensor networks: modeling and improvement perspectives. In *Proceedings of the Design, Automation and Test in Europe*, (Vol. 1), (pp. 196 - 201). IEEE Press.

Cavalcanti, D., Schmitt, R., & Soomro, A. (2007). *Performance analysis of 802.15.4 and 802.11e for body sensor network applications*. Paper presented at the 4th International Workshop on Wearable and Implantable Body Sensor Networks (BSN 2007). Aachen, Germany.

Chevrollier, N., & Golmie, N. (2005). *On the use of wireless network technologies in healthcare environments*. Paper presented at the 5th Workshop on Applications and Services in Wireless Networks (ASWN 2005). Paris, France.

Chipcon, A. S. (2004). *SmartRF. CC2420 - 2.4 GHz IEEE 802.15.4/Zigbee RF transceiver, CC2420 data sheet*. Retrieved from http://inst.eecs.berkeley.edu/~cs150/Documents/CC2420.pdf.

Draft, IEEE. 802.15.4b™/D2. (2005). *Draft revision for standard for information technology part 15.4b: Wireless medium access control (MAC) and physical layer (PHY) specifications for low-rate wireless personal area networks (WPANs)*. New York, NY: IEEE Press.

Eklund, J. M., Hansen, T. R., Sprinkle, J., & Sastry, S. (2005). *Information technology for assisted living at home: Building a wireless infrastructure for assisted living*. Paper presented at the 27th Annual International Conference of the IEEE Engineering in Medicine and Biology Society. Shanghai, China.

Gang, L., Krishnamachari, B., & Raghavendra, C. S. (2004). Performance evaluation of the IEEE 802.15.4 MAC for low-rate low-power wireless networks. In *Proceedings of the IEEE International Conference on Performance, Computing and Communications*, (pp. 701 - 706). Phoenix, AZ: IEEE Press.

Golmie, N., Cypher, D., & Rebala, O. (2005). Performance analysis of low-rate wireless technologies for medical applications. *Elsevier Computer Communications, 28*(10), 1266–1275.

HealthService24 Project. (2009). *Website.* Retrieved from http://www.healthservice24.com/.

IEEE. 802.15.4 Std. (2003). *Wireless medium access control (MAC) and physical layer (PHY) specification for low-rate wireless personal area networks (LR-WPANs).* New York, NY: IEEE Press.

Jovanov, E., Milenkovic, A., Otto, C., & de Groen, P. C. (2005). A wireless body area network of intelligent motion sensors for computer assisted physical rehabilitation. *Journal of Neuroengineering and Rehabilitation, 2*(1), 6. doi:10.1186/1743-0003-2-6

Li, H., & Tan, J. (2005). An ultra-low-power medium access control protocol for body sensor network. In *Proceedings of the Engineering in Medicine and Biology Society Annual International Conference (IEEE-EMBS)*, (pp. 2451 - 2454). IEEE Press.

Lo, B. P. L., & Yang, G. Z. (2005). Key technical challenges and current implementations of body sensor networks. In *Proceedings of the 2nd International Workshop on Wearable and Implantable Body Sensor Networks*, (pp. 1-5). London, UK: IEEE.

Maharshi, A., Tong, L., & Swami, A. (2003). Cross-layer designs of multichannel reservation MAC under rayleigh fading. *IEEE Transactions on Signal Processing, 51*(8), 2054–2067. doi:10.1109/TSP.2003.814465

Malan, D., Fulford-Jones, T., Welsh, M., & Moulton, S. (2004). Codeblue: An ad hoc sensor network infrastructure for emergency medical care. In *Proceedings of the 1st International Workshop on Wearable and Implantable Body Sensor Networks*, (pp. 55-58). London, UK: IEEE.

Mišic, J., Shafi, S., & Mišic, V. B. (2006). Performance of a beacon enabled IEEE 802.15.4 cluster with downlink and uplink traffic. *IEEE Transactions on Parallel and Distributed Systems, 17*, 361–376. doi:10.1109/TPDS.2006.54

MobiHealth Project. (2004). *Website.* Retrieved from http://www.mobihealth.org/.

MyHeart Project. (2006). *Website.* Retrieved from http://www.hitech-projects.com/euprojects/myheart/.

Otal, B. (2010). *Optimization of wireless ambient and body sensor networks for medical applications.* PhD Dissertation. Catalunya, Spain: Universitat Politècnica de Catalunya (UPC).

Otal, B., Alonso, L., & Verikoukis, C. (2009). Highly reliable energy-saving MAC for wireless body sensor setworks in healthcare systems. *IEEE Journal on Selected Areas in Communications, 27*(4), 553–565. doi:10.1109/JSAC.2009.090516

Otal, B., Alonso, L., & Verikoukis, C. (2010). *Design and analysis of an energy saving distributed MAC mechanism for wireless body sensor networks.* EURASIP Journal on Wireless Communication and Networking.

Otal, B., & Habetha, J. (2005). *Power saving efficiency of a novel packet aggregation scheme for high-throughput WLAN stations at different data rates*. Paper presented at the IEEE Vehicular Technology Conference. Stockholm, Sweden.

Park, T. R., Kim, T. H., Choi, J. Y., Choi, S., & Kwon, W. H. (2005). Throughput and energy consumption analysis of IEEE 802.15.4 slotted CSMA/CA. *Electronics Letters, 41*(18), 1017–1019. doi:10.1049/el:20051662

Pollin, S., Ergen, M., Ergen, S., Bougard, B., Der Perre, L., & Moerman, I. (2008). Performance analysis of slotted carrier sense IEEE 802.15.4 medium access layer. *IEEE Transactions on Wireless Communications, 7*(9), 3359–3371. doi:10.1109/TWC.2008.060057

Ragil, C. (Ed.). (2005). Striving for cableless monitoring. *Philips Medical Perspective Magazine, 8*, 24 - 25.

Shyu, M.-L., Chen, S.-C., & Luo, H. (2002). Optimal bandwidth allocation scheme with delay awareness in multimedia transmission. In *Proceedings of ICME, 2002*, 37–540.

Tong, L., Zhao, Q., & Mergen, G. (2001). Multi-packet reception in random access wireless networks: From signal processing to optimal medium access control. *IEEE Communications Magazine, 39*(11), 108–112. doi:10.1109/35.965367

Wang, X. (2004). Wide-band TD-CDMA MAC with minimum-power allocation and rate- and BER-scheduling for wireless multimedia networks. *IEEE/ACM Transactions on Networking, 12*(1), 103–116. doi:10.1109/TNET.2003.822663

Woo, A., Madden, S., & Govindan, R. (2004). Networking support for query processing in sensor networks. *Communications of the ACM, 47*(6), 47–50. doi:10.1145/990680.990706

Xu, W., & Campbell, G. (1992). A near perfect stable random access protocol for a broadcast channel. In *Proceedings of the IEEE International Conference Comunications (ICC)*, (pp. 370–374). Chicago, IL: IEEE Press.

Yang, G.-Z. (Ed.). (2006). *Body sensor networks*. London, UK: Springer-Verlag. doi:10.1007/1-84628-484-8

Yuen, W.-H., Lee, H., & Andersen, T. D. (2002). A simple and effective cross layer networking system for mobile ad hoc networks. In *Proceedings of PIMRC, 2002*, 1952–1956.

Chapter 3
Smart Clothing for Health Care

Nuno M. Garcia
*Instituto de Telecomunicações, Portugal
& University of Beira Interior, Portugal &
Lusophone University of Humanities and
Technologies, Portugal*

Isabel G. Trindade
University of Beira Interior, Portugal

Rui Miguel
University of Beira Interior, Portugal

Paula Sofia Sousa
*Instituto de Telecomunicações, Portugal &
University of Beira Interior, Portugal*

José Lucas
University of Beira Interior, Portugal

ABSTRACT

The use of wearable technologies in medicine and health care has become of important in order to considerably improve benefits for patients and health service providers. Within telemedicine, biomedical clothing plays a crucial role. The main technology advances and the research of the Textile and Paper Materials Research Unit (UMTP) and of the Assisted Living Computing and Telecommunications Laboratory (ALLab) teams, in the area, will be addressed. Issues that remain unsolved will be presented. The chapter presents an overview of the key concepts for telemedicine and the role of textile electrodes and their integration in smart clothing. The development of software algorithms that specifically handle signals that are collected using biomedical clothing, integrating resiliency and a proper set of alarms, is presented and discussed in the context of classical biomedical signal processing. Finally, biomedical clothing design will be discussed in social, psychological, and esthetical contexts.

INTRODUCTION

Telemedicine is not a new concept. In fact, the first telemedicine experiments took place around the mid 20th century (Grigsby & Sanders, 1998), and its development is tightly connected to the development of the telecommunications networks, and more recently, to the development of the Internet.

DOI: 10.4018/978-1-4666-0888-7.ch003

More recently, the concept of telemedicine is no longer viewed as simply the act of providing medical acts to a distant patient, and thus involving a doctor or a physician on one side of the communication network and on the other side, a patient or a person who requires medical assistance. Telemedicine is now perceived more widely as the act of providing health care by means of a telecommunication network, possibly using specialized devices such as sensors or actuators, maybe not even requiring the physical presence of a physician or a health care practitioner.

This chapter provides a focused review of the state of the art on the issue of clothing that integrates ECG sensors, and discusses some of the developments made on these areas by the research groups at UMTP / University of Beira Interior and from the Assisted Living Computing and Telecommunications Laboratory from the *Instituto de Telecomunicações* (Assisted Living Computing and Telecommunications Laboratory, 2010).

After this initial section where the motivation for this subject has been presented, a Background section presents some of the most relevant research and projects in this area. The following section contains an overview of the concept for telemedicine. A section describing the motivation for the approach of smart clothing to a class of circulatory system diseases follows. Sections describing the construction and the evaluation of textile electrodes, and its integration in smart clothes precede a section where an argument for the need of new resilient and adaptative algorithms is discussed. Issues related to the design of biomedical clothing as an argument for user adoption are presented. Finally, future trends are suggested and conclusions are drawn.

BACKGROUND

Since the year 2000, the European Union invested over 500M€ (De Lombaerde & Van Langenhouve, 2011) in Research and Development (R&D) projects, on intelligent clothing or smart garments, due to its strategic importance for potential savings in the health care national systems and in the improvement of the quality of life for the society. In Europe, in particular, the increasingly large segment of elderly population demands for wearable technologies in Medicine and Health Care. Several European Projects, involving Industrials and Research Centres were financed (*e.g.* http://www.clevertex.net, http://www.proetex.org, http://

www.systex.org, http://www.mobiserv.eu, http://www.psycheproject.org, http://veritas-project.eu). From EU funded projects such as MyHeart (Harris & Habetha, 2007), the main achievements consist of knitted T-shirts, and of seamless and textile electrodes to monitor in real-time Electrocardiograms (ECG) using a 5-lead configuration (Paradiso, Loriga, & Taccini, 2005). The T-shirts also integrate textile sensors to monitor pulmonary and abdominal ventilation and body movement. Muscle activity monitoring has also been demonstrated. Nowadays, many spin-off companies from universities have been formed, *e.g.* in Italy (http://www.smartex.it), in Finland (http://www.meagemg.com), in the United Kingdom (http://smartlifetech.com), and in Portugal (http://www.biodevices.pt).

Nevertheless, while wearable technologies are becoming a mainstream commodity for sports (consider the commercial products from Polar or from Adidas, such as the bra and the wrist strap), longer time is still to come for clothing that monitors the vital signals in health care. Research and development in the area have not stopped to increase, and nowadays there are trials being done in many European hospitals to improve the efficiency of the solutions, the comfort of patients and the trust of health care providers.

To acquire know-how in these emerging technologies is important. Not only because of the challenges that still have to be overcome, but also mostly because of the expected impact these technologies will have in a near future for increasingly ageing populations in Europe, in the United States and in some countries from Asia and the Oceania. Among the issues that remain to be solved, the following are being addressed by the UMTP research group: overall reliability for signals captured while walking, standing or sleeping; signal isolation, to allow as little interference from artifacts and cross-talk from other signals being monitored; clothing architecture and design, to allow its adoption from users and to make it as comfortable as possible, while also to make it appealing to use and to maintain.

The article by Pantelopoulos and Borbakis (2010a), summarizes the variety of approaches that are being taken to achieve wearable monitoring systems for health care. The main physiological signals monitored are Electrocardiogram (ECG), including heart beat rate measurements, respiration, oxygen saturation, blood pressure, temperature, and posture and muscle activity by surface Electromyography (EMG). The sensors used can be divided in three groups: 1) textile sensors, which comprehend knitted and fabric based sensors; 2) electronic sensors embedded into clothing; and 3) sensor motes, which are sensors with microprocessor units and wireless communication capability. The activity at UMTP has been focused in the development of sensors of the first group, integrated in clothing.

In what concerns how the wearable devices are felt by the users, many challenges still need to be overcome. Some of the aspects to be addressed for the clothing concern standardized sizes, type of fibres and its structure, and finally, ergonomics and aesthetics. At UMTP some work has been done on inclusive clothing, for children with psychomotor handicap (Pires & Miguel, 2009).

It is foreseeable that the users that will benefit the most from wearing clothes with integrated ECG monitoring are elderly people. Thus, the clothing design in itself is quite a challenge, as this group of users will have different concerns and requirements than younger users do (McCann, Hurford, & Martin, 2005). Furthermore, being the users people with chronic or potentially chronic cardiovascular diseases, it is very important that the monitoring itself is as little intrusive as possible while making the users feel secure.

TELEMEDICINE AND TELE-HEALTH CARE

To fully understand the concept of biomedical clothing, one needs to define what is currently understood by telemedicine, or as stated before, remotely provided health care services.

The development of the Internet in the past few years has enabled the use of a set of features that allow for faster communications, accessible from a variety of points and scenarios, including mobile scenarios through the use of technologies that shall be presented and discussed in the next sections. As communications became faster, more accessible to users in more places, and even accessible to mobile users, the notion that these communication infrastructures could be used to convey medical or health related data to a health care provider became appealing to users, to health care providers, and even to governments who see in these technologies a manner to alleviate the already heavy health systems budgets.

Currently, the telemedicine concept involves the following components:

- a user who benefits from the solution (and thus, a user who has a problem or a necessity),
- a health care provider who can supply the relevant information to the user, and possibly manage the users' medical data,
- the telecommunications infrastructure, usually set up in a non-exclusive manner, *i.e.*, a telecommunications infrastructure which can transmit data between the end user medical devices and the health care provider premises, usually being this infrastructure the Internet,
- and finally, a set of devices at the end user location whose function is to collect the user's relevant medical or environmental data, and to transmit that data to a local proxy device or directly to the health care premises equipment.

Figure 1 shows a scheme for a typical telehealthcare system. The components discussed previously can be found as follows:

Figure 1. Typical remote health care communications scheme

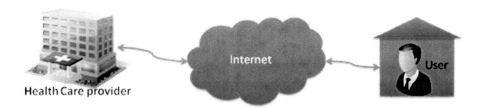

- the user, here depicted at the right of the figure. The user's setup may include mobile or fixed sensors and/or actuators, e.g. room temperature sensors or bodily temperature sensors;
- the Internet and its connections to the interested parties within the system,
- the health care provider, being this a company, a hospital or simply, a physician's practice.

Elaborating a bit further on each of these components, it is possible to define what is the concept of biomedical clothing and what role it must assume in the tele-healthcare scenario.

The health care provider is a structure that is able to perform a number of tasks that are relevant to the system, and which final goal is to enhance or improve the health or quality of life of its service subscribers, here referred to as users. These functions, from an information science point of view consist of:

- the creation and maintenance of the information system infrastructure that supports the operations of the structure,
- the collection, recording, and maintenance of the data from the users, including the compliance with the laws and regulations that are enforced in the structure legal and societal environment,
- the processing of the collected data as to provide the expected answers to the users, also in view of the current laws and regulations.

As a major difference from the initial telemedicine systems, the processing of the collected data may be done automatically by a system without the direct action of a technician (being this a physician or some other health care practitioner), for example, when the system raises an alarm if some threshold has been crossed.

An example of such functions would be the following: XPTO HealthCare provides a health care service that allows users to submit their weight using an online application. XPTO HealthCare is committed to alert the user if his or her weight surpasses the value that has previously been agreed as a goal, considering his or hers physiological condition, the season of the year (working season, holidays, and so on), and some other variables (*e.g.*, intention to increase or decrease the weight, foreseen amount of exercise, *etc.*). XPTO HealthCare needs to create an information system that is able to implement these complex algorithms, but also to provide the necessary input (*e.g.* the webpage where the user submits his or her reading) and output (*e.g.* the messaging service to alert the user) needed to provide the task that was initially contracted.

The computational platform used by XPTO HealthCare will certainly include a number of computers, telecommunication devices, storage devices and others, either at the organization facilities or outsourced, and the software needed to run and operate such devices, for example, operating systems, database managers, *etc.*. The software that integrates the rules that implement the health care monitoring of each user must also comply with current laws and regulations, for example, by assuring that the users' data is not disclosed to other users or that sensible confidential data is not asked for nor registered at the company's databases at all.

At the user's premises, the sensors for this example can be extremely simple—a regular off-the-shelf scale and a computer connected to the Internet is sufficient to read the user's weight and to provide the means to register the data into the XPTO HealthCare website.

The technological communications infrastructure is usually the Internet, currently a pervasive and always available infrastructure that provides a mean to transmit content from one machine to another.

Although this is a simple health care scenario, it integrates all the components of the concept. A much more complex scenario may be devised when the number and nature of the sensors and actuators in the user premises increases and varies, and when the number of rules and interactions that the service provider integrates increases. For example, the user's home or the user's wearable devices may integrate a mean to assess the amount of daily exercise for a particular user (Felizardo, 2010), and this data may be sent in an automatic manner to the health care provider, which in turn may want to warn the user if the amount of exercise is not compatible with the goals that the user wants to achieve. Increasing the degree of complexity, the health care provider may want to correlate a specific user's data with a significant set of data, either belonging to a relevant subset of the population or with previous usage patterns.

The collection of data with the purpose of integration and use in algorithms that perform data mining in larger databases may, this way, provide an additional degree of information to the user, now viewed as another sample in a set that contains the history and expected outcome of many other users' previously stored records. The scheme shown in Figure 1 may be added of several other players. For example, the Health

Care Provider may want to contact directly other stakeholders, such as emergency services, the hospital, the user's physician or the user's closest relatives (a scenario that is interesting if the user is an elder or a disabled person). On the user's side, the array of devices and actuators may also play a more active role, for example is the Health Care Provider is capable of changing the parameters or sensors it is interested in record, or the reading rate, or even if it wants to assess the activity of the user in a particular time of the day. The user may also want to be able to contact directly his or her physician, or family or the local health care personal assistant through the eHealth platform.

From the telecommunications infrastructure, often perceived as the Internet, the significant technologies that support telemedicine are:

• access networks that use broad band technologies such as high speed optical networks, *e.g.* networks that are build using the Fibre To The Home (FTTH) paradigm (or Fibre To The *x*, usually referred to as FTTx, where x stands for Home, Premises, Building, *etc.*); in such optical networks, users have access to data links that deliver some 100 Mb/s (roughly 100 millions of bits per second) of download speed, being the upload speed usually lower;

• mobile communications such as 3G, 3.5G or 4G networks, being the last currently on an early stage of implementation; the 4G requirements defines a 100 Mb/s bandwidth for high speed nodes such as users in trains, and 1 Gb/s for lower speed nodes such as stationary or walking users;

• high speed transport networks, being these the networks that stand in the core of Internet communications. The Internet core networks support the transmission of data packets from one end to the other of the Internet cloud, *e.g.* from one user in San Francisco to the health care provider offices in Lisbon. The high-speed transport networks links can reach several Tera bits per second (Tb/s), for example considering current optical routers implementing WDM (Wavelength Division Multiplexing). The high-speed core networks that support the Internet are extremely important, not only because of its inherent reliability, but also because of its ability to efficiently transport high volume data such as multimedia data (*e.g.* data generated at a video-conference).

The equipments at the user premises may be classified in two major categories, according to their placement and use. If the equipments are installed at the user's home (being here the notion of "home" very broad), the equipments are classified as fixed. Otherwise, if the equipments are to be used by the user even when he or she is moving and outside the home, they are said to be mobile.

On another aspect, if the equipments are devised to measure a specific signal, *e.g.* the temperature of the room, or the user's blood pressure, they are classified as sensors. Otherwise, if the equipments are devised to perform a specific action, such as closing the blinds of the windows to prevent the house from overheating, these are classified as actuators. A device such as a robot, which may perform active tasks but to do so needs to read some data from the environment, includes sensors and actuators.

Sensors (and to some extent, actuators) may be wearable or not, in the sense that when a device is wearable it is designed to be carried by the users as part of his or her clothes or accessories. For example, a motion detection device that is placed around the neck is a wearable device.

Biomedical clothes are wearable devices that include sensors that read biomedical data, such as temperature, movement, heart signals, breathing signals, and so on. As these devices are wearable, there is a strong concern on the usability of such devices, being the issue of fashion, ease of use, and of comfort, of extreme importance, some users valuing one property more than another.

In fact, it is well known that one of the barriers for the deployment of telemedicine is the low adoption rate of the solutions by end users, but this is something that needs further reflection and thus, it will be addressed later.

Mobile devices such as smart phones or to some extent laptops (*e.g.* tablet computers) can also be perceived as wearable devices, if the device has some sensing and or actuating capabilities and or if the device serves as a gateway device between the sensors and actuators actually wear and the Home gateway.

Figure 2 shows a scheme for a sample application where the mobile device serves as a personal gateway between the sensors and the home gateway. This figure shows the two gateways in the Home Environment: the Home Gateway, who is responsible for the transmission of data from the home to the Internet, and the Personal Gateway, showed as "PG" close to the User, responsible for interfacing the data to and from the user's sensors and actuators to the closest gateway available, *e.g.* the Home Gateway. Sample devices shown in this figure are the thermometers for the environment and the body temperatures, the heart beat sensor installed in the user's wearable devices (a bracelet, a vest, or some other wearable device), a scale, and a Home Computer.

The relevant functions of the Home Gateway are:

- to identify and communicate with the user's fixed sensors and actuators,
- to allow a secure channel to convey data between the Home Environment and the gateway at the Health Care Provider facilities,

and

- to allow regular and secure communication with other devices and hosts in the Internet. Similarly, the relevant functions of the Personal Gateway are:
- to identify and communicate with the user's mobile sensors and actuators,
- to recognize a trusted gateway and to manage the list of trusted gateways,

Figure 2. Sample scheme showing details of the home environment in a telemedicine scenario

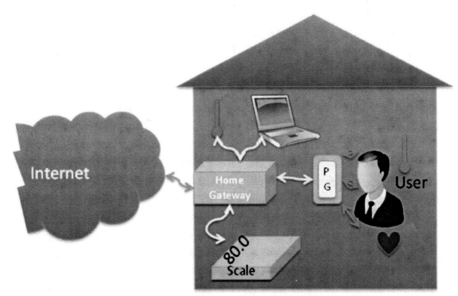

Home Environment

•   to allow a secure channel to convey data between the User's Environment and the Home Gateway or some other trustable gateway (*e.g.* the Health Care Provider gateway or the Hospital Gateway).

These relevant functionalities do not limit the definition of the Home and Personal Gateways, and several other functions may be implemented in order to allow extended features of the system. Yet, the main focus of both gateways is their ability to automatically recognize and communicate with a wide diversity of sensors and actuators, and to provide a secure mean of transmission of the data from and to these devices.

Some sensors require a specific set of operating conditions, for example, the sensor to measure the heartbeat must be configured and placed in a manner that it actually contacts the surface of the skin in the body where heartbeats are recognizable. To implement this and other sensors whose placement is critical for its regular operation, researchers have proposed the creation of sensorized clothes, which fall into the wider

category of the biomedical wearable devices. In fact, biomedical wearable devices are devices such as a chest band, or a bracelet, or even a necklace (NASA Tech Briefs, 2011). Yet, to achieve a higher degree of acceptance from the users, including a higher degree of comfort, wearable textile devices that resemble as much as possible regular clothes are the favoured configuration (Trindade, et al., 2010).

Efforts have been made to create smart clothing to address problems in areas that are key to the well being of the elder and disabled population, mostly in the so-called developed countries. Such is the case of some diseases of the circulatory system, discussed in the following section.

CIRCULAR SYSTEM DISEASES

The circular (or circulatory) system is one of the most important systems of the human organism as it carries blood to all parts of the body. This blood carries in nutrients, oxygen and water, necessary to life and cell metabolism, as in turn carries out the products of this metabolism, which are not needed and eliminated.

The circulatory system consists in the heart and the blood vessels—arteries, veins, and capillaries. The function of the heart is to pump the blood, the arteries direct the blood to all parts of the body, where through capillaries the exchange of gases and nutrients occur, and the veins return the blood to the heart and a new cycle begins.

As all systems in the organism, the circular system is also susceptible to factors and diseases that influence its correct function, leading to the compromise of the activity of certain organs. The factors that can lead to malfunctioning of the circular system are mainly aging and incorrect habits that prevail especially in developed countries society.

Over time, a degenerative process occurs resulting in hardening and thickening of the arteries walls (arteriosclerosis). The walls lose their elasticity, which is fundamental to their contraction and appropriate distribution of blood. The main causes of arteriosclerosis are advanced age, and among others, some life-style related factors, such as a diet rich in cholesterol and saturated fats, poor exercise habits and smoking.

Associated with arteriosclerosis is often atherosclerosis. Atherosclerosis is a chronic inflammatory disease in which occurs the formation of plaques inside blood vessels. The atherosclerotic plaques are composed primarily by lipids and fibrous tissue that forms in the blood vessel wall, and gradually leads to decreasing the blood vessel diameter. The main risk factors of atherosclerosis are hypertension, lack of physical activity and obesity, smoking and alcoholism, among others.

The average life expectancy has increased due to developments in the available diagnostic and treatment methods, resulting in an increasing incidence of these diseases, which are the leading cause of death in developed countries.

The more common cardiovascular diseases are: hypertensive; acute myocardial infarction; other ischaemic diseases; pulmonary circulation and other heart diseases; embolism, thrombosis and other diseases of arteries, arterioles, and capillaries.

Table 1 shows some statistics from the World Health Organization for Developed countries like France, UK, Portugal, and USA.

The cardiovascular diseases listed in the table are mainly detected with Electrocardiograms (ECG) and with blood pressure measurements. The electrocardiogram consists mainly in the registration of the heart behaviour, observed from various plans and points of the body. In general, specialists propose the use of 12-lead ECG where twelve electrodes are placed in specific locations of the body, in contact with the human skin (Malmivuo & Plonsey, 1995).

Table 1. World Health Organization's statistics for the number of deaths caused by circular system diseases in UK, France, Portugal, and USA

Diseases vs. Percentage of Deaths	United Kingdom	France	Portugal	USA
Hypertensive	0,46%	1,55%	1,11%	2,34%
Acute myocardial infarction	7,58%	4,16%	6,26%	6,17%
Other ischaemic heart diseases	9,78%	3,54%	2,56%	12,04%
Pulmonary circulation and other heart disease	4,61%	10,29%	7,74%	6,97%
Cerebrovascular	9,90%	6,43%	17,51%	5,87%
Total 1	32,34%	25,96%	35,18%	33,38%
Overall of circular system	**35,81%**	**28,44%**	**37,59%**	**35,16%**

The ECG is then performed with sensing electrodes that, through the skin, capture the electrical signals produced by the heart activity. The type of signal depends upon the location of the electrodes and how their signals are treated or processed from the signal process point of view. The heart activity generates electrical waves that are mainly periodic and are structured in a way called the P-QRS-T complex, as shown in Figure 3.

Other circulatory system measurement is the blood pressure. Regular measurements of the blood pressure detect if a person suffers of hypertensive or hypotensive disease. The hypertension is usually measured by assessing the detection of the heartbeat of the person when a pressure is applied to the limb where the measurement is made, for example in the upper arm or in the finger. The blood pressure measurements are composed by two values, corresponding to the systolic and to the diastolic stages of the heart movement.

Nowadays, X-rays and ultra-sound imaging techniques are also useful in diagnosis of the circular system diseases. As imaging is more used in anatomical and interventional cardiology, ECG is used in functional cardiology. Yet, in the context of smart clothing, the X-rays and many other imaging health technologies are for now out of the scope of application and use to wearable devices and clothes.

There is no cure for most of these cardiovascular diseases as most of them are directly related to life style and nutrition factors and ageing. It is up to each individual to ensure for a healthy condition and adopt habits and behaviours of a healthy lifestyle.

Therefore, the development of new methods and techniques of diagnosis have in vision a better and more personalized monitoring, focusing mainly on prevention. Smart clothes can have a primal role in monitoring life styles, and consequently helping to advise the user and shape such life styles.

USING TEXTILE ELECTRODES IN SENSORIZED CLOTHES

To capture a biosignal, such as the signal generated by the heart, or an Electromyography (EMG) signal, the sensor must include an adequate number of electrodes that stay in contact with the surface of the skin, as to allow the measurement of the very small difference of electric potential between two or more specific areas of the body. These very small differences in electric potential are typically in the order of some tenths of mili-Volt and are generated by the muscular activation. The further away from the skin and the smaller the muscle,

Figure 3. A typical ECG trace showing P, QRS, and T waves

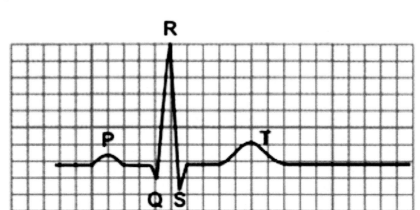

the more difficult it is to detect and measure the activity of such muscle.

To increase the accuracy of such measurements, the noise must be limited to a minimum, and this is often achieved by using self-adhesive electrodes, possibly impregnated with a conductive gel that improves the quality of the signal. In Trindade et al. (2010) the authors have presented manufacturing techniques used in textile sensors and the comparison of EMG signals using self-adhesive metallic electrodes impregnated with conductive gel and considering dry textile electrodes further discussed in the following section.

It is considered that the signal has noise and/ or artefacts when the electrodes fail to perform accurate measurements, either by limitation of the type of signal (*e.g.* trying to measure the activity of a muscle that is activated conjointly with other muscles), or by limitations imposed by the measurement scenario (e.g. when the user is moving). For example, the sensorized garment build by BioDevices (Biodevices SA, 2010) is capable of recording full ECG signals using up to five lead ECG sensor, and for that it uses self-adhesive gel impregnated electrodes.

Considering the use of sensorized clothes as tools that allow cardiac signal monitoring, the need for a full ECG quality signal often imposes a number of restrictions on the architecture of such garment, for example, that the user is immobile or that the user is wearing a garment whose electrodes are as immune as possible to the user's motion. These considerations limit not only the application scenarios of the clothes, but also impose an important adoption barrier to end users, since the correct application of the electrodes in its proper places may be a non-trivial task for a user that is not a health professional, let alone for a user that is somehow motion-handicapped.

If the signal requirements are more relaxed, for example, if the user only wants to know its own heart rate, the architecture of the garment may be more user-friendly. In fact, there are a large number of applications, which require little more

than the user's heart rate, such as for example the ones concerning its application in the area of sports training.

As with most new implementations of health care solutions, the community has verified a significant barrier to adoption from the users. The underlying reasons to the adoption barrier are not yet well studied, but one can suppose that these are related to difficulties and discomfort caused by the garment and the perception that the personal benefits brought by the clothes are not enough to create in the user the necessary enthusiasm regarding its regular usage.

Trying to eliminate the adoption barrier, researchers from the UMTP have previously proposed and manufactured a garment including integrated electrodes (Trindade, et al., 2010) (see Figure 5). This T-shirt looks as much as possible to a regular T-Shirt, mostly because it does not need the intervention of the user to install and connect standard auto-adhesive electrodes. These standard electrodes usually connect via a snap connector to the electronics in charge of the capture of the signal and its posterior processing and transmission.

Yet, the replacement of the auto-adhesive electrodes with integrated textile electrodes, while increasing the comfort and hopefully the ease of adoption, pose a trade off as they decrease the quality of the signal because they are more prone to signal noise and user motion generated artefacts. Further research currently ongoing UMTP /UBI is trying to narrow this gap.

TYPES OF TEXTILE ELECTRODES FOR BIOMEDICAL CLOTHING TO CIRCULAR SYSTEM DISEASES

The research field is going on and several research groups have already demonstrated a relevant application of the wearable technology and how its potential impact is remarkable in clinic practices concerning physical and rehabilitation treatments. Presently, the main use of clinic techniques resides

Figure 5. Pictures of the vest built by the textile and paper materials research unit (UMTP), University of Beira Interior (Covilhã, Portugal), showing the vest (picture at the left), the housing system for the data sink unit (outside the pouch, picture at the middle), the sink unit inside the pouch located at the back of the vest (picture at the right); the electrodes and the cables are not visible because they are integrated (embroidered) in the vest.

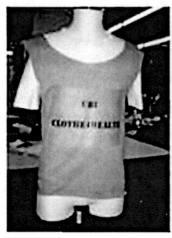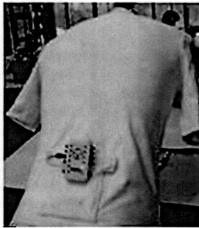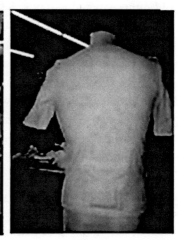

on methods that embed devices into smart clothing and/or textiles in the patient's body (Bonato, 2005).

Smart textiles can be described as textiles that can feel *stimuli* from the environment, react and adapt themselves to these *stimuli*, by integrating devices or specific textile apparatus that allow the realization of new functionalities in the textile structure (Hertleer, Troquo, Rogier, & Langenhove, 2008; Rodrigues, Miguel, Reis, Araújo, & Lucas, 2008).

The development of functional textile products has as solutions the integration of special materials (change of phase, shape memory materials, microencapsulated chemicals, and conductive yarns) and/or electronics and micro-systems.

Integration is not straightforward due to parameters such as functionality, aesthetics, comfort (thermo, physiological, flexibility, and mobility), durability, and ease of care. Generally, the following integration levels are considered:

• Low: electronic components are mounted on a garment, this is, they are integrated in a wearable accessory (ribbon, belt, or bag). This level has no manufacturing difficulties, but the acceptance and range of use scenarios are limited;

• Medium: components are integrated in garments. Conductors, connectors, and electronic devices are integrated into specific functional elements (pockets and "channels"). There are not many manufacturing difficulties and market segments do exist;

• High: conductors, connectors, sensors, and electronic devices are made by textile materials fully integrated in the clothing. They present many practical and technological problems, but have many potentialities.

The textile support represents the first level of functionality of a wearable garment system, as it constitutes the infrastructure to incorporate the basic functions, such as energy and information transmission and sensorial capability.

Fibres and yarns with specialized electrophysical properties can be integrated and used as basic elements to produce woven or knitted functional textile systems (Rodrigues, et al., 2009; Scilingo, et al., 2005). This produced woven textile structure may use cotton yarns with metallic filaments which assure the conductive medium between fabric extremities (for later connection) and em-

Figure 4. a) and b), pictures of embroidery textile electrodes in plain-weave fabrics, before and after cotton removal, respectively; c) picture showing the BioPlux portable unit connected to standard electrodes applied on a human arm. In the background, a computer screen with arm muscle activity (S-EMG) signals.

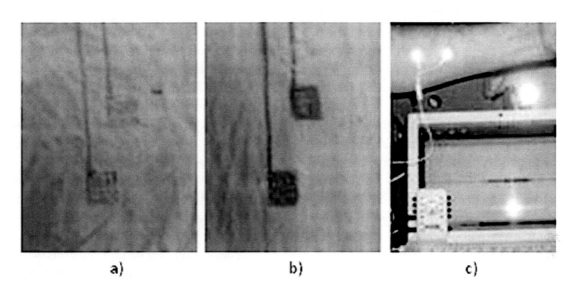

a)   b)   c)

broidered electrodes at the inner fabric surface, which define the detecting surface position. The main objective in the development of a wearable clothing is to have a high integration level structure to keep the most important advantages inherent to the characteristics of conventional textiles: mechanical behaviour, mobility, comfort, and ease of care, among others. The woven textile structure development is based on fabric engineering, which constitutes the technological basis for biomedical clothing.

At UMTP, first developments towards textile sensors and electrically connectors consisted in the use of yarns composed one monofilament of Stainless Steel (SS) twisted around by three cotton threads (Trindade, et al., 2010).

Figure 4 shows a set of two textile electrodes, made by means of embroidery, using cotton/SS years. The textile electrodes were integrated in a sleeve prototype and Surface Eletromiography (SEMG) measurements were recorded with a BioPlux device as shown in the same figure. The picture at the left in Figure 4 shows the electrodes just after they have been embroidered; it

is also visible the transmission yarns, vertically, connecting one edge of the electrode to the area where the electronic device will be connected (not visible). The picture in the centre has two additional manufacturing steps apart from the embroidery and the placement of the transmitting wires; first, the cotton was removed by the application of a solvent solution, *e.g.* a mild acid washing solution that dissolves the cotton, leaving the stitched SS filaments unexposed; this picture also shows a protection applied to the wires that transmit the signal to the connection with the BioPlux sensor.

The knowledge about the technology of structures between warp and weft yarns and float overlapping is fundamental for the positioning and integration of conductive yarns in the fabric. The float overlapping in simple fabrics comprises the partial embedding of smaller floats into larger ones, when they are centred. In fabric constructions, this overlapping allows different aesthetic and technological effects (for example, different properties in each fabric side when using distinct materials).

The use of a warp and weft woven structure as textile support allows creating a fabric that, relatively to other structures, does not lose the textile characteristics and presents better mechanical behaviour: cohesion, deformation, recuperation. These characteristics allow to obtain a higher electrode positional rigidity, as well as to develop other types of electrodes, namely by printing.

The fabrics produced with electrically conductive yarns exhibit mechanical properties similar to those of fabrics produced without the conductive yarns. The FAST System, whose name means Fabric Assurance by Simple Testing, evaluates thickness, determines the bending rigidity, the extensibility and the dimensional stability of a fabric. This system can also determine the formability and shear rigidity of fabrics. The tested fabric parameters were compression, bending rigidity, extensibility, shear rigidity, and formability. The comparison is made with fabrics without metallic yarns. The fabrics with metallic yarns show an insignificant change in thickness, it is slightly higher than fabrics without metallic yarns. Concerning the bending rigidity and extensibility, changes are noticed between both fabrics, but of less importance. The small variations observed in shear rigidity results lead to conclude that metallic yarns in certain proportions do not influence shear rigidity (Rodrigues, et al., 2008).

According to Dall'Acqua, *et al.* (2004), the affinity of different types of fibres, yarns and fabrics with doped polymers allows production of textile composites improving the electrical properties (Rodrigues, et al., 2009).

Intelligent clothing integrating textile sensors should be comfortable, non-intrusive, appealing in aspect, and long lasting. It is essential that the defined textile characteristics are maintained, and all materials used in its manufacture must be biocompatible, so not to create unwanted physiologic or biological reactions to its user.

MANUFACTURING TECHNIQUES AND METHODS USED IN BIOMEDICAL CLOTHING

Biomedical clothing is a concept of garment that integrates textile sensors and textile interconnections, to capture in real-time specific physiological signals of the human body and have them recorded in, *e.g.*, a Personal Digital Assistant (PDA) or another type of data recording equipment and consequently transmitted to a health care office. Most biomedical clothing developments consist in shirts and vests for either sport training or ambulatory or home-based health care, integrating sensors for cardiac and respiratory vital signals monitoring.

The development of small size sensors that can be connected to the body or part of clothing, *e.g.* by embedding or integrating its elements, open a large number of possibilities to monitor patients during long periods of time. This is particularly relevant to the practice of physical and rehabilitation treatments. The wearable technology allows the clinical staff to treat the data, acquired at home or by direct observations relating to the impact of clinic interventions in mobility, thus reaching a higher independence level and better quality of life (Bonato, 2005).

The textile support represents the first level of functionality of a wearable garment system, as it constitutes the infrastructure to incorporate the basic functions, such as energy and information transmission and sensorial capability (Plux SA, 2011; Rodrigues, et al., 2008).

The manufacture of the electrodes in such garment is now presented. Figure 4 and Figure 5 shows the details of the prototype and the prototype that results from the process described below.

The plain-weave fabrics that are used as support for the textile electrodes are made of 45% wool and 55% polyester. In each fabric strip, two rectangular shape electrodes are produced, using a stitching machine to create an embroidery pattern. Each electrode is made with two sewing passages, using a stainless steel with cotton (SS/cotton) yarn supplied by Dyntex Korea (2011). The yarn consisted of two cotton plies twisted around a SS filament with 30 μm in diameter. The SS filament is non-corrosive and has good break resistance. Two stitching passages were used in the embroidery pattern making, to assure that if a thread was broken in the process, the electrode could be finished, by continuing the stitching from the point it was interrupted. Moreover, this is viable from the manufacture point of view and the two layers provide the electrodes with higher robustness and lower electrical resistance. Polyester (PET) thread was used for tacking. Hence, one face of the plain weave strip shows two nearly identical embroidery electrodes of cotton and the other face shows polyester.

Near each embroidery electrode male snap fasteners are stitched. The male snap fasteners are suitable to connect the textile electrodes to the terminals of the signal processing electronic module, where the signal filtering and amplification is performed.

Each square electrode has an area each of $1 cm^2$ and uses a distance between the centre of each electrode defined by y_{e-e} = distance along the length of the muscle fibres and x_{e-e} = distance along the width of the muscle. In the T-shirt used to perform the ECG, three electrodes with similar area and x_{e-e} = 2cm are used. The plain-weave fabrics suffer very little dimensional variation, under applied stress, keeping the distance between electrodes nearly unchanged.

The fabric strip with the embroidery electrodes was immersed in a 70% concentration sulfuric acid aqueous solution bath at a temperature of 40 ^{0}C for 15 minutes. After the chemical treatment, the cotton fibres were completely removed from the electrodes, exposing the SS filaments. Consequently, one face of each electrode becomes electrically conductive while the polyester side is not. The plain-weave strips were then sewed to the elastic knits of lycra that shape the clothing. The elastic knitting provides applied pressure to the electrodes against the skin, promoting good electrical contact.

For the signal acquisition and recording, a commercial wireless portable unit (BioPlux [Plux SA, 2011]) is connected to the textile electrodes, through snap fasteners and interconnects of twisted cotton/SS threads.

The BioPlux signal processing module (electronic proximity module), where the signal collection, filtering and amplification are performed, is very compact (about 1mm x 3mm x 5mm) and lightweight and can be easily confined to a hem. The module has four shielded cables; two entering the electronic module, with female snap fasteners terminals to connect to standard bipolar electrodes; two leaving the module, with four pin terminals to plug to two of the 8-channels BioPlux wireless portable unit. Notice that in the textile embodiment, the metallic male snap fasteners stitched to the plain weave fabric are fastened to the two terminals entering the electronic proximity module. In the module, the signals are filtered and amplified by a factor of 1000 and connected through one cable to the portable unit, which transmits the signals as data at a rate of 1kHz, via wireless, to a PC within a spatial radius of about 10 meters.

The heartbeat rate can be monitored by a T-shirt made of lycra. The T-shirt is covered by a stylish cotton cover. The portable unit is held inside a pocket. In the HEARTBEAT RATE measurement, the BioPlux uses three electrodes and three cables to connect the electronic proximity module of the BioPlux to the textile interconnects through snap fasteners. Because the T-shirt is made with a lycra knitting that applies low pressure and exhibits low resilient properties, there is a need to apply a threshold pressure to the electrodes against the skin to prevent too high noise levels. The pressure achieved and maintained over time is very dependent upon the elastic knitting that makes the clothing.

As this is a prototype it is necessary to compare the signals obtained with the textile electrodes with the signals obtained with standard electrodes. It is observed that the signal amplitude and shape are very similar in both experiments, but the noise level, observed in the baseline signal is higher in the experiments with textile electrodes than in those with standard ones. Some of this noise may be due to environment electromagnetic radiation and electrostatic charge of the electrodes, so it is necessary to integrate the scheme for signal electromagnetic shielding. The electrostatic charge of the electrodes disappears when the human touches a large metallic surface, which works as an electrical ground.

The cardiac signals obtained with the T-shirt while standing up are different from the signals obtained with standard electrodes. Because the T-shirt is made with a lycra knitting that applies low pressure and exhibits low resilient properties, two issues occur. Firstly, the verified contact between the textile electrodes and the skin was low, causing a noise level that is high when compared to the signal level, so the experiments had to be performed with the volunteer applying pressure with his hand over the region where the electrodes were. Secondly, while the pressure applied by hand was enough to provide a signal comparable to that obtained with standard electrodes in terms of amplitude and noise level, the same is not obtained by only narrowing the T-shirt, *i.e.* the need to specifically design the T-shirt in a manner to increase the pressure in specific points was identified. In this test, while the signal obtained is good enough to obtain the heart beat rate, the noise level is considerably higher than in the other two experiments. In addition, after some time, the noise level would become too high, making impossible to detect the signal, and forcing the test user to again, apply a threshold pressure to the electrodes against the skin to regain acceptable noise levels. The pressure achieved and maintained over time is very dependent upon the elastic knitting that makes the clothing, and thus there is the need to devise the garment having in consideration the necessary pressure between the electrodes and

the skin to promote a good collection point for the signals.

If the volunteer starts walking, the cardiac signals obtained with the textile electrode in the T-shirt exhibit strong artifacts. In accordance with literature, artifacts caused by motion of the person wearing the intelligent garment are always present and require specific algorithms to be minimized. However, the heart beat rate can still be measured as the cardiac peaks are still resolved and not masked by the artifacts.

The signal isolation regarding ambient interference must be integrated. In addition, a combination of filtering hardware and/or software to remove artifacts and ambient interference should be explored and applied.

RESILIENT AND ADAPTATIVE HEARTBEAT DETECTION ALGORITHM

According to Malmivuo and Plonsey (1995), 90% of the heart's electrical activity can be explained with a dipole source model, and to this purpose, it is sufficient to measure three independent components. Although the results obtained from a 12-lead are more complete and allow a full ECG curve plot, for the purpose of researching new ECG signal processing algorithms, the simplified three lead version was used.

Using a three lead ECG sensor, researchers at ALLab and at UMTP developed a new type of heart-beat detection algorithm that may be used when the subject is moving, and adequate to ECG signal captured by textile electrodes, *i.e.* when the electrodes are not in perfect adherence with the subject's skin (Garcia, et al., 2011). The remaining part of this section is an extension of the work published in Garcia *et al.* (2011).

The motivation for this new class of algorithms is derived from the existence of a new type of electrodes. For the classical scenario, using auto-adhesive electrodes, a number of approaches have been proposed to solve the problem of creating a wearable device or a sensorized vest that allows to monitor a person's heart beat rate, or even better, to monitor a person's full cardiac signal by mean of an Electrocardiography (ECG) machine, *e.g.* the ones published by Pantelopoulos and Bourbakis (2010b) and Paradiso *et al.* (2005).

Other projects regarding the creation of wearable devices are for example the MyHeart project (Harris & Habetha, 2007) which approaches five different application areas. Although the start of this project goes back to 2003, one of its work-packages was focused on the development of on-body electronics that can be integrated into functional textiles with the goal of producing intelligent clothes.

The category under which these types of devices fall is quite wide. For example, if the device is wearable but not integrated into a vest, then it is usually called a device, such as the ones produced by Polar *e.g.* Polar Electro Oy (2006). If the device is integrated into a vest and includes sensors and electrodes, it is called a sensorized vest, such as the one produced by BioDevices (Biodevices SA, 2010).

Furthermore, if the device or vest is supposed to perform some medical task, such as generate alarms, or measure data that is critical to the maintenance of the state of health or life of the user, then it is called a medical device or a medical sensorized vest. Interested readers may refer to Couto and Garcia (2001) to find under which class of devices a given vest is classified under the European Union regulations.

Typically, a sensorized vest includes at least the following components:

- the vest itself,
- the electrodes which are in contact with the body or the mean in order to read the signal into electrical form, or the sensors that need to measure the signal near the user's body,
- the electronic module that processes the signal collected by the sensing electrodes, and finally

- a transmitter/receiver and/or recording unit.

In the photos shown in Figure 5, it is possible to see the vest, the electronic unit that processes and transmits the collected signals (outside and inside the protective pouch on the back of the vest), and the sensors (here attached to regular electrodes). The wearable electronic unit used was the BioPlux (Plux SA, 2011).

To better understand the need to a resilient heartbeat detection algorithm, we may want to visualize the differences of the recorded signal while using standard pre-gelled auto-adhesive electrodes and clothe-integrated textile electrodes. Figure 6 shows a set of ECG signals captured with a set of standard auto-adhesive pre-gelled electrodes. The sensor and the transmission unit used in this setup was the BioPlux Research shown in Figure 5. The electrodes are placed according to the three lead pre-cordial position.

The same electrodes and transmission unit was used with a set of textile embroidered electrodes shown in Figure 4. The textile electrodes are integrated into the vest as to be placed over the skin of the subject at the same location as the previous standard electrodes.

Both Figure 6 and Figure 7 show signals collected when the user is standing but not moving. It is clearly visible that although the user is immobile, the signal collected with textile electrodes shows a less clear (more irregular) base line when compared to the signal captured with standard electrodes. Nevertheless, in Figure 7 the heartbeat peaks are easily detectable, proving that textile-integrated electrodes can be used in such scenarios.

While Figure 6 and Figure 7 show the signals collected when the user is standing still, Figure 8 and Figure 9 show the signals collected when the user is jumping, for respectively, signals captured with standard electrodes and signals captured with textile electrodes.

It is clear that when the subject is moving, the signal shows increased noise and artifacts. The

Figure 6. Signal captured using auto-adhesive standard pre-gelled electrodes. The figure at the top shows a detail of roughly 2 seconds of the signal. The figure at the bottom shows a larger of roughly 30 seconds. The signal is shown without y-axis units, as these should be interpreted as arbitrary units.

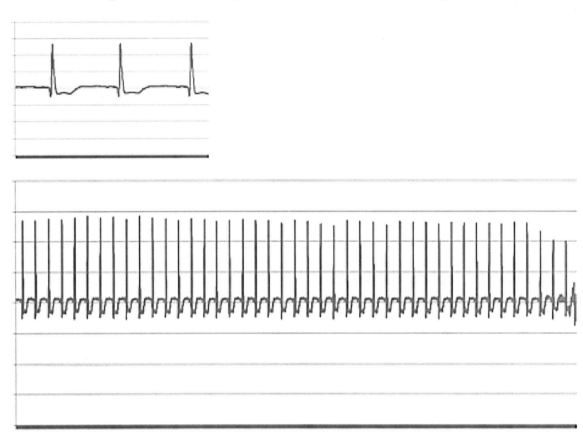

Figure 7. Signal captured using embroidered textile electrodes. The figure shows a sample signal of roughly 30 seconds. The signal is shown without y-axis units, as these should be interpreted as arbitrary units.

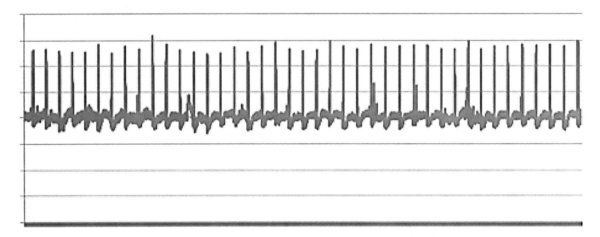

Figure 8. Signal captured using auto-adhesive standard pre-gelled electrodes. The figure shows a detail of roughly 30 seconds of the signal when the user is jumping. The signal is shown without y-axis units, as these should be interpreted as arbitrary units.

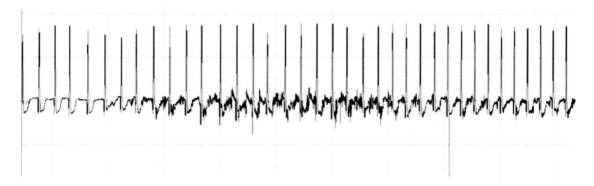

number and type of noise and artifacts is related to the type of movement and proportional to the intensity of this movement, and is introduced in the signal by the lack of solidarity between the textile electrode and the user's skin. The presence of these artifacts is unwanted and it introduces uncertainty to standard heart beat detection algorithms such as the ones in Afonso, Tompkins, Nguyen, and Shen (1999), Cristov (2004), and Pan and Tompkins (1985).

Yet, the process that generates the signals does not change in nature just because the subject has started moving. Therefore, it is necessary to devise a new algorithm that takes into account the signals captured by less-efficient but more comfortable

electrodes, by creating means to handle the noise and artifacts in the signal and integrating a degree of uncertainty of the measurement and a degree of prediction of the signal itself.

The signals shown in Figure 7 and in Figure 9 allow the visual analysis of the difference between signals collected while resting and moving when using embroidered textile electrodes. The detection of the heartbeat in ECG signal while in a rest position is very much straightforward, and several approaches have been made to this purpose as previously presented.

It is known that the ECG signal has a distinctive shape, usually termed the PQRST complex (Malmivuo & Plonsey, 1995) (see Figure 3). It is

Figure 9. Signal captured using textile embroidered electrodes. The figure shows a detail of roughly 30 seconds of the signal when the user is jumping. The signal is shown without y-axis units, as these should be interpreted as arbitrary units.

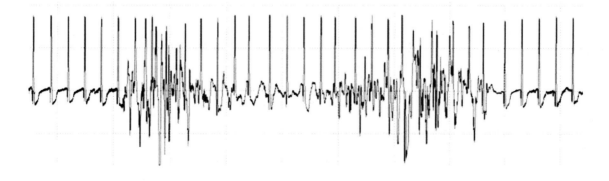

also known that for any individual, the heartbeat rate can vary greatly, from some 29 beats per minute (bpm), as recorded on the cyclist Miguel Indurain (Jeukendrup & Diemen, 1998) to some 220 bpm, in the case of some Olympic athletes.

This additional piece of knowledge on the signal shape and expected behavior can be integrated into the algorithm, *i.e.*, the algorithm will work based on a prediction of what are the expected limits for the evolution of the next heart beat.

The base algorithm works as follows: the initial *n* signal values are used to create an average base line, which will serve as a threshold to detect the peak representing a heartbeat. After detecting a heartbeat, the algorithm skips the following *m* signal values, as it is known that after a heartbeat normally there is a period that corresponds to the remainder of the PQRST wave (the ST segment). After the *m* samples have been read, the algorithm starts again to look for a new peak above

the threshold, in the mean time, update with the information of the mean value for the baseline. Both *n* and *m* can be defined accordingly to the ECG sampling rate. Figure 10 shows the flowchart for the algorithm, for a signal that disregards the existence of errors.

When the signal is too noisy, the algorithm detects the first peak above the base line, but also detects nearby peaks that could also be candidates for the location of the heartbeat. In this case, the algorithm chooses the first occurrence of the heartbeat and raises an alarm to an initial level, indicating that the measurement was performed with some degree of error. In the subsequent readings, and subject to a time parameter that states how long should an alarm last, the algorithm raises or decreases the alarm levels if the signal is analyzed as having errors or not.

The algorithm foresees four degrees of alarms and one degree of regular measurement, *i.e.*,

Figure 10. Basic flowchart for the algorithm when the signal has no noise or artifacts

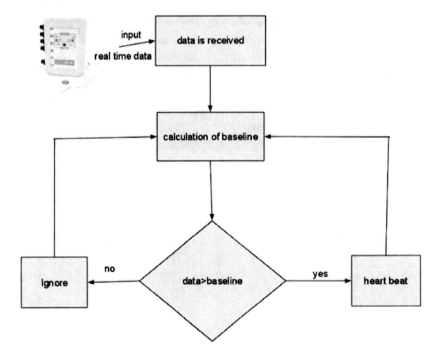

Figure 11. State diagram for the alarm sequence part of the algorithm

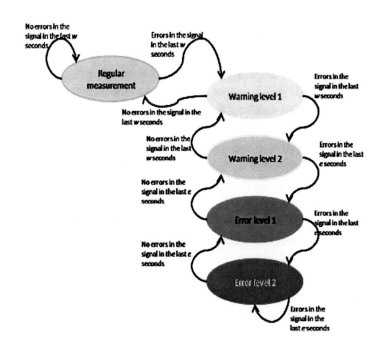

measurement without error. The initial state is regular measurement. Figure 11 shows the state diagram for the resilient and adaptative algorithm. This diagram shows how the alarm levels raise from the no-alarm state to the Warning Level 1, Warning Level 2, Error Level 1, and Error Level 2, if the signal is interpreted as having errors. Also noteworthy is the fact that the concept of error is different between the Warning Level 1 and 2 and the Error Level 1 and 2. In the case of Warning Level 1 and 2, the concept of error is associated with the co-existence of multiple possible heartbeat locations and a plateau location, what makes it possible to detect a base line from which the heartbeat is detectable. For the signal to raise to the status of Error, it means that there is no significant difference between the base-line value and the heat-beat value. If the system detects an error of this type, it still will escalate the warning levels before it reaches the Error state.

Smart clothes integrating textile electrodes will need to develop and validate new signal processing algorithms, in particular if, when compared to standard use-case scenarios, the clothe embodies some type of difference in view of these standard use-cases. For example, if the signal transmission is achieved by means of textile conductive yarns instead of electrical standard shielded cables, and / or the signal is collected using textile electrodes instead of skin adhesive pre-gelled electrode, and so on.

This new class of algorithms will need to integrate the knowledge previously acquired on the type of signal being read, as a mean to lessen the impact of the uncertainty and error brought by the less efficient electrodes and textile circuitry elements.

BIOMEDICAL CLOTHING DESIGN

Design, in general, is defined as simultaneously a creative process and a solution to a problem. Likewise, also the Clothing Design can work not only as a fashion element, but also as a way of intervening in the life of people who wear the clothes, for example those whose psychomotor skills are weakened, as is the case of children with psychomotor development delays. In this case, functional, therapeutic, and playful clothing, to contribute to the improvement of the life quality of these children, was conceived and manufactured.

Yet for other users, the clothes need to be engineered to be as similar to regular clothes as possible. The integration of electronic components such as sensors and personal gateways poses integration and usability important challenges. For example, in terms of functionality regarding the attachment of separable elements, either functional or aesthetic, Velcro® is the conventional material that works best in this context, although magnets have also demonstrated a great effectiveness and acceptance by the inquired parents and therapists. In what concerns the sensory stimulation, the most immediate elements, like bright colors, lights, sounds, and textures are those which are more successful with children. The conclusions reached with prototypes designed for children indicate that modular clothing, which allows varied and customizable aesthetic aspects and the selection of sensory stimulation elements, which are customizable to each child and to his particular therapeutic needs, is the solution that works the best.

Either referring to adult or to young users, to elderly or to handicapped users, or to healthy users that simply need to be monitored for a short period of time, the key issue for the efficiency of health care solutions integrating smart clothes, is the adoption of such solutions by the end users.

If the user fails to perceive the advantages of adopting the solution, independently of its usefulness and innovation, the solution becomes useless and therefore, inefficient.

Thus, adoption is truly the hurdle to overcome in the case of the use of Smart Clothing in Health Care scenarios. And it is also key because of the nature of the stakeholders interested in its success. The stakeholders are, first and foremost, the Health Care operators who reap the financial and social benefits associated with the increase of quality of life of a specific segment of the population; the Health Care operators may be, for example, an insurance company or a state or company Health Care system; these stakeholder promote research and development of innovative and efficient solutions, many times creating funding programs for research. Second and obviously, the stakeholder is the user who profits directly from the smart clothe usage, either because the smart clothes allow the users' to enjoy better health, or it contributes for a better and more accurate diagnostic, or otherwise contributes for a betterment of the user's quality of life. Other indirect stakeholders are the user's circle of family and friends. Yet, although they may be of major influence as they can contribute to the user's adoption of the solution, it is best to consider the user's decision as the point where all the social and psychological influences take shape.

Aesthetics and fashion are an important tool to use in promoting the adoption of a smart clothe (McCann, Hurford, & Martin, 2005). Therefore, from an aesthetical perspective, the clothes must be designed and engineered in a manner that allows them to comply with:

- the functional and non-functional requisites;
- the user's personal aesthetic preferences; and
- the user's personal functional preferences.

The functional and non-functional requisites or requirements are the list of functions or tasks that the smart clothe must perform or support, for example, a smart clothe such as the one depicted in Figure 5 must capture and transmit the user's ECG signal using a three electrode pre-cordial placement (functional requirement) and must be washable (non-functional requirement).

In a generic manner, the aesthetic and functional preferences of "The User" (as the entity that is representative of the group of users) are harder to pinpoint, although for each user these

Figure 12. Complexity of smart clothes and wearable technologies (adapted from Hurford et al. (2006)

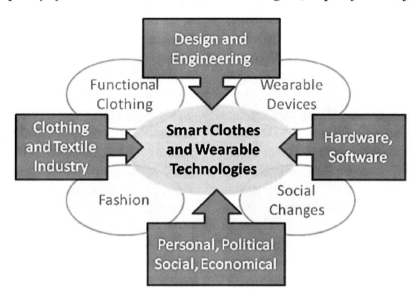

are straightforwardly defined as his/her personal preferences regarding the aesthetic and the functionality of the clothes.

Hurford *et al.* (2006) present a scheme that shows the complex weave of interactions that influence the field of Smart Clothes and Wearable Technology, shown in Figure 12 (adapted). This scheme depicts the four areas that intervene in the definition of a Smart Clothe solution, namely Design and Engineering, Hardware and Software, the Clothing and Textile Industries, and the Personal, Political, Social, and Economical factors, being these the ones that range from the personal choices to the laws and regulations. This scheme also shows different areas that result from and provide interaction to the process of defining a Smart Clothing solution, namely: Wearable Devices, Functional Clothing, Fashion, and Social Changes, being the later the one that represents the impact that changes in society have in this definition, in particular the changes that are motivated by hardware and software innovation.

The scheme on Figure 12 brings yet another variable to consider in the complex weave of interrelations that influence the user's adoption of the solution: the software. Initially, smart clothing solutions required little or no interaction between the user and the solution. With the increased development of functionalities and thus, the creation of more complex solutions, the probability for the user-software interaction becomes bigger. The issue of software usability is widely researched and studied for varied groups of users and this discussion falls outside the scope of this chapter. Thus, keeping in perspective the success of a Smart Clothing solution, there are other areas that deserve great attention, in the area of the engineering and design of the software, namely, the existence of user friendly, intuitive, adaptable interfaces, the use of data transmission protocols that are compatible with a mobile personal gateway in a variety of scenarios, and adaptable algorithms that are capable to provide reliable results despite of adverse usage situations.

FUTURE TRENDS

There are a number of technologies, which recently have been proposed for the Smart Clothing in the Health Care area. On the area of textile with electronics integration, we have witnessed recently interesting developments on the integration of antennas in textiles (Kubler, Derigent, Thomas, & Rondeau, 2011). A higher degree of integration of Radio Frequency Identification (RFID) tags allows an increased number of applications and usage scenarios. On a similar area, the creation of electronic devices using textiles is an area that promises to enlarge the scope of Smart Clothing. For example, the construction of textile antennas (Osman, et al., 2011), or textile sensors (Catrysse, et al., 2011; Jur, Sweet, Oldham, & Parsons, 2011).

It is expectable that the convergence *phenomena* will again be observed in the area of Smart Clothing for Health Care, as the scheme in Figure 12 suggests, creating solutions whose degree of integration is higher, with wider scenarios of application and allowing for the intervention of other areas of science such as Data Mining, Artificial Intelligence, Robotics, and so on, in a path that will lead to the creation of the Internet of Health Things.

There are also a number of problems that still need to be solved. In a generic manner, and without any particular order, one family of problems are the need to devise a sound business model that can be implemented in a transversal manner. Another type of problem is related to the hindered opportunity to use all the medical data in a manner that allows data mining and advanced artificial intelligence algorithms to cross-relate data and to infer new trends and provide insightful and coherent information. For example, it is impossible to create a worldwide database of medical data, mostly because regional and national laws and regulations often forbid personal data to be stored outside political boundaries. Finally, on another class of problems, and regarding the Internet of Health Things, the diverse technologies are not yet mature to coherently be integrated and provide a comprehensive solution that can be adopted pervasively.

CONCLUSION

We cannot stress enough the issue of user adoption as the single most important aspect for the success of a Smart Clothing solution in a Health Care scenario. Throughout this chapter, we have presented different aspects of currently ongoing research and its associated problems and expectations. We have focused mostly on the textile and hardware integration aspects, regarding a field of application related to circulatory systems diseases.

The ongoing research, integrating a variety of scientific areas, from management to engineering, from design to medicine, will undoubtedly produce new and efficient Smart Clothing solutions for Health Care scenarios.

REFERENCES

Afonso, V. X., Tompkins, W. J., Nguyen, T. Q., & Shen, L. (1999). ECG detection using filter banks. *IEEE Transactions on Bio-Medical Engineering, 46*(2), 192–202. doi:10.1109/10.740882

Assisted Living Computing and Telecommunications Laboratory. (2010). *ALLab @ instituto de telecomunicações.* Retrieved 7 April 2011, from http://allab.it.ubi.pt.

Biodevices, S. A. (2010). *Biodevices.* Retrieved 7 April 2011, from http://www.biodevices.pt.

Bonato, P. (2005). Advances in wearable technology and applications in physical medicine and rehabilitation. *Journal of Neuroengineering and Rehabilitation, 2*(2).

Catrysse, M., Puers, R., Hertleer, C., Langenhove, L. V., Egmond, H. V., & Matthys, D. (2011). Towards the integration of textile sensors in a wireless monitoring suit. *Sensors and Actuators. A, Physical, 113*(2-3), 302–311.

Couto, R. G., & Garcia, N. M. (2001). *CE marking - A synthesis of the conformance CE marking on medical devices*. White Paper. Covilhã, Portugal: Instituto de Telecomunicações.

Cristov, I. I. (2004). *Real time electrocardiogram QRS detection using combined adaptative threshold*. Retrieved 7 April 2011, from http://www.biomedical-engineering-online.com/content/3/1/28.

Dall'Acqua, L., Tonin, C., Peila, R., Ferrero, F., & Catellani, M. (2004). Performances and properties of intrinsic conductive cellulose–polypyrrole textiles. *Syntethic Materials*, *146*, 213–221.

De Lombaerde, P., & Van Langenhouve, L. (2011). Monitoring and evaluating the provision of (donor-funded) regional public goods. *Regions & Cohesion*, *1*, 101–123. doi:10.3167/reco.2011.010107

Dyntex Korea. (2011). *Dyntex Korea web site*. Retrieved 14 February 2011, from http://www.dyntex.co.kr.

Felizardo, V. (2010). *Validação do acelerómetro xyzplux para estimação do gasto energético com aquisição de dados de diversos parâmetros fisiológicos*. MSc Thesis. Covilhã, Portugal: University of Beira Interior. Retrieved from http://allab.it.ubi.pt/images/documents/disertacao_%20virginie.pdf.

Garcia, N. M., Tavares, P., Miguel, R., Trindade, I., Lucas, J., & Pereira, M. (2011). *Resilient heartbeat detection algorithm for signals captured by smart-textiles*. Paper presented at the AUTEX 2011 - 11th World Textile Conference. Mulhouse, France.

Grigsby, J., & Sanders, J. H. (1998). Telemedicine: Where it is and where it's going. *Annals of Internal Medicine*, *129*, 123–127.

Harris, M., & Habetha, J. (2007). The MyHeart project: A framework for personal healh care applications. *Computers in Cardiology*, *34*, 137–140.

Hertleer, C., Troquo, A., Rogier, H., & Langenhove, L. V. (2008). The use of textile materials to design wearable microstrip patch antennas. *Textile Research Journal*, *78*(8), 651–658. doi:10.1177/0040517507083726

Hurford, R., Martin, A., & Larsen, P. (2006). *Designing wearables*. Paper presented at the 10th IEEE International Symposium on Wearable Computers. Montreaux, Canada.

Jeukendrup, A., & Diemen, A. V. (1998). Heart rate monitoring during training and competition in cyclists. *Journal of Sports Sciences*, *16*(1), 91–99. doi:10.1080/026404198366722

Jur, J. S., Sweet, W. J. III, Oldham, C. J., & Parsons, G. N. (2011). Electronic textiles: Atomic layer deposition of conductive coatings on cotton, paper, and synthetic fibers: Conductivity analysis and functional chemical sensing using "all-fiber" capacitors. *Advanced Functional Materials*, *21*(11), 1948. doi:10.1002/adfm.201190035

Kubler, S., Derigent, W., Thomas, A., & Rondeau, É. (2011). *Prototyping of a communicating textile*. Paper presented at the International Conference on Industrial Engineering and Systems Management - IESM 2011. Metz, France.

Malmivuo, J., & Plonsey, R. (1995). *Bioelectromagnetism*. New York, NY: Oxford University Press.

McCann, J., Hurford, R., & Martin, A. (2005). *A design process for the development of innovative smart clothing that addresses end-user needs from technical, functional, aesthetic and cultural view points*. Paper presented at the Ninth IEEE International Symposium on Wearable Computers (ISWC 2005). Osaka, Japan.

Osman, M. A. R., Rahim, M. K. A., Azfar, M., Samsuri, N. A., Zubir, F., & Kamardin, K. (2011). Design, implementation and performance of ultrawideband textile antenna. *Progress in Electromagnetic Research B*, *27*, 307–325.

Pan, J., & Tompkins, W. J. (1985). A real-time QRS detection algorithm. *IEEE Transactions on Bio-Medical Engineering, 32*(3), 230–236. doi:10.1109/TBME.1985.325532

Pantelopoulos, A., & Borbakis, N. (2010a). A survey on wearable health care systems based on knitted integrated sensors. *IEEE Transactions on Systems, Man, and Cybernetics, 40*(1), 1–12. doi:10.1109/TSMCC.2009.2032660

Pantelopoulos, A., & Bourbakis, N. G. (2010b). A survey on wearable sensor-based systems for health monitoring and prognosis. *IEEE Transactions on Systems, Man and Cybernetics. Part C, Applications and Reviews, 40*, 1–12. doi:10.1109/TSMCC.2009.2032660

Paradiso, R., Loriga, G., & Taccini, N. (2005). A wearable health care system based on knitted integrated sensors. *IEEE Transactions on Information Technology in Biomedicine, 9*, 337–344. doi:10.1109/TITB.2005.854512

Pires, A., & Miguel, R. (2009). Design de vestuário para a estimulação sensorial de crianças com atrasos ao nível do desenvolvimento psicomotor. In *Proceedings of Congresso E_design – Visões para o Ensino na Europa nos Novos Contextos Ambientais e Económicos, CPD – Centro Português de Design.* Lisbon, Portugal: IEEE.

Plux, S. A. (2011). *bioPlux research.* Retrieved 14 February 2011, from http://www.plux.info/biopluxresearch.

Polar Electro Oy. (2006). *RS100 training computer - running & multisport - get active - heart rate monitors - polar electro - global English.* Retrieved 7 April 2011, from http://www.polar.fi/en/products/get_active/running_multisport/RS100.

Rodrigues, S., Miguel, R., Lucas, J., Gaiolas, C., Araújo, P., & Reis, N. (2009). *Wearable technology - Development of polypyrrole textile electrodes for electromyography.* Paper presented at the BIODEVICES 2009 - International Conference on Biomedical Electronics and Devices. Porto, Portugal.

Rodrigues, S., Miguel, R., Reis, N., Araújo, P., & Lucas, J. (2008). *Wearable technology for muscle activity monitoring.* Paper presented at the CONTROLO 2008 - 8th Portuguese Conference on Automatic Control. Vila Real, Portugal.

Scilingo, E. P., Gemignani, A., Paradiso, R., Taccini, N., Ghelarducci, B., & Rossi, D. D. (2005). Performance evaluation of sensing fabrics for monitoring physiological and biomechanical variables. *IEEE Transactions on Information Technology in Biomedicine, 9*(3), 345–352. doi:10.1109/TITB.2005.854506

Tech Briefs, N. A. S. A. (2011). *Electrocardiography (ECG) necklace.* Retrieved 13 June 2011, from http://www.techbriefs.com/component/content/article/10231.

Trindade, I., Lucas, J., Miguel, R., Alpuim, P., Carvalho, M., & Garcia, N. M. (2010). *Portable systems for health care.* Paper presented at the The IEEE 12th International Conference on e-Health Networking, Applications and Services (IEEE HealthCom 2010). Lyon, France.

Trindade, I. G., Pereira, M., Salvado, R., Lucas, J., Garcia, N. M., Silva, J. S., et al. (2010). *Intelligent clothing for health care.* Paper presented at the Symposium de Materiais e Processos Inovadores. Covilhã, Portugal.

Chapter 4
Measuring Specific Absorption Rate by using Standard Communications Equipment

Diana Bri
Universitat Politècnica de Valencia, Spain

Jaime Lloret
Universitat Politècnica de Valencia, Spain

Carlos Turro
Universitat Politècnica de Valencia, Spain

Miguel Garcia
Universitat Politècnica de Valencia, Spain

ABSTRACT

Specific Absorption Rate (SAR) is used to measure the body tissue exposure to electromagnetic fields. This chapter describes how SAR values can be estimated from a deployed Wireless Local Area Network (WLAN). We carried out this work using the Received Signal Strength (RSS) obtained from the access points. This parameter is easily obtained by an ordinary wireless network scanner. RSS variations are measured for a different number of people in the same room and without people. It will allow us to estimate how much energy is absorbed by a group of people and by a single person on average. Moreover, we have included the weight of the people in order to know the RSS lost by kilogram. These measurements were taken at the Higher Polytechnic School of Gandia, Universitat Politècnica de València, Spain, in two placements: the library and inside an anechoic camera.

INTRODUCTION

Today, the Electromagnetic Fields (EMF) caused by human technology represent one of the most common environmental features. Its growth is amazing because of the fast advances in the wireless technology. So, speculations and suspicions about the consequences on health are being spread among the population.

In response to this concern the World Health Organization (WHO) established the International EMF Project in 1996 (WHO, 2002). This project

DOI: 10.4018/978-1-4666-0888-7.ch004

Table 1. ETSI and FCC comparison

		Band (GHz)				
		2.4	5.15 – 5.25	5.25 – 5.35	5.470 – 5.725	5.725 – 5.825
ETSI						
	Power	100 mW	200 mW	200 mW	1000 mW	25 mW
	EIRP	20 dBm	22 dBm	22 dBm	30 dBm	14 dBm
FCC						
	Power	4000 mW	200 mW	1000 mW		P2MP – 4 W (36 dBm)
	EIRP	36 dBm	22 dBm	30 dBm		P2P – 200 W (53 dBm)

is focused to analyze the possible health effects of EMF in the frequency range from 0 to 300 GHz.

There are several public directives and recommendations referred to EMF in Europe. One of them is the directive 1999/5/EC of the Parliament and of the Council of 9 March 1999 on radio equipment and telecommunications terminal equipment (EC, 1999a). The one which is related to the human body exposure to EMF is the Council Recommendation of 12 July 1999 on the limitation of exposure of the general public to electromagnetic fields (0 Hz to 300 GHz) (EC, 1999b).

The basic restrictions on electromagnetic fields depend on frequency (EC, 1999b). These restrictions are specified by the following physical quantities and their main adverse effects on health:

- From 0 to 1 Hz, magnetic flux density for static magnetic fields (0 Hz) and current density for time-varying fields up to 1 Hz are taken into account. The objective is to prevent effects on the cardiovascular and central nervous system.
- From 1 Hz to 10 MHz, current density to prevent effects on nervous system functions is taken into account.
- From 100 kHz to 10 GHz, restrictions on SAR to prevent whole-body heat stress and

excessive localized heating of tissues is taken into account. In the range 100 kHz to 10 MHz, restrictions on both current density and SAR are provided.
- From 10 GHz to 300 GHz, basic restrictions on power density are provided to prevent heating in tissue at or near the body surface.

The objective of this chapter is to analyze the exposure of people to WLANs' radio frequency in the 2.4 GHz ISM band. In order to establish a security measurement, many countries have limited the transmitting power of the WLAN device according to the working frequency. Table 1 shows the transmitting power limitations for the European Telecommunications Standards Institute (ETSI) and for the Federal Communications Commission (FCC) for several radio frequencies.

But, the body exposure limits are given in terms of Specific Absorption Rate (SAR). This rate indicates the radio frequency energy absorption per unit mass of body tissue. Averaged SAR is calculated for the whole body or for some parts of the body (ICNIRP, 1998). It is expressed in watts per kilogram (W/kg). Whole body SAR measures are related to thermal effects caused by Radio Frequency (RF) exposure. On the other

Table 2. Basic restrictions for electric, magnetic and electromagnetic fields (0 Hz to 300 GHz)

Magnetic Range	Magnetic flux density (mT)	Current density (mA/m^2) (rms)	Whole body average SAR (W/kg)	Localised SAR (head and trunk) (W/kg)	Localised SAR (limbs) (W/kg)	Power density, S (W/m^2)
0 Hz	40	-	-	-	-	-
>0-1 Hz	-	8	-	-	-	-
1-4 Hz	-	8/f*	-	-	-	-
4-1000 Hz	-	2	-	-	-	-
1000 Hz -100 KHz	-	f/500	-	-	-	-
100 KHz-10 MHz	-	f/500	0.08	2	4	-
10 MHz-10 GHz	-	-	0.08	2	4	-
10 GHz-300 GHz	-	-	-	-	-	10

* f is the frequency in Hz

hand, local SAR values are used to assess and limit RF energy absorption in individual parts of the body; particularly in sensitive body parts sensitive parts like the head and ears, that is, soft body parts.

Specific Absorption Rate (SAR) appears in all mobile phones' technical specifications in order to establish the maximum allowable limit (SAR values, Nokia—SAR, Samsung—SAR). This parameter is set by the Directive 1999/5/EC of the European Parliament (EC, 1999a) and by the ICNIRP Guidelines (International Commission on Non-ionizing Radiation Protection) (ICNIRP, 1998).

Table 2, which has been obtained from reference (EC, 1999b), shows basic restrictions for electric, magnetic and electromagnetic fields (from 0 Hz to 300 GHz). The values for our case are those in the penultimate row. We can see that they are from 0.08 W/Kg for the whole body, 2W/

Kg for head and trunk, and at 4 W/Kg for limbs. These values are calculated over any six-minute period and 10 grams of body tissue.

In order to set abovementioned values uncertainties related to individual sensitivities, environmental conditions, and changeable characteristics of the population, like age or health, have been taken into account. SAR testing is conducted using a standard operation while the device transmits to certified maximum power level in all the tested frequencies bands (they were shown in Table 1). When a device is working, the real SAR level can be below the maximum value because devices are designed to use only the power required to reach the network. Necessary power can vary according to some factors such as the device antenna gain, the proximity to the base station or to other devices, the working frequency, etc. So, these factors will also influence on the SAR directly.

In this chapter we analyze the SAR of the human body when it is exposed to WLANs devices working at the 2.4GHz radio frequency ISM band. In order to make these measurements we will use a controlled indoor place and an uncontrolled environment where no variable can be fixed.

The main focus of this study is to know the Specific Absorption Rate of the human body exposed to wireless local area networks working at the 2.4GHz radio frequency ISM band. The SAR is calculated by measuring RSS in two different ways, on a WLAN working in an uncontrolled environment and on another WLAN deployed in a controlled environment.

This work is based on the comparison between RSS measured when there are people next to WLANs and when there is nobody. SAR is calculated from this comparison and it is taken into account several corporal features of human bodies next to WLANs deployed.

SAR calculated from WLAN devices provides valuable information to medical researchers. It lets to study the possible implications of WLANs on the population health and, if it was necessary, to establish new exposure limits in this kind of networks.

The chapter is structured as follows. The second section shows the most important SAR studies and the related works found in the literature. Moreover, the most used guidelines to study SAR around the world will be described. Next, in the third section, we discuss the composition of the human body and we explain how electromagnetic waves affect to each part of the body. We will also give details about the consequences. The analytical considerations to estimate SAR and the absorption of the human body are described in the fourth section. The fifth section explains how data are collected, where measures are done, and which software is used for data analysis in our first test bed. Furthermore, this section also shows the obtained results in graphs and provides the mean measures. Then, in section sixth, the second test bed is explained in the same way than the first

one. The difference between them is mainly the place where measures were taken. In the first one, it is an uncontrolled indoor environment, and in the second one, it is a controlled indoor. Finally, last section finishes the chapter, provides the conclusions summarizing the best results and collects the main ideas of this work.

BACKGROUND

Due to the importance of SAR in terms of public health, the literature in this field is quite abundant. There are some papers and studies that present experimental researches or simulations to analyze the influence of human body in electromagnetic waves propagation, mainly the body shadowing on wireless propagation.

Bahillo et al. (2010) assess how human body affects on electromagnetic field in the current localization systems based on RSS. A RSS meter is always held by a person, so this paper is based on the idea that it involves errors in RSS measures. Currently, these errors are not taken into account. In order to carry out this study, a human body is simulated with FDTD (of finite-difference time-domain) method. The simulated frequencies are 900 MHz, 1800 MHz, and 2400 MHz, and for different angles in azimuth (from 0 to 180 degrees) because the orientation of the RSS meter can be varied. Simulations show the power level of the incident wave of the wireless RSS meter before and after the human body. The results illustrate a significant variation between both measures. It proves the power absorption in presence of a body. Then, this conclusion is corroborated with an experimental measure in an outdoor environment and a real human body. This paper concludes that the RSS meter gives 15 dB less (on average) than the incident wave when the human is giving his back to the emitter, but, in contrast, the RSS meter gives is the same dBs as the incident wave when the human is facing it.

Another interesting work was presented by Karma K. Eudon in 2008 (Eudon, 2008). It analyzes the human shadowing effect on video streaming over IEEE 802.11b. The video streaming quality is measured in function of the human traffic in different indoor locations and varying distances from the access point. Results obtained conclude that the more human traffic the more degradation in the quality of the video occurs.

In the medical field, there is a work published that studies the influence of the electromagnetic field and SAR values by implanting in the head a kind active medical device called cochlear implant (Parazzini, et al., 2010). Then, they simulate a head model with and without a cochlear implant during exposure to WiFi frequencies. Next, both results are compared. Vertical and horizontal polarizations of incident wave are considered for simulations. The conclusion is that close to the cochlear implant of the head, the electromagnetic field and the SAR distribution vary moderately. It is more significant in lower frequencies. However, average SAR values don't show variations between simulations with or without implant.

On the other hand, several important organizations have established guidelines where are collected all maximum exposure limits of radio frequency energy for human. These documents are very necessary for the society, and especially for manufacturers of electronic devices and health researchers. For example, the Swiss Federal Office of Public Health (BAG) asked to The Foundation for Research on Information Technologies in Society (IT'IS) to perform a study on the exposure to electromagnetic fields from wireless data communication devices up to 6 GHz (Kühn & Kuster, 2006). The IEEE C95.1 standard (IEEE, 1999) offers recommendations about the maximum exposure limits to guarantee safety and health for people exposed to electromagnetic fields between 3 KHz to 300GHz. It explains each related parameter in detail, comments safety factors, measurement procedures, etc. for two kinds of environments: controlled and uncontrolled. Others

important references are the Recommendations of the National Council on Radiation Protection and Measurements (NCRP) in the USA (NCRP, 1986) and the National Radiation Protection Board (NRPB) in the United Kingdom (NRPB, 1993). Finally, in the USA the Federal Communications Commission (FCC) wrote a guideline (FCC, 1997) based on the recommendations of the NCRP. It is focused to protect workers and population in general from RF fields. According to the National Environmental Policy Act of 1969, the FCC has legal responsibilities to do it, so it guarantees that the wireless devices marked by it comply with the required exposure limits. European and other countries have followed their own directive and regulation (EC, 1999a; ICNIRP, 1998).

All guidelines differentiate between exposure limits for the general population in an uncontrolled environment and for workers in a controlled environment. In general, in an uncontrolled environment the limits are much smaller than in a controlled environment. Another important key of these guidelines is to distinguish between exposure to whole-body and to a particular region because these values change considerably. All the guidelines aforementioned conclude that the exposure to RF energy under the recommended SAR limits is safe.

In this chapter we are going to estimate the average signal level absorbed by a person in a real scenario in a different manner than the previous works. That is, we are going to measure the SAR by a person in two indoor environments by measuring the RSS.

Human Body and Effects of Electromagnetic Waves on It

In this section, the human body's composition and the effects of the Electromagnetic (EM) waves are going to be studied. First, we will analyze the composition of the body. In this part we are going to see that the body is mainly composed of soft elements and liquids. Then, some effects of EM waves over the human body will be described and we will see how these effects are produced.

Human Body Composition

The human body's composition is the sum of various tissues and systems that make up the human body. This differs from the morphological anatomy and it forms the chemical anatomy (Heymsfield, et al., 1996).

In order to determine the human body composition, there are methods based on direct chemical analysis of human body parts. They are most accurate, but they have a big disadvantage: they cannot be applied during the living period. The knowledge of the chemical anatomy facilitates the understanding of many processes, especially those that generate changes in tissue composition or in some parts of the body, and it often helps to explain the pathophysiological mechanisms.

The human body composition can be inferred by indirect methods, which are based on the estimation of the human body's density and volume. By measuring the weight under water, and then applying the Archimedes' principle we can calculate both values.

The theoretical model of the "5 level" of the human body composition, allows more than 30 determinations (Wang, et al., 1992). The five levels are:

- Atomic level
- Molecular level
- Cellular level
- Tissue-systems level
- Body level

Atomic Level

Oxygen is the most abundant atom in the human body. The % of the main elements in a human body is as follows Oxygen (61%), Carbon (23%), Hydrogen (10%), Nitrogen (2.6%) and Calcium (1.6%).

Molecular Level

Water is the 60% of body weight. It is the most abundant chemical compounds, followed by proteins and lipids. There is a 26% of Extracellular water and 34% of Intracellular water. Lipids form 20% of the body weight (17.9% is non-essential fat and 2.1% is essential). There is 15% of protein and 5.3% of minerals.

Cellular Level

The total cell mass of an adult is 1018 cells. There are 4 classes of cells:

- Connectives (adipocytes, osteoclasts, osteoblasts)
- Epithelial cells
- Nerve
- Muscle

Tissue-Systems Level

The tissue-systems level includes:

- Muscle tissue. Skeletal muscle is between 30% and 40% of body weight.
- Mesenchyme tissues. Bone tissue is 7.1%, blood is 7.9%, connective tissue and adipose tissue, which can be subcutaneous (11%), visceral (7.1%), interstitial (1.4%), and bone marrow (2.1%).
- Epithelial tissues. They are formed by skin (3.7%), liver (2.6%), gastrointestinal tract (1.7%), and lungs (1.4%).
- Nervous tissue: It is the central and periphery nervous system. Central nervous system is around 2%.

Body Level

The division of the body level is:

- Head

- Neck
- Arms
- Trunk
- Legs

Electromagnetic Effects in the Human Body

Since the introduction of mobile phones in the mid-1980s, many researchers have investigated the exposure of the biological tissue to electromagnetic waves. Radio frequency energy can be harmful due to the ability of to heat rapidly the biological tissue (Lin, 2003). In this section we will see how this heating is produced in the human body.

From the medical point of view, high frequency electromagnetic oscillations do not cause depolarization of nerve fibers. In spite of that, because high frequency waves have quite high alternations, they traverse muscular structures, but the muscles are not excited. High frequency waves produce heat inside the body. In contrast, low frequency waves have major effects, but they are not studied in this chapter because WLANs work at high frequency.

All these electromagnetic waves penetrate easily through the skin, which is not a big obstacle. Besides, they heat more the functional areas that have aqueous component (i.e. soft tissues and organs) than fatty parts. Although, all waves produce heat inside the body, the heat will be different according to its penetration and the way to spread the produced heat.

High frequency waves act on the body in the same manner than when electrical current flows through the organizational structures. They can penetrate the human body through a triple mechanism:

- Conduction current: it is the most simple and typical way of conduction in bodies and it is used by the continuous current. The most important effect of this mecha-
nism is the production of heat through the Joule's law.
- Displacement current: high frequency waves are able to pass through dielectric bodies. In order to understand it, we must think that the molecules potentially are electrical dipole, which become a real dipole when they have an electric field and the electrical charges are oriented.
- Induction current: high frequency current can induce a current in the same frequency. These waves pass through the body as conduction current.

The molecules under the influence of an electromagnetic field have a polarity change of many millions of times per second. So its performance depends on its specific frequency.

Inside the human body, the most abundant molecule is the water (about 60% of body weight). Although the water molecule is electrically neutral, it has a distribution of charge that resembles a dipole. That is, it has more positive charge for hydrogen atoms and more negative charge for the oxygen atoms. This molecule has an appearance similar to a 120° angle, where the oxygen molecule is in the vertex and the hydrogen is placed in each side.

Taking into account that hydrogen molecules are placed beside the positive field and the negative field is on the other side, the electromagnetic field begins to act on water molecules. The hydrogen atoms are rejected by the charges of the same sign, and attracted by opposite charges. However, the oxygen atom are rejected by the negative charges and attracted by positive charges.

Overall, the water molecule tends to rotate in order to be placed in the opposite way, so its positive poles face up to the negative charges, and the negatives face up to the positives.

Because the frequency changes so quickly, when this rotation movement starts, the situation of the fields is opposite. On the right, it will be the negative pole of field and on the left it will be the positive one. Thus, the water molecule begins to turn around in the opposite direction to the previous event. Finally, in this molecule, its charges are close to the field of the opposite polarity. This phenomenon is repeated with each new polarity change, again and again. The water molecules start a series of successive rotations, so the molecules rub against each other. This friction causes a warming effect on the molecules and their own heating.

In summary, the action of the electromagnetic field using high frequency waves causes friction and produces heating in the water molecules. The internal organs (muscles, soft organs, entrails, etc.) are composed primarily of water, and therefore they are heated. However, this heat does not come from outside. It is interesting to know that compared with other organs, the skin and the body fats are not easily heated when they are radiated by electromagnetic waves.

This shaking of the molecules causes different effects on the human body. Tattersall *et al.* (2001) appoints the increase of the temperature and the reduction of the blood pressure, as general effects. Other effects reported by Thom (1996) are an outstanding fatigue and the necessity of sleeping, in response to the total body heating. It is clear that these effects occur when a body is irradiated for a large time. Thom concludes that the cumulative effect of many irradiations during a long time can be dangerous.

After the first years of wireless communications appearance, some people began to suffer these symptoms. It usually occurs when people live or stay a long time close to the transmitters. Most common symptoms are anxiety, fatigue, depression, headaches, and insomnia.

Today, the current equipment of high frequency radiation produces less undesirable effects because they have improved along the years and more precautions are taken into account when developing the transmitters. For this reason, the places chosen to locate the high-frequency equipment is as far as possible from places where there are risky people, as for example hospital, schools, parks, etc., or others places where there are many people for long periods of time.

The level of heat caused in the molecules when the waves go through the body, depends on the frequency wave and the incident angle. Several studies have obtained this conclusion. Moreover, some researchers have studied the heat level in each element of the human body (Merckel, 1972). In the Table 3, we observe the heat level ranges from 0 to 5, where 0 means no heat and 5 means high heat. According to Table 3, we can see that waves mainly affect muscles (4) and body fat (3). So, people with more muscles and/or body fat absorb more electromagnetic field.

In our case, we use wireless equipment that work at the 2.4GHz radio frequency band and thus a wavelength of 12.5 cm. At this wavelength, the energy produced by the high frequency is

Table 3. Heating human body parts for several types of waves

	FAT	MUSCLE	Periosteum	BONE
Short Wave – Capacitor Field	4	2	1	1
Short Wave – Selenoidal Field	1.5	5	1	1
Short Wave – Selenoidal & Circuplode	0	5	2	2
UHF Waves – Selenoidal Field	1	4	1	1
UHF Waves – Throught Field	2	4	2	2
Microwave	3	4	0	0

particularly well absorbed by the body tissues. This happens because they have a high percentage of water. These microwaves go through the subcutaneous fat with low losses then, in the muscles and organs with much blood, they are transformed into heat. This phenomenon also happens in the skin. Obviously, this increase of the temperature in the body not is desirable.

Short term exposure to very high levels of RF radiation has caused cataracts and temporary sterility (caused by changes in sperm count and sperm mobility), in rabbits. Some other causes may occur after the exposure of testis to high-level RF radiation. Mice and rabbits have been employed in most of the experimental investigations on biological effects of RF exposure (Lin, 2003).

Furthermore, an epidemiological study of cancer illness has discovered that the main cancers associated with EMF exposure are leukemia, nervous system tumors, lymphoma, and breast cancer. They mainly happen among children living in residential settings with EMF and adults in occupational settings with EMF (Karunarathna, et al., 2005).

Other effects of EMF exposure are the depression as well as the fatigue, irritation, and headaches. Epidemiological studies have found higher ratio of depression-like symptoms and higher rates of suicide among people living near transmission lines. On the other hand, adverse pregnancy outcome, including miscarriages, still birth, congenital deformities, and illness at birth have been associated with maternal occupational exposure to electromagnetic fields. Moreover, man exposure to electromagnetic fields has also been linked to reduce fertility, lower the number of born males compared to females, congenital malformations and teratogenic effects expressed in the form of childhood cancer. In vivo studies with rats showed that their exposure to high electromagnetic waves reduced plasma testosterone concentrations and reduced sperm viability (California EMF Program, 2001).

Analytical Considerations

In this section, we will include all analytical considerations that should be taken into account when the RSS is decreased, because of the presence of the human body, and the equations that relate the SAR with other parameters.

In any given time and place, the RSS values received from a device in a wireless network depend on a large number of unpredictable factors. Specifically, in a WLAN 802.11 network, small changes in position or direction may result in high differences in RSS. Moreover, similar effects can happen even if the wireless devices remain static, due to the presence of moving objects that may interfere in the access point to station propagation.

It is clear that the first factor influencing RSS values obtained by a wireless device is the distance between emitter and receiver, as this distance causes attenuation in RSS values. In free space we can easily computed as the standard path loss equation, but in real deployments we must take account of the material being traversed by the radio waves and its signal absorption.

So, previously to have any idea about the energy scattered by the presence of living beings it is necessary to determine beforehand the sort of dependence present among those RSS values and the distance between the emitter and the receiver. Usually this has been known as path loss, and it is modeled to be inversely proportional to the distance between the emitter and the receiver raised to a certain exponent. This exponent is known as path loss exponent (Mazuelas, et al., 2009), path loss factor (Hashemi, 1993), or path loss gradient (Qi, 2003).

Other factors that affect RSS values are the multipath or fast fading and the shadowing or slow fading (Li, 2006). These two factors can be modeled with Rayleigh or Rician and log-normal distributions (Mazuelas, et al., 2009). Therefore, RSS values can be modeled finally by means of the Friis transmission formula (Hashemi, 1993).

$$P_R = \frac{G_t G_r}{4\pi} \cdot P_t \cdot \frac{g^2 \cdot \gamma}{d^n} \qquad (1)$$

where P_t is the transmitted power, G_t and G_r are the transmitter and receiver gains, respectively, d is the distance between transmitter and receiver, n is the attenuation variation index with the distance ($n=2$ in the air), and g and γ are the parameters that conform the Rayleigh/Rician and lognormal distributions, respectively.

In many models the effect of the losses due to multipath effect is added (Valenzuela, 1993) (Frühwirth, 1996). But, averaging over certain time interval we can eliminate the fast fading term, due to multipath loss (Liu, et al., 2006). Thus the propagation losses can be modeled by the expression (2), where the

$$L\ (dB) = Lo - 10 \cdot n \cdot log(d) - K \cdot SAR \qquad (2)$$

Where Lo is the power losses (in dB) at a distance of 1 meter (e.g. 40.2 dB at 2.44 GHz frequency), K is the number of people in the room, and SAR is the mean SAR of the people inside the room. All the other parameters have been defined previously.

But these propagation losses occur for each access point in the room, so the absorbed RSS will depend on the SAR and the number of people in the room, the number of access points deployed in the room, and on the distance to the wireless devices.

The FDTD (finite-difference time-domain) modeling technique (Taflove, 1998) is the preferred method for making SAR calculations. This differential formulation allows users to divide the model space into very small cells, which provides excellent resolution of tissue in the human body. Other computational methods are unable to model the tissue structure to a resolution that is accurate enough for such calculations.

So, using the FDTD technique we can obtain the e-field components in any area we desire to model and the distribution of the local SAR values can be calculated directly from the electric field distribution, which results expression (3) (Tinniswood, et al., 1998; Khalatbari, et al., 2006).

$$SAR = \frac{\sigma \cdot E_{max}^2}{2 \cdot p} \qquad (3)$$

Where σ is the conductivity on the desired cell of the FDTD domain and p is the density of the sample.

The value will depend heavily on the geometry of the part of the body that is exposed to the RF energy and on the exact location and geometry of the RF source. The SAR value is then measured at the location that has the highest absorption rate in the entire head, which in the case of a mobile phone is often as close to the device's antenna as possible.

In far field conditions, WBA-SAR (Whole Body Averaged SAR) has been successfully used as an easy estimator for SAR. As shown in previous studies (Hirata, et al., 2010), it is reasonable to consider the human body approximately as a half-wave dipole. The resonance frequency can be reasonably estimated from the height of the human subjects. The analogy of a half-wave dipole and human body models at their respective resonance frequency was confirmed in (Gadhi, et al., 1995).

Let us summarize the fundamental characteristics of the halfwave dipole antenna. For the current distribution on the antenna $I(z)$ and the maximum current I_0 [A], the effective height of the antenna L_e [m] is given by equation (4) (Kraus, et al., 2002).

$$L_e = \frac{1}{I_0} \int_0^L I(z)dz \qquad (4)$$

Where, L is the physical height of the antenna. The effective height of the half-wave dipole is given by the following equation (5) (Kraus, et al., 2002).

$$L_e = \frac{\lambda}{\pi} \cong 0.636L \qquad (5)$$

For an antenna of known effective height, the induced voltage V_o [V] is given by multiplying the effective height by the incident electric field or incident power density S_{inc} [W/m2], that will be related with the signal power received and the effective section of the human body under the angle of incidence of the signal. It is shown in equation (6).

$$V_o = \sqrt{120\pi \cdot S_{inc} \cdot L_e} \qquad (6)$$

So, we can estimate the induced voltage in the antenna and obtain an equation to estimate the WBA-SAR in a human body model by equation (7).

$$WBSAR \cong 7.52 \cdot S_{inc} \cdot \frac{H^2}{W} = 7.52 \cdot \frac{S_{inc}}{B} \qquad (7)$$

Where W is the weight of the human, and $B = W/H^2$ [kg/m2] is the body mass index (BMI). From last equation we can simply estimate the WBA-SAR in terms of the RSS power, the BMI of the human body, and the angle of incidence of the signal.

Data Collection and Analysis

Next, two different ways are shown to calculate the SAR. Test bed 1 is based on RSS measured according to number of people next to WLAN inside the library at the Higher Polytechnic School of Gandia, Polytechnic University of Valencia, and their weights. This WLAN is deployed in a real environment and so, it is an uncontrolled environment. We do not manage any variable as

for example, number of people, their position in the library, etc. In contrast, test bed 2 is based on a WLAN deployed for us in an anechoic camera, so it is does a controlled environment. In this case, calculation of SAR is based on RSS measured again, but now it depends on specific features of human bodies which are inside anechoic camera and their positions.

Test Bed 1

In order to analyze the electromagnetic radiation absorbed by the people, we have measured the signal level variations in an indoor wireless local area network IEEE 802.11g. This wireless network works at the 2.4 GHz ISM band. In order to do it we used a wireless network scanner called Vistumbler (Vistumbler Website). This program permits to detect all wireless access points reached and indicates which are available and which are not. It allows to measure the Media Access Control (MAC) address of each AP, the RSS (in % and in dB) from each one, kind of authentication used, etc. In this work we will pay attention to the RSS parameter.

The measurements have been taken in the wireless local area network of the Higher Polytechnic School of Gandia, Polytechnic University of Valencia. The chosen place is the library which is placed inside of one of the building of the campus. Library presents good features to do these measurements because people are studying or reading in silence, and the movement in this place is minimal.

The measurements have been taken by a laptop with a wireless card Atheros 802.11b/g/n. After scanning all wireless networks, data was exported to an excel file. In order to obtain the most accurate results, while the computer is scanning wireless networks it was disconnected from all access points. We gathered the RSS every second during 250 seconds. Once data have been already imported to an excel file, the main statistical parameters have been calculated (see Table 4)

Table 4. Statistical measures in the library

	0 persons	**11 persons**	**34 persons**
Maximum RSS value (dB)	-30	-30	-30
Minimum RSS value (dB)	-31	-33	-33
Average RSS value (dB)	-30.01158301	-30.01571709	-30.62544803
Average weight (Kg)	-	65.09090909	64.32352941

Figure 1. RSS without people

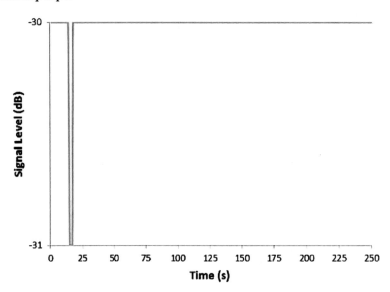

Figure 2. RSS with 11 persons

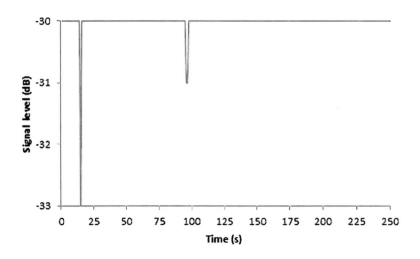

Figure 3. RSS with 34 persons

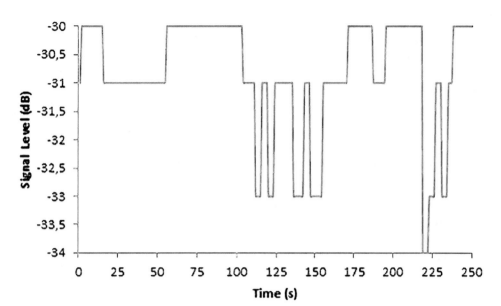

and the time evolution has been represented (see Figures 1-3).

The library is the biggest room of the building. It has five central long tables and five side tables on both sides. Moreover, although this room has coverage from several access points, there is one principal access point inside the room. So, our measurements are taken from this one.

First measurements were taken at 8 am without any person inside the room, the second one were collected at 9 pm with 11 people seated, and the last one at 11 pm with 34 people. The data has been gathered over a period of 250 seconds, because this time is enough to see results and accurate mean values. Finally, we gathered the weight of each person inside the room.

In Table 4, the main statistical results of our test bed are shown (maximum RSS, minimum RSS and average RSS [in dB], and average weight in kg).

Because the transmitting power of the access point in this place reached 100mW, we considered that -30 dB is equivalent to a signal level of 100%.

Although between zero and eleven persons there are no significant differences, we can see that the RSS is considerably reduced when the number of people is increased up to 34 persons.

Next graphs show the signal level evolution for all cases. It proves that there are more inferior peaks with eleven people (see Figure 2), and with thirty-four people (see Figure 3) than when library is empty (see Figure 1).

In Figure 1, the RSS in dB along the time, when there is not any person, is represented. RSS value is -30 dB most of the time except in the 18th second that the RSS is decreased up to -31 dB. As there is only one inferior peak, a continuous linear tendency can be considered. We can see that when there is not any person, the RSS reaches its maximum value. So, it is deduced the absorbed RSS will be considered zero.

In Figure 2, the RSS in dB along the time, when there are eleven persons placed in the same room where the measurements were taken, is represented. All these people were not connected with a computer or any type of device to the WLAN. They were studying. We can see in Figure 2, that their bodies absorb some RSS because the RSS mean value is lower. The RSS evolution presents a linear tendency in -30 dB, but in this case there are two inferior peaks: the first one in the 18th second and the second one in the 99th. We can see that the RSS absorption is not still very significant.

In Figure 3, we can see the RSS evolution when there are 34 persons in the library. In this case the RSS is rampant. In this case, when there are many people in the room, the RSS absorption is very significant. It has the lowest inferior peak at 222th second with a value of -34 dB. There are some intermediate values of -31 dB and -33 dB. So, from these three figures, we can conclude that the more people in the room the more RSS absorbed. There is higher SAR in this last scenario.

We have calculated the SAR using two different ways. On the one hand, we have estimated the average absorbed RSS per person, and, on the hand, we have estimated the average absorbed RSS per Kg. Table 5 shows the SAR values obtained in the WLAN.

The variation of the RSS of the wireless channels and the radio interference when there are people in the room and when they are not, let us know how much energy is absorbed by them.

Test Bed 2

In this part of this chapter, we have analyzed the specific absorption rate in a controlled environment, in contrast to the previous scenario where no variable was controlled.

We used an anechoic chamber in order to have a controlled environment. This kind of room is designed to avoid reflections of both sound and electromagnetic waves (Ono, et al., 1996). Test bed 2 has been done in the anechoic chamber of the Higher Polytechnic School of Gandia, Polytechnic University of Valencia. It has been built to study the sound waves so it is insulated acoustically. Although, acoustic waves are not important for us, in this case, this anechoic chamber is also insulated from external frequency (especially those of wireless local area networks). No WLAN can be detected inside it. Thus, this chamber is useful to perform this study because it avoids possible interferences from outside. In this way, the variations of the wireless signal strength will be given only due to the presence of human bodies inside the chamber.

Anechoic chambers are composed of structures insulted acoustically, or electromagnetically, from the outside. They are built of brick walls. Besides, inner walls are lined with wedged formations

Table 5. SAR calculation

	11 persons	34 persons
Average RSS (dB)	-30.01571709	-30.62544803
Absorbed average RSS (dB)	0.01571709	0.625448003
Average weight (Kg)	65.09090909	64.32352941
SAR (absorbed signal level (dB) / number of people)	0.001428826	0.018395530
SAR (absorbed signal level (dB)/ Kg)	0.000241463	0.009723471

which absorb acoustic or electromagnetic waves. Thus, anechoic chambers create a reflection free space. These wedges are made of different materials such as foam, fiber glass, rock, wool, etc. The most important feature of these materials is to avoid any reflection.

Absorption level of each chamber depends on the length of wedges. Besides, the dimensions of the chamber are chosen according to two variables: dimensions of devices which are going to be tested and the frequency range of the transmitted signals. So, to know how and for what the anechoic chamber is going to be used is essential in order to build it.

Originally anechoic chambers were used in the acoustics field in order to minimize the reflections of the chamber. But now, these chambers are also used to reduce reflection and external noise in radio frequencies. In the last years, they have improved their features (Hemming, 2002).

An ideal anechoic chamber is a room completely free of acoustic reverberations. Any sound projected into the enclosure, and at any frequency, is completely absorbed. Effectiveness of an anechoic chamber is measured in dB of rejection, i.e. the ratio of direct sound and reflected sound within an enclosure.

Our analysis was performed in the Sound waves anechoic chamber of the Higher Polytechnic School of Gandia, Polytechnic University of Valencia.

In order to know the SAR of a human body inside this room, we set up a wireless local area network inside this place using an access point. Then, we measured the RSS received by the wireless interface card of a laptop. This laptop uses a wireless network scanner called Vistumbler to know received signal level (we have used the same procedure than in the analysis if test bed 1).

We have used the Linksys Wireless-G broadband router, model WRT54G, as access point. It was used to build the wireless local area network necessary for this study. This router includes dedicated hardware devices featuring a built-in

network adapter, a high gain antennas kit and one radio transmitter (Linksys Datasheet). It works in the 2.4GHz radio frequency band (IEEE 802.11b, IEEE 802.11g or both can be chosen) and it can be configured in infrastructure mode. We have chosen this router because the transmitting power can be changed by the user and, in this study we need to choose the lowest transmitting power. The influence of people's presence on the wireless signal will be better reflected in the signal strength when there is low transmitting power. Minimum output power is 0 dBm (1 mw), so this is the transmitting power that we have configured. We will call this router "access point" during the rest of the chapter, because we will only use this function of the device. The laptop used to receive the signal level of the WLAN is the same than the one used in the study performed in test bed 1.

The high gain antennas kit provides an omnidirectional design for 360 degrees. It is composed by two high gain antennas for R-TNC connectors and one antenna stabilizer. This is the model HGA7T. Its maximum gain is 7 dBi and its maximum voltage standing wave ratio is 1.92 Volts with a nominal impedance of 50 Ohms. Besides, it provides a linear vertical polarization.

According to features of the previous antenna and its radiation pattern, we have calculated the near and the far-field region. It lets us know in which exact point of the anechoic camera should be located the human bodies that are going to be studied.

Space surrounding an antenna is subdivided into three regions (Balanis, 2005): the reactive near-field region, the radiating near-field region and the far-field region.

The near-field region is divided into the reactive near-field and the radiating near-field. The reactive near-field region is the region close to the antenna. It is too complex to predict because the relationship between the electromagnetic and magnetic field is very changeable. In each a location one of them can dominate and only for a short distance, the opposite is the predominant. So, in this region the reactive component of the near-field region can give ambiguous or undetermined results when measures are taken in this region.

In contrast, the radiating near-field region, also called the Fresnel region, has not got reactive field components from the source antenna. The relationship between the electromagnetic and magnetic field is more predictable, but this relationship is still complex and different to the far-field. In this region, there are still some localized energy fluctuations.

On the other hand, in the far-field region, referred as Fraunhofer region, the angular distribution of the electromagnetic field is independent of the distance to the antenna. That is, the field has a regular distribution of electric field strength and magnetic field strength in a plane perpendicular to the propagation direction. In other words, the wave is locally plain. However, the amplitude of the electromagnetic field decreases according to the inverse with the distance, i.e. the transmission power decreases as the square of the distance from the antenna.

Distances of these regions (IEEE, 2003) can be calculated by formulas (8), (9), and (10). They are the most commonly used. Formula 8 is useful to know the limiting distance which the reactive near-field region is spread to.

$$r < R_1 = 0{,}62 \cdot \sqrt{\frac{d_{máx}^3}{\lambda}} \qquad (8)$$

The r parameter is the distance to the antenna source, R_1 is the boundary limit between the reactive and the radiating near-field, and d_{max} is the maximum dimension of the used antenna. The wavelength λ depends on the frequency f and the speed of light c according to the formula $\lambda = c/f$. Because $c = 3 \cdot 10^8$ m/s and $f = 2.4$GHz for the antenna, λ is 12.5cm.

Dimensions of our antenna kit is 14 mm width and 130 mm height, so its d_{max} is 13 cm. With this value, R_1 is equal to 8.22 cm.

Next, the distance of the radiating near-field is calculated using formula 9.

$$R_1 < r < R_2 = \frac{2d_{máx}^2}{\lambda} \qquad (9)$$

Now, we can estimare R_2 because variables are known: $R_2 = 27.04$ cm.

As we see in formula 10, from R_2 to higher values, there is the the the far-field region.

$$r > R_2 \qquad (10)$$

In conclusion, the field regions for our antenna are the following:

- The reactive near-field region: From r=0 cm to R_1= 8.22 cm
- The radiating near-field region: From R_1=8.22 cm to R_2=27.04 cm
- The far-field region: From R_2=27.04 cm

Signal Measurements at Test Bed 2

To analyze the human body's SAR, we have chosen four people, two women and two men, each one with a different body structure. We need to study with different persons because the body mass index, the height and weight, and even the body stucture of each one will be parameters than will affect the measurements, as we will show very soon.

The first man (man1) weights 81 kg and has a height of 185 cm. He has an athletic and strong constitution. He has a high muscle mass. His body mass index is 23.6 kg/m². The second man (man2) weights 69 kg and has a height of 179 cm. He has a skinny structure and so a high bone mass. His body mass index is 21.53 kg/m². The first woman (woman1) has a height of 169 cm and a weight of 77.8 kg. She has a wide constitution with a high body mass. Her body mass index is 27.24 kg/m². The second woman (woman2) has a height of 160 cm and a weight of 52 kg. She has a slim constitution with a normal body mass. Her body mass index is 20.31 kg/m².

Each one of these persons has come to the anechoic camera individually and has stood for 5 minutes in five different positions, while the laptop was taking measurements with the wireless network scanner. We can see in Figure 4 the position of the latop and the position of the access point in the anachoic chamber. The five positions of the persons are depicted with red crosses.

The first position (L1) is the closest to the access point's antenna, just 6 centimeters away, so it is in the reactive near-field region, but not in the direct path between the access point and the signal meter. We chose that point to simulate the usage of a mobile wifi device in the pocket of a user. With that idea in our mind we chose the second point (L2) in the reactive near-field region, but in the line of sight between the access point and the laptop.

The third position (L3) is close to the access point, just 25 centimeters of the antenna, to simu-

late a user holding a mobile device in his hand, but already in the radiating near-field region.

The fourth position (L4) is at the midpoint of the direct path between the access point and the meter but, in this case, without interfering with the sight between them to simulate signal received from other users' devices and infrastructure access points. That point is in the far-field region at 1 meter from antenna. The fifth position (L5) is adjacent to the laptop meter, obviouslly in the far-field region, and simulate a user receiving signal with his laptop from an access point.

From our previous discussions we expect that the body mass of the user will have a direct impact in the signal received, and as we discussed previously, on the SAR for that user. Also we expect more consistent results in the far field measurement points than in the near-field ones.

In Figure 5, we show the RSS for each person when is located in position 1, just one centimeter away from the access point's antenna. Here the expected signal in -30dB, so any difference from

Figure 4. Scheme of the anachoic chamber's stage used to take measurements

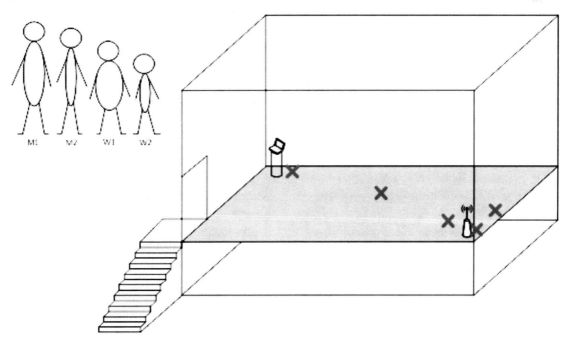

Figure 5. RSS at L1, one centimeter away from the access point

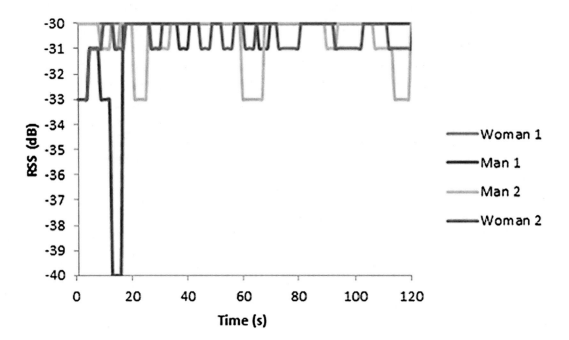

that measurement will be a consequence of the interaction of the person in the anecoic chamber.

In this location, the person studied is in the reactive near-field region and it involves that results can be confusing. In fact, Woman 1 does not present any absorption in this location and the signal level is constant in -30 dB all the time for her. In contrast, the Man 1 has an spectaular absoprtion before the second twenty, and the signal is reduced to -40 dB. However, the rest of time his absorption is much lower. On the other hand, results for the Woman 2 and the Man 2 are more coherent. The Man 2 as has a higher weight than the Woman 2, he presents a greater absorption of the signal, but within a consistent range of values.

In Figure 6, we average the received signal level by the laptop of the Figure 5 for each person. Here we can conclude than results are not logical if we take into account the weight of each person. This is because in the reactive near-field region,

the electromagnetic field is highly unstable, and so the received signal.

In Figure 7 we show the results from the second measurement point. Here we are still in the reactive near-field region, but we detect much different signal levels than in our previous setup, as we ae acting like a wall between the access point and the laptop.

In Figure 7 RSS evolution is similar for all people but with different ranges of values. When the Woman 1 is in the second location, her RSS is the lowest one. Therefore, it is considered that she presents a higher absorption of the wireless signal. Although she has a lower weight than the Man 1, her consitution is much wider. So, as in position L2 people act like a wall, and she has a body mass index higher, her absorption is greater.

On the other hand, the second lower measurement is from Man 1, then the Man 2 and finally, the second woman. These results are directly

Figure 6. Average RSS at L1

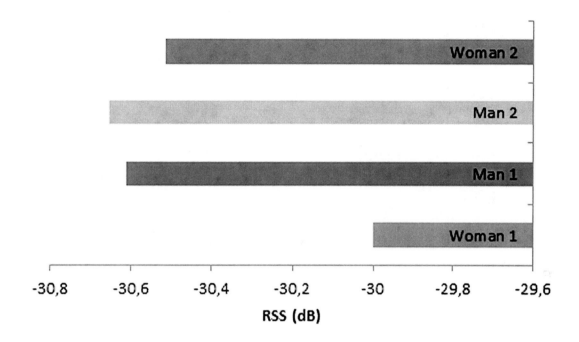

Figure 7. RSS at L2

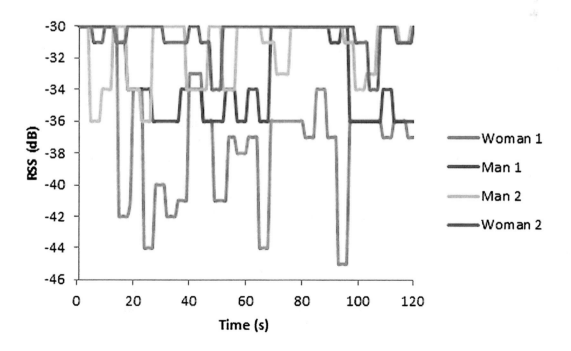

Figure 8. Average RSS at L2

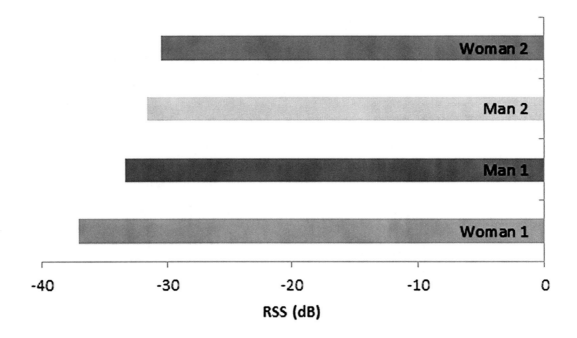

related to body mass index of each person. Figure 8 presents the average RSS for each user at L2.

The average signal level gathered when the woman 1 is in the second place for 5 minutes, is about -37 dB, about -33 dB when the first man is inside, -31 dB for the second man, and -30.52 dB when the woman 2 is present.

At L3 we are in safer ground. Simulating a mobile device in our hand we are still into the radiating near-field region but the electromagnetic field is a more stable.

In Figure 9 we show the signal received in the laptop when our four testers are at L3, 25 cm away from the access point. In that case, Man 1 has the most absorbing profile and so the received RSS level at the laptop shows lower peaks. At L3 is more important the total weight than the body mass index. This is so because here, signal does not necessarily have to go through the body to reach the laptop. The following person more absorbent is the Woman 2, she has the second higher total

weight. Next, she is followed closely by the Man 2, and again the Woman 2 is the least absorbent.

The average RSS value is shown in Figure 10.

The average RSS level when man1 is inside the chamber in the third position, is -35.22 dB, when woman1 is -32.9 dB, -32.7 dB for man2, and -31.2 dB when woman2 is inside the chamber.

Now, results in the fourth position (L4) are analyzed. In this location, we are in the far-field region one meter away from both the acces point and the laptop. L4 is close to the midpoint of the direct path between the access point and the meter but the direct sight among them is free. So, in this case, people do not act as a obstacle but as an absorbent object, in the same way that in the locations one and three.

As we can see in Figure 11, again the received RSS when Man1 is in this position is the lowest, so here he is the most absorbent too. Next, the second lower RSS level is obtained when Woman1 is in the anachoic chamber. Finally, man2 and woman 2 are the least absorbent because their weights are

Figure 9. RSS at L3.

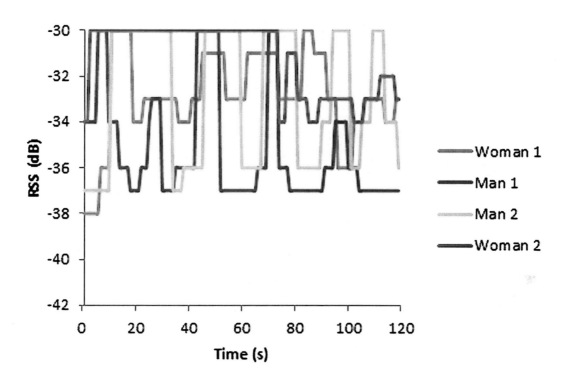

Figure 10. Average RSS for the third location (L3)

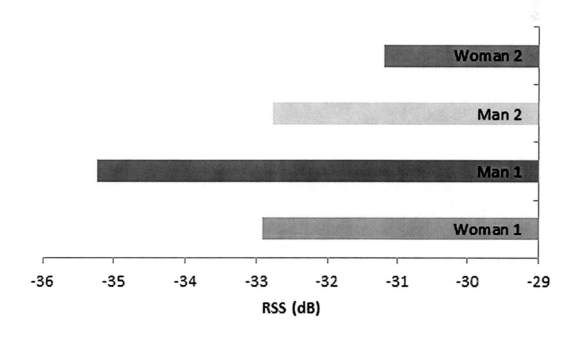

Figure 11. RSS at L4, in the middle of the room

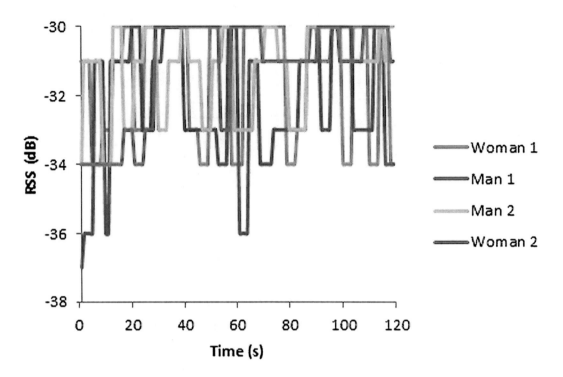

Figure 12. Average RSS at the fourth location (L4)

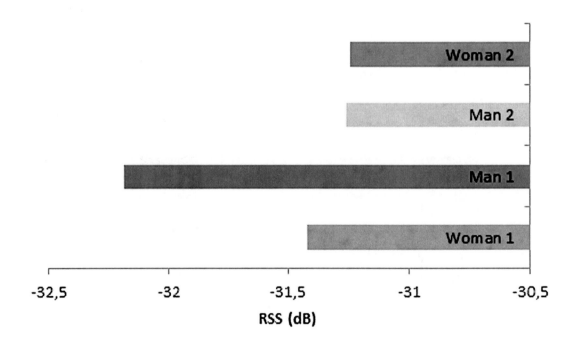

the lowest. They show a similar absorption in this point (see Figure 12).

Figure 12 shows that the absorption of wireless signal due to the presence of people is lower in this location than in the previous one and so the received average RSS level is higher. In this case, when Man1 is present in the chamber, the RSS level is -32.18 dB on average, when woman1 is inside, the RSS is -31.42 dB on average, and about -31.2 dB for man2 and woman2.

Finally, we have considered the fifth position to simulate a user receiving signal from an access point and also to check if near the laptop's antenna the human bodies have any significant feature regarding the absoption. People are to 10 centimeters from the laptop and obviouslly they are in the far-field region. Results obtained are shown in Figure 13 and they are very similar to the third and fourth location.

Although in Figure 13 Man2 presents lower peaks in the RSS level evolution, on average he is just the second lower with -32.7 dB (see Figure 14). These lower peaks may be due to some movement of the person. As it can be seen in Figure 14, Man1 is the most absorbent person with a RSS average level of -33.87 dB, Woman1 is next with -33.1 dB average, and the last one is Woman2 with an average RSS of -32 dB.

SAR Estimations

Now we have estimated the SAR by person and location, according to his total weight and his body mass index. It has been calculated for all locations except for the first one. This is so because as we mentioned before, results on that location are not stable enough to make any prediction. On the other hand, although the second location is in the reactive near-field too, as people act as a wall, it does have been considered.

We can see the SAR calculation for the second location in the Table 6. In this location, the absorption of the wireless signal is due to the body

mass index, and the SAR calculated according to this parameter is the most representative one.

At L2 SAR for Woman1 is the highest one with a value of 0.260 dB/Kg/m². This is because her body mass index is the highest too. As in this location (in front of the access point), signal has to go through this higher body mass, the effect of her kind of body is more absorbent because, her constitution is quite wide, so it is more difficult for the electromagnetic wave goes through it and it causes power losses in the wireless signal. In this location, she is the one that presents her highest SAR level, and it is the highest in all cases and for all persons.

For the same reason, SAR in dB/Kg is also the highest for woman1; it is 0.091 dB/Kg.

The second SAR more significant level is the obtained by man1. He has a SAR level of 0.143 dB/Kg/m². SAR in dB/Kg for him is 0.042.

Next comes woman2 and man2, as have an inferior weight and body mass index. They present lower absorption levels because their constitutions the slimmer. According his body index mass, SAR for the man2 is 0.074 dB/Kg/m², and taking into account his total weight is 0.023dB/Kg. On the other hand, woman2 absorbs 0.026 dB/Kg/m² and her SAR level is 0.010 dB/Kg. So, she is the least absorbent person.

Now, in Table 7 we show the SAR values in the third location.

As we can see, in the third location L3, man2 is more absorbent than the rest of persons. Here, persons are next to the access point's antenna, exactly 25 centimeters, but not in the direct path (and there in not any reflected path, as we are in an anechoic chamber). So as man2 has a higher total weight, he has higher absorption. His absorption has been 0.221 dB/Kg/m² and 0.064 dB/Kg.

Here, the second more absorbent person is man2, with a SAR value of 0.129 dB/Kg/m² and 0.040 dB/Kg. Woman2 presents very similar values to him, 0.107 dB/Kg/m² and 0.037 dB/Kg. In this location, this is so because the more influential body feature here is the people's height.

Figure 13. RSS evolution at L5, close to the laptop

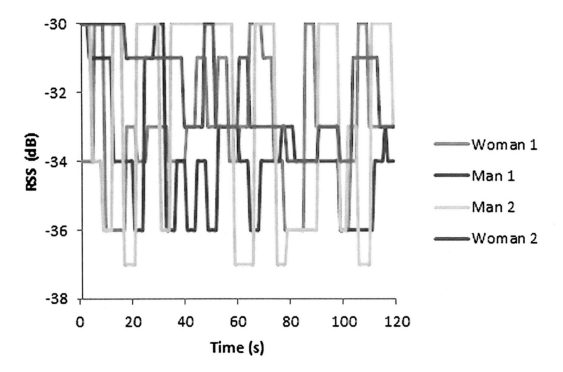

Figure 14. Average RSS at L5, close to the laptop

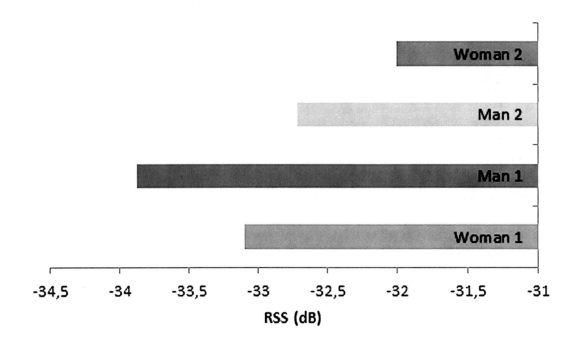

Table 6. SAR calculations for the second location L2

	Woman 1	Man 1	Man 2	Woman 2
Average RSS (dB)	-37.09	-33.37	-31.59	-30.52
Absorbed average RSS (dB)	7.09	3.37	1.59	0.52
Total weight (Kg)	77.8	81	69	52
Body Mass Index (Kg/m^2)	27.24	23.6	21.53	20.31
SAR (absorbed signal level / Kg)	0.091	0.042	0.023	0.010
SAR (absorbed signal level / Kg/m^2)	0.260	0.143	0.074	0.026

Table 7. SAR calculations for the third location L3

	Woman 1	Man 1	Man 2	Woman 2
Average RSS (dB)	-32.90	-35.22	-32.77	-31.20
Absorbed average RSS (dB)	2.90	5.22	2.77	1.20
total weight (Kg)	77.8	81	69	52
Body Mass Index (Kg/m^2)	27.24	23.6	21.53	20.31
SAR (absorbed signal level / Kg)	0.037	0.064	0.040	0.023
SAR (absorbed signal level / Kg/m^2)	0.107	0.221	0.129	0.059

Table 8. SAR calculations for the fourth location L4

	Woman 1	**Man 1**	**Man 2**	**Woman 2**
Average RSS (dB)	-31.42	-32.18	-31.26	-31.24
Absorbed average RSS (dB)	1.420	2.18	1.26	1.24
total weight (Kg)	77.8	81	69	52
Body Mass Index (Kg/m²)	27.24	23.6	21.53	20.31
SAR (absorbed signal level / Kg)	0.018	0.027	0.018	0.024
SAR (absorbed signal level / Kg/m²)	0.052	0.092	0.058	0.061

The reason for that is that the higher the impact surface is, the higher absorption is caused. This is the reason for which the woman 2 is again the least abosrbent, because she is the shortest of all of them. She has an absorption of 0.059 dB/Kg/m² and 0.023 dB/Kg.

Table 8 presents absorption levels for each person according their body mass indexes and their weights at the midpoint between the laptop meter and the access point, L4, one meter of each one but without interfering in their direct sight.

In general, SAR values in the fourth location are the lowest of all our measurements. This location is at a midpoint of the chamber and the influence on the electromagnetic waves is less important. Absorption of wireless signal due to the presence of people is the lowest. In this case, results are a little ambiguous, because they do not depends on the weight, height, body index mass or constitution of the analyzed people. Although the absorbed average RSS does is coherent because the person who weighs more, the more signal level absorbs, in contrast in SAR level does is not so. Man 1 is the most absorbent in this point, then

woman 2 is the second one and finally, woman 1 and man 2 have the minimum SAR levels.

To conclude the SAR calculations, we are going to show results for the last location L5, next to the laptop and in the other side of the anechoic chamber, in Table 9.

In this case, SAR levels are coherent with body features of the analyzed people. Here the person who has the highest absorption is man 1. His SAR is 0.164 dB/Kg/m² and 0.048dB/Kg. Both his weight and his height are the highest. Next, man 2 is the second more absorbent person in terms of dB/Kg/m² with a value of 0.126. That is, if we considerer the body mass index, man 2 is the second more absorbent, although his body index mass is lower than woman 1. In constrast, according to the total weight, woman 1 is the second more absorbent with 0.039 dB/Kg. It can be considered that both of them have similar SAR values if we compare them in the same terms, that is, in dB/Kg or in dB/Kg/m². Man 2 has a SAR value of 0.039 dB/Kg and woman 1 absorbs 0.114 dB/Kg/m². Finally, as in the rest of cases except in the fourth

Table 9. SAR calculations for the fifth location L5

	Woman 1	*Man 1*	*Man 2*	*Woman 2*
Average RSS (dB)	-33.10	-33.87	-32.71	-32.00
Absorbed average RSS (dB)	3.10	3.87	2.71	2.00
total weight (Kg)	77.8	81	69	52
Body Mass Index (Kg/m^2)	27.24	23.6	21.53	20.31
SAR (absorbed signal level / Kg)	0.040	0.048	0.039	0.039
SAR (absorbed signal level / Kg/m^2)	0.114	0.164	0.126	0.099

location, woman 2 is the least absorbent. She has the lowest weight, height and body index mass.

FUTURE RESEARCH DIRECTIONS

The main contribution of this chapter has been provided the SAR levels which are absorbed by the human bodies exposed to wireless signals in the 2.4 GHz frequency band. It is related directly to RSS level and the number of people next to wireless signal. Moreover, we have shown that this absorption depends on the weight, the height, and the constitution of each human body. Due to the direct relationship between the number of people and the RSS, the more people inside the WLAN environment, the more RSS is absorbed. So, in a future work we should develop an adaptable network protocol, which takes into account this feature. Results are also useful for the network designers. They may take this effect into account in order to design the WLAN appropriately. Besides, this study shows to the research community which is the specific absorption rate of WLANs

working at 2.4 GHz. So, it will also let medical researchers to study the possible implications of WLANs on the population health.

Knowing the SAR on average, we will be able to estimate the number of users just measuring the RSS. In order to carry out this experiment, we should know the RSS level in each room when they are empty (without people). Then, according to RSS decreases we will be able to predict how many people are in a room. In this future work, we should analyze if RSS has an unusual behavior when a lot of people are connected to WLAN.

Finally, with the obtained data in this chapter and more conclusions that will be extract with other own works, we will be able to analyze how affect the presence of people next to a network into access points' coverage.

CONCLUSION

In this chapter, we have monitored a real wireless local area network using a wireless network scanner in order to know which SAR is given in an indoor uncontrolled environment. The place used to take the measurements was the library of the Higher Polytechnic School of Gandia, Polytechnic University of Valencia. We chose this location because the people inside were seated and there was very few movement. Moreover, there were not people using laptops or any type of devices connected to the WLAN, so the fluctuations of the RSS was only because of the signal absorption of the people. It was the best place in order to avoid any external effect to the RSS.

In this analysis, the RSS has been measured for different number of people during 250 seconds. Then, we performed a statistical analysis with the measurements obtained. It is proved that the presence of people influence the RSS in an indoor environment when a WLAN is working.

Finally, we estimated the Specific Abortion Rate (SAR) using the measurements taken in terms of the absorbed RSS per number of people and of the absorbed RSS per kilogram.

Then we have done a similar work, but in an indoor controlled environment. We have chosen an anechoic chamber both for the absence of reflected signal and because is a fairly good faraday chamber and so we can rid of unwanted EM interferences. So the only one active WLAN has been built for us inside the chamber with a wireless router to do this study. There the absorption profile of 4 persons (two men and two women), with different body features, has been analyzed.

Results show that people's location influence very much in absorption level of the wireless signal. Besides, taking into account the field region of the electromagnetic field is fundamental to obtain coherent measurements. In the near-field region, results are more significant when people are in the radiating near-field than when people are in the reactive near-field. Besides, access points should not be in front of or behind very near of people because, in this case, people act as walls and there are more power losses. So, it is always better that among access points and devices connected to it such as laptops, phones, etc. there are not any person. Moreover, in the far-field region, depending on the distance which people are from access point, they absorb more or less signal.

It is necessary emphasizing that people in both test beds were not moving. They were seated in the first test bed in the library and the four people analyzed on the second test bed were stand up. Movement of users gives results more difficult to analyze. The most significant result from both test beds is that there s a direct relationship between the body features of people and the SAR and that people with higher weight, height and body mass index absorb more wireless signal than people with lower body characteristics.

Results in the second test bed are similar to the first one in an uncontrolled indoor, but SAR values calculated are more accurate. However, the first test bed is more realistic because in a real environment any variable cannot be controlled. Anyway, the coincidence in results from the two test beds validates the SAR estimates obtained from real indoor environments.

Also we have found that is very difficult to make real world measurements of SAR in the near-field area, so from, the communications engineer point of view, would be wise to develop devices that aren't too close to human being, to avoid any potential problem due to SAR.

Finally, medical researchers can use this work to know which level of signal is absorbed by human bodies exposed to the 2.4 Ghz radio frequency band used by WLANs. So this work can help to develop medical studies to establish safe exposition limits for this kind of networks, especially in the far-field radiating area.

REFERENCES

Bahillo, A., Prieto, J., Mazuelas, S., Lorenzo, R. M., Fernández, P., & Abril, E. J. (2010). E-field assessment errors caused by the human body on localization systems. In *Proceedings of the IEEE 71th Vehicular Technology Conference*, (pp. 1-5). Taipei, Taiwan: IEEE Press.

Balanis, C. A. (2005). *Antenna theory analysis and design*. New York, NY: John Wiley & Sons Inc.

California, EMF Program. (2001). *An evaluation of the possible risks from electric and magnetic fields (EMFs) from power lines, internal wiring, electrical occupations and appliances*. Draft 3. Oakland, CA: California Department of Health Services.

Eudon, K. K. (2008). *Video streaming over 802.11b in the presence of fading due to human traffic and Bluetooth interference*. MSc Thesis. New Brunswick, Canada: University of New Brunswick.

European Commission. (1999a). *Directive 1999/5/EC of the European parliament and of the council on radio equipment and telecommunications terminal equipment and the mutual recognition of their conformity*. Geneva, Switzerland: Official Journal of the European Communities.

European Commission. (1999b). *Council recommendation 1999/519/EC on the limitation of exposure of the general public to electromagnetic fields (0 Hz to 300 GHz)*. Geneva, Switzerland: Official Journal of the European Communities.

FCC. (1997). *Evaluating compliance with FCC-specified guidelines for human exposure to radio-frequency electromagnetic fields*. OET Bulletin 65. Washington, DC: FCC.

Frühwirth, T., Molwitz, J. R., & Brisset, P. (1996). Planning cordless business communication systems. *IEEE Expert Magazine. Special Track on Intelligent Telecommunications*, *11*(1), 50–55.

Gandhi, O. P., & Aslan, E. (1995). *Human equivalent antenna for electromagnetic fields*. US Patent no.5394164. Washington, DC: US Patent Office.

GuidelinesICNIRP (1998). Guidelines for limiting exposure to time-varying electric, magnetic, and electromagnetic fields. *Health Physics*, *74*(4), 494–522.

Hashemi, H. (1993). The indoor radio propagation channel. *Proceedings of the IEEE*, *81*(7), 943–968. doi:10.1109/5.231342

Hemming, L. H. (2002). *Electromagnetic anechoic chambers: A fundamental design and specification guide*. New York, NY: John Wiley & Sons Inc.

Heymsfield, S. B., & Wang, Z. (1996). Human body composition: Conceptual advances. In *Progress in Obesity Research* (pp. 245–257). London, UK: John Libbey & Co.

Hirata, A., Fujiwara, O., Nagaoka, T., & Watanabe, S. (2010). Estimation of whole-body average SAR in human models due to plane-wave exposure at resonance frequency. *IEEE Transactions on Electromagnetic Compatibility*, *52*(1), 41–48. doi:10.1109/TEMC.2009.2035613

IEEE. (1999). *IEEE C95.1-1991: Safety levels with respect to human exposure to radio frequency electromagnetic fields, 3 KHz to 300 GHz*. New York, NY: IEEE Press.

IEEE. (2003). *ANSI/IEEE standard 149-1965, revision of standard 149-1979 test procedures for antennas*. New York, NY: IEEE Press.

Karunarathna, M. A. A., & Dayawana, J. (2005). Human exposure to RF radiation in Sri Lanka. *Sri Lankan Journal of Physics*, *6*, 19–32.

Khalatbari, S., Sardari, D., Mirzaee, A. A., & Sadafi, H. A. (2006). Calculating SAR in two models of the human head exposed to mobile phones radiations at 900 and 1800 MHz. *PIERS Online*, *2*(1), 104–109. doi:10.2529/PIERS050905190653

Kraus, J. D., & Marhefka, R. J. (2002). *Antennas for all applications* (3rd ed.). New York, NY: McGraw-Hill.

Kühn, S., & Kuster, N. (2006). *Development of procedures for the EMF exposure evaluation of wireless devices in home and office environments supplement 1: Close-to-body and base station wireless data communication devices.* Zurich, Switzerland: The Foundation for Research on Information Technologies in Society (IT'IS).

Li, X. (2006). RSS-based location estimation with unknown pathloss model. *IEEE Transactions on Wireless Communications, 5*(12), 3626–3633. doi:10.1109/TWC.2006.256985

Lin, J. C. (2003). Biological bases of current guidelines for human exposure to radio-frequency radiation. *IEEE Antennas and Propagation Magazine, 45*(3).

Lin, J. C. (2003). Microwave cataracts and personal communication radiation. *IEEE Microwave, 4,* 26–32.

Linksys by Cisco. (2011). *Wireless-G broadband router WRT54GL.* Retrieved from http.//www.linksysbycisco.com/UK/en/products/WRT54GL.

Liu, B.-C., Lin, K.-H., & Wu, J.-C. (2006). Analysis of hyperbolic and circular positioning algorithms using stationary signal strength difference measurements in wireless communications. *IEEE Transactions on Vehicular Technology, 55*(2), 499–509. doi:10.1109/TVT.2005.863405

Mazuelas, S., Bahillo, A., Lorenzo, R., Fernandez, P., Lago, F., & Garcia, E. (2009). Robust indoor positioning provided by real-time RSSI values in unmodified WLAN networks. *IEEE Journal of Selected Topics in Signal Processing, 3*(5), 821–831. doi:10.1109/JSTSP.2009.2029191

MD National Council on Radiation Protection and Measurements. (1986). *Biological effects and exposure criteria for radio frequency electromagnetic fields. Report 86.* Washington, DC: MD National Council on Radiation Protection and Measurements.

Merckel, C. (1972). Microwave and man - The direct and indirect hazards, and the precautions. *California Medicine, 117*(1), 20–24.

National Radiological Protection Board. (1993). Board statement on restrictions on human exposure to static and time-varying electromagnetic fields. *Documents of the PRPB, 4*(5).

Nokia. (2011). *SAR information.* Retrieved from http://sar.nokia.com/sar/index.jsp.

Ono, N., Hayashi, Y., Kisuki, A., & Ikeda, Y. (1996). *Anechoic chamber and wave absorber patent.* US Patent no.5.510.792. Washington, DC: US Patent Office.

Parazzini, M., Sibella, F., Paglialonga, A., & Ravazzani, P. (2010). Assessment of the exposure to WLAN frequencies of a head model with a cochlear implant. *Bioelectromagnetics, 31*(7), 546–555. doi:10.1002/bem.20601

Qi, Y. (2003). *Wireless geolocation in a non-line-of-sight environment.* Ph.D. Dissertation. Princeton, NJ: Princeton University.

Samsung. (2011). *SAR information.* Retrieved from http://www.samsung.com/uk/support/sar/sarMain.do?prd_mdl_name=SCH-I510.

Taflove, A. (1998). *Advances in computational electromagnetics: The finite difference time domain method.* London, UK: Artech House.

Tattersall, J. E. H., Scott, I. R., Wood, S. J., Nettell, J. J., Bevir, M. K., & Wang, Z. (2001). Effects of low intensity radiofrequency electromagnetic fields on electrical activity in rat hippocampal slices. *Brain Research, 904*(1), 43–53. doi:10.1016/S0006-8993(01)02434-9

Thom, H. (1996). *Introduction to shortwave and microwave therapy.* Springfield, IL: Charles C. Thomas.

Tinniswood, A. D., & Gandhi, O. P. (1998). Computations of SAR distributions for two anatomically based models of the human head using CAD files of commercial telephones and the parallelized FDTD code. *IEEE Transactions on Antennas and Propagation, 46,* 829–833. doi:10.1109/8.686769

Valenzuela, R. A. (1993). A ray tracing approach to predicting indoor wireless transmission. In *Proceedings of the IEEE Vehicular Technology Conference,* (pp. 214–218). Secaucus, NJ: IEEE Press.

Values, S. A. R. (2011). *The complete SAR list for all phones (Europe).* Retrieved from http://www.sarvalues.com/eu-complete.html.

Vistumbler. (2011). *Website.* Retrieved from http://www.vistumbler.net/.

Wang, Z. M., Pierson, R. Jr, & Heymsfield, S. B. (1992). The five-level model: A new approach to organizing body-composition research. *The American Journal of Clinical Nutrition, 56,* 19–25.

WHO. (2002). *Establishing a dialogue on risks from electromagnetic fields.* Retrieved from http://www.who.int/entity/peh-emf/publications/en/emf_final_300dpi_ALL.pdf.

KEY TERMS AND DEFINITIONS

Anechoic Chamber: It is a room designed to stop reflections of either sound or electromagnetic waves. Besides, it is insulated from exterior sources of noise. So, it is an insulated space and without reflections of infinite dimension.

Body Mass Index (BMI): It is defined as the individual's body weight divided by the square of his or her height. So, it is measured in terms of kg/m^2.

Electromagnetic Waves: They carry energy from a place to another one travelling through space. Electromagnetic radiation is classified according to the frequency of its wave. They carry information by varying a combination of the amplitude, frequency and phase of the wave within a frequency band.

RSS (Received Signal Strength): It is a measurement of the power level received from a wireless signal by an antenna.

SAR (Specific Absorption Rate): It is defined as the power absorbed by the body when it is exposed to a radio frequency (RF) electromagnetic field. It is measured as the power absorbed per mass of tissue and has units of watts per kilogram (W/kg).

WBA-SAR (Whole Body Averaged SAR): It is defined as the SAR measured over the whole body on averaged. It has units of watts per kilogram (W/kg).

Wireless Network Scanner: It is a software program used as instrument to scan networks. It is based on finding wireless access points and on extracting several parameters of the scanned networks such as speak signal, MAC address, status, type of authentication, etc.

WLAN (Wireless Local Area Network): It is a type of computer network that connects computers and devices without cables. It uses some wireless distribution method as spread-spectrum or OFDM radio. Besides, it usually provides a connection through an access point to the wider internet. It is deployed in a limited geographical area.

Chapter 5
Overview of Biomedical Engineering

Ahmad Taher Azar
Modern Science and Arts University (MSA), Egypt

ABSTRACT

Biomedical Engineering is a branch that unites engineering methods with biological and medical sciences in order to enhance the quality of our lives. It focuses on understanding intricate systems of living organisms, and on technology development, algorithms, methods, and advanced medical knowledge, while enhancing the conveyance and success of clinical medicine. With engineering principles, biomedical engineering improves the procedures and devices to overcome health care and medical problems by combining both biology and medicine with engineering principals. In the field of Biomedical Engineering, engineers usually need to have background knowledge from such different fields of engineering as electronics, mechanical, and chemical engineering. Specialties in this field like bioinstrumentation, biomechanics, biomaterials, medical imagining, clinical engineering, bioinformatics, telemedicine and rehabilitation engineering, which will be introduced in this chapter together with an overview of the field of biomedical engineering.

INTRODUCTION

The Whitaker Foundation (2011) defines Biomedical Engineering as:

"Biomedical engineering is a discipline that advances knowledge in engineering, biology, and

medicine, and improves human health through cross disciplinary activities that integrate the engineering sciences with the biomedical sciences and clinical practice. It includes: 1) the acquisition of new knowledge and understanding of living systems through the innovative and substantive application of experimental and analytical techniques based on the engineering sciences; 2) the development of new devices, algorithms,

DOI: 10.4018/978-1-4666-0888-7.ch005

processes, and systems that advance biology and medicine and improve medical practice and health care delivery."

The Biomedical Engineering Society (1996) states the following definitions for biomedical engineering as part of their career-guidance document:

"A Biomedical Engineer uses traditional engineering expertise to analyze and solve problems in biology and medicine, providing an overall enhancement of health care. Students choose the biomedical engineering field to be of service to people, to partake of the excitement of working with living systems, and to apply advanced technology to the complex problems of medical care. The biomedical engineer works with other health care professionals including physicians, nurses, therapists, and technicians. Biomedical engineers may be called upon in a wide range of capacities: to design instruments, devices, and software, to bring together knowledge from many technical sources to develop new procedures, or to conduct research needed to solve clinical problems."

Biomedical engineers working within a hospital or clinic are more properly called clinical engineers, but this theoretical distinction is not always observed in practice, and many professionals working within hospitals today continue to be called biomedical engineers. Biomedical Engineers must have excellent analytical skills, as well as problem-detection and problem-solving skills. They should work well independently, but also be able to work well a member of a team. Having good written and verbal communication skills is also becoming more important, and Biomedical Engineers should also plan to constantly update their training and knowledge by reading current literature and attending conferences and seminars on their specialist subjects (http://www.guidetocareereducation.com/careers/biomedical engineering). For Biomedical Researchers, the focus is often on adding to the store of knowledge of their specialist subject, rather than on creating new products and items. The knowledge they discover can be used in the development of biomedical products, or in other areas of medicine, for example to improve treatment methods and speed up patient recovery. Creativity is an important attribute for Biomedical Researchers. For them, the focus of their work is on new ways of understanding the human body and the types of engineering and mechanical devices that can improve medical equipment and patient treatments. In addition, they should have good problem-solving and analytical skills, as well as good written and verbal communication skills.

HISTORY OF BIOMEDICAL ENGINEERING

The history of biomedical engineering involves a sequential and iterative process of discovery and invention: new tools for studying the human body leading to a deeper understanding of body function leading to the invention of improved tools for repair and study of the human body, and so forth (Saltzman, 2009). Table 1 summarizes some major milestones in the Biomedical Engineering Field.

Biomedical Engineering originated during World War II. In 1947, after World War II, administrative committees were established by the Institute for Radio Engineers and the American Institute for Electrical Engineers (forerunner of the Institute of Electrical and Electronics Engineers IEEE]) to study biological and medical areas related to engineering (Garfield, 1987). In 1948, the first conference of engineering in medicine and biology was established in the United States, under the sponsoring of the Institute of Radio Engineers, the American Institute for Electrical Engineering, and the Instrument Society of America (Requena-Carrion & Leder, 2009).

Since the formation of Institute of Electrical and Electronics Engineers (IEEE) in 1963, the

Table 1. Major milestones in biomedical engineering

1895	Conrad Roentgen (German) discovered the X-Ray using gas discharge tubes.
1896	Henry Becquerel (French) discovered X-rays were emitted from uranium ore. Two of his students, Pierre and Marie Curie, traced the radiation to the element radium.
1901	Roentgen received the Nobel Prize for discovery of X-rays.
1903	William Eindhoven discovered the electrocardiogram (ECG).
1927	Drinker respirator
1929	Hans Berger discovers the Electroencephalogram (EEG).
1930's	X-rays were being used to visualize most organ systems using radio-opaque materials, refrigeration, permitted blood banks.
Mid 1930's-early 1940's	Antibiotics, sulphanilamide, and penicillin, reduced cross-infection in hospitals.
1940's	Cardiac catheterization.
1950's	electron microscope.
1950's-1960	Nuclear medicine.
1953	Cardiopulmonary bypass (heart-lung machine).
1970's	CT, MRI imaging systems.
1975	Whitaker Foundation was established.
1980's	Gamma Camera, Positron Emission Tomography (PET) and SPECT.
1997	First Indigenous Endo vascular Coronary Stent (Kalam-Raju Stent) was developed by Care Foundation.

first issue of *IEEE Transactions on Biomedical Engineering* was published by IEEE Engineering in Medicine and Biology Society (EMBS). In 1968, the Biomedical Engineering Society was formed to give "equal status to representatives of both biomedical and engineering interests and promote the increase of biomedical engineering knowledge and its utilization (Schwan, 1984; Garfield, 1987). In 1972, the Biomedical Engineering Society started publishing the Annals of Biomedical Engineering. Today there are additional societies such as the Association for the Advancement of Medical Instrumentation (AAMI), American Institute for Medical and Biological Engineering (AIMBE), the International Federation for Medical and Biological Engineering, International Society of Biomechanics (ISB), the Society for Biomaterials, the Bioelectromagnetics Society and the National Institute of Biomedical Imaging and Bioengineering (Hendee, et al., 2002). The definition and the main objectives of these socities are included in the Appendix A.

In 1975, The Whitaker Foundation was established. The foundation has primarily supported interdisciplinary medical research and education, with the principal focus being on biomedical engineering. The foundation has become the nation's largest private benefactor of biomedical engineering (http://www.whitaker.org/). The Foundation also supported the enhancement or establishment of educational programs in biomedical engineering, especially encouraging the formation of departments (Katona, 2006). In the same year, a special issue of IEEE Transactions on Biomedical Engineering was published including general topics related to the foundation of the biomedical engineering (Harmon, 1975; Jacobs, 1975; Weed, 1975); biomedical engineering and health care (Brown, 1975; Mylrea & Siverston, 1975); biomedical engineering educational (Johns, 1975; Schwartz & Long, 1975; Moritz & Huntsman, 1975; Cox, et al., 1975; Peura, et al., 1975; Detwiler, et al., 1975; Torzyn, et al., 1975) and the development of the biomedical industry (Kahn, 1975).

A history of the development of the academic field was written by Peter Katona, president of the Whitaker Foundation (Katona, 2002). According to Katona, the first formal academic programs were established at The Johns Hopkins University, the University of Pennsylvania, the University of Rochester, and Drexel University in the 1950s when they received training grants for biomedical engineering from the National Institutes of Health (NIH). At Johns Hopkins this action ultimately led in 1970 to the establishment of the Biomedical Engineering (BME) Department in the School of Medicine (Massey & Johns, 1981). In the Arab world, BME started as a conjunction between medicine, engineering, and basic sciences. The first BME undergraduate programme was founded at Cairo University in 1976 (http://www.eng.cu.edu.eg/dept/en/sbe/index.htm). The programme integrated knowledge from two pre-existing programmes of Biomechanics and Bio-electronics into a stand-alone BME Department under the umbrella of the Faculty of Engineering.

In 1980, the undergraduate BME program was established in the Whiting School of Engineering, thus drawing on the strengths of both schools. It is now the largest undergraduate program in the Whiting School. Approximately more than 170 graduate programs in bioengineering, biomedical engineering, biological engineering, and biotechnology are listed in Peterson's guide (Peterson's, 2011; Harris, et al., 2002). The numbers of students enrolled in biomedical engineering degree programs are shown in Figure 1 as reported in Saltzman (2009).

MAIN DUTIES OF BIOMEDICAL ENGINEER AND CLINICAL ENGINEER

Main Duties of Biomedical Engineer

Graduates of biomedical engineering can be employed in a range of sectors, whether educational, industrial, or hospitals. Job opportunities in the field are as follows:

- Participate in the design of research and diagnostic instruments, medical equipment's manufacturing, facility's construction, diagnostic standards development or implementation and testing of new devices.
- Work as special products consultants for hospitals, informatics and diagnostic protocols development and designing, cooperate with hospitals and other related sectors.
- Biochemical process evaluation and design for doing medical compounds or components
- Teaching and researching in the field, because biomedical engineering combines different engineering areas, researches are usually performed by engineering together with researchers from different area like dentistry, nursing, pharmaceutical sciences, etc.
- Development of inspection protocols, codes and safety standards, they can review and evaluate new products, take place in academic activates and participating with public regarding this matter.
- Resolve situations with medical equipment when clinical staff find difficulties in the use of the medical devices, acquiring alternate equipment or solutions and contacting the dealers for term or loan negotiation.
- Guarantee solutions to any medical problem that may occur, by analyzing procedures and policies, identifying set ups or the part key pattern that would cause such a problem and affect the performance, stating the changes to staff, applying these procedure revision and following up in case the same problem occur again.
- Manage, lead, and improve significant projects that are meant to develop existing care delivery system like the ICU charting device and the laser devices.

Figure 1. The numbers of students enrolled in biomedical engineering degree program (adapted from Saltzman, 2009) (reprinted with the permission of Cambridge University Press)

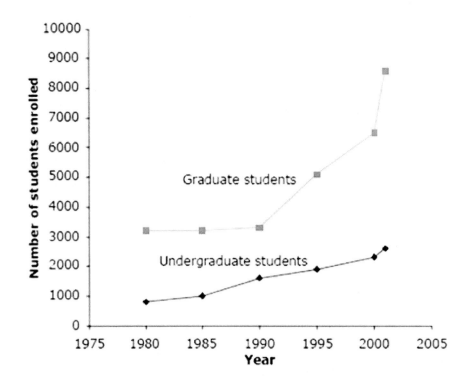

- Perform investigations in cases of a patient injury or service distortion that may affect patient's care by securing all proofs, conducting an interview with everyone involved in the incident and preparing summary of the incident and advices for any change, in case of device failure, engineers work with manufacturers to decide the right action to be taken and follow up with both user and manufacturer to make sure the changes are applied correctly.
- Engineers can also assist users with capital equipment planning, this can be done by providing equipment information about their conditions and serviceability, translate their needs into technical statement in order to analyze how the new purchase will affect the operating cost.
- Reviewing trade articles for medical equipment and surveying its market, re-

tain continuous awareness of health care technology trends and development, surfing the web and remain in a contact with dealers.
- Assessment arrangement of contract plan to make sure of the chosen selection. Being in contact with users and dealers for services discussions as contract options, equipment trainings, spare parts availabilities, and the time for response. Controlling teams to make sure that all devices and equipment meet their needs, recommend purchases for users and having the responsibility to install and integrate the new technologies.
- Provide training, consultancy, and advice to users, the operation manual and their safety and effectiveness for preserving the organisation's funding.
- Developing regulations for the department and its operating procedure in order

to enhance the operation efficiency in the department.

- Reduce medical risks by keeping the system to observe device's notices and provide certain recommendations.
- Observe spending and report for budget, whether contract or supply budget for the responsible area.

Main Duties of Clinical Engineer

Clinical Engineering is a new field that rapidly expanding which is developed as a result of the changing needs of the health-care career (Oakes, 1975). It has an active nature, which attracts the ones who enjoy new challenges of a developing field. Clinical Engineering plays an important role in development and propositions of amenities, technology and its methods as they are connected to health care delivery. It goes back to late 1960s when engineers were persuaded to enter this field in response to the electrical safety of patients in hospitals and clinics.

The term "Clinical Engineering" was first published in 1969 in a paper by Landoll and Caceres (1969), and from here a new engineering field was born and hospitals started establishing a centralized departments for clinical engineering but soon it soon it became clear that electrical safety failure constituted small part of the whole problem reported by the medical devices in hospitals or clinics. During that time, these devices were not completely understood nor maintained properly. Visual inspections often showed frayed wires, broken knobs, or liquid spills. Some equipment was not serviced according to the recommendations of the manufacturer and did not perform according to their specifications. Complete inspection for the performance was carried by the mid 1970s before and after using, which then became usual and logical procedures were developed (Newhouse, et al., 1989). Departments of clinical engineering became then the logical support core of all medical technologies and having the

responsibility for all systems that are being used in any clinical environment as well as the training centre for equipment users for the use and safety (Bronzino, 2000).

Inside the clinical engineering program form, there are three divisions (Webster & Cook, 1979). The first is the service and maintenance division that is responsible for all duties related to medical equipment as soon as it is in the clinic or hospital. This include also the safety and performance incoming inspection, training, preventive maintenance, implementation and repair. Director of service and maintenance is usually a clinical engineer substantial organizational skill. Repair duties are separated from preventive maintenance duties within this division. Biomedical equipment technicians with significant managerial experience normally lead these duties. So that there are independent crosschecks on the quality of preventive maintenance functions and repair, it is important that they are separated from each other. This will guarantee that the preventive maintenance unit is not disturbed to carry out repairs that have propensity to super code the preventive maintenance duties. Avoiding this will promote preventive maintenance to an initial department function— preventing the medical equipment from failing.

Engineering is the second main sector with the responsibility for problem solving; the engineering sector is responsible for service planning, renovations, purchasing of medical equipment, training programs, assistance in initiating policies for clinical environments (ex. Purchase protocols), custom equipment development, computer applications, service review and support for maintenance sector, and generally to solve real life problems. In order to create an interdisciplinary support group in this sector, speciality support need to be acquired as needed covering fundamental engineering and science fields, including experts in mechanical, electronics, and chemical Engineering, physics, computer science, physiology, biochemistry, and medicine for identifying the main field. The number of experts to achieve this function changes the management system and not the whole basic structure. Specialist engineers and scientists are chosen based on their forte skills in their field, so not all of the scientists and engineers can presume administrative duties, they are encouraged to expand their skills for medical environment applications.

The third sector in the clinical engineering department is the administrative and clerical staff (Webster & Cook, 1979). Only one sector is used for all administrative and clerical support to reduce the prospective of identical files and records. Within a computer database, there should be one of each: equipment control file system, computer system with common database, technical manual library, and one filling system. Engineers and technicians can be assigned the clerical help. Training of the clerical team is as essential as it is for engineers and technicians, with regard to the diverse tasks within the department. One missing clerical member can disable the department, because this one may be the only one who is familiar with the filing system. This management method is the best way, although it is hard to implement the right away, but in the long run it is considered the best. It is essential that tasks and duties are general for biomedical engineering job description development and the same for that of the clinical engineering, so that the director of the program can use trained employees in various tasks.

In the 21st century, the focus of Clinical Engineering is shifting towards clinical systems integration, with a concentration in patient safety (Zambuto, 2004). Clinical Engineering brings biomedical engineering to the clinical setting and can be an alternative career for biomedical engineers (Flexman, 2007). Clinical Engineer in most medical environments monitors one or more biomedical technicians for equipment repairing and providing maintenance. Clinical Engineers started to have considerable tasks within hospitals and clinics. Those tasks of clinical engineers may include the following:

- Technical support provision for equipment through systems of healthcare, providing maintenance, preserving parts record, carrying out customer area rounds, and taking part in one-call rotation.
- Recording test results and actions using software applications.
- Participate in project petitions as the purchase of a new product, bid specifications development, vendor proposals analysis, plan for installations, testing acceptance and renovations, upgrading, or disposing medical equipment.
- Pre-emptive maintenance schedule development; providing training for the technical team on procedures to be followed for scheduled maintenance on equipment within the department.
- Department development participation and continuous quality enhancement to the use of patient care related devices.
- Assist with evaluation of the outcome of the department against quality standards and generate reports based on that; this includes complete quality verifications.
- Analysis of equipment performance and incident investigation.
- Developing built in equipment services for patient care and device safety to present them to the clinical team and provide training for patient care equipment users.
- Review safety and emergency procedures and how to use patient care equipment.
- Review safety alerts for patient equipment and consider notices and take necessary steps to make sure that the defected equipment is tested or not anymore in service.
- Comparing patient care equipment and under consideration devices for purchase to develop an assessment criteria.
- Provide assistance for the head of the department and the engineering management team in the assessment and administration of technical matters as they do their tasks

Figure 2. Sub-disciplines of biomedical engineering

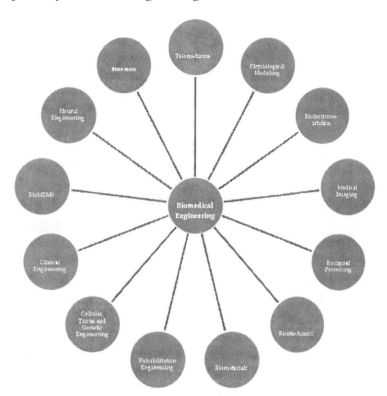

and duties as long as it is related to maintenance, reparation of patient care devices, and technical support in general.

In case of a break down in the clinical engineering program, which is the most distinct area that is backed up by the biomedical technicians. Compared to biomedical or clinical engineers, technicians work under a more instant stress. Emergency and stressful situation are more likely to happen in service and maintenance. Choosing biomedical technicians is very critical because they are often encountered with on the floor situations like medical devices failure. Hence, they should be chosen for professional qualities as biomedical and clinical engineers. Considering the difference between biomedical equipment technician and clinical or biomedical engineer is crucial as a career selection. There should be substantial assessment used with respect to experience and educational background compared to professionalism and quality in selecting biomedical or clinical engineer and biomedical equipment technicians.

BIOMEDICAL ENGINEERING SPECIALIZATIONS

Engineers of Biomedicine study a range of human health related problems (see Figure 2). Concepts like quantitative human physiology and mathematical analysis are important to all biomedical engineers. However, some of them study systems related to the understanding of circuits and electrical signals, mechanics or chemistry, and that is why biomedical engineering is appropriately split into sub categories, these subcategories shows kind of tools that are to be used to solve the problem. Another way of seeing what biomedical engineering is about is understanding the differences and similarities between those subcategories.

Biomedical/Physiological Modelling

Biomedical engineers have pioneered development of physiological models, as they are specialists in physiology and mathematics. To help them understand and anticipate behaviour of a system, they make mathematical models of their systems. In order to describe the engineering plan, methods and tools that are used to acquire an inclusive understanding of the functions of living organisms, the term Physiological modelling is used. To resemble dynamic biomedical systems, physiological modelling involves using computer simulations, discrete mathematics, and numerical methods (Marmarelis, 2004). Not only this but also to support and fortify experimental conclusions and to provide more precise models of behaviour to image systems. One of the most important results of biomedical engineering are the mathematical models of blood flow in small vessels, these models still direct the evolution of tissue-engineered blood vessels and cardiovascular biomaterials.

The growth of physiological modelling and simulation gets more important to biomedical engineering because of their numerous uses (Johnson, 2000). First, mathematical modelling is considered to be an important implement for complex biophysical systems investigation. Second, computer architecture advancement made the level of complexity model practical to apply the computational paradigm to complex biophysical systems. Third, possible operating scenarios can be examined by the doctors before they enter the operation room, and clarify solutions to challenges during the operation time and reduce time spend in the operation room, hence, reducing patient's stress and costs. Fourth, that it allows investigating suspicious scenarios by creating this physical model for subject experiments under study, which let researchers to oversee anatomies and pathologies instead of a general model. Depending on the application requirements, models can be mirror-imaged, scaled, or manipulated.

Bioinstrumentation

Bioinstrumentations involves biological variable measurements, this assists the physicians in treatment and diagnosis of their patients (Khandpur, 2004). In order to operate the equipment, electronics and measurement techniques are necessary. Computers are necessary also for handling the data; a computer can process a large quantity of information in medical imagining system. Electronic instruments are essential to hospitals, as blood pressure monitors, in order to provide continuous and valid feedback on ill patient's health status. Over the past 20 years, biomedical instruments have become more multifaceted as microelectronics has evolved more complicated techniques and materials. Functions that used to be performed on supercomputers can now be done on microchips that are tiny enough to be embedded. Some instruments such as cardiac pacemakers have been implanted for a long time but now they are multifunctional, which has given a great assist in human health care. Delivering electrical simulation is used to treat other diseases like Parkinson's and other neurological disorders by other similar instruments. New things will be done in the future by instrument implementation such as delivering drugs and monitoring local tissue states, sending detailed information on internet function outside the body (Saltzman, 2009).

In order to study signals, most bioinstrumentation systems are made of components that sense those signals, amplify and record them in a noticeable form like current, force, and pressure (see Figure 3).

A device must electrically stimulate tissues in order to obtain a biological event for recording. Stimulators excite the tissues and allow the operator to control the stimulus frequency, amplitude, and duration. Electrodes and input transducers are the two types of input devices; they notice certain changes and transmit electrical signals along a wire to the amplifier. Input device is a simple electrode because the signal that is being

Figure 3. The basic elements of a biological recording system

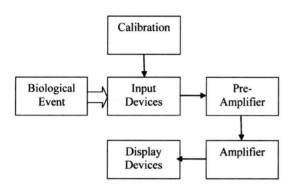

recorded is an electrical signal. First, this signal is detected by the electrode, sent to the amplifier to strengthen it, and then it can be shown on the monitor.

The term Electrode refers to the part that is in contact with cells or tissues that is responsible for detection and stimulation, while the term Lead refers to the wire between the electrode and amplifier and computer (bioinstrumentation), in which both of them are used to conduct electrical current to and from the body cells and tissues. Depending on the current, magnitude and location on cells or tissues, electrodes may take different shapes. They also should be good electrical conductors and nontoxic to body tissues. Electrodes are usually made of inert metals that good electrical conductors like gold, nickel silver alloy, palladium, or platinum. Because not all signals can be electrical, others can be mechanical (ex. muscle movement), they first should be converted to electrical signals and then be sent to the amplifier. This happens by devices that convert one form of energy to another, in our case a mechanical signal to an electrical signal; these devices are called transducers.

System's components must be adjusted so that a measured input output relationship is known, this process is called Calibration. It is not possible to change system's output into a relevant representation without this information. Elec-

trical signals generated by input transducers or detected by the electrodes are strengthened by the amplifiers, which is very important step because biological signals are usually very small and can't be measured without amplification. This output signal is amplified until it is measurable. Users can usually regulate the signal amplification same as regulating the volume of a radio.

Signals must be shown in a way to be examined after they are being amplified. Signals can be displayed on display devices in a variety of forms like dials, digital meters, light panels, or loudspeakers. Displaying electrical signals graphically as deflections of a line moving on a computer monitor is the most complicated yet most frequently used display device in the physiology labs. Hence, it is essential to extend the visual application from recorded data to the maximum amount of information within the data.

Biosensors

Sensors, a device that detects, measure and change one type of signal to another. Biosensors are but for the analysis of biomaterial samples, Biosensors are used in order to understand their bio composition, function, and structure, biosensors as any sensor, convert a biological response into an electrical signal. Biosensors are made of a biological recognition component connected directly to a signal transducer as shown in Figure 4. They are usually used for biological research and clinical medicine for measuring physiological variables and take a part in diagnostic medical applications. The milestones of biosensors are summarized in Table 2. Strict requirements must be taken into considerations on the design and use of biomedical sensors for accurate medical diagnostic procedures.

In biomedical applications, different kinds of sensors can be used (Neuman, 2000). The first time is the physical sensor, which is a device that gives data about a physical property within a system, such as mechanical, thermal, hydraulic,

Figure 4. The biosensor

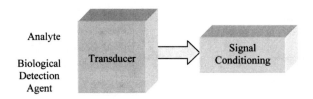

or geometric factors. Second is the chemical sensor, which converts the chemical information whether a sample's concentration or a total composition analysis into an analytical signal that can be used and processed by the computer. A chemical sensor is an essential component of an analyzer that performs various functions like signal processing, data processing, sampling, or sample transport. It works according to a plan as a function of time and it can be an important part of an automated system.

For chemical sensors, two main functional units are contained within, receptor and transducer. Others can include a separator. Chemical data are received to the receptor part and converted to a form of energy that could be measured by the transducer, and then the transducer transforms the energy carrying the data into classifieds, a

Table 2. Major milestones of biosensors (Joshi, 2006)

1916	First report on the immobilisation of proteins
1922	First glass pH electrode
1956	Prof. Clark, Father of biosensor concept, Invention of the oxygen electrode
1962	First description of a biosensor: an amperometric enzyme electrode for glucose.
1969	First potentiometer biosensor: urease immobilised on an ammonia electrode to detect urea.
1970	Invention of the Ion-selective Field Effect Transistor (ISFET)
1972/5	First commercial biosensor: Yellow Springs Instruments glucose biosensor
1975	First immunosensor
1976	First bedside artificial pancreas
1980	First fibre optic pH sensor for in vivo blood gases
1982	First Fibre Optic pH sensor for glucose
1983	First Surface Plasmon Resonance (SPR) immunosensor
1984	First mediated amperometric biosensor: ferrocene used with glucose oxidase for the detection of glucose
1987	Launch of the MediSense ExacTech™blood glucose biosensor
1990	Launch of the Pharmacia BIACore SPR-based biosensor system
1992	i-STAT launches hand-held blood analyser
1996	Glucocard launced
1996	Abbott acquires MediSense for $867 million
1998	Launch of LifeScan FastTake blood glucose biosensor
1998	Merger of Roche and Boehringer Mannheim to form Roche Diagnostics
2001	LifeScan purchases Inverness Medical's glucose testing business for $1.3billion

separate major sensor category. The chemical sensors include biological recognition reactions as enzyme-substrate, antigen-antibody, or ligand-receptor in order to recognize complicated biochemical molecules. Bio-analytic sensors are given high sensitivity and specificity in biochemical substance recognition and identification.

Medical Imaging

Medicine has been revolutionized by Biomedical imagining technology. Technologies as conventional radiographic imaging, CT, MRI, and ultrasonic imaging give access to physicians to reliable and safe ways for collecting medical images, providing a non-invasive method to picture the body from the inside (Semmlow, 2004; Bankman, 2000). These imaging devices can be used to recognize uncommon things inside the human body like tumours, broken bones or a leaking blood vessel.

X-ray is one of the most common types of imagining, in which radiations are used to take a static image of a certain area of the body. Although x radiations are considered to be dangerous and it's a risk being exposed to it, the risk is considered to be stochastic depending on its use, but it's probable to cause a death of individuals exposing to it. Hence, the patient's benefits should be greater than risk of the exposing damage (Nokes, et al., 1995).

Biomedical engineers have been pioneers in the construction and design of new imagining machines, the creation of medical imaging approaches using these machines and the analysis of imaging data.

Imaging quality improves each year, which means a more precise disease diagnosing and a better health care. Currently, imaging techniques provide data on tissue anatomy, but in the future it will provide information about the function of tissues as well, which will result in studying the progress of a disease and helping in new treatments development. In the nest subsections, short description of CT scan and MRI will be discussed.

Computed Tomography (CT)

The CT scanner is revolutionary in that it does not record an image in the conventional way. There is no image receptor, such as film, or image intensifier tube. In a CT scanner, a collimated X-ray beam is directed on the patient, and the attenuated remnant radiation is measured by a detector whose response is transmitted to a computer. The computer consider the location of the patient and the spatial relationship of the X-ray beam to the region of interest. It analyzes the signal from the detector so that a visual image can be reconstructed and displayed on a television monitor. The image can then be photographed for later evaluation and file. The computer reconstruction of the cross-sectional anatomy is accomplished with mathematical equations adapted for computer processing called algorithm. The difference in operating characteristics and image quality is far greater over the range of CT scanners than for a comparable top-to-bottom range of conventional radiographic equipment. It is particularly important to perform a careful evaluation before purchasing a CT unit and to maintain the system continuously during use. Improper CT monitoring and maintenance produce poor images that may result missed diagnosis.

Magnetic Resonance Imaging (MRI)

Hornak (2011) defines MRI as:

"Magnetic Resonance Imaging (MRI) is an imaging technique used primarily in medical settings to produce high quality images of the inside of the human body. MRI is based on the principles of Nuclear Magnetic Resonance (NMR), a spectroscopic technique used by scientists to obtain microscopic chemical and physical information about molecules. The technique was called magnetic resonance imaging rather than Nuclear Magnetic Resonance Imaging (NMRI) because of the negative connotations associated with the

word nuclear in the late 1970's. MRI started out as a tomographic imaging technique, that is it produced an image of the NMR signal in a thin slice through the human body. MRI has advanced beyond a tomographic imaging technique to a volume imaging technique."

Brief history of MRI is also defined by Hornak (2011) as:

"Felix Bloch and Edward Purcell, both of whom were awarded the Nobel Prize in 1952, discovered the magnetic resonance phenomenon independently in 1946. In the period between 1950 and 1970, NMR was developed and used for chemical and physical molecular analysis. In 1971 Raymond Damadian showed that the nuclear magnetic relaxation times of tissues and tumors differed, thus motivating scientists to consider magnetic resonance for the detection of disease (Damadian, 1971). In 1973 the x-ray-based Computerized Tomography (CT) was introduced by Hounsfield (1973). This date is important to the MRI timeline because it showed hospitals were willing to spend large amounts of money for medical imaging hardware. Magnetic resonance imaging was first demonstrated on small test tube samples that same year by Paul Lauterbur (1973). He used a back projection technique similar to that used in CT. In 1975, Richard Ernst proposed magnetic resonance imaging using phase and frequency encoding, and the Fourier Transform (Kumar, et al., 1975). This technique is the basis of current MRI techniques. A few years later, in 1977, Raymond Damadian demonstrated MRI called field-focusing nuclear magnetic resonance. In this same year, Peter Mansfield developed the Echo-Planar Imaging (EPI) technique (Mansfield, 1977). This technique will be developed in later years to produce images at video rates (30 ms / image). Edelstein and co-workers demonstrated imaging of the body using Ernst's technique in 1980. A single image could be acquired in approximately five minutes

by this technique. By 1986, the imaging time was reduced to about five seconds, without sacrificing too much image quality. The same year people were developing the NMR microscope, which allowed approximately 10 μm resolution on approximately one cm samples. In 1987 echo-planar imaging was used to perform real-time movie imaging of a single cardiac cycle (Chapman, et al., 1987). In this same year Charles Dumoulin was perfecting Magnetic Resonance Angiography (MRA), which allowed imaging of flowing blood without the use of contrast agents (Dumoulin, Souza, Hart, 1987). In 1991, Richard Ernst was rewarded for his achievements in pulsed Fourier Transform NMR and MRI with the Nobel Prize in Chemistry. In 1992, functional MRI (fMRI) was developed (Bandettini, et al., 1992). This technique allows the mapping of the function of the various regions of the human brain. Five years earlier, many clinicians thought echo-planar imaging's primary applications was to be in real-time cardiac imaging. The development of fMRI opened up a new application for EPI in mapping the regions of the brain responsible for thought and motor control. In 1994, researchers at the State University of New York at Stony Brook and Princeton University demonstrated the imaging of hyperpolarized ^{129}Xe gas for respiration studies (Albert, et al., 1994). In 2003, Paul C. Lauterbur of the University of Illinois and Sir Peter Mansfield of the University of Nottingham were awarded the Nobel Prize in Medicine for their discoveries concerning magnetic resonance imaging. MRI is clearly a young, but growing science."

According to Hornak (2011):

"Magnetic resonance imaging is based on the absorption and emission of energy in the radio frequency range of the electromagnetic spectrum. It is clear from the attenuation spectrum of the human body why x-rays are used, but why did it take so long to develop imaging with radio waves, especially with health concerns associated with *ionizing radiation such as x-rays? Many scientists were taught that you cannot image objects smaller than the wavelength of the energy being used to image. MRI gets around this limitation by producing images based on spatial variations in the phase and frequency of the radio frequency energy being absorbed and emitted by the imaged object. Currently, there are approximately six major clinical MRI Original Equipment Manufacturers (OEMs). In addition to these clinical OEMs, there are two major experimental MRI OEMs. Other MRI related subsystem manufacturers include RF coil, contrast agents, compatible devices, RF amps, and magnets."*

Appendix B contains tables of some of the major manufacturers of MRI devices.

Biosignal Processing

According to Northrop, Biosignals are biological signals are biological signals space-time records of a biological event as heartbeats or a contracting muscle (Northrop, 2003). Biosignals contain useful data that describe the physiological mechanism of a system or a certain biological event, because signals produced during these biological events can be measured and analysed, whether they are electrical, chemical or mechanical, which helps in medical diagnosis (Cerutti, et al., 2011).

Biological signals can be obtained by different methods. In order to retrieve useful data, biosignals are analysed following data acquisition. Amplification, filtering, digitization, processing, and storage, all of which are considered the basic methods of signal analysis, can be applied to various biosignals. Simple electronic circuits or digital computers can accomplish such techniques. Also sophisticated digital processing methods are common and can enhance the quality of data obtained remarkably such as signal averaging, wavelet analysis, and artificial intelligence techniques (Thompkins, 1993).

Biomechanics

Biomechanics exerts basic statics, dynamics, fluids, solids, thermodynamics, and continuum mechanics to biological or medical problems (Fung, 1996; Schneck & Bronzino, 2002). It also includes motion study, material deformation, flow within the body, and transport of chemical constituents across biological and synthetic media and membranes. Artificial hearts and heart valves, artificial joints replacements and the understanding of the functions of different body organs were developed by the progress of biomechanics. Complexity of biological organisms and systems helped widen the field of biomechanics.

Biomaterials

At the end of 1800s, the use of biomaterials rapidly increased, especially after the appearance of aseptic surgical technique by Dr. Joseph Lister in the 1860s. As late as eighteenth century, the first metal device to fix bone fracture was used, then in 1938, the first total hip replacement prosthesis was implanted, and in 1950s and 1960s, polymers were proposed for blood vessels and cornea replacements. At the time being, biomaterials are used throughout the human body, which consists of living tissue and artificial materials used for implementation (Ratner, et al., 2004). For the implant material design, understanding the behaviour and properties of living material is essential.

Appropriate material selection to be placed in the human body can be one of the hardest duties for biomedical engineers. Specific metal alloys, ceramics, polymers, and composites have been utilized as implantable materials. They must be nontoxic, non-carcinogenic, chemically inert, stable and mechanically strong enough to withstand the repeated forces of a lifetime, and in order to provide a true biological and mechanical match for the living tissues, new biomaterials contain living cells.

Rehabilitation Engineering

Since the late 1970s, there has been a great growth in technology application to improve problems encountered by disable people. Different terms have been used to describe this activity, this include prosthetics/orthotics, rehabilitation engineering, assistive technology, assistive device design, rehabilitation technology, and biomedical engineering. As this field was growing more, various terms were more commonly used, strengthened by their use in federal legislations, but the most common terms used now are assistive technology and rehabilitation engineering (Cook & Hussey, 2002). The two terms are not even though they are indistinguishably. According to James Reswick (1982), a pioneer in Rehabilitation Engineering, "Rehabilitation Engineering is the application of science and technology to enhance the handicaps of individuals with disabilities." On the other hand, assistive technology is considered as a rehabilitation engineering activity product. This relation is similar to health care as a practice of medicine product. In order to assist people with perceptive difficulties, rehabilitation engineers are developing hardware and software computer adaptation.

Cellular Tissue and Genetic Engineering

Tissue engineering is a field of biomedical engineering combining engineering with biology in order to create tissues or cellular products outside the human body or to rectify tissues inside the human body. It is obliged to be knowledgeable of various biological fields, like cell and molecular biology, physiology and system integration, stem cell proliferation and differentiation with lineage attributes extracellular matrix chemistry and compounds, and endocrinology (Lanza, et al., 2000). Tissue Engineering also demands knowledge in different engineering disciplines like biochemical, mechanical, polymer sciences, bioreactor design and application, mass transfer analysis of gas and liquid metabolites, and biomaterials.

Clinical applications will include other scientific fields as a translation of tissue engineering; to easy the acceptance and the use by clinicians of the novel engineered tissues.

The merging of these sciences has led to medicine field regeneration, in which at the moment it has two planned clinical aims: (1) cell reparation of damaged tissues through cell therapies, including injection or cell implementations or cellular removal-sometimes blending with scaffolding material, or (2) ex tissue formation to be used as grafts or extracorporeal organs in order to help or augment ailing in vivo organs. Within the next years, clinical trials with cell therapies or extracorporeal organs are projected as repair mechanisms for other tissues; at the moment it's underway for cartilage, bone, skin, neural, and liver tissues only (Enderle, et al., 2005). The success of the therapeutic modalities in the future will be defined by the scientific and economic issues.

Clinical Engineering

Clinical engineering is the application of technology to health care in clinical environments, as was described earlier. Along with physicians, nurses, and other hospital staff, clinical engineer is a member of a health care team. They are in charge of development and maintenance of computer medical instrumentation and equipment records database and for sophisticated materials use and purchase. Clinical engineers can work with physicians to customize instrumentation to the specified necessity of the physicians and the hospital. It usually includes instrument interfacing with computer systems and specific software for instrument control and data acquisition and analysis. They are also in charge with the application for up to date technology related to health care.

The economic, social, regulatory, and cultural dynamics factors are the main challenges of clinical engineering through which clinical engineers must successfully navigate (Grimes, 2003, 2004a).

Bioinformatics

Bioinformatics is the merging of biology and information technology (Lesk, 2002). This field include computational tools to manage, analyse and manipulate large collection of biological data. Bioinformatics has three constituents. (1) Database creation for enabling the storage of management of large collection of biological data. (2) Algorithm development to specify data sets relationships. (3) Biological data sets analysis and interpretation by using these tools, such as DNA, RNA and protein sequence, structure, gene expression profiles and biochemical pathways. In 1990s the term bioinformatics was first used, basically having the same meanings with the analysis and management of DNA, RNA and protein sequence data (Rashidi & Buehler, 2000). Later in the 1960s, computational tools for sequence analysis has been available but until advances in sequencing technology this was a minority interest, which led to a fast growth in the number of stored sequence in database as GenBank. At the moment, Bioinformatics has enlarged to include other types of biological data like protein structure, gene expression profiles and protein interactions. In which each field requires a particular database, algorithm and statistical methods.

BioMEMS

MEMS or Micro-Electro-Mechanical Systems are mechanical elements integration, sensors, actuators, and electronics on the same silicon substrate through micro fabrication technology. Micromechanical components are manufactured using compatible "micromachining" process that carve away parts of the silicon wafer particularly or add new layer to construct the mechanical and electromechanical instruments while the electronics are manufactured using integrated circuit process order. MEMS permit the establishment of smart products, increasing the computational capability of microelectronics with the recognition and control abilities of micro sensors and micro actuators and expanding the space of practical application and designs.

MEMS is a technology that allows the formation of smart products, increasing the computational capability of microelectronics with the recognition and control abilities of micro sensors and actuators to grow the area of possible designs and applications. Interest in MEMS is expanding rapidly in fields like biosensors, pacemakers, immunoisolation capsules, and drug delivery (Grayson, et al., 2004). The devices have a minimum of one property's dimension of (100 nm–200 μm), up to few mm. They may also be the objectives of nanotechnology, as well as the key element to larger equipment like medical imagining machines. MEMS devices can function whether inside or outside a living system, and have built in or external power supply. They can be smart systems with built in microprocessors, in which they may function as an open ended or a closed loop system. All devices can integrate together or with other modules and carry out one or more function connected by tubing or other conduits. The intrinsic attributes of BioMEMS pledge the production of small-scale, low-cost biomedical devices that can be a revolution in biomedical investigation. As a result, a primary key is researching the field, as well as related nanotechnology for medical applications as surgical instruments, tissue repair, artificial organs, diagnostic tools, and drug delivery systems.

Neural Engineering

Neural Engineering is an important research field in more than one branch of knowledge that sustain neuroscience and engineering techniques to analyse neurological functions and designing of solutions to problems accompanied with neurological limitations and dysfunction (Durand,

2007). Neural Engineering's number one aim is to provide rehabilitation solutions for nervous system disorders and to solve neuroscience problems.

Engineering and quantitative methodology's significance applied to the nervous system differences common fields in neurosciences from neural engineering. Combination between engineering and neuroscience differentiate neural engineering from other engineering fields as artificial neural networks. It is located just between and gathers from basic neuroscience and clinical neuroscience. Different features of research areas at the molecular, cellular and system levels are enclosed by neural engineering like experimental, computational theoretical, applied, and clinical. All these areas are properly initiated and have noticeable identification even though some of them may overlap like neuromodulation and neuroprostheses.

Telemedicine

"Medical information exchange between sites by means of electronic communications in order to improve the health of patients," is the definition of Telemedicine (Sood, et al., 2007). According to Greeks, the term "tele" means "at a distance," therefore, electronic communication means audio-visual telecommunication that allows duplex real time interaction between the physician and the patient.

Telemedicine is considered to be a productive and inexpensive substitute to the standard way of medical care (i.e. face-to-face). It is a fast progressive application of clinical medicine for consulting, and remote medical care in which data is transferred through Internet and other types of networks.

It can be as easy as a professional medical discussion over the phone or as complicated as a videoconference to carry on a real time consultation between a patient and a physician on two different continents.

Telemedicine is classified to three types, store and forward, interactive services, and remote monitoring (Oakley, 2006). All are old ways of consultation but are still required.

- Store and forward: All medical data including audio, video, images, reports are gathered and sent to a medical professional for diagnosis. The two, doctor and the patient, don't have to be both present at the time of the examination, as all data can be saved for examined later on.
- Interactive telemedicine: A real time communication between the patient and the doctor, which includes home visits, phone conversation, and internet interaction. Many examinations and check-ups are done by telemedicine. Telemedicine is affordable compared to face-to-face examination.
- Remote monitoring: which is also known as self-testing or self-monitoring technique. Physicians and doctors can monitor their patients with a lot of technological instruments. Persistent diseases such as heart diseases, asthma, or diabetes can be monitored and managed by this type of telemedicine. It can result in a better satisfaction and faster outcome. It's also a cost-effective method compared to traditional face-to-face monitoring.

When thinking of how to solve the problem of unreachable means of healthcare, telemedicine is the key. Telemedicine can perform various tasks together with basic healthcare services if implemented in a proper way. Quality of telemedicine has improved as information technology improves, which result in a cost reductions to a large extent. Still, considerations about the safety of patient's data or depending totally on such technologies are being raised. However, the wise use of it can save lives and reduce expenses.

CURRENT AND FUTURE DIRECTIONS OF BIOMEDICAL ENGINEERING

The foundation of the patient-monitoring concept within a medical environment was because of the biomedical instrumentation technology development to measure the chemical and physical data and signals released by the human body in a non-invasive way. It granted the development of medical care's quality. Moreover, medical imagining technology developed from one to three-dimensional measurement and became quicker. Meanwhile, saying that the medical imaging has entered the four-dimensional measurement is not an exaggeration. Not only medical imagining but also treatment technologies have progressed to nominal invasive techniques such as endoscopic surgery. Grand compilation techniques as image-guided computer-aided assisted surgery robot has been employed in medical applications since the end of the 20th century.

Extraordinary microscopic surgeries that are very sensitive and precise which cannot be carried out by a doctor can be possible through new systems and surgeon's skills combination. So, evolution of medicine is promoted concurrently by the progress in medical treatment technologies. Biomedical engineering progression in the 20th century has changed the idea of health care by transforming it from classical to cutting-edge care assisted by instrumentation and imaging, as the progress in anaesthesiology necessary in awake surgeries. The expectancy for more future developments in this area is because of the social desire to "improve and maintain a medical treatment of a high quality as well as health and welfare" (Kikuchi, 2007).

The progression of more powerful computer systems will assist in a better understanding of the human body's function and structure, and using such system will allow the evolution of a conceptual model of the entire biological continuum of the human organism based on imag-ing and visualization data, ranging from whole body to subcellular structure information. These systems will bring a new dimension to treatment and diagnosis. Bringing all diagnostic steps and therapies to non-invasive steps will be another challenge for biomedical engineers. Biomedical engineering development of both macro and micro body processes can eventually lead to more intrinsic and reliable diagnostic methodologies (Ghista, 2000).

More comfortable recovery, faster rehabilitation, shorter stays in hospitals, and health care expense reduction will all be lead with less invasive methods and devices. Evolution of better methods for joint disease access and surgery performance, as well as more dependable fixation of the artificial joints and better mechanical dedication will all be required for achievement of the objectives. Even re-growing a worn out joint by using the methods of tissue engineering or regeneration of stem cell after dispensing with mechanical artificial joints may also be possible. Enormously developed dynamic field is represented by the intelligent systems and technologies in rehabilitation engineering. For disabled people's well-being, these systems are very important. Challenges that will be awaiting for biomedical engineers is to develop these technologies. Examples of such technologies are: telemedicine, aids for people with visual, hearing, and speech impairments, artificial limbs, wheelchairs, tissue engineering for repairing brain damage after stroke and for regenerating nerves after spinal cord injuries, and electrical devices for the maintenance of continence.

Due to the rapid advancement in health care and the long-distance communication through telemedicine, in order to enhance diagnosis and treatment, increase access to suitable medicine and technologies, a prominent potential should prevail.

The central component of diagnosis will always be the simple X-ray and ultrasonic imagining, as they both are not expensive but only need to be customized for the local environment. Taking a current technology and producing an affordable, easier access in-field model would be the real challenge. Later, pocket-sized and inexpensive ultrasound images will be used like a stethoscope is now, which will surely save accident victim's lives. A sensor that is in a size of a pill already exists, in which, upon swallowing, it can report the internal body temperature as passing via intestinal tract. Other internal body conditions such as bleeding areas or distorted cells will be reported as well in the near future by the use of relative devices. Then later on, they can be directed to certain locations inside the body in which a disease exists and has to be cured. Emergency medicine's tendency is not special.

Since the drawing of the famous skeleton picture and its musculature by Leonardo da Vinci, Biomedical Engineering has come a long way. Medicine practice is totally reliant on the work of engineers, as engineering applications exist in every medicine area. Electronic patient records, super powerful electro medical instruments and tiny invasive technologies, they are just the start. New telemedicine and e-health care services provisions will be possible in the near future. Progression is speeding up and new challenges are waiting for biomedical engineers; there is no limit to the possibilities for their work in the practical medical revolution. Future engineers will certainly be working to develop things that cannot yet come to our minds.

CONCLUSION

During the previous century in most countries, quality of life and life expectancy have increased; an essential role has been played in this enrichment by the creation of reliable, safe, and cost-effective medical technologies. Significant Bio and Nano technologies are merged today in medical technologies. The latest medical technology and knowledge reward people with advanced health care. In the old days, medical instruments showed development every 10 years. The need of the public, now, is represented by a stable

provision of advanced health care. A combination of Bio and Nano technologies needs to be essentially established in the near future, generally "translation research" needs to be established to contain "engineering research and basic medicine." Product Realisation Research for clinical medicine contribution will be implemented by the outcome of the result.

REFERENCES

Albert, M. S., Cates, G. D., & Driehuys, B. (1994). Biological magnetic resonance imaging using laser-polarized ^{129}Xe. *Nature, 370*, 199–201. doi:10.1038/370199a0

American Institute for Medical and Biological Engineering. (2011). *Website.* Retrieved from http://www.aimbe.org.

Association for the Advancement of Medical Instrumentation (AAMI). (2011). *Website.* Retrieved from http://www.aami.org.

Bandettini, P. A., Wong, E. C., Hinks, R. S., Tikofsky, R. S., & Hyde, J. S. (1992). Time course EPI of human brain function during task activation. *Magnetic Resonance in Medicine, 25*, 390–397. doi:10.1002/mrm.1910250220

Bankman, I. (2000). *Handbook of medical imaging: Processing and analysis management.* San Diego, CA: Academic Press.

Biomedical Engineering Society. (1996). *Planning a career in biomedical engineering.* Retrieved from http://www.bmes.org/aws/BMES/pt/sp/be_faqs.

Biomedical Engineering Society (BMES). (2011). *Website.* Retrieved from http://www.bmes.org/aws/BMES/pt/sp/home_page.

Bronzino, J. D. (2000). Clinical engineering: Evolution of a discipline. In Bronzino, J. D. (Ed.), *The Biomedical Engineering Handbook* (2nd ed.). Boca Raton, FL: CRC Press LLC.

Brown, J. H. U. (1975). The biomedical engineer and the health care system. *IEEE Transactions on Bio-Medical Engineering, 22,* 95–99. doi:10.1109/TBME.1975.324425

Cerutti, S., Baselli, G., & Bianchi, A. (2011). Biomedical signal and image processing. *IEEE Pulse, 2*(3), 41–54. doi:10.1109/MPUL.2011.941522

Chapman, B., Turner, R., & Ordidge, R. J. (1987). Readl-time movie imaging from a single cardiac cycle by NMR. *Magnetic Resonance in Medicine, 5,* 246–254. doi:10.1002/mrm.1910050305

Cook, A. M., & Hussey, S. M. (2002). *Assistive technology: Principles and practice* (2nd ed.). St. Louis, MO: Mosby.

Cooper, R. A., Ohnabe, H., & Hobson, D. A. (2006). *An introduction to rehabilitation engineering.* Boca Raton, FL: CRC Press Taylor & Francis.

Cox, J. R. Jr, Pfeiffer, R. R., & Pickard, W. F. (1975). Experience with a training program in technology in health care. *IEEE Transactions on Bio-Medical Engineering, 22,* 129–134. doi:10.1109/TBME.1975.324432

Damadian, R. (1971). Tumor detection by nuclear magnetic resonance. *Science, 171,* 1151. doi:10.1126/science.171.3976.1151

Detwiler, J. S., Sanderson, A. C., & Vas, R. (1975). A clinically oriented bioengineering program for undergraduates. *IEEE Transactions on Bio-Medical Engineering, 22,* 140–145. doi:10.1109/TBME.1975.324434

Dumoulin, C. L., Souza, S. P., & Hart, H. R. (1987). Rapid scan magnetic resonance angiography. *Magnetic Resonance in Medicine, 5,* 238–245. doi:10.1002/mrm.1910050304

Durand, D. M. (2007). What is neural engineering? In *Journal Of Neural Engineering (Vol. 4).* Dordrecht, The Netherlands: IOP Publishing.

Enderle, J., Blanchard, S. M., & Bronzino, J. (2005). *Introduction to biomedical engineering* (2nd ed.). New York, NY: Academic Press.

Flexman, J. (2007). Alternative careers for biomedical engineers. *IEEE Engineering in Medicine and Biology Magazine, 26*(5), 10–11. doi:10.1109/EMB.2007.906029

Fung, Y. C. (1996). *Biomechanics* (2nd ed.). New York, NY: Springer-Verlag.

Garfield, E. (1987). Exploring the frontiers of biomedical-engineering - An overview of historical and current considerations. *Current Contents, 9*(10), 3–11.

Ghista, D. N. (2000). Biomedical engineering: Yesterday, today, and tomorrow. *IEEE Engineering in Medicine and Biology Magazine, 19*(6), 23–28. doi:10.1109/51.887243

Grayson, A. C. R., Shawgo, R. S., & Johnson, A. M. (2004). A biomems review: Mems technology for physiologically integrated devices. *Proceedings of the IEEE, 92*(1), 6–21. doi:10.1109/JPROC.2003.820534

Grimes, S. L. (2003). The future of clinical engineering: The challenge of change. *IEEE Engineering in Medicine and Biology Magazine, 22*(2), 91–99. doi:10.1109/MEMB.2003.1195702

Grimes, S. L. (2004). Clinical engineers: Stewards of healthcare technologies. *IEEE Engineering in Medicine and Biology Magazine, 34*(1), 5.

Grimes, S. L. (2004a). Clinical notes: Opportunities and challenges in clinical engineering. *IEEE Engineering in Medicine and Biology Magazine, 23*(2), 94–95. doi:10.1109/MEMB.2004.1310991

Grimes, S. L. (2004b). Clinical engineers: Stewards of healthcare technologies. *IEEE Engineering in Medicine and Biology Magazine, 23*(3), 56–58. doi:10.1109/MEMB.2004.1317982

Guide to Career Education. (2011). *Website*. Retrieved from http://www.guidetocareereducation.com/careers/biomedical-engineering.

Harmon, L. D. (1975). Biomedical engineering education: How to do what, with which, and to whom. *IEEE Transactions on Bio-Medical Engineering, 22*, 89–94. doi:10.1109/TBME.1975.324424

Harris, T. R., Bransford, J. D., & Brophy, S. P. (2002). Roles for learning sciences and learning technologies in biomedical engineering education: A review of recent advances. *Annual Review of Biomedical Engineering, 4*, 29–48. doi:10.1146/annurev.bioeng.4.091701.125502

Hendee, W. R., Chien, S., Maynard, C. D., & Dean, D. J. (2002). The national institute of biomedical imaging and bioengineering: History, status, and potential impact. *Annals of Biomedical Engineering, 30*(1), 2–10. doi:10.1114/1.1433491

Hornak, J. P. (2011). *The basics of MRI*. Retrieved from http://www.cis.rit.edu/htbooks/mri/.

Hounsfield, G. N. (1973). Computerized transverse axial scanning (tomography). *The British Journal of Radiology, 46*, 1016–1022. doi:10.1259/0007-1285-46-552-1016

IEEE. Engineering in Medicine and Biology Society. (2011). *Website*. Retrieved from http://www.embs.org.

International Society of Biomechanics (ISB). (2011). *Website*. Retrieved from http://isbweb.org.

Jacobs, J. E. (1975). The biomedical engineering quandary. *IEEE Transactions on Bio-Medical Engineering, 22*, 100–106. doi:10.1109/TBME.1975.324426

Johns, R. J. (1975). Current issues in biomedical engineering education. *IEEE Transactions on Bio-Medical Engineering, 22*, 107–110. doi:10.1109/TBME.1975.324427

Johnson, C. R. (2000). Numerical methods for bioelectric field problems. In Bronzino, J. D. (Ed.), *The Biomedical Engineering Handbook* (2nd ed.). Boca Raton, FL: CRC Press LLC.

Joshi, R. (2006). *Biosensors*. India: Isha Book.

Kahn, A. R. (1975). Biomedical engineering education for employment by industry. *IEEE Transactions on Bio-Medical Engineering, 22*, 147–149. doi:10.1109/TBME.1975.324436

Katona, P. G. (2002). The Whitaker foundation: The end will be just the beginning. *IEEE Transactions on Medical Imaging, 21*(8), 845–849. doi:10.1109/TMI.2002.803606

Katona, P. G. (2006). Biomedical engineering and the Whitaker foundation: A thirty-year partnership. *Annals of Biomedical Engineering, 34*(6), 904–916. doi:10.1007/s10439-006-9087-7

Khandpur, R. S. (2004). *Biomedical instrumentation: Technology and applications*. New York, NY: McGraw-Hill Professional.

Kikuchi, M. (2007). Status and future prospects of biomedical engineering: A Japanese perspective. *Biomedical Imaging and Intervention Journal, 3*(3), 1–6. doi:10.2349/biij.3.3.e37

Kumar, A. D., Welti, D., & Ernst, R. R. (1975). NMR Fourier zeugmatography. *Journal of Magnetic Resonance (San Diego, Calif.), 18*(1), 69–83.

Landoll, J. R., & Caceres, C. A. (1969). Automation of data acquisition in patient testing. *Proceedings of the IEEE, 57*(11), 1941–1953. doi:10.1109/PROC.1969.7440

Lanza, R., Langer, R., & Vacanti, J. (2000). *Principles of tissue engineering*. San Diego, CA: Academic Press, Inc.

Lauterbur, P. C. (1973). Image formation by induced local interactions: examples employing nuclear magnetic resonance. *Nature, 242,* 190–191. doi:10.1038/242190a0

Lesk, A. M. (2002). *Introduction to bioinformatics.* Oxford, UK: Oxford University Press.

Mansfield, P. (1977). Multi-planar image formation using NMR spin-echos. *Journal of Physics. C. Solid State Physics, 10,* 55–58. doi:10.1088/0022-3719/10/3/004

Marmarelis, V. Z. (2004). *Nonlinear dynamic modeling of physiological systems.* New York, NY: John Wiley InterScience.

Massey, J. T., & Johns, R. J. (1981). A short history of the collaborative biomedical program. *Johns Hopkins APL Technical Digest, 2,* 141–142.

McCally, R. L. (2005). The master's degree program in applied biomedical engineering. *Johns Hopkins APL Technical Digest, 26*(3), 214–218.

Moritz, W. E., & Huntsman, L. L. (1975). A collaborative approach to bioengineering education. *IEEE Transactions on Bio-Medical Engineering, 22,* 124–129. doi:10.1109/TBME.1975.324431

Mylrea, K. C., & Siverston, S. E. (1975). Biomedical engineering in health care—Potential vs reality. *IEEE Transactions on Bio-Medical Engineering, 22,* 114–118. doi:10.1109/TBME.1975.324429

Neuman, M. R. (2000). Biomedical sensors. In Bronzino, J. D. (Ed.), *The Biomedical Engineering Handbook* (2nd ed.). Boca Raton, FL: CRC Press LLC.

Newhouse, V. L., Bell, D. S., & Tackel, I. S. (1989). The future of clinical engineering in the 1990s. *Journal of Clinical Engineering, 14,* 417.

Nokes, L., Jennings, D., Flint, T., & Turton, B. (1995). *Introduction to medical electronics applications.* London, UK: Butterworth-Heinemann.

Northrop, R. B. (2003). *Signals and systems analysis in biomedical engineering.* Boca Raton, FL: CRC Press.

Oakes, J. B. (1975). Clinical engineering-The problems and promise. *Science, 190,* 239–242.

Oakley, A. (2006). *Introduction to telemedicine* (2nd ed.). London, UK: RSM Books.

Peterson's. (2011). *Graduate programs in engineering and applied sciences* (46th ed.). Princeton, NJ: Peterson.

Peura, R. A., Boyd, J. R., Shahnarian, A., Driscoll, W. G., & Wheeler, H. B. (1975). Organization and function of a hospital biomedical engineering internship program. *IEEE Transactions on Bio-Medical Engineering, 22,* 134–140. doi:10.1109/TBME.1975.324433

Rashidi, H. H., & Buehler, L. K. (2000). *Bioinformatics basics: Applications in biological science and medicine.* Boca Raton, FL: CRC Press.

Ratner, B. D., Hoffman, A. S., Schoen, F. J., & Lemons, J. E. (2004). *Biomaterials science: An introduction to materials in medicine* (2nd ed.). San Diego, CA: Academic Press.

Rehabilitation Engineering and Assistive Technology Society of North America (RESNA). (2011). *Website.* Retrieved from http://resna.org.

Requena-Carrion, J., & Leder, R. S. (2009). The natural history of the engineering in medicine and biology society from a modern perspective. In *Proceedings of the IEEE Engineering in Medicine and Biology Society Conference 2009,* (pp. 1086-1088). IEEE Press.

Saltzman, W. M. (2009). *Biomedical engineering.* Cambridge, UK: Cambridge University Press.

Schneck, D. J., & Bronzino, J. D. (2002). *Biomechanics: Principles and applications.* Boca Raton, FL: CRC Press. doi:10.1201/9781420040029

Schwan, H. P. (1984). The development of biomedical engineering: Historical comments and personal observations. *IEEE Transactions on Bio-Medical Engineering, 31*(12), 730–736. doi:10.1109/TBME.1984.325328

Schwartz, M. D. (1984). The emerging field of clinical engineering and its accomplishments. *IEEE Transactions on Bio-Medical Engineering, 31*(12), 743–748. doi:10.1109/TBME.1984.325233

Schwartz, M. D., & Long, F. M. (1975). A survey analysis of biomedical engineering education. *IEEE Transactions on Bio-Medical Engineering, 22*, 119–124. doi:10.1109/TBME.1975.324430

Semmlow, J. L. (2004). *Biosignal and medical image processing: MATLAB-based applications.* Boca Raton, FL: CRC Press Taylor & Francis.

Society for Biomaterials (SFB). (2011). *Website.* Retrieved from http://www.biomaterials.org/index.cfm.

Sood, S., Mbarika, V., Jugoo, S., Dookhy, R., Doarn, C. R., Prakash, N., & Merrell, R. C. (2007). What is telemedicine? A collection of 104 peer-reviewed perspectives and theoretical underpinnings. *Telemedicine Journal and e-Health, 13*(5), 573–590. doi:10.1089/tmj.2006.0073

The Whitaker Foundation. (2011). *A history of biomedical engineering (May 2002).* Retrieved from http://bmes.seas.wustl.edu/WhitakerArchives/glance/history.html.

Thompkins, W. J. (1993). *Biomedical digital signal processing.* Englewood Cliffs, NJ: Prentice-Hall.

Torzyn, N. T., McKinney, W. D., Abbott, E. L. Jr, Cook, A. M., & Gillott, D. H. (1975). Biomedical engineering program to upgrade biomedical equipment technicians. *IEEE Transactions on Bio-Medical Engineering, 22*, 145–147. doi:10.1109/TBME.1975.324435

Webster, J. G., & Cook, A. M. (1979). *Clinical engineering: Principles and practices.* Tanglewood Cliffs, NJ: Prentice Hall.

Weed, H. R. (1975). Biomedical engineering—Practice or research? *IEEE Transactions on Bio-Medical Engineering, 22*, 110–113. doi:10.1109/TBME.1975.324428

Zambuto, R. P. (2004). Clinical engineers in the 21st century. *IEEE Engineering in Medicine and Biology Magazine, 23*(3), 37–41. doi:10.1109/MEMB.2004.1317980

APPENDIX A: PROFESSIONAL SOCIETIES OF BIOMEDICAL ENGINEERING

American Institute for Medical and Biological Engineering (AIMBE)

In 1991, in order to initiate a clear inclusive identification for the biomedical field, the American Institute for Medical and Biological Engineering was founded creating a link between fundamentals of engineering with problems of biomedical science. It searches for serving and organizing a wide constituency from medical and biological scientists and practitioners to academic departments and industries.

Association for the Advancement of Medical Instrumentation (AAMI)

In 1967, the Association for the Advancement of Medical Instrumentation was founded, which is considered to be the principal professional organization for researchers, manufacturers and medical equipment operators. AAMI is a non-profit, voluntary organization that includes 6,000 members and 375 organizations, presenting more than 100 more than 100 committees of medical professionals, engineers, technicians, equipment manufacturers, researchers, and government regulators. It is also considered to be the number one source of medical equipment and technology information, which assist in industry standards development.

Technology practices, revisions, and updates are all researched by the AAMI. Its committees have substantial impact over the manufacture, training and use of medical equipment worldwide, as educational programs, which are one of the main focal points of the AAMI. It also supplies members' training by books, magazines, technical documentations, and software publishing, and certifies in wide range of specialities for medical technicians. A variety of conferences are being financed by the AAMI so that its members can exchange their knowledge and experience. Even though some practices and standards are not authorised by the government, the AAMI recommended ones are considered as industry standard. When specifying a defect or an action of violating someone or something, many medical facilities inspection site AAMI suggested practices and standards. AAMI membership is voluntary; however, it's highly admired within the medical instrumentation community.

Biomedical Engineering Society (BMES)

Biomedical Engineering Society was embraced in Illinois on the 1st of February in 1968 as retaliation to the demand to supply an equal status society to representatives of biomedical and engineering interests.

In 2004, BMES issued its "Historical Perspective" to celebrate a 35-year growth. BMES was established to provide service to students, academics, and professionals of biomedical engineering and bioengineering as a non-profit association. Its goal is to upgrade knowledge in the field of biomedical engineering around the world and its use for healthcare. At the beginning, the society's membership included 171 founding members and 89 charter members.

November 18th 1968 Houston, Texas, was the first meeting to be held by the BME Society simultaneously, with the 21st Annual Conference on Engineering in Medicine and Biology. Blacksburg, Virginia in 1990 was the first annual meeting of the BMES. And since that, BMES organize annual multiday scientific meeting with presentations and exhibits.

BMS hosts sessions, events, career services and pre-meeting workshops and courses for students, graduates, and professionals. It also publishes a monthly journal that is called the Annals of Biomedical Engineering (AMBE) and quarterly journal called Cellular Bio molecular Engineering (CMBE).

IEEE Engineering in Medicine and Biology Society (EMBS)

IEEE Engineering in Medicine and Biology Society is a branch of Institute of Electrical and Electronic Engineers (IEEE) and is considered to be the largest biomedical engineer's society in the world with 8,200 members from 70 different countries. Members benefit from access to the most fascinating people, practices, information, ideas, and opinion. Members do not have to be electrical engineers in specific but must be from sciences background like chemical, biochemistry, medicine, bioengineering, and biomedical engineering.

EMBS main interest includes applications of ideas and techniques from the physical and engineering to biology and medicine. It hosts major international conferences each year as well as regional ones. Transactions on Biomedical Engineering journal is published monthly, another Transactions on Neural Systems and Rehabilitation Engineering, Transactions on Information Technology in Biomedicine, and Transactions on Nano bioscience journal is published every three quarters and IEEE Engineering in Medicine and Biology Magazine that is published twice a month. Transactions on Medical Imaging, Transactions on Neural Networks, Transactions on Pattern Analysis, and Machine Intelligence are secondary publications are authored in collaboration with other societies.

Society for Biomaterials (SFB)

Society for Biomaterials (SFB) encourages advances in biomedical materials R&D by collaborative educational programs, clinical applications, and professional standards in the biomaterials discipline.

Scientists and engineers in the field of biomaterials study cells together with their components, complex tissues and organs and the way they interact with other materials and implanted prosthetic devices and how to improve and characterize the materials used for measuring, restoring and improving physiological functions and improve the quality of life. Researchers in this discipline started a chain of International Biomaterials Symposia concentrating predominantly on materials for reconstructive surgery in 1969. The more popular they became, the more the idea to start a devoted organization started to grow.

SFB was founded in April 1974 in order to encourage and advance research and develop biomaterial science. The first annual meeting was held in the facilities of Clemson University in Clemson, South Carolina in 26th of April 1975. Dr. C. William Hall, the society's founder was acknowledged with both an annual award and scholarship in his name. Within the discipline of biomaterials, SFB is the oldest scientific organization. SFB supports 13 Special Interest Groups (SIG) that supply forum for networking and new ideas within a focused environment in order to remain in the first place. It also improves student chapters in various universities like Clemson University, Michigan Tech University, the University of Florida, and the University of Memphis. The society presents some awards annually to faculty and students, not only this but it also nominates entitled individuals to the status of Fellow, Biomaterials Sciences, and Engineering. SFB remain to be a world's pioneer in the biomaterials discipline through annual meetings organizations that are held in the United States and participation in the quadrennial World Biomaterials Congress, which are designed for industry, academia, and clinicians to collect and talk about the latest progressions in the field. Publications include the journal of Biomedical Materials Research Part A and B—Applied Biomaterials and the Biomaterials Forum.

International Society of Biomechanics (ISB)

In order to encourage the study of biomechanics at the international rank, The International Society of Biomechanics (ISB) had to be founded in 1973. With a membership of scientists from different fields like anatomy, physiology, engineering (mechanical, industrial, aerospace, etc.), orthopaedics, rehabilitation medicine, sport science and medicine, ergonomics, electro-physiological kinesiology, and others.

Social activities involve organizing of biennial international congresses (which is considered to be the main activity for the society), publishing of congress proceedings and a biomechanics monograph chain, distributing a society newsletter, sponsoring meetings related to biomechanics and affiliation with the *Journal of Biomechanics*, the *Journal of Applied Biomechanics*, *Clinical Biomechanics*, the *Journal of Electromyography and Kinesiology*, and *Gait and Posture*. This contributes special chances for members to get a better understand of topics within the field and assist with professional contacts. The congresses are usually held in different countries in order to encourage the development of the field.

Rehabilitation Engineering and Assistive Technology Society of North America (RESNA)

RESNA was founded in August 1979 at a meeting of the Inter-Agency Conference on Rehabilitation Engineering for those involved in R&D, application of assistive technology, rehabilitation engineering, with the goal to enhance the lives of disabled people through the use of technology. Its membership is for rehabilitation professions, consumers and students, in which they are all committed to exchange knowledge and experience for the advancement of assistive technology, with over 1,400 members mainly from the United States and Canada. Toronto, June 1980 was the first official membership and board meeting simultaneously with an international conference on rehabilitation engineering, later in 1981 its first private conference was held in Washington DC in August 1981. In order to enhance wheelchair-testing standards, RESNA received additional federal assets to determine the number of people working and training needs in bestowing rehabilitation technology through state rehabilitation agencies, and a three-year award to improve culturally responsive training materials for facilitative technology followed by another three-year award to improve national instructions for education of providers and for continuous quality enhancement in facilitative technology. RESNA has 7 Special Interest Groups (SIG's) and 7 Professional Specialty Groups (PSG's).

APPENDIX B: SOME OF THE MAJOR MANUFACTURERS OF MRI DEVICES

Table B1. Clinical MRI Original Equipment Manufacturers (OEMs).

Esaote http://www.esaote.com/
Fonar http://www.fonar.com/
General Electric Healthcare http://www.gehealthcare.com/
Hitachi Medical Systems http://www.hitachimed.com/
Millennium Technology http://www.millennium.ca/
Odin Medical technologies http://www.odinmed.com/
Philips Healthcare http://www.healthcare.philips.com/
Siemens Healthcare https://www.smed.com/
Toshiba Medical Systems http://www.medical.toshiba.com/

Reprinted with permission of Hornak (2011)

Table B2. Experimental High Field MRI OEMs.

Agilent Technologies http://www.varianinc.com/
Bruker Biospin MRI http://www.bruker-biospin.com/

Reprinted with permission of Hornak (2011)

Table B3. Manufacturers of MRI Contrast Agents

Bracco Group http://www.bracco.com/
Bayer HealthCare Pharmaceuticals http://bayerimaging.com/
GE Imaging Agents http://www.geimagingagents.com/
Lantheus Medical Imaging http://www.radiopharm.com/
Sigma-Aldrich http://www.sigmaaldrich.com/

Reprinted with permission of Hornak (2011)

Table B4. MRI Compatible Device Manufacturers

Biophan Technologies http://www.biophan.com/
InVivo http://www.invivocorp.com/
Magmedix http://www.magmedix.com/
Medrad http://www.medrad.com/
MR Resources http://www.mrr.com/
Schiller http://www.schiller.ch/
SA Instruments http://www.i4sa.com/

Reprinted with permission of Hornak (2011)

Table B5. Magnet System Manufacturers

Bruker Biospin MRI http://www.bruker-biospin.com/
Magnex Scientific http://www.varianinc.com/
Resonance Research / Stern Magnetics http://www.rricorp.com/

Reprinted with permission of Hornak (2011)

Table B6. Gradient Supplies

Copley Controls http://www.copleycontrols.com/
Tesla Engineering http://www.tesla.co.uk/

Reprinted with permission of Hornak (2011)

Table B7. RF Amps

Communication Power Corporation http://cpcamps.com/
Advanced Energy http://www.advanced-energy.com/
Herley Medical Products http://www.herley.com/

Reprinted with permission of Hornak (2011)

Table B8. RF Coil Manufacturers

Advanced Imaging Research http://advimg.com/
Doty Scientific http://www.dotynmr.com/
GE Healthcare http://www.gehealthcare.com/
IGC Medical Advances http://www.medadv.com/
InVivo http://www.invivocorp.com/
Lammers Medical Technology http://www.lammersmedical.com/
Machnet B.V. http://www.machnet.nl/
MR Instruments http://www.mrinstruments.com/
Nova Medical http://novamedical.com/
RAPID Biomedical http://www.rapidbiomed.com/
Scanmed http://www.scanmed.com/
XL Resonance http://www.xlres.com/

Reprinted with permission of Hornak (2011)

Chapter 6
Critical Concepts in M–Health Technology Development:
Time, Space, and Mobility

Henrique M. G. Martins
University of Beira Interior, Portugal

ABSTRACT

This chapter is a theoretical in-depth review of three conceptual groups that serve as the fundamental basis for m-health technology development—both at hardware and software levels   as well as for technology adaptation to work/life practices, and for adoption and usage studies. Objectively the review will focus on the concepts of Time (clock, event, practice-based, and timeless time), experiences of time (subjective construction of the "past," "present," and "future," time aggregation/"episodification" frequency, rhythm, cycles, "spiraling," and mono-polichronicity), space, and mobility (namely physical mobility, remote versus local, modalities of travelling/visiting/ wandering, micro-mobility).

INTRODUCTION

The most significant difference between MICT and desktop-based ICT is the fact that the computing devices can move while retaining connectivity to networks or act as isolated computing devices. In both cases, MICT introduces a new dimension to Information Systems (IS)—mobility—and, thus, has the potential to disrupt spatial and temporal arrangements of both actors and their actions. Since spatial and temporal dimensions of the organisation of doctors' work practices have been shown to influence how they use pen-and-paper and desktop ICTs (Westbrook, et al., 2004; Martins, et al., 2005), and, since MICT can potentially change where and when work can be done, it seems valuable to explore some theories about time, space and mobility.

DOI: 10.4018/978-1-4666-0888-7.ch006

Orlikowski highlights the importance of looking at time in organizations (Orlikowski & Yates, 2002), and this is reinforced in the medical context by Strauss *et al.* (1997). Another reason why it is crucial to look at time is its intricate relationship with space and mobility. Time and space are intuitively connected in our everyday life experience. Giddens (1984) notes that movement in time always accompanies movement in space and, thus, that these are interrelated concepts which need to be studied together. Mol, however, has suggested that space can also be conceived as social topologies (Mol & Law, 1994) regardless of any physical dimension, and therefore understanding of workspace in such terms is a potentially additional tool to look at the use of MICT for work. Similarly, Castells (1996) suggests that "*spatial forms and processes are formed by the dynamics of the overall social structure.*" It is therefore important to understand space in order to understand action taking place, its location and position, and from thereon (Dix, 2000) actors' mobility modalities.

CONCEPTS OF TIME

The concept of time has not been stable though history as Lee and Liebenau (1999) describe. Time has also been studied in a variety of disciplines from mathematics, biology and psychology to anthropology and sociology (Orlikowski & Yates, 2002) as well as management and organizations (Bluedorn & Denhardt, 1988). There are several conceptualisations of time in the literature that are seen as shaping the way in which work, and more broadly all human activities, can be understood (George & Jones, 2000; Orlikowski & Yates, 2002). How we conceptualise time may in turn have implications for how we use other conceptual models, like those of space, mobility and even participants: be they individuals, groups or communities (George & Jones, 2000). This section does not aspire to be an exhaustive review of the

time literature but rather summarizes concepts of time and temporalities that have been claimed to be particularly related and relevant to the analysis of work and organizations.

"Clock-time" and "event time": Probably the most discussed division in conceptualisations of time is that of clock time against social or event time in its broadest sense. Several authors have written about clock time and event time (Bluedorn & Denhardt, 1988; Lee & Liebenau, 1999). A commonly held description of clock-time is provided by Lee who mentions clock-time is often conceptualised as "*homogeneous and divisible in structure, linear and uniform in its flow, objective and absolute, that is, existing independent of objects and events, measurable (or quantifiable), and as singular*" (Lee & Liebenau, 1999), thus, there would be one, and only one, "correct time." This conceptualisation has been dominant in contemporary society and derives more from the natural sciences than from sociological concerns. It has, however, a strong relation with two aspects in management and organization analysis. It relates with the notion of time as a resource—the "time is money" metaphor—which means time can be spent, saved, wasted, possessed, budgeted, used up and invested. People often understand time in financial terms in everyday life. In addition, due to the work of Marx and others, this conceptualisation explains the close relationship between time and productivity.

The concept of social time, or event time, as it is generally referred to, although more loosely defined, arose as an alternative perspective to the rigidity of "clock-time" that was felt to be inadequate for social analysis. Bluedorn and Denhardt present it as "fundamentally a social construction that varies tremendously between and within societies" (Bluedorn & Denhardt, 1988). Examples of this would be dinnertime or prime time TV, which may vary between groups of people in their duration and in when (with regards to clock-time) they happen although they retain a shared meaning within the particular groups of individuals. Under this perspective, time is a subjective essence constructed

Table 1. Summary of analytical constructs for analysing temporal organization of work

Concepts of time	Clock time
	Event time
	Practice based
	Timeless time
Experiences of time	Subjective construction of the "past," "present" and "future"
	Time aggregation/ "episodification"
	Frequency, Rhythm, Cycles, and "Spiralling"
	Mono-Polichronicity

via a "network of meanings" and it is experienced as heterogeneous in its duration and divisible in identifiable moments/epochs. As such, event time cannot be measured but only understood, and time becomes not the usual independent variable, but a problematic and researchable phenomenon of its own. To some extent, social time, as a concept independent of clock time seems to be unnatural and increasingly authors that typify temporality describe concept hybridisations and categories that share both types when they want to describe people's experiences of time (Table 1).

Practice based: In a recent contribution to the conceptualisation of time (Orlikowski & Yates, 2002), Orlikowski and Yates, claimed that *temporal structuring* may serve as a way to "bridge the subjective-objective dichotomy." Based on structuration theory (Giddens, 1984) and the "practice turn" Orlikowski and Yates propose that *"through their everyday action, actors produce and reproduce a variety of temporal structures which in turn shape the temporal rhythm and form of their ongoing practices."* This conceptualisation is considered superior for research and understating of organizational phenomena in the sense that it combines both previous perspectives and provides a practical orientation. Examples of such structures are: weekly meeting schedules, project deadlines or academic calendars. These have in common that:

"[P]eople establish and reinforce (implicitly or explicitly) those temporal structures as legitimate and useful organizing structures for their community. In turn, such legitimised temporal structures – while always potentially changeable because they are constituted in action – become taken for granted, serving as powerful templates for the timing and rhythm of members' social action within the community. Thus temporal structures are both a medium and the outcome of people's recurrent practices" (Orlikowski & Yates, 2002, p. 685)

According to this concept, time both shapes and is shaped by ongoing human action, thus it is not entirely objective or subjective, homogenous or heterogeneous, and cannot be measured against clock-time alone.

"Timeless time": Castells (1996) argues that due to information technology and the rise of a network society, a reconceptualization of time is needed This "timeless time" involves two types of perturbation: 1) *"Compressing the occurrence of phenomena, aiming at instantaneity,"* making time ephemeral, and, 2) *"introducing random discontinuity in the sequence of phenomena"* creating an undifferentiated eternal time.

Castells' notion of timeless time shares similarities to Harvey's work on post-modernity (Harvey, 1989), where he argues for the notion of instantaneous-time which he links to changes in the connections of time, space and technology. For Harvey an increasing time-space compression of physical and human processes and experiences are connected with an instantaneous IT-mediated mobility, which has been carried to extremes. As a result, time and space appear, literally, compressed. As people are "forced" to alter their representations of the world to themselves, they feel a sense of a shrinking space, as more is closer at any given instant of time.

Individuals' Experience of Time and Time Dimensions of Work

George and Jones (2000) discuss time along six "time dimensions" as aspects of time experience. One of the aspects raised by these authors is that the past, present and future are not isolated but are artificial constructs as people experience time as a *"continuation, connection and inseparability of the past, present and future."* Accordingly it may not be meaningful to dissect time into discrete, objective units to which we assign specific content. On the other hand, like individuals, groups and organizations may also have different collective experiences of time. Given that the subjective experience of time often differs from objective clock time, a rich understanding of how people experience work in organizations necessitates consideration of the subjective experience of time in organizations.

Another aspect of time experience is that of *"time aggregations,"* which are the ways people choose to aggregate their experience of time into an episode, or episodes, so they can give it meaning. The length of time a person chooses to bracket the phenomenon in question will affect the meaning attributed to it, and its relationship to other phenomena.

Another way to look at phenomena or activities' relationship with time is to take into account that most human activities occur with specific frequency, certain rhythms, and cycles. When an increase in the frequency of a phenomenon or activity arises, time may be experienced as accelerated. George and Jones (2000) term this *"Spiralling."*

In addition to how people experience time in their work, some authors believe it is also valuable to understand how they organize their work in relation to time. Hall (1983) identified two distinct orientations in peoples' inclinations towards preferred modes of organizing work over clock-time, monochronicity and polichronicity. Polychronicity means doing several things at once. This is seen to be associated with an orientation towards the present with less concern with timetables or procedures. Time is, thus, an inexhaustible resource, and interpersonal relations are as important as the work to be performed. Monochronicity, in contrast, means doing one thing at a time. There is a concentration or dedication to one particular task and time is seen as an exhaustible resource. Interpersonal relations are thus relegated to secondary importance, temporarily or permanently. Other authors (Benabou, 1999; Bluedorn, et al., 1999) have developed these concepts arguing that these are better understood as part of a *"chronicity"* spectrum, between mono and polychronicity.

Time: Summary of Analytical Constructs

Table 1 presents a summary of all concepts discussed and which are thought to be useful in explaining temporal patterns of work. In addition to the existence of certain patterns and experiences of time, these may change under the influence of IT. In other words, MICT could potentially provoke changes in the way people organize their activities over time, in whether these are accomplished simultaneously or not, and how time is itself experienced by people through their use of these novel technological artefacts.

SPACE, WORKPLACE, AND MOBILITY

Space and Place: Physical Spatiality

The terms space and place are often used in a more or less synonymous way. Some authors however, distinguish between them. Giddens, for example,

(Giddens, 1990, p. 18) refers to space as the abstract, asocial conceptualisation of geographical location, while place refers to social inhabited physicality. In pre-modern cultures, he argues, the connection between geographic space and place was mediated by "presence" and localised activities. Now, however, geographic space can increasingly be conceptualised and thought of as detached from its roots in the enactment of place. This is because relations with "absent" others (human and non-human) have increased, and at the same time, we are able to think of geographic spatiality in its abstraction. Escobar also describes space as *abstract, universal, homogeneous, modern,* and place as *local, grounded, and traditional* (Escobar, 2001). When contrasted with place, space becomes an abstract field in which trajectories of history, political, economy, technology, and social relations are mapped, like those of work practices, in on-going dynamic terms (Kelly, 2003). Place, on the other hand, refers to *"the experience of, and from, a particular location with some sense of boundaries, grounds, and links to everyday practice"* (Escobar, 2001). Kelly rearticulates this definition:

"place is the local, lived articulation of sense, body, identity, environment, and culture, a person is always in and of place. Place is captured in the intersubjective sharing of experience and social practice (...) places should be conceived as both produced by and productive of subjects" (Benabou, 1999, p. 2280).

Kelly's definition of place has the advantage that it accommodates other conceptualisations of space such as Taussig's (1997) *geographic imaginaries*, that describe how places become connected not only to real but also imagined social practices. Harrison and Dourish emphasise the importance of meaning in distinguishing place from space: a place is a *"space which is invested with understandings"* (Harrison & Dourish, 1996). A house becomes home when a certain meaningful interpretation is assigned to it, interestingly not all houses become homes, and not all people residing in a house may consider it to be their home. This example serves to show how the concept of place is socially constructed from a given spatiality. Since work in its broadest sense can be seen as a human activity by the same token, *workplaces* are all those spaces where work occurs. The concept and how we can understand the workplace then becomes highly dependent on how the space/spatiality where it occurs is itself conceptualised.

To be able to differentiate it from other spatialities, I refer to "physical space" when space is conceptualised according to physical/Euclidian/geographic spatiality. This is the most commonly used concept of space in work and organization studies, in which work occurs in a physical space, thus one could say in *"physical workplaces."* Alternative views on workplace could be suggested, however, departing from notions of social space (Mol & Law, 1994) which may be important for work done in collaboration between people located in different physical spaces.

Social Spatiality: Topologies of Regions and Networks

When talking about "the Social" Mol (Mol & Law, 1994) proposes, *"The social doesn't exist as a single spatial type. Rather, it performs several kinds of space."* She mentions two of these social spatiality topologies: regions and networks. Mol defines regions as *"the types of social spaces where activities, humans and objects are clustered together and where boundaries can be drawn, dividing those similar from those that are different."* An example of this could be hospital doctors' visits to their patients in a ward round. These social spaces can overlap with physical environments (e.g. a specific room) and Mol suggests that, in this case. *"The understandings of the work and its organization hold their shape by fixating to the workplace."* This means that, in cases of overlap, it is the practice of the work being carried out that helps to identify if it is "occurring" through social space (i.e., it could be happening in another physical setting) or if it has roots in that specific physical location as well, in which case it argued as happening in both a physical and social spatiality.

For Mol, another form of thinking about social spaces is through the use of a network metaphor, for her: *"Networks are types of social spaces where distances between objects, humans and activities are defined by their relations rather than their physical location. The relations of similarity, rather then physical closeness, create proximity in networks"* (Mol & Law, 1994) Following this definition work can be identified as happening within a network, by looking at the "objects" involved (both human and non-human), their characteristics and those of their relations. According to Law and Mol: *"Objects in a network have stable relations between each other (...) these objects have been described as "immutable mobiles" since they are mobile in Euclidean space, but static in a network topology (immutable)"* (Mol & Law, 1994). For example, movement of two individuals in physical spatiality might mean they can be potentially static in their relation at the level of the social spatiality, for example, of a network if they keep unchanged their relations to a central individual acting as hub of the social network, or when they keep their social bond stable. This example highlights why these social "spaces" are not dependent on Euclidian space. The opposite example is equally possible to conceive. Two individuals might move to, or occupy, the same physical location (for example a given meeting room) without that meaning any reduction in their social distance.

Location, Position, Dislocation, and Sense of Motion

To understand mobility, Dix suggests, there is a need to think about location and position. If to move is *"to change in position from one point to another,"* then, as Dix *et al.* (Dix, 2000) highlight,

the notion of mobility requires the notion of location/position within a given dimension. For physical space, in absolute terms, this means relocation from one geographical coordinate to another but there is still a need to conceptualise location and position in relation to other topographic elements/concepts. This is required not only for physical but also for other spatialities, if we are to understand movement between them.

According to Graham (1998), for physical space these topographical concepts are relatively established and include: point in space, co-presence and outside/inside. Parallel concepts for social spaces remain undeveloped despite claims that they are equally necessary to understand mobility. Authors like Esbjörnsson and Vesterlind (2002) and Green (2002), emphasise mobility through social time and space. Green (2002), for instance, argues that *"mobility means [that] people are able to retain continuity in their tasks and mental processes regardless of the physical separation and, to an extent, of time synchronization."*

Mol (Mol & Law, 1994) and Esbjörnsson and Vesterlind (2002) discuss dislocation towards and away from social regions or networks corresponding to an increase or reduction in the "sense of belonging." Motion in relation to social spaces is, thus, relational. A second form of dislocation, however, is when people move between the relative positions they occupy in networks or regions (Mol & Law, 1994) regardless of their physicality. Someone who was peripheral to a group can quickly become central as he/she "moves" to occupy a position that involves dealing with the entire group. For example, a contributor who becomes editor of an academic journal or someone who gradually becomes more influential without necessarily occupying a formal position as such. This form of mobility within social space is termed "contextual mobility" by Kakihara and Sørensen (2002) and is seen as being influenced by certain technologies (especially ICT). MICT have the potential to convey information and communication, which themselves are representatives and actors of specific social contexts, regardless of physical space. MICT thus enables certain contexts and information to become co-present, which would not otherwise, leading to context interactions that may be desirable or undesirable (Kakihara & Sørensen, 2002). Conversely, using MICT can mean certain contexts of interaction are not discontinued when participants are forced to physically move thus ensuring a continuation of tasks being carried out.

Physical Mobility

Regarding the movement of people (and "their" objects) a number of taxonomies of mobility are presented in the literature. These do not necessarily create exclusive or incompatible categories, and in practice, they often appear to be related.

Remote vs. Local Mobility

Bellotti and Bly (1996) suggest that local mobility, for example, people moving within a hospital department, should be differentiated from the traditional notion of mobility as movement between remotely located settings, which they call remote mobility. They argue that this distinction is valuable since people's support needs (for work for example) vary significantly and may even be contradictory between the two modalities. Perry *et al.* (2001) offer a definition of local mobility as *"within easy walking distance of the office, walking between rooms or buildings at a local site."* Bardram and Bossen (2003), in contrast, describe it as intermediate between face-to-face and remote situations: *"Local mobility as we understand it occupies the intermediate space between working together over distance on the one hand and working face-to-face in an office or a control room on the other."*

Wandering/Visiting/Travelling Modalities

Addressing how people move (walking or in vehicle) and also the time they spend in the "sta-

tionary locations," rather than simply the range of their movements, Kristoffersen and Ljungberg (2000) distinguish three "modalities" of mobility: travelling, visiting and wandering, each of which has distinct characteristics:

- *Travelling* is the process of going from one place to another, [often] in a vehicle;
- *Visiting* is spending time in one place for a prolonged period before moving on to another place;
- *Wandering* is extensive local mobility in a building or local bounded area in the sense that the person is walking around.

These different modalities need not to be mutually exclusive and there may be differences within them. Thus, some forms of travelling modality may affect the suitability of certain types of MICT device (e.g. a laptop may be usable while travelling on a train, while a person travelling by bicycle might prefer to carry a small PDA). Similarly the weight of a device becomes an issue in wandering modality, or a *visitor* might bring ICT devices to the place they visit, e.g., a laptop, tablet PC, handheld, or use an installed desktop device. These two taxonomies of mobility apply to people and, to some extent, could be used to think of objects moving in the physical space with them. Having discussed concepts of mobility that, for the most part, relate with physical movement of either objects or people, it is important to look at attempts by some authors to expand this concept to other spatialities and also to time.

What Moves? Non-Human Actors

Dix *et al.* argue that concepts of mobility need not be related only with mobility of human actors, although they recognise that humans and objects differ in terms of aspects like auto-propelled mobility, will and purpose (Dix, 2000). While their proposed taxonomy is actually aimed at mapping the mobility of computing devices/"software agents," encompassing objects and virtual entities, through both physical and virtual spaces it may be useful in understanding other IT actors, like desktop PCs, mobile computers, and software applications, that may be encountered by people in their work. In addition, although the remaining content of this section will focus more on developing concepts of human mobility, non-human actors' mobility is still important since humans, by their actions (movement in physical space, relationships interaction, and "cyberspace" navigation by use of online resources), may also move non-human actors. This is one of the ways in which Dix *et al.* suggest that devices can become mobile the other is when devices move under the control of certain inbuilt programs. They propose that a device can be classified as (Dix, 2000, p. 298):

- *fixed* - the device is not mobile at all (e.g., a terminal fixed in a particular location);
- *mobile* - may be moved by others (e.g., a PDA or wearable computer that is carried around);
- *autonomous* - may move under its own control (e.g., a robot).

As the device use may be influenced by its surroundings, they suggest that it is also relevant to consider the relationship between a given device and other devices or its environment. Accordingly, a device may fall into one of 3 categories:

- *free* - the computational device is independent of other devices, and its functionality is essentially self-contained.
- *embedded* - the device is part of a larger device
- *pervasive* - the functionality provided by the device is essentially spread throughout the environment.

Lastly, they suggest that devices need to be considered with regards to the extent to which it is bound to a particular individual or group. In this respect they can be:

- *personal* - the device is primarily focused on supporting one person
- *group* - the device supports members of a group such as a team
- *public*- the device is available to a wide group

Non-human objects are often moved between humans for a variety of purposes. While sending an object to someone by post for example would be included in this category, understanding that objects also move between people working in collaboration, often within short ranges is equally important. Luff and Heath present a view of objects' *micro-mobility* (Luff & Heath, 1998) as: *"the way in which the artefact may be mobilised and manipulated for various purposes around a relatively circumscribed, or "at hand" domain."* An example is a paper-based medical record that is used for both synchronous and asynchronous collaboration between both doctors and other professionals, and between the patient and the doctor, or a tablet PC manipulated over an exam room table desk between the physician and the patient. Micro-mobility refers to the interpersonal manipulation between at least two people: *local and detailed uses of objects-in-interaction..."* (Luff & Heath, 1998, p. 313) and thus it presupposes some sort of social interaction between the two (or more) people involved in manipulating the object, even if these interactions do not occur simultaneously. This seems important as *the way objects are moved, when or how fast, for example also transmits information about its contents or the nature of the relationship between those involved.* An example would be when a paper folder is dropped at someone's desk with a brisk movement and no introductory comment. The contextual nature captured by the concept of micro-mobility, thus allows it to be used not only to explore the movement of objects over short range, in frequent interactions, but also to capture some of the social intricacies of manipulating objects.

Table 2. Summary of constructs for analysing space and mobility in the workplace

	Physical Arena	Social Arena
Concepts related with space	Space Workplace	Space as regions Space as Networks
Concepts of Mobility	Physical mobility	Contextual mobility
Taxonomy Modalities of mobility	Remote *versus* Local Modalities of travelling/ visiting/wandering Micro-mobility	Dislocation to/from – "sense of belonging" Dislocation within - Changes in social position in relation to others and to the core of the region or hubs in the network

Space and Mobility: Summary of Analytical Constructs

Table 2 presents a summary of all concepts discussed about space and mobility and which may be useful to study spatial and mobility patterns of work. Not only do these concepts allow a careful consideration of the spatial characteristics of medical work, they also allow us to look at different modalities of mobility that may be involved as doctors carry out their work. This is important as technology, namely ICT, has been suggested as possibly affecting both the physical and social arenas of the spatial organization of work. In addition, MICT devices, have their own mobility modalities, that may correspond, or not, with that of human actors. Esbjörnsson (Esbjörnsson & Vesterlind, 2002) argues that the degree of correspondence may be related to usage levels and the perceived adequacy of these devices.

CONCLUSION

Main conclusions should be highlighted:

1. Understanding the different conceptualizations of time is very important for software design and application adaptability creation in order to secure best fit to existing work and social practices.
2. Expanding the notion that time episodes in practice are not just regulated by chronology and clock time, which is critical for more

dynamic application designs—not just for Mobile ICT usage but also equally for fixed desktop computing.

3. Mobility concepts are useful for the architecture of solutions in complex and dynamic work environments since, although the most significant difference between MICT and desktop-based ICT is the fact that the computing devices can move while retaining connectivity to networks, it is MICT ability to merge uneventfully with existing mobility practices that renders it acceptable for usage.

REFERENCES

Bardram, J. E., & Bossen, C. (2003). Moving to get ahead: Local mobility and collaborative work. In *Proceedings of the Eighth European Conference on Computer Supported Cooperative Work*. Helsinki, Finland: Kluwer Academic Publishers.

Bellotti, V., & Bly, S. (1996). Walking away from the desktop computer: Distributed collaboration and mobility in a product design team. In *Proceedings of ACM 1996 Conference on Computer Supported Cooperative Work*. ACM Press.

Benabou, C. (1999). Polychronicity and temporal dimensions of work in learning organizations. *Journal of Managerial Psychology, 14*(3/4), 257–268. doi:10.1108/02683949910263792

Bluedorn, A. C., & Denhardt, R. B. (1988). Time and organizations. *Journal of Management, 14*(2), 299–320. doi:10.1177/014920638801400209

Bluedorn, A. C., Kalliath, T. J., Strube, M. J., & Martin, G. D. (1999). Polychronicity and the inventory of polychronic values (IPV): The development of an instrument to measure a fundamental dimension in organizational culture. *Journal of Managerial Psychology, 14*(3/4), 205–230. doi:10.1108/02683949910263747

Castells, M. (1996). The information age: Economy, society and culture: *Vol. I. The rise of the network society*. Oxford, UK: Blackwell Publisher.

Dix, A. (2000). Exploiting space and location as a design framework for interactive mobile systems. *ACM Transactions on Computer-Human Interaction, 7*(3), 285–321. doi:10.1145/355324.355325

Esbjörnsson, M., & Vesterlind, D. (2002). *Mobility and social spatiality*. Paper presented at the Workshop Transforming Spaces: The Topological Turn in Technology Studies. Darmstadt, Germany.

Escobar, A. (2001). Culture sits in places: Reflections on globalism and subaltern strategies of localization. *Political Geography, 20*, 139–174. doi:10.1016/S0962-6298(00)00064-0

George, J. M., & Jones, G. R. (2000). The role of time in theory and theory building. *Journal of Management, 26*(4), 657–684.

Giddens, A. (1984). *The constitution of society*. Cambridge, UK: Polity Press.

Giddens, A. (1990). *The consequences of modernity*. Palo Alto, CA: Stanford University Press.

Graham, S. (1998). The end of geography or the explosion of place? Conceptualizing space, place and information technology. *Progress in Human Geography, 22*(2), 165–185. doi:10.1191/030913298671334137

Green, N. (2002). On the move: Technology, mobility, and the mediation of social time and space. *The Information Society, 18*, 281–292. doi:10.1080/01972240290075129

Hall, E. T. (1983). *The dance of life: The other dimension of time*. Garden City, NY: Anchor Press.

Harrison, S., & Dourish, P. (1996). Re-place-ing space: The roles of place and space in collaborative systems. In *Proceedings of CSCW 1996*. Cambridge, MA: ACM Press.

Harvey, D. (1989). *The Condition of postmodernity*. Oxford, UK: Blackwell.

Kakihara, M., & Sørensen, C. (2002). Mobility: An extended perspective. In *Proceedings of the Hawai's International Conference on System Sciences*. Big Island, Hawaii: IEEE Press.

Kelly, S. E. (2003). Bioethics and rural health: Theorizing place, space, and subjects. *Social Science & Medicine, 56*, 2277–2288. doi:10.1016/S0277-9536(02)00227-7

Kristoffersen, S., & Ljungberg, F. (2000). Mobility: From stationary to mobile work. In Braa, K., Sørensen, C., & Dahlbom, B. (Eds.), *Planet Internet* (pp. 41–64). Lund, Sweden: Studentliteratur.

Lee, H., & Liebenau, J. (1999). Time in organizational studies: Towards a new research direction. *Organization Studies, 20*(6), 1035–1058. doi:10.1177/0170840699206006

Luff, P., & Heath, C. (1998). Mobility in collaboration. In *Proceedings of ACM 1998 Conference on Computer Supported Cooperative Work*. Seattle, WA: ACM Press.

Martins, H. M. G., Nightingale, P., & Jones, M. R. (2005). *Any time, any place? Temporal and spatial organisation of doctors' computer usage in a UK hospital department*. Paper presented at the Healthcare Computing Conference. Harrogate, UK.

Mol, A., & Law, J. (1994). Regions, networks and fluids: Anaemia and social topology. *Social Studies of Science, 24,* 641–671. doi:10.1177/030631279402400402

Orlikowski, W. J., & Yates, J. (2002). It's about time: Temporal structuring in organizations. *Organization Science, 13*(6), 684–700. doi:10.1287/orsc.13.6.684.501

Perry, M., O'Hara, K., Sellen, A., Brown, B., & Harper, R. (2001). Dealing with mobility: Understanding access anytime, anywhere. *ACM Transactions on Computer-Human Interaction, 8*(4), 323–347. doi:10.1145/504704.504707

Strauss, A. L., Shizuko, F., Sucker, B., & Wiener, C. (1997). *Social organization of medical work.* New Brunswick, NJ: Transaction Publisher.

Taussig, K. S. (1997). Calvinism and chromosomes: Religion, the geograpical imaginary, and medical genetics in the Netherlands. *Science as Culture, 4*(29), 495–524. doi:10.1080/09505439709526483

Westbrook, J. I., Gosling, A. S., & Coiera, E. (2004). Do clinicians use online evidence to support patient care? A study of 55.000 clinicians. *Journal of the American Medical Informatics Association, 11*(2), 113–120. doi:10.1197/jamia. M1385

Chapter 7
mHealth:
A Passing Fad or Here to Stay?

Mowafa Househ
King Saud Bin Abdul Aziz University for Health Sciences, Saudi Arabia

Elizabeth Borycki
University of Victoria, Canada

Andre Kushniruk
University of Victoria, Canada

Sarah Alofaysan
King Saud Bin Abdul Aziz University for Health Sciences, Saudi Arabia

ABSTRACT

The mHealth field focuses on the use of mobile technologies to support hospital care, healthy behavior, patient monitoring, and educational awareness. It is a new field that is developing rapidly, with thousands of mHealth applications developed within the last two years alone. In this chapter, the authors discuss the current state of, and the opportunities and challenges within, the mHealth field. They also introduce the term Mobile Social Networking Healthcare (MSN-Healthcare), which they define as follows: "The use of mobile health applications that incorporate social networking tools to promote healthy behaviors and awareness among patient groups and communities." This concept has not been introduced in previous literature. This chapter is organized as follows: 1) introduction and background of mHealth; 2) opportunities for the implementation of mHealth in relation to chronic disease management, the education of health professionals, the needs of health professionals, and the decision-making process for patients and clinicians; 3) challenges concerning implementation and usability, information needs, and interactions with clinical work; 4) current application uses; and 5) future trends and conclusion.

INTRODUCTION

mHealth is a developing field that refers to the use of mobile information and communication technologies in healthcare. The universal use of mobile communication technologies within developed and developing countries makes it an economical and feasible solution in a healthcare environment. Current figures show that approximately five billion people utilize cellular phones around the world (Central Intelligence Agency, 2011), which is equivalent to 70% of the world

DOI: 10.4018/978-1-4666-0888-7.ch007

population (U.S. Census Bureau, 2011). Therefore, the potential for health education, training and awareness, remote monitoring, diagnostic treatment, communication between patients and providers, and epidemic outbreak tracking is further accentuated by the pervasive use of mobile health technologies around the world (Vital Wave Consulting, 2009).

In 2009, the United Nation's Vodafone Foundation Partnership produced a report showcasing over fifty mHealth projects from around the world. The report suggests that for mHealth to be successful, multi-sector collaboration between private and public enterprises is needed. Over the last couple of years, such partnerships have transpired and can be seen in today's conferences. For example, in 2010, mHealth summits were held in Washington, D.C. and Dubai, UAE. In 2011, several conferences will have been hosted mainly in the U.S. as well as in other parts of the world. These conferences provide opportunities for community members to network, collaborate, and exchange ideas concerning mHealth. The proliferation of such conferences and reports demonstrates the growing importance of this domain.

As with every new technology, there is a great deal of excitement concerning the potential of mHealth. It is our belief, however, that the benefits and challenges of mHealth need to be carefully evaluated. Researchers, policy makers, and individuals within technological organizations are trying to understand the potential of this field for patient care. There is much to learn about mHealth to determine if it is just another fad or a technology that is here to stay. Within this context, the purpose of this chapter is to provide policy makers, hospitals, clinicians, and academics with a more objective understanding of the opportunities, challenges, and benefits of mHealth.

Like previous innovations in health care, there are several factors can influence innovation within any field. In a paper describing the dissemination of innovation within healthcare, based on Everett Rogers's study concerning the diffusion of innovation, Berwick (2003) discussed three basic clusters that influence the spread of change within any institution. These three basic clusters are as follows: 1) the perceptions of the innovation; 2) the characteristics of the individuals who adopt the innovation; and 3) contextual factors such as leadership, incentives, or management. Berwick argues that innovation is used by individuals when it is perceived to benefit them. In time, the majority will follow suit in adopting the new innovation. Therefore, how healthcare policies and organizations support those early mHealth adopters will influence mHealth adoption within healthcare. In our opinion, the current state of mHealth adoption is in the early stages. The future level of mHealth adoption within healthcare will depend on factors such as its usefulness to clinicians and the consumer; support from healthcare organizations and the health informatics community; and the potential for companies to make a profit in the area.

This chapter focuses on the current state, opportunities, and challenges of the mHealth field. The organization of the book chapter is as follows: 1) a background section on mHealth; 2) opportunities for the implementation of mHealth in relation to chronic disease management, the education of health professionals, the needs of health professionals, and the decision-making process for patients and clinicians are described; 3) challenges concerning implementation and usability, information needs and interactions with clinical work; 4) summary of current application uses; and 5) future trends and conclusion.

BACKGROUND

In 2000, *unwired e-med* was the term used to describe what practitioners in the field refer to today as mHealth (Laxminarayan & Istepanian, 2000). It was not until 2003 that the authors Istepanian and Lacal coined the term mHealth and defined it as follows: "emerging mobile communications and network technologies for healthcare systems" (Istepanian, et al., 2006, p. 3; Istepanian & Lacal, 2003). Several comparable definitions have emerged since that time (Vital Wave Consulting, 2009; Knowledge for Health Organization, 2011; Mechael & Slonininsky, 2008).

With the growing importance of mHealth within the field of health informatics, recent debates about its place within the field have emerged. For example, the World Health Organization (WHO) and the United Nation Foundation depict mHealth as a subset of health informatics, which is an overarching definition related to the "use of information and communication technology for health" (Vital Wave Consulting, 2009; Mechael & Slonininsky, 2008). Other authors, however, have asserted that mHealth is a domain that is independent of health informatics due to its unique mass media potential, which can be used for the well-being of patients and potentially improving healthcare service delivery. As with any new field of research, such debates do occur. However, because mHealth is a relatively new research domain with insufficient evidence to demonstrate its effectiveness (Mechael & Slonininsky, 2008), we believe it is more important to focus on evaluating the impacts of mobile devices on health care service delivery, patient care, and health outcomes, rather than engage in unnecessary debates.

Furthermore, we classify mHealth as a subset of the health informatics domain, which, according to the Canadian Health Informatics Association (COACH), "involves the application of information technology to facilitate the creation and use of health related data, information and knowledge" (Canadian Health Informatics Association, 2011). We use this definition because it is an overarching definition of the various sub-disciplines within the health informatics domain, which we believe includes mHealth. This perspective is not meant to degrade the field, but rather place it within the context of an evolutionary process that its predecessors such as telemedicine have followed. We believe that defining mHealth in such a way

will provide for more lasting credibility in the field, encourage health informaticians to pursue mHealth research, and help garner the support of health informatics organizations. In the end, this will help the discipline of mHealth evolve into a recognizable and researchable sub-discipline within the overarching domain of health informatics.

Although there are emerging debates within the field, the potential benefits of mHealth are apparent. In the developing world, the WHO, the United Nations, and the National Institutes of Health (NIH) are promoting mHealth. For instance, in 2008, the United Nations Foundation, in association with Vodafone, produced a report outlining the role of mHealth in achieving the following three United Nations health millennium goals (Mechael & Slonininsky, 2008; United Nations, 2008):

- Reduce child mortality: reduce by two-thirds between 1990 and 2015
- Improve maternal health: reduce the maternal mortality ratio by three-fourths between 1990 and 2015
- Combat HIV/AIDS, malaria, and other diseases: halt the spread of these diseases by 2015 and then begin to reverse the spread of HIV/AIDS and the incidence of malaria and other major diseases

The United Nation's Vodaphone report discusses various projects that have been conducted in the developing world related to education and awareness of diseases, remote data collection, remote monitoring, communication with and training of health care workers, disease and epidemic outbreak tracking, and diagnostic and treatment support in relation to the millennium goals.

For example, the report outlines details of the Masilulke and Text to Change projects, which have been successful in utilizing Short-Message Service (SMS) for HIV/AIDS education. The educational awareness interventions included

SMS-based quizzes that were designed to encourage testing and counseling for HIV/AIDS. The report also outlines details of another project in Uganda where healthcare workers were given Personal Digital Assistant (PDAs) to collect health information within the field from a variety of ill patients. There were significant cost savings of 25% and increased job satisfaction with the ease and usefulness of the mHealth technology. For remote monitoring, Tuberculosis (TB) patients living in Thailand were provided with mobile phones. Healthcare workers called patients and reminded them to take their prescription medications. As a result of this intervention, medication compliance rates rose as high as 90%. More recently, an article in The Economist on mobile phone use in the developing world reports that new mHealth services are being used in Africa for drug safety, processing real-time information on illnesses, and helping healthcare workers gather information on newborns (Economist, 2011). These examples are only some of the examples of successful mHealth technologies that have been used in the developing world.

For years in the developed continents of Europe, North America, Australia and the country of Japan, mHealth technologies have been used in a variety of healthcare settings. A systematic review performed by Fjeldsoe et al. (2009), focusing on behavioral change interventions delivered by mobile phone SMS, reported that SMS interventions had positive behavioral outcomes related to preventative health behaviors (smoking cessation, physical activity, anti-obesity behavior modification) and clinical care studies (diabetes self-management, asthma self-management, hypertension medication compliance, and bulimia nervosa outpatient care). Other studies in the developed world have focused on the use of mHealth technology for health promotion. For example, a recent Australian study on the use of text messaging in relation to educational interventions for sexual health promotion found that the intervention yielded positive results (Gold, et al.,

2010). The authors reported that their positive, short, and relevant messages provided useful information to the participants, which helped them remember existing information and reduced their apprehension about getting tested for sexually transmitted diseases. Another recently published Australian study focused on the attitudes of patients concerning the use of mobile phones to monitor and manage depression, anxiety, and stress. The authors reported that patients were willing to use mobile phones to manage their health as long as their privacy and security were protected and the programs were easy to use (Parker, et al., 2010).

In summary, there is a significant potential for mHealth technologies in the developing and developed world to improve healthcare services and patient care. Most of the studies on mHealth, however, have focused on the developing world, and for good reason (Mechael & Slonininsky, 2008). In the developed world, receiving high quality health care services is a privilege that most citizens enjoy. Within the developing world, the quality of healthcare services is lacking. Because of the pervasive use of mobile technologies, healthcare institutions and workers can now reach the general public to promote and manage healthcare service delivery as outlined in the following quote:

In many parts of the world, epidemics and a shortage of healthcare workers continue to present grave challenges for governments and health providers. Yet in these same places, the explosive growth of mobile communications over the past decade offers a new hope for the promotion of quality healthcare. Among those who had previously been left behind by the 'digital divide,' billions now have access to reliable technology. There is a growing body of evidence that demonstrates the potential of mobile communications to radically improve healthcare services—even in some of the most remote and resource-poor environments [Qtd. In Vital Wave Consulting]

The proliferation and adoption of mobile phone technologies within the developing world has created an opportunity for governments and healthcare institutions to reach millions of people who otherwise would have been out of reach. Even though many of the studies today in both the developed and developing world focus on mobile phones as a primary mHealth intervention, it is only one of the many mHealth technologies in use today. mHealth technologies are classified into the following categories (Mechael & Slonininsky, 2008):

1. Mobile Phones: technological communication devices that connect to wireless communication networks through radio or satellite transmissions. Much of the mobile phone use today in both the developing and developed world is based on SMS text messaging services (The Economist, 2006).

2. Smart Phones: mobile phones with advanced features such as Wi-Fi capability, touch screens, Bluetooth, and QWERTY (Standard English computer keyboard) (Nusca, 2009). The Apple iPhone is an example of a smart phone. Today, they are primarily used to access, input, and process healthcare information. They are also used for educational purposes.

3. Mobile Telehealth Devices: stand-alone technology or an add-on to a mobile or smart phone. They help clinicians observe and diagnose patients on a more regular basis through constant patient monitoring.

4. MP3 Players: a technology that carries large amounts of data in the form of sound and video. An example of such a technology is the Apple iPod. Such technologies can disseminate health information in the form of sound files or sound with video (e.g., podcasts), but they have not been widely used within the healthcare community.

5. Mobile Computing: focuses on both software and hardware that allow individuals to access network services anytime and anywhere. The Apple iPad is an example of mobile computing hardware with thousands of software applications available for its users. Many of the current applications for mobile computing devices focus on education, clinical practice guidelines, podcasts, electronic medical records, and other health-related applications. Mobile computing unites MP3, mobile telehealth devices, and smart phones into one cohesive device.

With the advent of the various forms of mHealth technologies, there is a growing need, in both the developed and developing world, to understand the potential impacts of mHealth on healthcare service delivery and health outcomes. However, this chapter does not focus on evaluating the impacts of mHealth on health service delivery and health outcomes; given the novelty of this domain, we believe such analyses are premature. Instead, we specifically explore the opportunities for mHealth in relation to chronic disease management; the education of healthcare professionals; the needs of and the ability to communicate with healthcare professionals; and the decision-making process for patients. We believe that these are currently the relevant issues. This chapter also examines some of the challenges that have not been discussed in detail in the literature, such as issues concerning usability, the information needs of clinicians and interactions with clinical work. We also review some of the current applications for mobile computing because we believe much of the future investment in mHealth will focus on this particularly growing area (Mechael & Slonininsky, 2008). In summary, exploring this new and emerging field and providing insight into the current state, opportunities, and challenges within this domain are the motivations behind this chapter.

OPPORTUNITIES FOR mHEALTH

As the field of mHealth begins to take shape, there are several areas in which mHealth can make a difference. Specifically, we believe these include chronic disease management; the education of healthcare professionals; the needs of and the ability to communicate with healthcare professionals; and the support indecision-making process.

Chronic Disease Management

Chronic diseases, such as heart disease, diabetes, cancer, and asthma, are the major causes of death and disability worldwide (World Health Organization, 2011). In 2005 alone, an estimated 35 million people died from chronic diseases (World Health Organization, 2011b). In Canada, which is one of the leading countries in healthcare service delivery, 89% of all deaths are the result of a chronic disease, and an estimated 231,000 (and growing) people die each year (World Health Organization, 2011). Other disturbing statistics published by the World Bank show that chronic disease, especially heart disease will become the top killer in South Asian countries (Mason, 2011). The Director of the Center for Chronic Disease Control in India summarized the global risks due to globalization and economic transition as follows:

It took almost 200 years for the U.S. and the U.K. to reach this high state of cardiac disease, which

we are reaching in 40 or 50 years or so because of the rapid economic transition that's occurring, and all the other changes that are happening within one's life span.

The causes of chronic disease are known and can be prevented (World Health Organization, 2011). Research shows that there are socioeconomic, cultural, political, and environmental factors such as globalization, urbanization and aging populations that are increasing the risk of chronic disease development (see Figure 1). In addition, there are common modifiable (unhealthy diet, physical inactivity, tobacco use) and non-modifiable (age and heredity) risk factors that can lead to intermediate chronic disease risk factors such as elevated blood pressure, elevated blood glucose, high cholesterol, and being overweight or obese. Over time, any combination of these factors can lead to heart disease, stroke, cancer, chronic respiratory disease, and diabetes. According to researchers, however, approximately 80%, of premature heart disease, type 2 diabetes and stroke, as well as 40% all incidences of cancer, can be prevented through regular exercise, the avoidance of tobacco products, and a healthy diet (World Health Organization, 2011). Figure 1 illustrates the risk factors that can cause chronic disease.

Figure 1. World Health Organization factors that can cause chronic disease (World Health Organization, 2011)

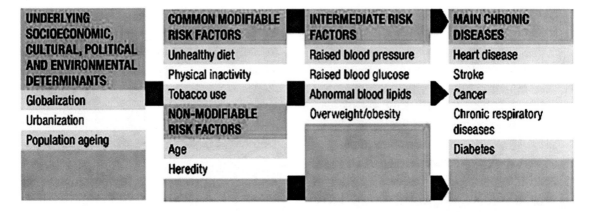

To combat this growing problem, the WHO has set a worldwide goal of reducing deaths from chronic disease by 2% annually. This reduction will improve global standards of living and save billions of dollars worldwide (World Health Organization, 2011). mHealth has been identified as an intervention that can assist the WHO in reaching its target (Lyall, 2010). Regrettably, the mHealth literature on chronic disease prevention and management is scarce, and the existing research has been primarily focused on text messaging (SMS) interventions. For example, a 2009 systematic review that focused on behavioral change interventions delivered through mobile phones revealed that out of 33 studies, only 14 studies met the inclusion criteria. Four of the studies focused on preventative behaviors, such as exercise, healthy eating, and smoking cessation. The remaining 10 studies focused on management of diabetes, hypertension, and asthma. The results of the systematic review were interesting in that it showed promising results in relation to altering short-term behavioral outcomes. The review also mentioned the need to improve the quality of the studies within this domain.

mHealth applications for the Apple iPad and iPhone that can help with the growing problems relating to chronic disease are being created at a rapid pace. According to a recent article by Mobile Health News, over 200 new Apple iPhone and iPad chronic disease management and prevention applications were launched between February and September of 2010. Over 50% of these applications focused on diabetes management. Only a few applications made the top 1,000 of the most widely used applications (Lyall, 2010). Other reports claim that by the year 2014, the dollars spent on chronic disease management, especially when it involves patient monitoring, will increase to $2 billion. Over 50% of the investment will be in heart disease management, followed by other chronic diseases, such as asthma, COPD, and diabetes (Cox, 2010). These developments will help generate awareness about the importance of mHealth technologies in the prevention and management of chronic disease.

In summary, there are many opportunities for policy makers, healthcare organizations, and academics to invest in mHealth applications to prevent and manage chronic disease. The mHealth field, specifically when it comes to chronic diseases, is still in the pilot phase. It is clear, however, that more mHealth software applications and technologies are being created in this area. Early indications show that the opportunities for mHealth to influence how chronic diseases are managed will continue to be promising.

Health Professional Education and Patient Education

Health Professional Education

A recent whitepaper on the summary of the global mHealth market from 2010 to 2015 reported that patient education and the education of healthcare professionals are becoming important areas of growth (Research2Guidance, 2010). In the past, face-to-face, telephone conferencing, video conferencing, and web-conferencing have been important technological tools for the education of both patients and healthcare professionals. To illustrate, Lau and Hayward (2000) employed a variety of technologies in a virtual network to promote education for healthcare professionals. The investigators recruited 25 healthcare professionals from 17 different Canadian regions to participate in a seven-week training program designed to develop skills in health policy, management, economics, research methods, data analysis, and computer technology. The subjects had access to a variety of technologies (web-conferencing, e-mail, newsgroups, document management, and internet access) that enabled the development of skills, the sharing information, and the ability to communicate and collaborate with one another. After analyzing their research results, the authors offered 10 recommendations for building successful professional education virtual networks. The building of relationships through support and the inclusion of external members in such networks can lead to greater information exchange, greater exchange of ideas, improved problem solving, and counseling support for decision-making groups. The authors noted that the technologies were especially helpful for groups working in remote communities because it helped foster communication linkages and information exchange with members in other areas.

Another study published in 2003 focused on the use of video conferencing for Continuing Medical Education (CME) in practice-based small groups. The study evaluated the feasibility, acceptability, effectiveness, and costs of the small group CME model through video conferencing. The study found that video conferencing was generally accepted by the participants in the study, although there were issues with audio and video quality (Allen, Sargeant, Mann, Fleming, Premi, 2003). These two studies are examples of the many types of technologies used within the health professional educational community.

Only recently has there been a growing interest in mHealth for the education of healthcare professionals. For the past 10 years, the medical faculty at the University of Pittsburgh has worked on the construction of the Global Health Network Super course Project. The project contains over 4,500 online lectures with over 50,000 participants from 174 countries (Linkov, LaPorte, Padilla, & Shubnikov, 2010). The project has employed a variety of internet-based methods for the education and recruitment of experts on cancer from around the world. The project has recently started to use mHealth technologies, such as mobile phones and smart phones, for educational purposes. The project uses SMS to send educational messages to its users. Mobile computers and smart phones can access their vast educational multi-media network. There is a dearth of available research focused on mHealth relative to the education of healthcare professionals. However, a growing

number of technological applications are being developed for this field. The future holds much promise for mHealth within this particular domain.

Patient Education

According to the U.S. Department of Health and Human Services, patient education is a key component of healthcare delivery services, especially when it comes to the management and prevention of disease (U.S. Department of Health and Human Services, 1996). This can be defined as a process whereby the patient takes on the responsibility of engaging in preventative behavior while communicating with the clinician throughout the care process (U.S. Department of Health and Human Services, 1996). The objective of patient education is to modify patient behavior in order to improve their overall health. According to the literature, patient education has been most effective in behavioral health changes relating to weight control, use of contraceptives, and encouraging exercise. Most of the studies, however, have focused on compliance with medication and preventative therapeutic regimens (U.S. Department of Health and Human Services, 1996). Some of the patient education services offered at major healthcare organizations such as the Canadian University Health Network (UHN) are:

- Preparing patients and families for surgical, medical and diagnostic procedures
- Helping patients and their families manage their diseases and conditions
- Supporting patients in making informed decisions concerning their health and health care (UHN, 2011)

Some of the UHN patient education materials are currently offered through the internet and through the in-hospital computer multi-media system. However, these services are not currently offered through mobile technologies (UHN, 2011). Similarly, other institutions such as St.

Jude Children's Research Hospital in Memphis, Tennessee, are internationally recognized for their patient education website, which is centered upon pediatric oncology and other catastrophic diseases (St. Jude Children's Research Hospital, 2011). The website offers high quality content such as games, brochures, multimedia presentations and other materials to support patient education. However, these services are not currently offered through mobile technologies (St. Jude Children's Research Hospital, 2011).

Only recently has there been a growing interest in conducting research on the impact of mHealth technologies on patient education, especially concerning health prevention and disease management. A review study that analyzed the impact of various technologies, including mobile phones, on diabetes patient education found that mHealth technologies improved the frequency of educational interactions between the patient and healthcare professionals. In their review, only two mHealth studies met their study inclusion criteria. One mHealth study included in the review, "Sweet Talk," used the text messaging educational information that was based on social cognitive theory. The program provides reminders, user feedback, and information and tips on self-management tasks, such as diet, exercise, blood glucose testing and how to inject insulin. The other study focused on the use of SMS and General Packet Radio Service (GPRS). GPRS allows for a greater volume of shared data that can be used with multi-media presentations and other applications, for data collection and for the educational support of diabetic patients. While the mHealth studies improved patient education, the authors suggested that more mHealth research is needed (Adams, et al., 2011).

A recent article published in the New England Journal of Medicine studied the use of the telephone as a device to improve clinician and patient communication and to improve patient satisfaction with preventative healthcare services (Wennberg, et al, 2010). In this stratified, randomized study comprising 174,120 participants, subjects were assigned to a coached educational support group or a non-coached patient support group. Both groups used the telephone to communicate. The study found that after one year, medical costs and hospital admissions were significantly reduced. In another patient education study, a healthcare organization sent text messages to dermatology patients for both educational and medication reminder purposes. The study found that there were significant improvements in patient health outcomes as a result of the mHealth intervention (McGee, 2010).

In summary, mHealth education for both patients and healthcare professionals shows promise. However, more studies are needed to determine the impacts of mHealth interventions on health outcomes over time. This can be accomplished through further research on and the evaluation of the new mHealth patient and health professional education software and hardware technologies that are currently being developed.

MEETING HEALTH PROFESSIONAL INFORMATION NEEDS AND SUPPORTING DECISION-MAKING

An important issue for health professionals (e.g., physicians, nurses, physiotherapists, occupational therapists, and social workers) is the ability to access information as needed from any location at any time. For healthcare professionals, the ability to retrieve information as needed is important because the quality of decision-making may suffer in its absence (Borycki, et al., 2009a). Since the introduction of computers into healthcare settings, such as hospitals, clinics and home care settings, healthcare professionals have shown that portable devices can be useful in providing evidence-based information. Portable devices allow clinicians to access a patient's health-related information (e.g., laboratory and diagnostic imaging test results) at any time and location. The devices are also useful in the decision-making process. Such information supports the informational requirements of healthcare professionals and also assists in the decision-making process concerning both treatments and interventions (Honeybourne, et al., 2006).

In hospitals around the world, healthcare professionals employ information technology as a means of creating mental models of both patients and the organizations where patients receive care. A mental model of a patient enables healthcare professionals to understand the nature of the patient's condition and more closely monitor the patient for any deterioration or improvement in their condition in response to treatment and intervention. Healthcare professionals must also have an understanding of the organization (e.g., hospital) where the patient is located, so the healthcare professional can monitor the organizational processes that provide the information used in patient care-related decision-making (Borycki, et al., 2009a, 2009b). For example, a physician who orders an urgent lab or diagnostic imaging test at a particular institution needs to know how quickly the results will be available. The physician can then check for test results using mHealth to remotely access the patient's electronic health record at the appropriate time. When the test is completed and the physician receives the information, the physician can then make timely decisions concerning treatment, especially in cases where urgent care is required. In organizations that have focused their information technology strategies upon computer work stations healthcare professionals are tethered to a single location within the healthcare facility even though they may be needed elsewhere (Shortliffe & Ciminio, 2006). In organizations that have implemented wireless carts, research has shown that the mobility of the clinician can be impaired because the wireless carts can be cumbersome or difficult to move from one location to another or into a patient's room (Koppel, Wetterneck, Telles & Karsh, 2008).

mHealth has been introduced as a solution to many of these problems, providing healthcare professionals with ubiquitous real-time access to information via light weight devices that can be moved throughout a health care facility. For the healthcare professional, this means having their informational needs met at any time at any location in the form of ubiquitous and seamless access to information via mHealth wireless devices: (a) clinicians can access information concerning evidence-based treatment approaches and interventions (Honeybourne, et al., 2006) and (b) they can access information concerning the patient's current health status (Borycki, et al. 2009b). mHealth devices are now used by health professionals to search for information to support decision-making (i.e., drug-related information or information from the latest research article) (Honeybourne, et al., 2006). In addition, mHealth supports decision making through alerts and reminders that appear on the mobile device about specific patients and their conditions. mHealth also has the capacity to remotely monitor patients through their devices (e.g., cell phones, smart phones) by connecting data from sensors on the patient with data monitoring centers. Some of this preliminary work on the remote monitoring of patients suggests that such advanced patient support capabilities can be disseminated on a large scale using mHealth. mHealth is a very new phenomenon in terms of its use in healthcare settings to support healthcare professional information needs. A number of projects are currently underway to determine how access to 2D images or video transmissions (e.g., ultrasound images) during patient emergencies via mobile devices would affect patient outcomes (Kyriacou, et al. 2009). In addition, allowing patients remote access to their own data through mHealth will change the way that healthcare is deployed. For example, Personal Health Records (PHRs) allow patients and ordinary citizens to review their own patient data and to electronically receive advice and support. Such applications are becoming increasingly available using smart phones and tablet PCs for access to key information (such as patient allergies) at any time or location. Work is currently underway to determine the best methods and approaches for providing support for such real-time decision making (in the form of guidelines and patient alerts and reminders) to health professionals and patients alike.

More research is needed to determine the effectiveness of using this approach to support health professional decision making during patient emergencies. Furthermore, research is needed to determine if providing information in real-time will have an effect upon patient outcomes. Lastly, there is a need to explore how the form of the mHealth device impacts the decision making of healthcare professionals. Research conducted by Kushniruk et al. (2005) suggested that mHealth devices must be rigorously tested to determine if screen size has an impact upon the ability of the device to convey sufficient information to the healthcare professional to support decision-making rather than to introduce new types of errors arising from the attributes of the technology. For example, some of the results of this research suggest that mHealth device screen size may influence the rate of medical errors for some types of activities. In the future, as the number of mHealth devices used in healthcare settings (e.g., hospitals) grows, mHealth applications should be developed to support the communication and exchange of information between members of the healthcare team. Much of the research on mHealth has focused on the initial usage of mHealth devices by patients. Future research should analyze the impact of real-time wireless ubiquitous access upon team and inter-professional work to determine how mHealth may affect healthcare professional teamwork. Researchers should study patient care processes and outcomes to analyze the changes that arise from the introduction of mHealth devices. mHealth has the potential to provide considerable support to the healthcare professional (e.g., physician and nurse) through real-time access to information related to patient care. Research is needed to better understand the potential benefits

and pitfalls of the technology, where patient care processes and outcomes are concerned and where mHealth may support inter-professional work.

CHALLENGES AND ISSUES WITH mHEALTH

The possibilities for integrating mHealth into complex healthcare practices depend upon the convergence and integration of health information technologies into a complex networked healthcare environment. There are two dimensions to mHealth: the technical dimension and the human dimension. The technical developments concerning mHealth are proceeding extremely well with a subsequent rapid decrease in cost, an increase in global coverage, and an increase in the number of applications available to the users of mHealth. From a technical perspective, this has included the widespread use of wireless networks, remote monitoring, the widespread uptake of mobile technologies and an increase in the potential for connecting remote devices to centralized high-performance computing centers (e.g., for conducting remote analysis of a patient's health needs or condition via mHealth). Despite this incredible potential, there are a number of challenges and obstacles that must be addressed before mHealth becomes routinely integrated into the work of healthcare professionals and patient health care (Kushniruk & Borycki, 2007). Perhaps the greatest challenge to the integration of mHealth into the complex medical and healthcare professional workflow is the "human factor." As mHealth applications saturate the market with stand-alone apps that can be used by both patients and healthcare professionals (a number of which are described in the latter part of this chapter), the need to integrate and connect mHealth to more complex systems and technological advances that are occurring at a national and global level will become critical. One central technology that mHealth must become integrated with is the Electronic Health Record

(EHR). The EHR is an electronic repository of patient data that will allow for entry and retrieval of data electronically as well as integration with technologies such as decision support and the interoperable sharing of health data. Central to this integration will be the need to improve our understanding of complex work activities and practices to design mHealth applications that fit seamlessly into and support the complex activities involved in health care. The initial attempt to integrate mHealth with electronic health record indicates that there are a number of limitations to current approaches (Chen, et al., 2003). The more complex activities of healthcare practice (e.g., providing support for medication administration in complex work environments) were more difficult to support through the use of mobile smart phone applications compared to other stand-alone health-related activities. Indeed, as mHealth applications become more pervasive, an improved understanding of how they will fit into complex workflows will be needed.

Methods for testing the usability and practicality of mHealth for complex health processes will require an improved understanding of both user needs and healthcare workflows. An improved evaluation of the use of these technologies will be required. Kushniruk and Borycki (2007) described the adaptation of approaches drawn from usability engineering to analyze mHealth applications that provide a range of support for both healthcare professionals and patients. For example, the heuristic evaluation can assess and predict potential user problems. Usability testing methods allow for both the observation and analysis of users as they interact with mHealth in complex work situations. A more complex analysis involves the development of "clinical simulations," where the testing takes place in either highly realistic situations or within actual clinical settings ("in situ" testing). The issues related to the development of effective mHealth for use by patients and healthcare professionals include the following: (1) the need for the device to be sensitive and aware of the context by the device (in order to provide advice or information that is relevant to the user's current work situation), (2) the need for ease of use and rapid learning of the device functions, (3) the need for appropriate integration into work tasks, and (4) the ability to switch into different modes and modalities of use.

Another major issue in the application of mHealth for use in healthcare settings is security and privacy (Kushniruk & Borycki, 2007). A number of healthcare organizations have found that the current encryption and security approaches for many mHealth applications inadequately protect the privacy and confidentiality of healthcare data. The development of secure data transmission and storage procedures is necessary before mHealth becomes a common feature of the healthcare profession.

THE CURRENT STATE OF APPLICATION USE

Because we live in the midst of a technological revolution, we must become more aware of the technological benefits and how such benefits impact our overall quality of life. In the last five years, there has been a tremendous technological explosion, especially in the field of mobile technologies. The worldwide growth in mobile technology has created a booming market for handheld devices, such as smart phones and tablets. Handheld technologies have affected and influenced business and medical practices as well as professional and individual lifestyles (John, 2011). The integration of the mobile phone technology with an ultra-portable computer, touch screens, browsers, multimedia players, cameras and state-of-the-art applications developed for medicine, physics, general health, languages, social networking, and more has added a great deal of improvement in many aspects. In the medical sector, for example, this integration has given clinicians the capability to amalgamate their medical information and communication resources into one compact handheld device, which makes their professional life much easier. On the other hand, mobile phones with these capabilities would assist the real-time monitoring and handling of personal health as well as increasing the health knowledge base of the society.

The rapid growth in the smart phone and tablet industry is a result of the increased competition in the market to provide consumers with a new generation of well-defined, cost-effective, high performance and easy-to-use handheld devices that are mostly Apple, Android, BlackBerry or Windows based operating systems. There are many prominent handheld devices offer different technical specifications, features, and platforms, such as the Apple iPhone and iPad, Samsung Galaxy Pad, BlackBerry Playbook, and HP Slate, to name just a few. Handheld devices are expected to replace laptops and personal computers due to the widespread adoption of these products by consumers. At the International Consumer Electronic Show, each year cutting-edge technologies are exhibited at the largest annual international technology show in the United States. According to the organizers of the show, "the handhelds and tablets market is expected to be big with more than 80 new tablets in stores later this year" (Consumer Electronic Show, 2011). Clearly, the great competitiveness in the market will increase opportunities for acceptance and implementation of handheld devices as consumers have more choices. The explosion in tablet and smart phone technologies and their widespread acceptance will lead to a similar revolution in handheld applications, especially in the health and medical realms.

The new generation of handhelds and mobile technologies has become increasingly adaptable to the needs and preferences of individuals and professionals. Individually, customized applications are available for installation, and many professionals consider these applications to be individual survival kits. These small applications (or "apps," as they are known) satisfy a wide range of general daily needs such as storing contact information, calculating numbers, or converting currency. In addition to assisting with these tasks, however, applications are now directed toward the more specific needs inherent monitoring individual health care, the management of chronic diseases and the enhancement of communication between patients and their healthcare providers. Most importantly, these handheld devices and applications have the potential to significantly impact the daily work flow of healthcare professionals by saving time and effort as well as increasing the quality of the healthcare outcomes through more accurate decision making. This technology also allows healthcare professionals to access a variety of major medical applications regardless of locations, extending the reach and mobility of healthcare professionals and increases the information accessibility. A recent study shows that 64% of physicians in the United States own smart phones, and more than half of these physicians use these devices for administrative work, continuing medical education and monitoring of patients remotely; this percent is expected to rise to 81% in 2012 (Manhattan Research, 2009).

With the growing adoption of handhelds and their applications (medical- and health-related applications) in medical communities, third parties are developing a large number of paid and free applications. These applications are available in the app stores of the operating systems for each device, such as Android Market, Blackberry App World, the Apple App Store, the Ovi Store, Samsung Apps, and Windows Marketplace, to name just a few. Most of the current applications are directed toward patients, clinicians, and healthcare professionals. Many of the newly developed applications, however, are aimed toward disease management, self-monitoring and control, and other clinical and educational applications. According to Rhea (2010), "The 319-bed Hospital of Central Connecticut has developed an iPhone application that allows patients to look up emergency room wait times." On the other hand, UPMC, one of the leading nonprofit health systems in the United States, is investing in the development of a security-enabled application that permits physicians to access patients' Electronic Health Records (EHRs) through their BlackBerrys. This application will provide physicians with the most recent information concerning their patients, including laboratory results, vital signs, medications and allergies even when they are off-campus (Rhea, 2010; eHealthServer, 2010).

Up till now, the design and development of health, clinical and medical applications is gaining an immense amount of attention from the media, application developers and the individuals and organizations interested in the advantages of mobile health care and the improvement in healthcare outcomes. LookTel, for example, was one of the most outstanding applications presented at the fifth annual international CTIA WIRELESS competition in 2010. LookTel received the first place prize in the latest technological solutions and mobile applications competition (CTIA, 2010). This application allows the visually impaired to quickly and easily scan and recognize objects, such as medication bottles, in order to read prescriptions in real time without connecting to the internet. Because of the value of this service, the LookTel application is currently sponsored by the National Eye Institute (NEI) of the National Institutes of Health (NIH).

Analysts expect that the two industry giants, Apple and Google, will seize control of the mobile applications and handheld device market. Apple still retains a larger share of the market than Google and is still the main inspirer of handheld devices and the applications they use. According to John (2011), "the outburst in tablets market is mainly inspired by Apple runaway success." iPhone, iPad and their applications are dominating the smart phone market, with more than 160 million users worldwide and more than 400,000 downloadable applications (Apple, 2011). The Apple applications market is rapidly growing, and third parties developers are submitting thou-

sands of new ideas and applications each month. Recently, Apple Inc. (2011) announced that more than 10 billion apps had been downloaded from its revolutionary App Store. The Apple App Store is the largest online media and application seller in the world, with over than 70% of the online market. Jack Kent (2011) reported that "In terms of mobile application stores, Apple remains far ahead of the competition, with the other stores so far." For these reasons, the Apple iPhone and iPad are more frequently adopted by medical professionals, rather than the other competitive handhelds, because of the ease of access to personal information, medical applications, clinical data, and other medical resources (Richard, et al., 2010). The success of Apple has forced the manufacturers of other smart phones, such as the Palm Pre, to make their devices compatible with Apple applications (Charny & Cheng, 2009).

However, many professionals are critical of the iPhone and iPad because they do not support Flash. Thus, some websites are not accessible through Apple's technology. Not allowing Flash on Apple's handhelds devices, however, shields the iPhone and iPad from a number of online threats, such as computer viruses and other vulnerabilities. The vulnerability of smart phones has been studied by Laurence Zipson (2010). His research shows that BlackBerry's low level of security has allowed for the hosting of some unofficial applications that later prove to be spyware. The same study warned Apple users to avoid Flash because it would make their iPhones and iPads increasingly vulnerable to malware. The study states that the Android platform is widely known as a hacker's haven. As a result of such research, we believe that Apple handheld devices are the safest choice for healthcare adoption due to their built-in security and privacy capabilities, which is a central concern for health care facilities. In Toronto's Mount Sinai Hospital, the iPhone has been fully integrated into the hospital's day-to-day practices and operations (Apple Inc., 2011). This integration includes in-place and in-house iPhone applications that provide clinicians with secure access to patient information. This revolution of medical practice at Mount Sinai hospital highlights the potential of the iPhone, iPad, and their applications in healthcare facilities.

As previously stated, the Apple App Store has launched more than 400,000 applications in its first 3 years of operation. The App Store contains more than 4,731 medically oriented applications and more than 7,340 healthcare monitoring and fitness applications (App Store, 2011). Apple products such as the iPhone, the iPad, and their applications have a proven efficiency, competence and proficiency in the mHealth industry. While the current state of medical and health applications on the market is generally covered, we have also selected some medical specialties applications based on their popularity within specific fields. According to the App Store (2011), the most popular medical and healthcare applications are as follows:

- For Clinician Decision Support: **eProcrates** and **Medscape.**
- For CME: **MedicalRadio, Pubsearch,** and **iRadiology.**
- For Chronic Disease Management and Self-Monitoring: **HeartWise, iAsthma in Control, iArthritis, Medic PHR,** and **Lost it!**
- For Patient Education: **iFirstAid.**
- For Professional/Specialist Education: **NeuroMind.**
- For Patient/Healthcare Professional Communication: **Universal Doctor Speaker.**

Table 1 describes the most popular applications in the App Store in different medical and health categories. Most of these applications grant the handheld user, whether patient, physician, clinician, or medical student, with a wide range of services that are useful in decision making, continuing medical education, self-monitoring,

education of patients, and healthcare communication with patients. Noticeably, the total number of downloads of the health- and medical-related applications is considered high, with more than 200,000 downloads for **Medscape** and 60,000 downloads for **MedicalRadio.** However, both applications are well known among the healthcare professionals; **Medscape** is intended to provide diagnostic support at the point of care, whereas **MedicalRadio** is meant to distribute real-time streaming of world-class Continuing Medical Education (CME) content to healthcare professionals. In 2010, **Medscape** was the top downloaded medical applications for healthcare professionals. On the other hand, the high number of ratings submitted for the health and medical applications show the popularity of this trend among users. For example, **Lost it!**, which is an effective weight-monitoring application, has received more than 302,356 ratings. In addition, **eProcrates** which is the most popularly downloaded medical application for drug reference, with more than 100,000 users on the iPhone, has received more than 44,471 ratings on the App Store. Based on users' ratings and reviews, there is great excitement about the features that can be provided in mobile applications. The amalgamation of the mobility of the users with the characteristics provided in these applications has greatly influenced the acceptance of these mobile applications. **UniversalDoctorSpeaker**, for example, is an application created to facilitate communication between patients and healthcare professionals in multilingual contexts. **UniversalDoctorSpeaker** aids the patient by reducing the language barrier; this is especially helpful to the patients travelling abroad for medication. Other characteristics of these applications include the capacity to access health services regardless of patient location and the ability to target a specific category of needs. **iAsthma in Control**, for example, is an application designed to attract kids with its delightful cartoon drawings that educate them on how to manage and control their asthma

Table 1. The most popular mHealth applications in the app store

Application Name	App Store Category	Sub-Category	Comments	Rating	Downloads
Lost it!	Healthcare	Self-Monitoring	Weight Monitoring	302,356 ratings	N/A
eProcrates	Medical	Clinician Decision Support	Drug Reference	44,471 ratings	N/A
Medscape	Medical	Clinician Decision Support	Point-of-Care Diagnostic Support	17,617 ratings	200,000+
iFirstAid	Healthcare	Patient Education	--	6,900 ratings	7,000+
HeartWise	Medical	Chronic Disease Management	Blood Pressure Monitoring	2,004 ratings	N/A
Pubsearch	Medical	CME	--	905 ratings	N/A
MedicalRadio	Medical	CME	--	502 ratings	60,000+
iRadiology	Medical	CME	Clinicians' Education	492 ratings	N/A
NeuroMind	Medical	Professional Education	Neurosurgical Education	279 ratings	54,000+
Universal Doctor Speaker	Medical	Patient/Health Care Professional Communication	--	97 ratings	N/A
iAsthma in Control	Medical	Chronic Disease Management	Managing Asthma for Children	80 ratings	N/A
iArthritis	Healthcare	Chronic Disease Management	--	11 ratings	N/A
Medic PHR	Healthcare	Self-Monitoring	--	5 ratings	N/A

attacks. (Refer to Appendix A for a detailed description of each application).

The development of medical and health applications is still in its early stages, but great advancement is expected in this area due to the increased demands in healthcare as well as the continued industrial development and innovation. Nowadays, many technological innovations are leveraging to impact on our health. Healthcare mobility has been enhanced by the innovation of new, small pieces of technology (gadgets) that have increased the value of mobile phones as a healthcare device. These gadgets can be linked to the patients' iPhone or iPad to help them monitor their health on a regular basis wherever they are. The typical glucose meter used by diabetic patients to measure their blood glucose level can be replaced by the new innovation of mobile iBGStar meter. iBGStar is a blood glucose meter that connects to the iPhone or iPad easily and permits the diabetic patient to take a blood drop and analyze it accurately, instantly sharing it with the healthcare professional. We believe that the innovation in health and medicine in the upcoming years will be powered by the ability of the handheld mobile devices and their applications to transform into diagnostic and self-monitoring devices.

DISCUSSION SECTION

The purpose of this chapter was to review the current state of, opportunities and challenges within the field of mHealth. Based on the findings of our review, we believe that the field of mHealth is currently in its early stages. The field, however, is rapidly expanding, especially in the developing world. The future adoption of mHealth applications within healthcare will largely depend on how useful it becomes to healthcare professionals and consumers. If it is found useful, this will drive both industry and healthcare organizations to invest in mHealth; otherwise, it may be at risk of becoming just another fad. mHealth researchers will play a large role in determining the usefulness, effectiveness, and impact of mHealth by evaluating the applications and the technologies within both inpatient and outpatient settings. The role of the researcher will help determine the types of positive or negative impacts mHealth has within healthcare, especially within patient care. The state of the current research has focused on the novelty of the technology by simply describing mHealth applications or technologies. Future studies must investigate the impact of mHealth on patients and physician behavior, quality of care, decision-making, and healthcare outcomes.

This chapter discussed the details and state of mHealth in relation to chronic disease management, the education of patients and healthcare professionals, the decision-making process for patients and clinicians, and the various challenges concerning implementation and usability within healthcare settings. For chronic disease management, research shows that mHealth applications can assist in the monitoring and influencing of patient behavior. However, more studies with better designs are needed to reach stronger conclusions concerning the long-term impact of mHealth applications on chronic disease management. There are a variety of applications that have been developed for the education of healthcare professionals and consumers, but again, these applications and the devices they run on must be further researched to determine their impact on both patient and healthcare professional education.

The types of information needed by healthcare professionals to support decision-making were also presented in this chapter. The literature shows that research should be conducted on mHealth devices to determine if issues, such as screen size, have an impact on the ability of the device to convey sufficient information to the healthcare professional. The concern is that the screen size may influence decisions, thus impacting patient care, especially in relation to medical errors. Much of the research has focused on the patient's usage of devices, but more research is needed on device use by healthcare professionals, especially interprofessional communication between various healthcare clinicians in the hospital environment. Usability studies to investigate the impact of mHealth in these settings are needed.

Various mHealth technologies and applications were also presented. There were several technologies that were highlighted in this chapter, such as mobile phones, smart phones, mobile tele-health devices, MP3 players, and mobile computing hardware. Several applications were also presented that are related to clinical decision support, CME, chronic disease management, patient education, specialist education, and patient and healthcare professional communication. Overall, there seems to be proliferation of mobile devices and applications being introduced into the market today. More research is needed on the usability of such technologies and applications to assess their impact on patient care, healthcare education, and decision-making. In general, mHealth is a new area of research. With the passage of time and rigorous evaluation, the impacts of the technologies and their related applications can be analyzed. It will take years of dedicated research within the area using a variety of approaches to evaluate the impact of mHealth technologies and applications on healthcare.

FUTURE TRENDS AND CONCLUSION

Based on the review of the literature and various mHealth applications, we believe that the future of mHealth will evolve from applications focusing on individuals to those that incorporate an element of social networking to promote healthy behaviors in groups. Today, social networking is playing a large role within the daily lives of individuals and has revolutionized the way interactions are taking place globally. Social media networking sites, such as Facebook, have many health-related support groups that provide educational and emotional support for individuals. The creation of mHealth programs that incorporate elements of social networking for patients can help promote group and community health. Therefore, in this chapter, we proposed the use of the acronym MSN-Health to describe the emerging field of mobile social networking healthcare. Research on the topic of mobile social networking health is only beginning to emerge; we have not found any use of the acronym MSN-Health in the health, technology, or health informatics literature. We define MSN-Healthcare as follows: "The use of mobile health applications that incorporate social networking tools to promote healthy behaviors and awareness among patient groups and communities." As the mHealth research domain evolves, we believe that MSN-Healthcare will play an important role in the field of mHealth research and the development of applications within this domain.

We also believe that, as the mHealth domain begins to mature, more emphasis will be placed on the evaluation of mHealth applications and their impact on patient care. To date, the evaluation of mHealth interventions is lacking because the focus has been on the development of the applications and not on the evaluation of their effects. As the mobile technology and mHealth application market expands, we believe that many of the applications will focus on patient education, monitoring, and management. Other applications will focus on the use of mHealth applications as an extension of the electronic medical record, which will allow clinicians to view patient information and share them with their patients at the bedside or in the office.

Finally, we believe that mHealth will develop into a more recognized research domain within the health informatics field, similar to the development of telemedicine. This development will require the creation and evaluation of applications and the development of educational programs dedicated to this specialization. Given the pervasiveness of mobile technologies within the developed and developing world, we believe that mHealth will become a more recognized and more established domain area than telemedicine within only a few years.

Is mHealth a fad or here to stay? In this chapter, we focused on the current state of and the opportunities and challenges within the field of mHealth. The chapter began with a description of the background of mHealth and then discussed the opportunities for mHealth with a specific focus on chronic disease management, the education of healthcare professionals, the ability to address the needs of healthcare professional, and the support of the decision-making process for patients. The chapter then analyzed the challenges for mHealth in relation to usability issues, information needs, and interactions with clinical work. A detailed discussion was provided on the current application uses. Finally, future trends within the field were mentioned, and we coined and defined the term MSN-Healthcare.

Based on our review of the current and future state of mHealth, we believe that mHealth in both the developed and developing world will play a strong role in supporting hospital care, healthy behavior, patient monitoring and educational awareness. mHealth will be the next phase of evolution within the health informatics field and will have dramatic impacts on the research, educational, technological, and clinical aspects of healthcare.

REFERENCES

Adams, A., Dale, J., Griffiths, F., Martin, S., Powell, J., Sturt, J., & Sutcliffe, P. (2011). Systematic review of communication technologies to promote access and engagement of young people with diabetes into healthcare. *BMC Endocrine Disorders, 11*(1).

Allen, M., Sargeant, J., Mann, K., Fleming, M., & Premi, J. (2003). Videoconferencing for practice-based small-group continuing medical education: Feasibility, acceptability, effectiveness, and cost. *The Journal of Continuing Education in the Health Professions, 23*(1), 38–47. doi:10.1002/chp.1340230107

Apple. (2011). *Apple's app store downloads top 10 billion.* Retrieved February 16, 2011, from http://www.apple.com/pr/library/2011/01/22appstore.html.

Apple Inc. (2011). *iPhone provides vital link to medical records.* Retrieved February 16, 2011, from http://www.apple.com/iphone/business/profiles/mt-sinai/.

Borycki, E. M., Lemieux-Charles, L., Nagle, L., & Eysenbach, G. (2009a). Evaluating the impact of hybrid electronic-paper environments upon novice nurse information seeking. *Methods of Information in Medicine, 48*(2), 137–143. Retrieved from http://dx.doi.org/10.3414/ME9222

Borycki, E. M., Lemieux-Charles, L., Nagle, L., & Eysenbach, G. (2009b). Novice nurse information needs in paper and hybrid electronic-paper environments: A qualitative analysis. *Studies in Health Technology and Informatics, 150,* 913–917.

Canadian Health Informatics Association. (2011). *COACH definition of health informatics: Health informatics (HI) is the intersection of clinical, IM/IT and management practices to achieve better health.* Retrieved January 30, 2011, from http://coachorg.com/health_informatics.

Central Intelligence Agency. (2011). *The world factbook.* Washington, DC: CIA. Retrieved January 28, 2011, from https://www.cia.gov/library/publications/the-world-factbook/index.html.

Charny, B., & Cheng, R. (2009). Palm's pre to access itunes. *The Wall Street Journal.* Retrieved February 16, 2011, from http://online.wsj.com/article/SB124353594043063537.html?mod=googlewsj.

Chen, E. S., Mednonca, E., McKnight, L., Stetson, P., Lei, J., & Cimino, J. (2003). PalmCIS: A wireless handheld application for satisfying clinician information needs. *Journal of the American Medical Informatics Association, 11*(1), 19–28. doi:10.1197/jamia.M1387

Consumer Electronic Show. (2011). *2011 international CES wows world with innovation and optimism.* Retrieved February 5, 2011, from http://www.cesweb.org/news/rssNews.asp.

Cox, A. (2010). *mHealth: What scope is there in the remote monitoring market for chronic diseases?* Retrieved February 14, 2011, from http://www.juniperresearch.com/analyst-xpress-blog/2010/08/23/mHealth-what-scope-is-there-in-the-remote-monitoring-market-for-chronic-diseases/.

Dolan, B. (2009). *ReachMD: 60,000+ downloads for CME app.* Retrieved February 21, 2011, from http://mobihealthnews.com/2990/reachmd-60000-downloads-for-cme-app/.

Dolan, B. (2009). *WebMD: Medscape mobile, 200,000+ downloads.* Retrieved February 21, 2011, from http://mobihealthnews.com/5307/webmd-medcape-mobile-has-200000-downloads/.

Economist. (2011). *Mobile services in poor countries: Not just talk.* Retrieved January 30, 2011, from http://www.economist.com/node/18008202.

eHealthServer. (2010). *UPMC brings key patient records to the bedside using blackberry smart phones*. Retrieved February 23, 2011, from http://www.ehealthserver.com/research-and-development/442-upmc-brings-key-patient-records-to-the-bedside-using-blackberry-smart-phones.

Epocrates. (2011). *Website*. Retrieved February 9, 2011, from http://itunes.apple.com/us/app/epocrates/id281935788?mt=8#.

Fjeldsoe, B. S., Marshall, A. L., & Miller, Y. D. (2009). Behavior change interventions delivered by mobile telephone short-message service. *American Journal of Preventive Medicine, 36*(2), 165–173. doi:10.1016/j.amepre.2008.09.040

3gdoctor. (2010). *mHealth is the leverage of mobile, the newest mass media, to improve health*. Retrieved January 30, 2010, from http://3gdoctor.wordpress.com/2010/03/22/the-definition-of-mHealth/.

Gold, J., Lim, M. S., Hellard, M. E., Hocking, J. S., & Keogh, L. (2010). What's in a message? Delivering sexual health promotion to young people in Australia via text messaging. *BMC Public Health, 10*, 792. doi:10.1186/1471-2458-10-792

HeartWise Blood Pressure Tracker. (2010). *Website*. Retrieved February 22, 2011, from http://itunes.apple.com/us/app/heartwise-blood-pressure-tracker/id311716888?mt=8#.

HeartWise Blood Pressure Tracker for iPad. (2010). *Website*. Retrieved February 22, 2011, from http://itunes.apple.com/us/app/heartwise-blood-pressure-tracker/id364899989?mt=8#.

Honeybourne, C., Sutton, S., & Ward, L. (2006). Knowledge in palm of your hands: PDAs in the clinical setting. *Health Information Library Journal, 23*(1), 51-59. Retrieved from http://www.ncbi.nlm.nih.gov/pubmed/16466499.

iArthritis. (2009). *Website*. Retrieved February 22, 2011, from http://itunes.apple.com/us/app/iarthritis/id322993302?mt=8.

iAsthma in Control. (2010). *Website*. Retrieved February 22, 2011, from http://itunes.apple.com/us/app/iasthma-in-control/id329847125?mt=8#.

iFirstAid. (2011). *Website*. Retrieved February 22, 2011, from http://itunes.apple.com/us/app/ifirstaid-lite/id295238909?mt=8#.

iRadiology. (2009). *Website*. Retrieved February 22, 2011, from http://itunes.apple.com/us/app/iradiology/id346440355?mt=8.

Istepanian, R., & Lacal, J. (2003). Emerging mobile communication technologies for health: Some imperative notes on m-health. In *Proceedings of the 25th Silver 59 Anniversary International Conference of the IEEE Engineering in Medicine and Biology Society*. Cancun, Mexico: IEEE Press.

Istepanian, R., Laxminarayan, S., & Pattichis, C. S. (Eds.). (2006). *M-Health*. New York, NY: Springer. doi:10.1007/b137697

John, I. (2011). *Tablets steal the show in Las Vegas*. Retrieved February 5, 2011, from http://www.khaleejtimes.com/biz/inside.asp?xfile=/data/business/2011/January/business_January271.xml&section=business.

Knowledge for Health Organization. (2011). *What is mhealth?* Retrieved January 30, 2011, from http://www.k4health.org/toolkits/mHealth.

Koppel, R., Wetterneck, T., Telles, J. L., & Karsh, B. T. (2008). Workarounds to barcode medication administration systems: Their occurrences, causes and threats to patient safety. *Journal of the American Medical Informatics Association, 15*(4), 408–423. doi:10.1197/jamia.M2616

Kubben, P. (2011). *Website*. Retrieved February 27, 2011, from http://blog.digitalneurosurgeon.com/?p=1116.

Kushniruk, A., & Borycki, E. (2007). Human factors and usability of healthcare systems. In Bardram, J., Mihailidis, A., & Wan, D. (Eds.), *Pervasive Computing in Healthcare* (pp. 191–215). Boca Raton, FL: CRC Press. doi:10.1201/9781420005332.ch8

Kushniruk, A. W., Triola, M. M., Borycki, E. M., Stein, B., & Kannry, J. L. (2005). Technology induced error and usability: The relationship between usability problems and prescription errors when using a handheld application. *International Journal of Medical Informatics, 74*(7-8), 519–526. doi:10.1016/j.ijmedinf.2005.01.003

Kyriacou, E. C., Pattichis, C. S., & Pattichis, M. S. (2009). An overview of recent health care supported systems for eemergency and mhealth applications. In *Proceedings from the IEEE English Medical Biological Society*, (pp. 1246-1249). IEEE Press.

Lau, F., & Hayward, R. (2000). Building a virtual network in a community health research training program. *Journal of the American Medical Informatics Association, 7*(4), 361–377. Retrieved from http://www.ncbi.nlm.nih.gov/pmc/articles/ PMC61441/ doi:10.1136/jamia.2000.0070361

Laxminarayan, S., & Istepanian, R. S. (2000). Unwired e-med: The next generation of wireless and internet telemedicine systems. *IEEE Transactions on Information Technology in Biomedicine, 4*(3), 189–193. doi:10.1109/TITB.2000.5956074

Linkov, F., LaPorte, R., Padilla, N., & Shubnikov, E. (2010). Global networking of cancer and NCD professionals using internet technologies: The supercourse and mhealth applications. *Journal of Preventive Medicine and Public Health = Yebang Uihakhoe Chi, 43*(6), 472–478. Retrieved from http://www.ncbi.nlm.nih.gov/pubmed/21139407 doi:10.3961/jpmph.2010.43.6.472

Lost it!(2011). *Website.* Retrieved February 22, 2011, from http://itunes.apple.com/us/app/lose-it/ id297368629?mt=8#.

Lyall, M. (2010). *Chronic diseases need attention of mHealth apps developers.* Retrieved February 14, 2011, from http://www.knowabouthealth.com/ chronic-diseases-need-attention-of-mHealth-apps-developers/7339/.

Manhattan Research. (2009). *Physician smart phone adoption rate to reach 81% in 2012.* Retrieved February 21, 2011, from http://www.man-hattanresearch.com/newsroom/Press_Releases/ physician-smartphones-2012.aspx.

Mason, M. (2011). *South Asians hit with heart attacks earlier than rest of world: Heart disease top killer.* Retrieved February 14, 2011, from http://www.google.com/hostednews/canadian-press/article/ALeqM5jR6gAxqnoC9T-KNq-Ck5XbOXbkeA?docId=5895164.

McGee, M. K. (2010). *Text messages boost patient outcomes.* Retrieved February 14, 2011, from http://www.informationweek.com/news/ healthcare/mobile-wireless/showArticle.jhtml?a rticleID=227500893&subSection=News.

Mechael, P., & Slonininsky, D. (Eds.). (2008). *Towards the development of an mhealth strategy: A literature review.* New York, NY: The World Health Organization. Retrieved from http://mo-bileactive.org/files/file_uploads/WHOHealthRe-viewUpdatedAug222008_TEXT.pdf.

Medic, P. H. R. (2010). *Website.* Retrieved February 22, 2011, from http://itunes.apple.com/us/app/ medic-phr/id336885531?mt=8.

Medscape. (2010). *Website.* Retrieved February 9, 2011, from http://itunes.apple.com/us/app/ medscape/id321367289?mt=8#.

NeuroMind. (2010). *Website.* Retrieved February 22, 2011, from http://itunes.apple.com/us/app/ neuromind/id353386909?mt=8#.

Neurosurgeon, D. (2011). *Blog.* Retrieved February 22, 2011, from http://blog.digitalncurosur-geon.com/?page_id=639.

Nusca, A. (2009). *Smartphone vs. feature phone arms race heats up: Which did you buy?* Retrieved January 30, 2011, from http://www.zdnet.com/blog/gadgetreviews/smartphone-vs-feature-phone-arms-race-heats-up-which-did-you-buy/6836.

Oehler, R. L., Smith, K., & Toney, J. F. (2010). Infectious diseases resources for the iphone. *Clinical Infectious Diseases, 50*(9), 1268–1274. doi:10.1086/651602

Parker, G., Proudfoot, J., Hadzi, P. D., Manicavasagar, V., Adler, E., & Whitton, A. (2010). Community attitudes to the appropriation of mobile phones for monitoring and managing depression, anxiety, and stress. *Journal of Medical Internet Research, 12*(5).

Pubsearch. (2010). *Website.* Retrieved February 22, 2011, from http://itunes.apple.com/us/app/pubsearch/id287239420?mt=8#.

Research2Guideance. (2010). *Mobile health market report 2010-2015.* Retrieved February 14, 2011, from http://www.research2guidance.com/shop/index.php/mHealth-report.

Rhea, S. (2010). Going mobile: Wireless devices and technology bring surge in advanced applications for health monitoring and treatment, but legal and privacy issues remain. *Modern Healthcare, 40*(18), 28–30. Retrieved from http://www.ncbi.nlm.nih.gov/pubmed/20480559

Shortliffe, E. H., & Ciminio, J. J. (2006). *Biomedical informatics: Computer applications in health care and biomedicine.* New York, NY: Springer Verlag.

St. Jude Children's Research Hospital. (2011). *How Cure4Kids can help.* Retrieved February 14, 2011, from https://www.cure4kids.org/ums/home/.

Store, A. (2011). *Website.* Retrieved February 22, 2011, from http://itunes.apple.com/us/genre/ios-medical/id6020?mt=8.

Technology, H. M. (2010). Mobile on the rise. *ProQuest Medical Library, 31*(3), 8.

The CTIA Wireless Association. (2010). *CTIA announces 2010 e-tech awards winners.* Retrieved February 16, 2011, from http://www.ctia.org/media/press/body.cfm/prid/1939.

The Economist. (2006). *The medical uses of mobile phones show they can be good for your health.* Retrieved January 30, 2011, from http://www.economist.com/node/5655105.

United Nations. (2008). *The millennium development goals report.* Retrieved from http://www.un.org/millenniumgoals/pdf/The%20Millennium%20Development%20Goals%20Report%202008.pdf.

Universal Doctor Speaker. (2010). *Website.* Retrieved February 22, 2011, from http://itunes.apple.com/us/app/universal-doctor-speaker-for/id364812043?mt=8.

University Health Network. (2011). *Patient education: Improving health through education.* Retrieved February 14, 2011, from http://www.uhn.ca/patients_&_visitors/health_info/topics/pen/index.asp.

U.S Census Bureau. (2011). *International database-World population summary.* Retrieved January 10, 2011, from http://www.census.gov/ipc/www/idb/worldpopinfo.php.

US Centers for Disease Control and Prevention. (2004). *About chronic disease: Definition, overall burden, and cost effectiveness of prevention.* Washington, DC: National Center for Chronic Disease Prevention and Health Promotion. Retrieved June 27, 2011, from http://www.cdc.gov/chronicdisease/about/index.htm.

US Department of Health and Human Services. (1996). *Guide to clinical preventive services: Report o the U.S. preventive services task force* (2nd ed.). Washington, DC: US Preventive Services Task Force.

Vital Wave Consulting. (2009). *mHealth for development: The opportunity of mobile technology for healthcare in the developing world.* Washington, DC: UN Foundation-Vodafone Foundation Partnership. Retrieved form http://www.globalproblems-globalsolutions-files.org/unf_website/assets/publications/technology/mHealth/ mHealth_for_Development_full.pdf.

Webopedia. (2010). *Mobile phone.* Retrieved January 30, 2010, from http://www.webopedia.com/TERM/M/mobile_phone.html.

Wennberg, D., , Bennett, G., O'Malley, S., Lang, L., & Marr, A., (2010). Randomized trial of a telephone care-management strategy. *The New England Journal of Medicine, 363,* 1245–1255. Retrieved from http://www.nejm.org/doi/full/10.1056/NEJMsa0902321 doi:10.1056/NEJMsa0902321

Whitney, L. (2011). *Report: Apple remains king of app-store market.* Retrieved February 16, 2011, from http://news.cnet.com/8301-13579_3-20032012-37.html.

World Health Organization. (2011a). *Facing the facts: The impact of chronic disease in Canada.* Retrieved February 14, 2011, from http://www.who.int/chp/chronic_disease_report/media/CANADA.pdf.

World Health Organization. (2011b). *Preventing chronic diseases: A vital investment.* Retrieved February 14, 2011, from http://www.who.int/chp/chronic_disease_report/English%20compressed.ppt.

Zipson, L. (2010). Smartphone vulnerabilities. In *Network Security Pre-Press.* Oxford, UK: Mayfield Press.

ADDITIONAL READING

Agar, J. (2004). *Constant touch: A global history of the mobile phone.* Cambridge, UK: Icon Books.

Al-Hakim, L. (2007). *Web mobile-based applications for healthcare management.* Hershey, PA: IGI Global. doi:10.4018/978-1-59140-658-7

Anderson, G., Asare, S. D., Eyitayo, A. O., Eyitayo, O. T., Mpoeleng, D., & Nkgau, T. (2007)... *Information Storage and Retrieval Techniques for Mobile Healthcare, 2*(12), 1096–1100.

BJ. F., & Richard, A. (Eds). (2009). *Texting 4 health: A simple, powerful way to change lives.* Healdsburg, CA: Captology Media.

Curioso, W. H., & Kurth, A. E. (2007). Access, use and perceptions regarding Internet, cell phones and PDAs as a means for health promotion for people living with HIV in Peru. *BMC Medical Informatics and Decision Making, 7*(1), 24. doi:10.1186/1472-6947-7-24

Free, C., Phillips, G., Felix, L., Galli, L., Patel, V., & Edwards, P. (2010). The effectiveness of m-health technologies for improving health and health services: A systematic review protocol. *BMC Research Notes, 3*(1), 250. doi:10.1186/1756-0500-3-250

Istepanian, R., & Lacal, J. (2003). Emerging mobile communication technologies for health: Some imperative notes on m-health. In *Proceedings of the 25th Silver 59 Anniversary International Conference of the IEEE Engineering in Medicine and Biology Society.* Cancun, Mexico: IEEE Press.

Istepanian, R. S. H., Jovanov, E., & Zhang, Y. T. (2004). Introduction to the special section on m-health: Beyond seamless mobility and global wireless health-care connectivity. *IEEE Transactions on Information Technology in Biomedicine, 8*(4), 405–414. doi:10.1109/TITB.2004.840019

Jordan-Marsh, M. (2010). *Health technology literacy: A transdisciplinary framework for consumer-oriented practice*. New York, NY: Jones & Bartlett Learning.

Kaplan, W. A. (2006). Can the ubiquitous power of mobile phones be used to improve health outcomes in developing countries? *Globalization and Health, 2*(9), 1–14.

Korhonen, I., Parkka, J., & Van Gils, M. (2003). Health monitoring in the home of the future. *IEEE Engineering in Medicine and Biology Magazine, 22*(3), 66–73. doi:10.1109/MEMB.2003.1213628

Mechael, P. (2009). The case for mhealth in developing countries. *MIT Innovations Journal, 4*(1), 103-118. Retrieved from http://www.mitpress-journals.org/doi/pdf/10.1162/itgg.2009.4.1.103.

Mechael, P. N. (2007). *Toward a development of mhealth strategy: Literature review*. Retrieved June 27, 2011 from http://mobileactive.org/files/file_uploads/WHOHealthReviewUpdatedAug222008_TEXT.pdf.

Mei, H. (2007). Smart distribution of bio-signal processing tasks in m-health. In *Proceedings of the On the Move to Meaningful Internet Systems 2007: OTM 2007 Workshops*, (pp. 284-293). Vilamoura, Portugal: Springer Verlag.

Micheli-Tzanakou, E., Altieri, R., Incardona, F., Kirkilis, H., & Ricci, R. (2006). Mobi-dev: Mobile devices for healthcare applications. In Istepanian, R. S. H., Laxminarayan, S., & Pattichis, C. S. (Eds.), *M-Health* (pp. 163–175). New York, NY: Springer.

Micheli-Tzanakou, E., Jones, V., Halteren, A., Dokovsky, N., Koprinkov, G., & Peuscher, J. … Herzog, R. (2006). Mobihealth: Mobile services for health professionals. In R. S. H. Istepanian, S. Laxminarayan, & C. S. Pattichis (Eds.), *M-Health,* (pp. 237-246). New York, NY: Springer.

Micheli-Tzanakou, E., Jones, V., Shashar, N., Shaphrut, O., Lavigne, K., & Rienks, R. … Widya, I. (2006). Remote monitoring for healthcare and for safety in extreme environments. In R. S. H. Istepanian, S. Laxminarayan, & C. S. Pattichis (Eds.), *M-Health,* (pp. 561-573). New York, NY: Springer.

Miller, F. P., Vandome, A. F., & McBrewster, J. (2010). *mHealth*. New York, NY: VDM Publishing House Ltd.

Mirza, F., Norris, T., & Stockdale, R. (2008). Mobile technologies and the holistic management of chronic diseases. *Health Informatics Journal, 14*(4), 309–321. doi:10.1177/1460458208096559

Norris, A. C., Stockdale, R. S., & Sharma, S. (2009). A strategic approach to m-health. *Health Informatics Journal, 15*(3), 244–253. doi:10.1177/1460458209337445

Olla, P., & Tan, J. (2009). *Mobile Health Solutions for Biomedical Applications*. Hershey, PA: IGI Global. doi:10.4018/978-1-60566-332-6

Park, S., & Jayaraman, S. (2003). Enhancing the quality of life through wearable technology. *IEEE Engineering in Medicine and Biology Magazine, 22*(3), 41–48. doi:10.1109/MEMB.2003.1213625

Sutcliffe, P., Martin, S., Sturt, J., Powell, J., Griffiths, F., Adams, A., & Dale, J. (2011). Systematic review of communication technologies to promote access and engagement of young people with diabetes into healthcare. *BMC Endocrine Disorders, 11*(1), 1. doi:10.1186/1472-6823-11-1

The Earth Institute. (2010). *Barriers and gaps affecting mhealth in low and middle income countries: mHealth alliance*. Retrieved June 27, 2011 from http://cghed.ei.columbia.edu/sitefiles/file/mHealthBarriersWhitePaperFINAL.pdf.

Wagner, E. (2008). Realizing the promises of mobile learning. *Journal of Computing in Higher Education*, *20*(2), 4–14. doi:10.1007/s12528-008-9008-x

Wu, R. C., & Straus, S. E. (2006). Evidence for handheld electronic medical records in improving care: A systematic review. *BMC Medical Informatics and Decision Making*, *6*(1), 26. doi:10.1186/1472-6947-6-26

KEY TERMS AND DEFINITIONS

App Store: An online mobile applications store that contains a wide variety of mobile applications for a particular operating system, such as Android Market, Blackberry App World, and the Apple App Store.

Chronic Disease: A disease that lasts for a long period and is rarely cured completely, such as heart disease, diabetes, and arthritis (US Centre for Disease Control and Prevention, 2004).

Handheld Device: A portable device that is small and light enough to be operated while held in the hands, such as iPhone, iPad, HP Slate, and BlackBerry Playbook.

Health Professional Education: The process of communicating and sharing health information among healthcare professionals as well as developing and building their skills.

mHealth: "The emerging mobile communications and network technologies for healthcare systems" (Istepanian, et al., 2006, p. 3; Istepanian & Lacal, 2003).

MSN-Healthcare: The use of mobile health applications that include social networking tools to promote healthy behaviors and awareness.

Patient Education: The process of educating and engaging patients in preventive behavior with the objective of modifying the patients' behavior and improving their overall health.

Social Networking: The share of interests, activities, information, and photos between people who are socially connected with each other.

Usability: The ease of use and learnability of mHealth applications and technologies among healthcare professionals and patients, measured by specific testing and evaluation methods to observe, predict and examine both user needs and healthcare workflows.

APPENDIX A

eProcrates is one of the most popularly downloaded application for drug reference, with more than 100,000 users on the iPhone and almost 750,000 users on other devices worldwide (Epocrates, 2011; Mobile apps on rise, 2010). Generally, ePocrates provides an enormous amount of information on thousands of drugs such as drug cost, dosages, and drug mechanisms of action. Moreover, it provides a comprehensive search tool where users can search in different diseases, drugs, and infectious diseases databases. One of the most popular features offered ePocrates is the drug-drug interaction database, which is especially useful for monitoring drug use in geriatric patients and patients with chronic diseases who may be on multiple drugs simultaneously. This application also allows quick access to thousands of drug monographs and formularies and can identify a drug by its appearance or its imprint code through the pill identifier tool. ePocrates quickly gained a large market share because it saved physicians time and money by offering them with all the key functions free of charge, unlike the other competitors. ePocrates (2011) reported that "ePocrates helps physicians save time; over 40% reports saving 20 minutes or more a day." According to ePocrates (2011), the overall number of customer ratings for this application is greater than 44,471.

Medscape is the top downloaded medical app for healthcare professionals in 2010 (Medscape, 2010). Medscape is a point-of-care diagnostic support application that helps healthcare professionals to re-search diagnostic criteria based upon organ, system, symptoms or disease with speed and confidence at the point-of-care. Medscape has been downloaded more than 200,000 times since it was launched in July 2009 (Dolan, 2009). This application offers a comprehensive drug reference, specialty-specific medical news, and a drug interactions checker for any combination of drugs, herbals and supplements. Medscape also has diseases and conditions reference and treatment guides, which are enhanced with videos and pictures. Medscape also provides healthcare professionals with features that support CME and medical literature searches. According to Medscape (2010), customers have submitted more than 17,617 ratings for this application.

MedicalRadio delivers world-class CME content to healthcare professionals in real-time streaming from an XM satellite radio station. ReachMd, the company that developed this application, is one of the leading companies in medical education and information for medical professionals. MedicalRadio was downloaded 3,000 times during its first week in the iPhone App Store, and it has since been downloaded 60,000 times (Dolan, 2009). MedicalRadio covers a broad range of topics for both general practitioners in healthcare and specialists. It also provides a free list of accessible and searchable medical podcasts that are weekly uploaded and updated. The major benefit of this application is that it allows users to take exams on the iPhone or iPad directly after finishing the CME/CE podcasts lessons.

Medic PHR is a directed informational tool that allows patients to input their daily health information to produce an artificial historical trend that outlines their overall health situation. Specifically, Medic PHR is a mobile repository for personal health information. Weight, glucose level, blood pressure and pulse, temperature, body fat, height, sleeping hours and dietary habits are an example of the data that can be entered into the Medic PHR application. This information can also be shared through text or as graphs with other healthcare providers, insurance companies and hospitals. The Medic PHR application offers patients the ability to self-monitor their health through graphical chart summaries and e-mailing their information and results in an organized form. Also, the Medic PHR application offers patients with user-friendly interfaces that reduce the time spent on data entry, as well as, the ability to convert units of measurement (e.g., lbs., kg). According to MedicPHR (2010), customers have rated this application more than 5 times.

Pubsearch is another valuable application for all healthcare professionals and medical students. Pubsearch provides quick and easy access to millions of medical research papers and journals that are indexed in PubMed. As a result of the popularity of this application, the next version was implemented to support the organization of searches into a favorite articles list. According to Pubsearch (2010), customers have rated this application more than 905 times.

iRadiology is an educational application designed to assist medical students and residents in developing their skills in interpreting X-rays, CT, and MRIs. iRadiology has catalogued more than 500 radiology cases. These radiology cases are derived from the well-known teaching website managed by Dr. Gillian Lieberman, an Associate Professor and Director of Medical Student Education at Harvard University. iRadiology assists residents in reviewing many radiology cases during their daily rounds or while on clinical rotations. The application provides the ability to zoom in, rotate, and scroll around the image to improve the resident's radiological interpretative skills. The images are organized by organ systems and by pathological entity, and each image is accompanied by an extensive explanation of the radiological and pathological findings. According to iRadiology (2009), customers have submitted more than 492 ratings for this application.

HeartWise is the easiest and most effective application for the self-monitoring of blood pressure. HeartWise has the ability to alert the patient when it is time to take a blood pressure measurement or medication. In December 2009, HeartWise was awarded the best medical application for heart monitoring on the iPhone (HeartWise, 2010). The HeartWise application assists patients with the recording and tracking of blood pressure, heart rate, and weight through a streamlined and elegant multi-language interface. This application automatically calculates arterial pressure, systolic blood pressure, pulse pressure, and Body Mass Index (BMI). These data can be exported to other sources or printed out in a formatted report. Similarly, HeartWise can import any personal health data or measurements that already exist in other applications. The most important characteristic of this application is the fast analysis and visualization of the patient's data, statistics and trends, which allows the patient to follow the fluctuation of his/her blood pressure and other measurements on a daily basis and over time. However, customers have rated this application more than 2,004 times (HeartWise, 2010; HeartWise for iPad, 2010).

Lost it! is an effective weight monitoring application that assists users in losing weight and maintaining a healthy life style. Lost it! allows the user to set goals and establish daily calorie counts within the user's calorie budget. A recent study shows that 85% of the active users have lost an average of 12 lbs. (Lost it, 2011). This application has many great features. It provides a comprehensive database of meals, calories, activities, and calories burned for each activity. The database is regularly updated to permit the user to add new foods or exercises. Lost it! can also track nutrients, such as protein, carbohydrates, fats, and calcium. The data are presented within a simple and attractive dashboard that can be shared with, for example, a dietician, or used for personal weight monitoring. Currently, Lose It! is the most popular weight loss application in the App Store, with more than 302,356 ratings (Lost it, 2011).

iFirstAid is an emergency first aid assistant application. The iFirstAid is designed to make recalling first aid procedures as easy as possible when needed. The iFirstAid application includes all crucial first aid topics such as CPR, bleeding, burns, choking and poisoning. This application provides police, fire and ambulance information center numbers for 99 countries. The first aid topics in this application are authored by Ella Tyler, an international first aid expert (iFirstAid, 2011). Customers have rated this application 6,900 times (iFirstAid, 2011).

iAsthma is a daily medical application designed for assisting children in the management of all aspects of their asthma. Asthma is a chronic disease that mostly affects children. For that reason, the Asthma Center at the Cincinnati Children's Hospital developed this application to improve children's knowledge concerning their condition. iAsthma teaches children how to manage their asthma and what the symptoms of an impending attack are. In addition, iAsthma reminds children to take their inhaler medication. According to iAsthma (2010), customers have rated this application 80 times.

iArthritis is a user-friendly arthritis pain record-keeping application intended to help arthritis patients monitor and keep track of changes in their pain (e.g., severe, mild, awful and moderate) over time. In addition to maintaining a detailed log of their pain history, the current and historical pain information can be visualized through a simple and attractive dashboard that provides further insight into the causes of pain and how to control it. The iArthritis application also helps patients track the effectiveness of their medications. Customers, however, have rated this application 11 times (iArthritis, 2009).

UniversalDoctorSpeaker is an application that facilitates the communication between patients and healthcare professionals who are not speaking the same language. This application is a part of Universal Doctor Project aimed at facilitating healthcare communication in multilingual contexts. Specifically, patients can explain the health situation in their own language by writing it down in the application. The application will then translate what the patient has described concerning their health into the language of the physician. The application can also translate physician information back to the patient. However, customers have rated this application 97 times (Universal Doctor Speaker, 2010).

NeuroMind is an excellent neurosurgical application that is used globally as a resource for medical students, neurology residents, and neurosurgeons. According to Kubben (2011), the total number of NeuroMind application downloaded is greater than 54,000. The United States reported the highest number of NeuroMind downloads, accounting for 35% of the world downloads (Digital Neurosurgeon, 2011). NeuroMind contains a wide range of neurological information such as basic neuro-anatomy, anatomical images, differential diagnosis and the WHO Safe Surgery checklist items. This application is the top ranked neurosurgical application for the iPhone and the iPad, with more than 279 rates (NeuroMind, 2010).

Chapter 8
Evaluation of Quality of Context Information in U-Health Smart Homes

José Bringel Filho
University of Evry Val d'Essonne (UEVE), France

Nazim Agoulmine
University of Evry Val d'Essonne (UEVE), France

ABSTRACT

Ubiquitous Health (U-Health) smart homes are intelligent spaces capable of observing and correctly recognizing the activities and health statuses of their inhabitants (context) to provide the appropriate support to achieve an overall sense of health and well-being in their inhabitants' daily lives. With the intrinsic heterogeneity and large number of sources of context information, aggregating and reasoning on low-quality raw sensed data may result in conflicting and erroneous evaluations of situations, affecting directly the reliability of the U-Health systems. In this environment, the evaluation and verification of Quality of Context (QoC) information plays a central role in improving the consistency and correctness of context-aware U-Health applications. Therefore, the objective of this chapter is to highlight the impact of QoC on the correct behavior of U-Health systems, and introduce and analyze the existing approaches of modeling, evaluating, and using QoC to improve its context-aware decision-making support.

INTRODUCTION

Two main factors are pushing towards the development and deployment of U-Health smart homes: 1) the worldwide increase of people that require for daily care (e.g., elders, people with chronic diseases or disabilities) that comes with an increase need for human costly services to assist them; 2) health providers and government's willingness to reduce the high costs for assisting them in specialized hospitals and institutions. In the specific case of world population ageing, recent studies[1] show that the growth rate of older population (1.9%) is significantly higher than that of the total population

DOI: 10.4018/978-1-4666-0888-7.ch008

(1.2%). For instance, the older U.S. population is numbered in 39.6 million (2009)[2], about one in every eight Americans (12.9%), and it will be about 72.1 million in 2030.

The development of U-Health and Ambient Assisted Living (AAL) systems (Belbachir, et al., 2010) is an important action to enable people requiring continuous care to live independently in their own homes (Kim, et al., 2010). See in Orwat (2010) a survey with a large number of U-Health solutions. Recent advances in wireless technologies (e.g., Bluetooth, RFID, ZigBee, 3G, 4G), in sensors/actuators (Dengler, et al., 2007; Matthews, et al., 2007) (e.g., unobtrusive physiological sensors), and the convergence of home broadband access with the Digital TV (DTV) (Oliveira, et al., 2010) expand the usage span of U-health systems in real scenarios. Unobtrusive physiological sensors (Adami, et al., 2003; Hagler, et al., 2010; Matthews, et al., 2007) and mobile technologies can be integrated to monitor human biological conditions for remote diagnostic of diseases (Dongsoo, et al., 2009), detect falls (Sixsmith, 2004), to treat life-threatening situations (Bottazzi, et al., 2006; Fry, 2005), to improve quality of life and to lower health care costs (Wang, et al., 2010). For instance, a elderly can be continuously monitored by a sensor-rich jacket[3] (e.g., blood pressure, heart rate, SpO_2[4], CO[5], breath rate) that communicates with a smartphone (e.g., via Bluetooth, Wifi) to send the collected data to a remote monitoring system using a 3G connection. This physiological information can yet be combined with data sensed from the environment (e.g., motion sensor, location sensor, thermometer) and in-home objects that interact with inhabitants (e.g., home appliances, sensor-rich chairs[6] and mattress[7]) in order to recognize their activities, providing accurate remote medical assistance (e.g., verifying if the patient is following correctly the medical advices and detecting abnormal behaviors). Indeed, U-Health systems can actively contribute to identify and prevent life-threatening situations, reducing the number of chronic disease deaths (Orwat, et al., 2008). Another possible application scenario of U-Health system is the health monitoring of communities for emergency preparedness and governance decision-making support, such as the control of outbreaks and epidemics (Oliveira, et al., 2010).

However, the success of such systems is closely linked to their ability to correctly determining the patient's activities and their critical biological conditions, named *health context*, for providing medical staff reliable information to take context-aware decisions. Based on Dey's definition of context (Dey, 1999) and on our definition previously presented in (Oliveira, et al., 2010), we define health context *as any information that can be used to characterize the situation of monitored people and the environment around them, which is considered relevant for the decision-making support in U-Health systems*. In fact, due to the nature of sensor-based long-term monitoring environments, health context is inherently imperfect since it may be incorrect, ambiguous, inconsistent, or unknown (Henricksen, 2002). This problem is intensified mainly by the large amount of sensors and context providers distributed in the environment with possibly different quality levels (Buchholz, et al., 2003; Filho, et al., 2010). In addition, aggregating, deriving, and reasoning on low-quality raw sensed data may reach conflicting and erroneous higher-level health status (Filho, et al., 2010). Also, the quality of context information may be reduced by applying privacy control on private context data in order to enforce ethical guidelines (Jantunen, et al., 2010) and to protect the privacy of patients (Filho, et al., 2010; Layouni, et al., 2009; Sheikh, et al., 2008).

Therefore, U-Health systems should be able to assess the Quality of Context information (Buchholz, et al., 2003) and verify its multi-dimensional aspects (e.g., precision, correctness, up-to-dateness) before using it. This is to reduce the probability of propagating errors in the reasoning and decision-making support of U-Health context-aware applications. Providing inconsistent and erroneous health context to the upper management layers of U-Health systems may have a direct impact on context-dependent decisions taken by the medical staff (e.g., caregivers, physicians, nurses) on any intelligent system. The need for quality control of raw sensed data was emphasized by Arnrich (2010), where they discussed the trade-off between patient's comfort and signal quality. For instance, an unobtrusive dry ECG electrodes embedded into clothes could offer a higher level of comfort and user acceptance than classical wet electrodes (Muhlsteff, 2004), however with lower signal quality. Arnrich, et al. (2010) pointed out the need for applying automatic quality control mechanisms on raw sensed data, such as running error compensation algorithms (Gibbs, 2005; Ottenbacker, 2008; Schumm, et al., 2010), e.g., error detection in ECG signal based on changes in the electrode-skin impedance or on accelerometers. Moreover, they argue that it is useful to indicate the quality of health context data as input for later data interpretation and decision-making support, reinforcing the need for quality assessment and control.

Although the existence of QoC assessment proposals for ubiquitous and pervasive systems (Filho, et al., 2010; Manzoor, et al., 2009; Sheikh, et al., 2007), QoC in U-Health systems has not been studied in depth, except for (Villalonga, et al., 2009) where the authors discussed the impact of QoC in wearable activity recognition systems. This chapter aims to discuss the use of QoC for improving U-Health systems, providing tools for controlling the quality of context information used for making decisions.

Theoretical Framework for U-Health Systems

In order to facilitate understanding of the discussions in this chapter, we present a theoretical framework that generalizes the main management functionalities of context-aware U-Health systems. We do not intentionally focus on a spe-cific application scenario (e.g., remote or local monitoring and diagnosis) in order to keep the generality of the framework.

This framework aims to highlight how, when, and where the quality of context could impact the correct behavior of U-Health systems. As previously stated, U-health systems need to assess and use QoC to reduce the likelihood of making incorrect decisions that could jeopardize patient's health. By analyzing the architecture of several U-health systems (Adami, et al., 2003; Belbachir, et al., 2010; Bottazzi, et al., 2006; Dongsoo, et al., 2009; Durresi, et al., 2008; Fry, 2005; Hansen, et al., 2006; Jantunen, et al., 2010; Layouni, et al., 2009; Orwat, et al., 2008; Sixsmith, 2004), we observe that the attempts to propose quality control of context information is still incipient. Most of existing contributions in U-Health systems consider that the collected context information is accurate and reliable for decision-making support. Figure 1 illustrates the theoretical framework for context-aware U-Health systems. For the sake of simplicity, we split the U-Health system in three main management layers, which communicate with each other in order to provide support to decision-making in medical applications: 1) *sensor layer*; 2) *system layer*; and 3) *decision-making layer*.

Let us mention that it is very important to consider QoC in the various management layers of any U-Health systems. For instance, QoC could be used for: 1) selecting context sources (e.g., sensors, context providers) from redundant sources, rejecting raw sensed data that does not reach the minimum quality level fixed by sensor-level QoC thresholds (i.e., eliminating ambiguity); 2) supporting system-level QoC thresholds, providing only health context information that meet these quality requirements to the U-Health applications (e.g., remote monitoring and emergency systems); 3) supporting rule-level QoC thresholds, reducing the probability of making incorrect context-dependent decisions.

The *Sensor layer* is composed by all physical (e.g., ECG sensor) and logical (e.g., Digital TV ap-

Figure 1. Theoretical framework for u-health systems

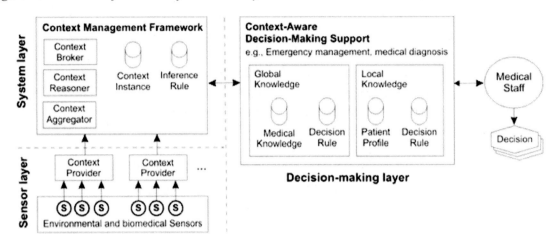

plication or mobile applications asking the patient about his/her body temperature and symptoms) sensors in charge of gathering environmental and biomedical information of observed inhabitants, as well as their interaction with in-home appliances for recognizing their activities. At sensing time, the system may gather some QoC parameters that will be used for evaluating the quality of sensed information, such as timestamp. In this layer, another entity, called context provider, may exist (e.g., a smartphone, a DTV set-top-box or a hardware unit with several embedded sensors), in charge of aggregating one or more raw sensed data. The context provider could verify multi-dimension quality thresholds in order to select raw sensed data from redundant context sources or to reject low-quality data. Moreover, QoC can be used in this layer to verify the reliability of context sources, requiring maintenance intervention in the sensing infrastructure (e.g., recalibration, replacement of sensors, etc). Then, the collected raw data enriched with some quality information will be transferred to the context management framework (i.e., context aggregator) at the *system layer*.

The *system layer* is in charge of the main context management functionalities, such as aggregating, inferring, deriving, obfuscating for protecting the privacy of patients (Oliveira, et al., 2010), and providing context information to the *decision-*

making layer. The context aggregator merges the collected raw data from the various sensors/context providers distributed in the environment and in/on the body of observed inhabitants, following a well-defined context model, such as ontology-based (Filho, et al., 2010) or key-value models (Strang, 2004). Then, the aggregated raw data is stored in the *context instance database* for future use. Usually raw sensed data should be refined or combined with other sensed information through inference and derivation methods before being used by the system (*context reasoning*). For example, signals from ECG sensors can be analyzed by pattern detecting algorithms for discovering any anomaly that can increase the risk of sudden death (Paoletti, 2006).

In addition, inference methods could be deployed in U-Health systems for recognizing inhabitant's activities. For instance, in an ontology-based system an SWRL (Semantic Web Rule Language)[8] rule could be used to infer that an inhabitant is eating if he/she is in the kitchen (e.g., using location information from RFID/Wifi based systems), he/she used the microwave (e.g., using embedded sensors in home appliances) and is sitting on the chair (e.g., using embedded sensors on the chair or accelerometers on his/her body). In this layer, the system needs to assess and verify the quality of raw sensed data for correctly infer-

Exhibit 1. Flow Diagram 1

$$Knowledge_{g,l} + health\ context \xrightarrow{Activate} Decision\_rule(s)_{g,l} \xrightarrow{Provide} Decision\ support$$

ring/deriving new high-level context information (e.g., activity). Moreover, the resulting high-level context information should be re-evaluated with regard to a set of well-defined quality aspects in order to automatically indicate the signal quality as an input for context interpretation and use for decision-making (Such, 2006).

Finally, U-health services and applications are constructed on the context management framework (*decision-making layer*), such as emergency management (Bottazzi, et al., 2006; Fry, 2005), self and remote monitoring (Dengler, et al., 2007; Hagler, et al., 2010; Jantunen, et al., 2010; Lupu, et al., 2008; Mattews, 2007), and medical diagnosis systems (Hansen, et al., 2006; Orwat, et al., 2008), which use context information to improve their decision-making support through the contextualization of knowledge. Generally, U-Health services have two knowledge bases as the main core of decision-making support: 1) global knowledge and 2) local knowledge. The global knowledge represents facts from the medical domain, described in an understandable format, which is associated with each type of supported decisions (e.g., diagnostic, disease treatments) and is valid regardless of the observed people. Although the decision rules defined on the global knowledge have a global scope of applicability, this kind of knowledge should be contextualized in order to provide better support for decision-making.

Unlike the global knowledge, the local knowledge represents facts (e.g., medical records, patient profile) associated with each monitored patient. In this case, the decision rules have a reduced and specific scope of applicability, i.e., each patient has a set of specific decision rules that may be activated by the system based on its local knowledge. Then, the medical staff interacts with the decision-making support layer (e.g., by using friendly interfaces), taking decisions based on the global and local decision rules activated by health context information associated with observed patients. The context-aware decision-making support for U-Health systems is generalized by Exhibit 1, where *g* and *l* indices represent the global and local scope associated with the knowledge and decision rules, respectively.

The local and global knowledge are combined with health context by the decision-making layer in order to activate local and global decision rules, providing medical staff decision-making support. From our viewpoint, it is important to verify the quality of health context used by the system before taking any context-dependent decision, i.e., before activating global or local decision rules.

Therefore, we modify the diagram 1 to introduce the QoC as depicted in the Exhibit 2.

We can conclude that U-Health systems need mechanisms to assessing and using QoC in each one of the three management layers, i.e., sensor, system, and decision-making layers. In order to

Exhibit 2. Flow Diagram 2

$$Knowledge_{g,l} + \left(health\ context, QoC\right) \xrightarrow{Activate} Decision\_rule(s)_{g,l} \xrightarrow{Provide} Decision\ support$$

meet this requirement, the following of this chapter presents several states of art approaches. Then it presents a semantic-based solution that uses OWL-DL ontologies[9] for modeling, evaluating, enriching, and using QoC to improve the decision-making support of U-Health systems. The proposed semantic-based approach is generic and technology-independent, so it could be reused and integrated with any existing U-Health system.

The remainder of this chapter is organized as follows: Section 2 presents the background (QoC definitions, modeling, and evaluating approaches). Section 3 discusses the use of QoC for improving context-based decisions in U-Health systems. This section also presents our semantic-based approach for modeling, evaluating, and using QoC. Section 4 presents some examples of using QoC to improve context-aware systems. Section 5 discusses the presented existing approaches for modeling, evaluating, and using QoC information. Finally, Section 6 concludes the chapter.

BACKGROUND

U-health systems expect that context information used by its context-aware decision-making support is correct and reliable. This is a strong assumption that may not be true all the time. As a consequence, these systems could face problems when using context information due to the unawareness about the quality of information—QoC (Buchholz, et al., 2003). In fact, health context information has an innate characteristic of imperfection and its quality is highly influenced by the way it is acquired (Henricksen, 2002). As previously discussed, U-Health systems may have various sources of context information distributed in the environment and the quality of sensed data is an important differentiator. Indeed, raw sensed data can be affected by many error sources, which are described in the following (Henricksen, 2002; Krause, 2005):

- **Unavailability of context:** context information might be unavailable or unknown by the system. For instance, if a U-health monitoring service does not receive ECG signals of observed inhabitants, it will be unable to detect life-threatening situations based on ECG signals;
- **Inapplicability of context:** context information might be out-dated or inapplicable to the current situation. For example, out-dated ECG signals are not useful for health emergency services, but it should be kept by the system for composing the medical record of a observed patient for later use;
- **Physical restriction of sensors:** physical constraints, comfort level, unobtrusiveness, and external influences, like temperature and humidity, might affect the accuracy of raw sensed data;
- **Context refinement:** wrong or inaccurate context information might be derived from other inaccurate low-level context information, propagating errors in the upper layers;
- **Malicious context provider:** malicious context providers might distribute wrong context data to U-health services, affecting directly any context-based decision made using that misinformation;
- **Ambiguity of context:** context information is often ambiguous. For instance, a smart home may have two or various sensors gathering the same type of information (e.g., ECG sensors on the bed and on the sensor-rich jacket). In this case, the system should decide which one is correct and reliable for decision-making;
- **Privacy of context:** privacy requirements of inhabitants with to regard their context might affect the detail level of context information disclosed in the U-Health system.

Henricksen, (2002) argues that context may be imperfect when: 1) context fails to reflect the true state of the real entity (e.g., inhabitants, patients) that it describes (incorrect); 2) context contains contradictory information (e.g., the current activity of an inhabitant detected by system is *sleeping*, whereas her indoor location indicates that he is in the kitchen); 3) context can be incomplete if some aspects of the situation are unknown by the system (e.g., the ECG signal is unavailable once the ECG sensor is off). Moreover, they argue the need for taking into account quality dimensions when modeling and using context information (Indulska, et al., 2003).

One of the first papers about Quality of Context (QoC) has been written by Buchholdz (2003). In this paper, the authors define the concept of quality of context *as any information that describes the quality of information that is used as context information*. Moreover, Buchholdz (2003) propose the following set of five QoC dimensions as the most important quality aspects associated with context information: precision, probability of correctness, trust-worthiness, resolution, and up-to-dateness. According to Buchholz, et al. (2003), the concept Quality of Context (QoC) differs from the concepts *Quality of Services (QoS)* and *Quality of Devices (QoD)*, since context information can exist without the presence of services and physical sensors. For instance, an inhabitant might provide manually his/her health situation (e.g., symptoms) by filling it in a user-friendly interface of a digital TV application. In this case, the situational data is completely independent of services/sensors and therefore the quality aspects are inherent to this information, i.e., QoC refers to information and neither to the process nor the hardware component that possibly provide the information. In fact, two similar objects representing a type of context information (e.g., ECG signal) related to the same entity (e.g., an inhabitant of a smart home) obtained from the same context source at different times can differ in terms of their precision, probability of correctness, trust-worthiness, up-to-dateness, etc.

Kim (2006) have extended the list of QoC dimensions based on data quality aspects, including accuracy, completeness, representation consistency, and access security. The characteristics of sensors, the situation of measurement, the values expressed by the context information object itself, and the granularity of the representation format have also been identified by Krause (2005) as data sources for determining the QoC. In the aim of relating quality dimensions with the value-added to the information for a context-sensitive application, Krause (2005) have defined the following notion of QoC: *Quality of Context (QoC) is any inherent information that describes context information and can be used to determine the worth of the information for a specific application. This includes information about the provisioning process the information has undergone (history, age), but not estimations about future provisioning steps it might run through.* This definition distinguishes the QoC objectives from the application-dependent worth of context information.

In fact, QoC is used to estimate the worth of context information for a context-dependent application. This definition also impacts the relation between the concepts QoC and QoS. For instance, Quality agreements established between a U-Health service and a context management infrastructure about future provisioning steps of context information are related to QoS, whereas information about the actual reached QoS in the provisioning steps could become part of the QoC. Therefore, QoC can be impacted at any step of context provisioning.

Manzoor, et al. (2008) have classified QoC into two groups: QoC source and QoC parameters. According to their viewpoint, QoC sources are quantities sensed from the environment or gathered from configuration files. However, QoC source values are not appropriate for use and should be transformed into higher-level values named QoC parameters. Then, context information should be associated with these QoC parameters and provided to context consumers, such as U-Health

Figure 2. The main operations of QoC evaluation

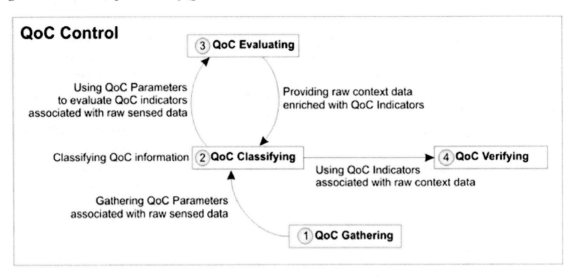

systems. Filho, et al. (2010) makes a similar classification, however they consider QoC source as QoC parameters that are used for evaluating QoC indicators. They define QoC Indicators (QoCI) as *any well-defined quality aspect that can be evaluated and used to describe the quality of context information*. For instance, we can evaluate the QoCI precision associated with ECG signals and body temperature of inhabitants. QoC Parameters (QoCP) are defined by them *as any information sensed from the environment that can be used to measure QoC indicators*. For instance, *captureTime, currentTime*, and *lifeTime* are QoCP used to measure the QoCI up-to-dateness using the method proposed by Manzoor, et al. (2008). Therefore, QoCI represent quality interpretations on QoCP according to a well-defined aspect (e.g., precision, accuracy) and their values are most likely to be used by context-aware U-health systems than QoCP.

As previously discussed, we observe the need for modeling, measuring, and integrating QoC assessment methods in U-Health systems. From our viewpoint, the integration of all steps of gathering, classifying, evaluating, and verifying quality aspects of context information corresponds to the concept named QoC control. We define QoC control as *"a set of operations performed by context-aware systems and applications in order to provide means of evaluating and verifying the quality of context information used for context-sensitive decision-making."* Figure 2 presents the main QoC control operations that should be addressed by U-Health systems.

In order to implement QoC control, U-health systems need to perform the following operations: 1) *QoC gathering:* sensing/profiling QoC parameters from the environment for evaluating QoC indicator; 2) *QoC Classifying*: representing QoC parameters and QoC indicators in an format understandable by the management layers of U-Health systems; 3) *QoC Evaluating:* assessment of QoC indicators by using QoC measuring methods applied on QoC parameters; 4) *QoC verifying:* verifying the values of QoC indicators associated with context used by context-dependent systems. We can note that QoC should be linked to context data delivered to U-health systems consuming that information. Thus, it should be included in context models and handled by context management frameworks.

In the next sections, we present the set of most important QoC indicators and QoC parameters that could be used for QoC control. Moreover, we present the existing approaches for modeling and evaluating QoC that could be integrated in U-Health systems.

QoC Indicators (QoCI)

Table 1 presents the set of the most important QoC indicators proposed in the existing work (Buchholz, et al., 2003; Filho, et al., 2010; Kim, 2006; Manzoor, et al., 2008; Sheikh, et al., 2007) to characterize context information from quality dimensions. We classify QoC indicators according to its scope of use, which could be *generic* or *specific*. Generic QoC indicators are relevant for improving the vast majority of context-sensitive systems, applications and services (e.g., U-Health systems) whereas specific QoC indicators are relevant only for some specific context-aware application domains. For instance, *significance* (Manzoor, et al., 2009) and *accessSecurity* (Filho, et al., 2010) are specific QoC indicators that may be used for changing priority when delivering

Table 1. QoC indicators

QoC indicator	Description	Scope
Probability of correctness (Brgulja, 2010; Buchholz, et al., 2003; Sheikh, et al., 2007)	It denotes the probability that a piece of context information is correct.	Generic
Trustworthiness (Buchholz, et al., 2003; Grossmann, et al., 2009; Manzoor, et al., 2008; Neisse, et al., 2008)	It indicates the belief the system has in the correctness of a context information.	Generic
Resolution (Buchholz, et al., 2003; Filho, et al., 2010)	It denotes the spatial granularity in which a sensed data was captured to represent a real world entity.	Generic
Temporal resolution (Sheikh, et al., 2007)	The period of time to which a single instance of context information is applicable.	Generic
Spatial resolution (Sheikh, et al., 2007)	The precision with which the physical area, to which an instance of context information is applicable, is expressed.	Generic
Up-to-dateness (Buchholz, et al., 2003; Filho, et al., 2010)	It describes the age of context information.	Generic
Precision (Buchholz, et al., 2003; Filho, et al., 2010; Judd, 2003; Sheikh, et al., 2007)	It describes how exactly the provided context information mirrors the reality.	Generic
Accuracy (Kim, 2006)	It is the degree of closeness of the context information value to the real world situation.	Generic
Completeness (Filho, et al., 2010; Kim, 2006)	It indicates the degree with which the attributes of the context are known by the system.	Generic
Significance (Manzoor, et al., 2008)	It indicates the worth or the preciousness of context information in a specific situation.	Specific
Sensitiveness (Filho, et al., 2010)	It describes how critical the context information is with regarding the privacy of observed user.	Specific
Access-security (Filho, et al., 2010, Kim, 2006)	It indicates the probability with which the context data was securely delivered to the context consumers.	Specific
Availability	It indicates the degree with which the context information is available when requested by context consumers.	Specific

context elements (e.g., emergency monitoring) and for indicating if a context element was transferred securely to U-health services, respectively.

It is easy to observe that some QoC indicators overlap when carefully analyzing their definitions. For example, resolution and spatial resolution represent the same idea although they have been used by different authors. Moreover, we observe that resolution and precision are also similar concepts. In fact, as in general any context element (e.g., temperature, humidity) is associated with location information then the precision of that location data represents the spatial resolution of the other context dimensions. However, we need to review the set of QoC indicators in order to verify the QoCI overlaps before proposing a new QoC model. We discuss in detail these existing overlaps in Section 3.

QoC Parameters (QoCP)

Table 2 presents the set of QoC parameters proposed in Bu, et al. (2006), Filho, et al. (2010), Kim (2006), Manzoor, et al. (2008), Sheikh, et al. (2007), and Villalonga, et al. (2009). Each QoC parameter is associated with its corresponding QoC indicator which could be derived from it. Moreover, there exist some general QoC parameters that characterize the context information, but which are not used to evaluate any QoC indicators (e.g., *sourceState*).

Table 3 presents a classification of QoC parameters with regarding the management level(s) in which they could be acquired (i.e., sensor, system, and application/decision-making level) and the corresponding set of possible gathering method(s) used to provide them to U-health systems.

QoCI Measurement Methods

Quality of context is a multi-dimensional concept that can be evaluated in an objective or subjective way. For instance, the precision of location information could be objectively determined us-

ing a numeric value in the same unit as context information, or in a subjective way such as high or low precision. The QoC assessment can be defined *as the process of assigning numerical or categorical values to quality dimensions in a given setting.* In this section, we describe some QoC measurement methods proposed to evaluate the set of QoCI using the QoCP.

Despite its importance (Buchholz, et al., 2003; Filho, et al., 2010; Henricksen, 2002; Krause, 2005; Kim, 2006; Manzoor, et al., 2008), few works (Filho, et al., 2010; Kim, 2006; Manzoor, et al., 2008) have focused on QoC measurement methods. Moreover, most of these studies (Kim, 2006; Manzoor, et al., 2008) propose to evaluate quality only on raw context information. Indeed, they do not consider that raw context data might be used to infer/derivate new higher-level context information and/or changed when enforcing privacy policies of users, which could invalidate the measured QoCI values. For instance, what are the QoC aspects charactering the address of users (i.e., country, city, street, and number) derived from GPS coordinates? What is the precision of the disclosed indoor location of users? Furthermore, no attention has been paid to QoC measurement methods to characterize the context information from privacy and security perspectives. In order to meet these requirements, Filho (2010) proposed several methods to verify the quality of inferred/derived context information, which are discussed.

In order to represent QoC in a form that it could be easily used/understood by context-aware services and to keep a uniform representation of QoC measurement values in the context provisioning process, it is appropriate to measure QoC indicators as a decimal that can take values in the range [0, 1]. Maximum value 1 means that QoC indicator is in complete compliance to the given quality aspect while the minimum value 0 means total nonconformity to the quality aspect. From the viewpoint of context management architecture, it should maximize the values of QoC indicators in order to provide context information with better

Table 2. QoC parameters and QoC indicators

QoC parameter	Description	QoC indicator
sourceState (Manzoor, et al., 2008)	It indicates whether the source of information is dynamic (e.g., a GPS sensor embedded in a smartphone) or static (e.g., temperature sensor in a room).	General information
sourceCategory (Manzoor, et al., 2008)	It indicates the category of the source of the context information (e.g., sensed, profiled, derived, inferred, and static).	General information
measurementUnit (Manzoor, et al., 2008)	It describes the numerical precision of context information.	General information Precision
sourceLocation (Manzoor, et al., 2008)	It represents the location of the source of a context element.	Trustworthiness (Manzoor, et al., 2008)
entityLocation (Manzoor, et al., 2008)	It represents the location of the observed entity.	Trustworthiness (Manzoor, et al., 2008)
currentDistance (Manzoor, et al., 2008)	It represents the current distance between the observed entity and the source of a context element (sensor).	Trustworthiness (Manzoor, et al., 2008)
maximumDistance (Manzoor, et al., 2008)	It is the maximum distance for which we can trust the observation of a source of context information.	Trustworthiness (Manzoor, et al., 2008)
sensorDataAccuracy (Manzoor, et al., 2008)	It is the accuracy with which a sensor can collect a context element.	Trustworthiness Accuracy
numberOfDataValues (Kim, 2006)	It is the total observed data values of a continuous context element.	Accuracy (Kim, 2006)
averageOfDataValues (Kim, 2006)	It is the average of the observed data values of a continuous context element.	Accuracy (Kim, 2006)
RMSE (Kim, 2006)	It is the Root Mean Squared Error used to calculate errors in continuous context elements.	accuracy (Kim, 2006)
confidenceUpperLimit confidenceLowerLimit (Kim, 2006)	They are the upper and lower limits defining a confidence interval, which estimates the true value of a context element.	accuracy (Kim, 2006)
numberOfAvailableAttributes (Kim, 2006)	It is the number of available attributes in the system.	Completeness (Kim, 2006)
totalNumberOfReadings (Kim, 2006)	It is the total number of attribute readings.	Completeness (Kim, 2006)
weightOfAttribute (Manzoor, et al., 2008)	It is the weight of a context element.	Completeness (Manzoor, et al., 2008)
numberOfAnsweredRequest (Filho, et al., 2010)	It is the number of requests answered with a valid context information.	Completeness Availability (Filho, et al., 2010)
numberOfRequest (Filho, et al., 2010)	It is the total number of requests performed on the context information.	Completeness Availability (Filho, et al., 2010)
windowOfObservation	It is the number of latest sensor readings considered to evaluate the availability of a context information.	Availability
currentCriticalValue (Manzoor, et al., 2008)	It indicates the relevance of a information to a specific scenario.	Significance (Manzoor, et al., 2008)
maximumCriticalValue (Manzoor, et al., 2008)	It indicates the maximum critical value that can be assigned to a context element.	Significance (Manzoor, et al., 2008)

continued on following page

Table 2. Continued

QoC parameter	Description	QoC indicator
measurementTime (Manzoor, et al., 2008)	It is the time (timestamp) at which a context information is measured.	Up-to-dateness (Manzoor, et al., 2008)
Lifetime (Manzoor, et al., 2008), temporalResolution (Sheikh, et al., 2007)	It is the period of time after which context information becomes obsolete and it is necessary to take its value again.	Up-to-dateness (Manzoor, et al., 2008)
currentTime (Manzoor, et al., 2008)	The system current time in the moment where a context element is used.	Up-to-dateness (Manzoor, et al., 2008)
Latency (Villalonga, et al., 2009) delayTime (Bu, et al., 2006)	The time delay between the moment a situation happens in real word and the time when the situation is detected in the system.	General information Up-to-dateness
Freshness (Sheikh, et al., 2007) age (Manzoor, et al., 2008)	The time that elapses between the determination of a context element and its delivery to a context consumer.	Up-to-dateness (Manzoor, et al., 2008)
numberOfDisclosureLevel (Filho, et al., 2010)	It is the maximum disclosure level associated with a context element.	Sensitiveness (Filho, et al., 2010)
CurrentDisclosureLevel (Filho, et al., 2010)	It is the current disclosure level in which a context information is being transmitted.	Sensitiveness (Filho, et al., 2010)
sourceAccuracy (Filho, et al., 2010)	It is the accuracy of the source of context element. The source could be a physical/logical sensor, or a reasoning process.	Precision (Filho, et al., 2010)
currentDetailLevel (Filho, et al., 2010)	It is the current detail level in which a context element is being represented.	Precision (Filho, et al., 2010)
numberOfDetailLevel (Filho, et al., 2010)	It is the maximum detail level of a context element.	Precision (Filho, et al., 2010)

quality. From the viewpoint of context-dependent applications, it is important to verify the quality agreement between the provided context data and the required quality level in order to improve the correctness of context-dependent decisions.

Filho, et al. (2010) have assumed that for any tuple of context element (*CxtObj*) and QoC indicator (*QoCI*) supported by a context management framework, which is represented by (*CxtObj, QoCI*), there exists one sequence of deterministic steps (*Alg*) whose result is a real number in the interval [0, 1], where 0 and 1 represent the minimum and maximum quality degrees of *QoCI* related to the context information *CxtObj*, respectively. This definition is formalized in Exhibit 3 where $QoCP_{set}$ is the set of QoC parameters used to measure the associated $QoCI_i$, and x is the *QoCI* value obtained from the QoC measurement method *Alg*.

The obtained *QoCI* values can be yet represented by vague terms such as *low*, *normal* and *high*. In this case, the fuzzy set theory (Zadeh, 1965) can be applyied to define membership functions associated with each QoC indicators. The main idea is to represent *QoCI* values in a format that facilitates the understanding of *QoCI* quantitative values by the medical staff (e.g., *low*, *normal*, *high*) associated with a degree of membership. In fuzzy set theory, an element belongs to a fuzzy set with a certain possibility of membership. Therefore, *QoCI* is a typical example of such a fuzzy concept.

Considering that QoC only depends on the piece of context it relates to, the QoCI values are then associated with context information by the context management system and must not be modified during the information lifetime. This implies that all applications should receive the same context information with the same set of QoCI values. In the following, we present the existing approaches (Brgulja, 2010; Filho, et al., 2010; Kim, 2006; Manzoor, et al., 2008) to measure

Table 3. QoC parameters and its gathering methods

QoC parameter	Management level			Gathering method				
	Sensor	System	Application/ decision-making	Configuration file	System	Sensor	Calculated information	Log file
sourceState, maximumDistance	X			X				
sourceCategory	X	X		X				
sourceLocation, entityLocation, measurementUnit	X			X		X		
measurementTime	X					X		
latency, delayTime	X			X		X	X	
sensorDataAccuracy, sourceAccuracy	X			X		X	X	
currentDistance	X	X					X	
averageOfDataValues	X	X					X	
RMSE	X	X					X	
confidenceUpperLimit, confidenceLowerLimit	X	X					X	
freshness, age	X	X					X	
numberOfDataValues, numberOfAvailableAttributes	X	X						X
totalNumberOfReadings, numberOfAnsweredRequest, numberOfRequest	X	X						X
lifetime, temporalResolution	X	X	X	X				
weightOfAttribute, windowOfObservation, numberOfDisclosureLevel, currentCriticalValue, maximumCriticalValue, currentDisclosureLevel, numberOfDisclosureLevel, currentDetailLevel, numberOfDetailLevel		X	X	X				
currentTime		X	X		X			
sourceAccuracy	X	X			X		X	

Up-to-dateness, Trust-Worthiness, Completeness, Availability, Accuracy, Significance, Sensitiveness, and Precision.

Up-To-Dateness

Before presenting the existing measurement approaches for QoCI up-to-dateness, we need to discuss some related concepts proposed in the literature. Mazoor, et al. (2008) define the up-to-dateness *as the degree of rationalism to use a context object for a specific application at a given time*. Sheikh, et al. (2007) uses the term freshness in the place of up-to-dateness, defining it *as the time that elapses between the determination of a context element and its delivery to a requester*. According to Buchholz, et al. (2003) and Kim, et al. (2006), the Sheikh's freshness definition is

Exhibit 3. Definition

$$\forall \, (CxtObj, QoCI_i), \exists \, A\lg(QoCP_{set}) : x, x \in \Re, 0 \leq x \leq 1, 1 \leq i \leq number \ of \ QoCI$$

Figure 3. Relationship between up-to-dateness, fressness, age, delay time/latency, temporal resolution, and lifetime concepts

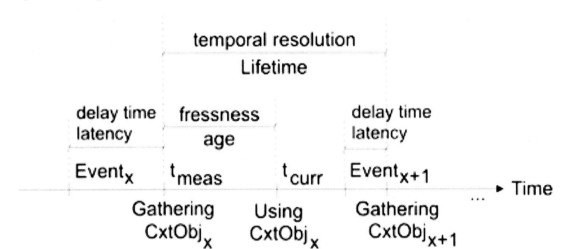

similar to the up-to-dateness concept, which is defined as the age of context information.

Sheikh, et al. (2007) uses another QoC indicator, named temporal resolution, which is defined *as the period of time to which a single instance of context information is applicable*, i.e., the period of time elapsed between two context gathering operations is the temporal resolution of that information. In fact, the temporal resolution has the same meaning as the QoC parameter *Lifetime* used by Manzoor, et al. (2008) to measure the up-to-dateness. Bu, et al. (2006) have used another concept, called delaytime, which is defined as the time interval between the time when the situation happens in real world and the time when the situation is recognized in the system. A similar definition is given by Villalonga, et al. (2009) for the term *Latency*, which is defined as the time delay between the time an activity is initiated and the time the activity is detected.

In light of these definitions, we can conclude that freshness and up-to-dateness are different concepts as up-to-dateness has a larger sense than freshness. On one hand, as stated by Manzoor, et al. (2008), up-to-dateness describes how current the context information is for an entity at a given time for making context-based decisions. On the other hand, freshness of a context element is the *age* of this information, which is a value used for determining the up-to-dateness according to a method proposed in (Manzoor, et al., 2008). Figure 3 gives a pictorial depiction of all concepts related to this QoC indicator.

To the best of our knowledge, in the existing work (Brgulja, 2010; Filho, et al., 2010; Kim, 2006; Manzoor, et al., 2008; Neisse, et al., 2008) that propose QoC measurement methods, there is only one solution to evaluate the up-to-dateness proposed by Manzoor, et al. (2008). Sheikh, et al. (2007) describe how to evaluate and use freshness (i.e., by getting the timestamp at sensing time and verifying the age of context element), but from our viewpoint it is a QoC parameter used to measure the up-to-dateness.

Manzoor, et al. (2008) have proposed to take into account the *Age* (i.e., the freshness) of context information and the *Lifetime* of that context information in order to calculate the value of up-to-dateness. The age of a context element represented by the object *CxtObj*, *Age(CxtObj)*, is calculated as the difference between the system current time in the moment where this CxtObj is used, t_{curr}, and the measurement time of that

Exhibit 4. Measuring up-to-dateness

$$U(CxtObj) = \begin{cases} 1 - \dfrac{Age(CxtObj)}{Lifetime(CxtObj)} : if \ Age(CxtObj) < Lifetime(CxtObj) \\ 0 : otherwise \end{cases}$$

context object, $t_{meas}(CxtObj)$, as specified in the following equation:

$$Age(CxtObj) = t_{curr} - t_{meas}(CxtObj)$$

Then, the up-to-dateness of the context object *CxtObj*, *U(CxtObj)*, is measured by Exhibit 4.

The value of up-to-dateness and, therefore, the validity of context object *CxtObj* decreases linearly as the age of that context object increases. The QoC parameter *Lifetime* is determined by taking into account specific requirements inherent to each context consumer (e.g., a U-Health service) and it can change depending on the type of context information. In a real implementation scenario, the QoC parameter *Lifetime* could be described, for example, using QoC configuration files defined by administrators of context provisioning infrastructures (global scope), or by administrators and users of context-aware services in the application/service layer (local scope).

However, the method proposed by Manzoor, et al. (2008) does not take into account the time of detection of a situation, i.e., the delay time (latency). Therefore, we propose a new method that takes into account the latency when evaluating the up-to-dateness of a context element, as specified in Exhibit 5.

Trust-Worthiness

Buchholz, et al. (2003) introduces a contradiction when they define trustworthiness. According to their definition, trustworthiness is used by the context provider to rate the quality of the actor from which the context provider initially received the context information. This definition is clearly opposed to the first definition of QoC, which states that QoC is about the information and not the process nor the hardware component that provides the information.

Therefore, trust-worthiness should indicate the belief in the correctness of context information. We identified two approaches to measure this indicator: 1) measuring the belief directly in the context information (Manzoor, et al., 2008); 2) measuring the truth that the context consumers have in the entity that provided the context information (Neisse, et al., 2008).

Manzoor, et al. (2008) have proposed a measuring method based on the first approach. They argue that trust-worthiness of a context object is highly affected by its spatial resolution, i.e., the distance between the sensor and the entity described by the context object. The farther the distance of a sensor to the entity the more the doubt in the correctness of information presented by that

Exhibit 5. Accounting for latency

$$U(CxtObj) = \begin{cases} 1 - \dfrac{\left[Age(CxtObj) + latency\right]}{Lifetime(CxtObj)} : if \left[Age(CxtObj) + latency\right] < Lifetime(CxtObj) \\ 0 : otherwise \end{cases}$$

context object. For example, unobtrusive sensors embedded in a mattress, such as ECG sensor, have a greater distance than if those who make direct contact with the patient's skin. Along with the *space resolution*, the *accuracy* with which the sensor collects context information also impacts the trust-worthiness of that information. Let the *accuracy* of the sensor data be δ, then the trustworthiness of context object *CxtObj*, *T(CxtObj)*, is defined by the following equation:

$$T(CxtObj) = \begin{cases} 1 - \dfrac{d(S,E)}{d_{\max}} \times \delta : if \ d(S,E) < d_{\max} \\ 0 : otherwise \end{cases}$$

where $d(S,E)$ is the distance between the sensor S that gathered the *CxtObj* about the entity E and d_{max} is the maximum distance for which we can trust the observation of this sensor. Every type of sensor will have different value of d_{max}. For example, d_{max} value for RFID reader for determining the location of inhabitants will be a lot more than the ECG sensors installed on the patient's body. Accuracy of a sensor, δ, could be provided by the fabricant or measured on the basis of historical analyses and statistical estimation methods, such as the presented by Kim, (2006). From our viewpoint, the second approach for measuring trustworthiness is not relevant to characterize the context information itself, but rather for describing the truth that we have in the context sources. Therefore, the method proposed by Neisse, et al. (2008) and Grossmann, et al. (2009) can be used to verify the belief in the context sources used to gathering the context information.

Accuracy

The accuracy of a context data is directly dependent of the accuracy of sensor and/or process (service) performed for obtaining it. Therefore, the more simple solution to measure the accuracy of a context data is considering the accuracy of the sensor or process performed for obtaining it as its indicator of accuracy. However, accuracy can be also statically determined by using historical analyse and statistical estimation methods. For instance, Kim, (2006) proposed a statistical estimation method to verify the accuracy. They define accuracy *"as the degree to which a context element is correct and reliable."* In fact, it is difficult or even impossible to know the correct value of discrete and continuous context data (i.e., the true value) without using a verification mechanism, such as validation performed by humans (i.e., historical analyse). Thus, Kim, (2006) estimated the confidence interval of context information generated by a sensor using a statistical estimation method. Then, a context value is considered as an accurate data if the value is within the confidence interval.

Kim, (2006) proposes the use of RMSE (Root Mean Squared Error)[10] to calculate errors. In case of continuous data, they use interval estimation method to calculate the confidence upper limit and confidence lower limit. The error of a sensor s_i, *RMSE(s_i)*, is defined by the following equation:

$$RMSE(s_i) = \sqrt{\frac{1}{N} \times \left[\sum_{j=1}^{N} (x_j - \bar{x})^2 \right]}$$

where N is the total observed data values of the context element, x_j is the observed data value, and $\bar{x}$ is the average of the observed data values. A confidence interval that estimates the true value of a sensor s_i, *TV(s_i)*, is the t-distribution with $v = N - 1$ degrees of freedom and V is the error. *TV (s_i)* is calculated by the following equation:

$$TV(s_i) = \left(\bar{x} - t(v,\alpha) \times \frac{\sqrt{V}}{N}, \bar{x} + t(v,\alpha) \times \frac{\sqrt{V}}{N} \right)$$

Completeness and Availability

Kim, (2006) defines completeness *"as the degree to which available context information are present."* It means that the nearest the value of completeness is to 1, the more information is available. Manzoor, et al. (2008) defines this QoC indicator *"as the quantity of information provided by a context object,"* which is different from the previous definition. Filho, et al. (2010) defines the QoCI completeness *"as the degree of availability with which the context information is provided to the context consumers."*

In (Kim, 2006) the completeness has been computed as the ratio of the number of attributes available (*AD*) in the context management system to the total number of attribute readings (*TD*). This concept is measured by the following equation:

$$C(CxtObj) = \frac{AD}{TD}$$

where *C(CxtObj)* is the completeness of a context information, *AD* is the number of available output values and *TD* is the total number of output values registered in the context management system.

Manzoor, et al. (2008) have enhanced this concept using weights for different attributes, as all attributes of a context object may not have the same importance in a given time. They proposed to measure the completeness of a context object as the ratio of the sum of the weights of available attributes of a context object to the sum of the weights of all the attributes of that context object. Completeness of context object *CxtObj*, *C(CxtObj)*, is evaluated by the following equation:

$$C(CxtObj) = \frac{\sum_{j=0}^{m} w_j(CxtObj)}{\sum_{i=0}^{n} w_i(CxtObj)}$$

where *m* is the number of the attributes of context object *CxtObj* that have been assigned a value and $w_j(CxtObj)$ represents the weight of the j_{th} attribute of *CxtObj* that has been assigned a value. Similarly, *n* is the total number of the attributes of context object *CxtObj* and $w_i(CxtObj)$ represents the weight of the i_{th} attribute of *CxtObj*. The value of completeness will be maximum, i.e., 1 if *n = m*. It means that all the attributes of context object *CxtObj* have been assigned a value.

Based on this measurement method, Filho, et al. (2010) proposed an approach to evaluate the completeness that indicates how the context information is complete, available, and up-to-date. They argue it is necessary to verify not only the completeness of a context data, but also if that information is up-to-date and available in the system at request time. According to their proposal, *CO(CxtObj)* and *U(CxtObj)* are the values of completeness and up-to-dateness related with the context object, respectively, which are obtained using the methods proposed by Manzoor, et al. (2008). *NumberOfAnsweredRequest* is the number of requests answered with a valid context information (i.e., *U(CxtObj) > 0* and *CxtObj≠ null*), and *NumberOfRequest* is the total number of requests performed on *CxtObj*, both obtained from log files. The completeness *C(CxtObj)* is measured by Exhibit 6.

The value 0 means that all requests on *CxtObj* were answered with a context data out-of-date

Exhibit 6. Measuring completeness of C(CxtObj)

$$C(CxtObj) = \begin{cases} CO(CxtObj) \times \dfrac{NumberOfAnswered\,Request}{NumberOf\,Request} & : if \begin{cases} U(CxtObj) > 0 \\ CxtObj \neq null \\ NumberOf\,Request > 0 \end{cases} \\ 0 : otherwise \end{cases}$$

Table 4. QoC indicators and examples of use in u-health systems

QoC Indicator	Similar to ...	Definition (Data quality) (Batini, et al., 2009)	Example of use in U-Health systems
Up-to-dateness	Timeliness (Batini, et al., 2009) Freshness and Temporal Resolution (Sheikh, et al., 2007) are QoC parameters	The extent to which context data are sufficiently up-to-date for a context-dependent service.	Verifying if the required set of context elements to make decisions is yet current and valid.
Completeness	Completeness (Batini, et al., 2009)	The extent to which context data is not missing and is of sufficient breadth and depth for a context-dependent service.	Verifying if the set of required context elements is available in the current context when making decisions.
Accuracy	Accuracy (Batini, et al., 2009)	It refers to the closeness of measured values, observations and estimations to the true value. It could be represented by the error rate of context sources.	Verifying if all required context elements used for decision-making support have accurate values.
Significance	Relevance (Batini, et al., 2009)	The extent to which context data is relevant in a specific situation.	In a critical situation, the more relevant context elements should be available to make decisions.
Probability of correctness	Free-of-error (Batini, et al., 2009)	The extent to context data is correct and reliable (it could be applied to simple context elements or to the entire context).	Verifying if the current context is correct before making any context-dependent decision.
Precision	Resolution (Batini, et al., 2009)	It describes how exactly the provided context information mirrors the reality. There are three kinds of precisions: statistical, numerical, and hierarchical.	Verifying if the context elements are described in a minimal required detail level to make decisions.
Availability	Availability (Batini, et al., 2009)	It indicates the degree with which the context information is available when requested by the system.	Verifying the availability of the sensor/context provider.

and/or the context information was unavailable (i.e., completeness = 0) at request time and 1 means that all requests were answered with a complete and valid context data.

In this work, however, we consider the availability of a context data as a independent QoC indicator that should be evaluated separately in order to provide means to identify gathering problems in the sensor layer (e.g., unavailability of sensors and context providers), i.e., we need a new specific method for the availability, disjointing the method to evaluate the completeness proposed in (Filho, et al., 2010). Therefore, we define the QoC indicator availability (see Table 4) as *the degree with which the context information is available in the system when requested by context consumers*. To evaluate the availability of a context information, let

windowOfObservation be the window size of latest sensor readings considered by the measurement method, *numberOfAnsweredReques t(CxtObj)* be the number of requests answered with a valid context information to the i_{th} sensor reading into the window (i.e., $U(CxtObj_i) > 0$ and $CxtObj_i \neq null$), and *numberOfRequest(CxtObj)* be the total number of request for the context information obtained in the i_{th} sensor reading into the window. Then, the availability of *CxtObj*, *AV(CxtObj)*, is measured by Exhibit 7 where *Number of Request(CxtObj)* > 0. The value 0 means that all requests on *CxtObj* were answered with an out-of-date context data and/or the context information was unavailable at request time and 1 means that all the latest requests into the window were answered with a current context data.

Significance

Manzoor, et al. (2008) defines this quality indicator as *"the worth or the preciousness of context information in a specific situation."* A context object with a high value of significance means that information will get immediate attention by the context management system and context consumer. According to Manzoor, et al. (2008), the significance of context object *CxtObj, S(CxtObj),* is evaluated by the following equation:

$$S(CxtObj) = \frac{CV\ (CxtObj)}{CV_{max}(CxtObj)}$$

where *CV(CxtObj)* is the current critical value of the context object *CxtObj*. This information should be gathered from a situation configuration file, which has the information about the critical values of each type of context information. $CV_{max}(CxtObj)$ is the maximum critical value that can be assigned to a context object of the type that is represented by *CxtObj*. In U-Health systems, this indicator is important to inform the upper layers about the significance of a context data according to the current situation, such as a sudden increase in blood pressure.

Sensitiveness

Filho, et al. (2010) proposed the QoCI sensitiveness, which is defined *"as the disclosure level of the context information at a given time."* The disclosure level of a context element can be changed by the context owners in order to enforce their privacy requirements. For instance, in a smart home patients may not wish your location be disclosed when he/she is in the bathroom.

To evaluate the QoCI sensitiveness, Filho, et al. (2010) consider that each type of context information has a well-defined hierarchy of the supported disclosure levels described in a configuration file. Then, they defined the *QoCP numberOfDisclosureLevel* as the maximum disclosure level associated with the *CxtObj* and *QoCP CurrentDisclosureLevel* as the current disclosure level of *CxtObj* with regarding the privacy requirements of the observed person. Then, the sensitiveness of *CxtObj, ST(CxtObj),* is evaluated by the following equation:

$$ST(CxtObj) = \frac{CurrentDisclosureLevel}{numberOfDisclosureLevel}$$

where *QoCP numberOfDisclosureLevel > 0*. The value 0 means that the context information is undisclosed and the value 1 means that the context information is being provided in the highest disclosure level. Therefore, the QoCI sensitiveness informs the context management layers and context consumers about the sensitivity of the context information, with regarding the privacy requirements of the observed person.

Precision

Filho, et al. (2010) defines the precision *as the level of details in which the context information is describing an entity of the real world.* They consider that context information is associated

Exhibit 7. Number of Request(CxtObj$_i$) > 0

$$A\,V(CxtObj) = \begin{cases} \prod_{i=1}^{WindowOfObservation} \dfrac{numberOfAnswered\,Request(CxtObj_i)}{numberOf\,Request(CxtObj_i)} & : if \begin{cases} U(CxtObj_i) > 0 \\ CxtObj_i \neq null \end{cases} \\ 0 : otherwise \end{cases}$$

with an orderly hierarchical scale, from the lower level to the higher level of details. For example, the indoor location of patients can be described at room level, which has higher precision level than described at floor level. When considering numeric values, such as body temperature, values described with three significant figures (e.g., 37.8° Celsius) is more precise than with two significant figures (i.e., 37° Celsius).

According to Filho, et al. (2010), the measurement of QoCI precision is a relation between the detail level of information and its maximum level of detail, multiplied by the accuracy of the method performed to obtain that information. Let *QoCP NumberOfDetailLevel* be the maximum level of detail for the *CxtObj* obtained from a configuration file, QoCP *SourceAccuracy* be the accuracy of the source of *CxtObj* (i.e., sensor, inferring or deriving operation), and *QoCP CurrentDetailLevel* be the current precision level of that *CxtObj*. The precision of *CxtObj* is measured by the following equation:

$$P(CxtObj) = \frac{CurrentDetailLevel}{NumberOfDetailLevel} \times SourceAccurracy$$

where *NumberOfDetailLevel > 0*. The value 0 means that the accuracy of the source of *CxtObj* is 0 (*SourceAccuracy = 0*) or the precision of this information has not yet been measured. The value 1 means that this information is described in the highest detail level and the accuracy of the source of context information is 1.

QoCI Associated with Raw, Inferred, and Derived Context Information

One or more raw context data may be used as input data by reasoning operations (e.g., deriving and inferring processes) in order to obtain new higher-level context information. For instance, ECG signal can be analyzed by feature extraction algorithms (Szczepański, et al., 2010) to detect abnormal rhythm patterns, such as bigeminy, tri-

geminy, and skipped beats. The detected rhythm pattern is a higher-level context data that characterizes the observed person from physiological dimension and the feature extraction algorithm is a derivation process applied on ECG signal (i.e., a raw context data).

We can clearly observe that the quality of detected rhythm pattern depends on the quality of ECG signal and the accuracy of performed derivation process. In fact, the quality aspects of the resulting context information (i.e., the derived or inferred context information) are strongly dependent on the quality of reasoning process and the quality of the set of raw context data used as input to obtain it.

The QoC parameter *sourceCategory* (Manzoor, et al., 2008) can be used to classify the context information according to the gathering method (e.g., sensed, derived, and inferred). Therefore, according to the type of gathering method it may be necessary to apply QoC aggregating methods to evaluate the quality of that information.

In order to measure the quality of inferred/derived context information, Filho, et al. (2010) proposed 4 (four) aggregating approaches: optimistic, pessimistic, average, and weighted average. To explain these methods, let *SCxtObj* be the set of *CxtObj* used as input data to infer/derive the new higher-level context information $CxtObj_{new}$, $QoCI_{i,j}$ be the value of the j_{th} QoC indicator associated with the i_{th} *CxtObj* used as input to obtain $CxtObj_{new}$, $SQoCI_i$ be the set of *QoCI* associated with the $CxtObj_i$ such that $QoCI \neq$ Accuracy, *n* and *m* be the number of elements in *SCxtObj* and *SQoCI*, respectively. Then, the QoCI accuracy of $CxtObj_{new}$, $AC(CxtObj_{new})$, is obtained by the following equation:

$$AC(CxtObj_{new}) = \prod_{i=1}^{n} AC(CxtObj_i) \times SourceAccuracy$$

where the *SourceAccuracy* is the accuracy of the source of the derived/inferred information. The accuracy of $CxtObj_{new}$ is measured in the same way for any aggregating method used to evaluate the quality of new higher-level context information. Then, to evaluate the remaining set of indicators QoCI, we should use one of the proposed methods as described in the following:

- **Optimistic approach**: Let $QoCI_{x,j}$ be the *highest value* of j_{th} QoCI associated with the x_{th} element from the set *SCxtObj*. Then, for each $QoCI_j \in SQoCI$, the $QoCI_{new,j} = QoCI_{x,j}, j \leq m$;
- **Pessimistic approach**: Let $QoCI_{x,j}$ be the *lowest value* of j_{th} QoCI associated with the x_{th} element from the set *SCxtObj*. Then, for each $QoCI_j \in SQoCI$, the $QoCI_{new,j} = QoCI_{x,j}, j \leq m$;
- **Average method**: For each $QoCI_j \in SQoCI$,

  the $QoCI_{new,j} = \dfrac{\sum\limits_{i=1}^{n} QoCI_{i,j}}{n}, j \leq m$;

- **Weighted average method**: Let w_i be the weight for the $CxtObj_i$. Then, for each $QoCI_j \in SQoCI$, the

  $$QoCI_{new,j} = \dfrac{\sum\limits_{i=1}^{n} QoCI_{i,j} \times w_i}{\sum\limits_{i=1}^{n} w_i}, j \leq m.$$

Modeling QoC

There are some challenges in modeling QoC, due mainly to the vagueness and subjectivity of the term quality. However, there is a wide range of well-defined concepts that try to describe in an objective or subjective way the quality of context information. Moreover, each one of these concepts can be described in many ways, for instance, the accuracy of ECG signal could be defined by the average error, the minimal error, the maximal error, or yet the probability distribution, i.e., for each QoC dimension and context type may we can apply one or more measurement methods.

Despite the importance of modeling quality information, few studies (Bu, et al., 2006; Filho, et al., 2010; Krause, 2005; Preuveneers, et al., 2006; Razzaque, et al., 2005; Tang, et al., 2007) have been carried out proposing QoC modeling process and QoC models. Razzaque, et al. (2005) proposed a QoC modeling process in order to help software engineers/developers in the task of modeling useful QoC for context-aware applications and services. The main steps of QoC modeling process are the following: *1) step 1:* using user's and application's requirements to determine the application view of context information and quality requirements; *2) step 2:* application's quality requirements are used to determine the quality parameters (subjective) for the application; *3) step 3:* with the parameter view, in this step we should determine the quality indicators (objective) for the application; *4) step 4:* with the quality view, the quality schema will be defined.

Krause, (2005) proposed a Context Meta-Model (CMM) for modeling context information that includes a base construct to represent quality aspects. Quality information is not of the same class as the context information value (QoC is represented by the metaclass *DatatypeClass*). However, QoC uses the same data constructs and transformation rules than context information. CMM is as information model inside the Java-based CoCo infrastructure (Buchholz, et al., 2004).

Manzoor, et al. (2009) proposed a XML-based approach for modeling quality information. They classify QoC information in two different groups: QoC sources (e.g., criticalValue) and QoC parameters (e.g., up-to-dateness). Unlike these authors, Preuveneers, et al. (2006) proposed an extension to OWL[11] documents for modeling context with support to quality information, exploiting the advantages of using ontologies, i.e., representation, sharing, reasoning, and semantic interoperability. In their approach, Quality of Context (QoC) parameters are modeled by means of two new property types: *QXObjectProperty* and *QXDatatypeProperty*. Both property types inherit from the *DatatypeProperty* and *ObjectProperty* OWL language constructs, as well as from a self-defined class *QualityExtension*, which models the QoC indicators.

Tang, et al. (2007) also proposed an ontology-based approach for modeling quality of information. Unlike Preuveneers, et al. (2006), they proposed an independent OWL-DL ontology for modeling QoC information. In this model, property class replaces the function of OWL property. Quality class is used by context information services to represent quality information with different QoC parameters. Then, Parameters classes are associated with the current situation.

Bu, et al. (2006) proposed a similar ontology-based model that represents only QoC indicators. In order to provide means of representing QoC indicators, QoC parameters, QoC aggregating methods, and QoC measurement methods, Filho, et al. (2010) proposed a new extended ontology-based model. The next section describes this model in detail.

USING QOC INFORMATION TO IMPROVE CONTEXT-BASED DECISIONS IN U-HEALTH SYSTEMS

As described earlier, QoC information can be used to improve each one of the three main management layers of U-Health systems: 1) sensor layer; 2) system layer; 3) decision-making layer. In fact, QoC can be used for:

- *Selecting reliable context source:* since it is possible to obtain the same context information from various sensors available in the environment (e.g., ECG signals from a sensor-rich jacket or from a smart mattress), QoC indicators associated with context information can be used to assist the system to select the most reliable context source from a set of similar context providers and sensors;

- *Filtering context data:* it is necessary to verify the quality of context information used to derive/infer new higher-level context information. In this case, QoC indicators associated with the set of context raw data may do not reach the required quality levels imposed by QoC threshold defined at system level;

- *Improving context-aware decisions:* each context element is associated with one or more QoC indicators that should meet QoC thresholds defined in the decision-making layer in order to control the quality of context.

We analyzed the set of QoC indicators presented in Table 4 and quality indicators from the data quality domain (Batini, et al., 2009) in order to indentify similarities between them and to propose a consistent set of QoC indicators. Table 4 presents the resulting set of QoC indicators and some examples of use in U-health systems.

U-health systems may use QoC indicators to improve any management layers. In this case, we need to differentiate each type of QoC threshold that could be defined in U-health systems according to the management layer where it will be applied. Table 5 presents the QoC threshold types and some examples of use in U-health systems.

In the next section we present our semantic-based approach for modeling, evaluating, and using QoC in U-Health systems.

Semantic-Based Approach for QoC Control in U-Health Systems

Figure 4 illustrates the architecture of our ConteXT Management Framework (*CxtMF*) that implements the proposed semantic-based approach for QoC control. *CxtMF* fully support QoC control, including the collection (gathering), measurement, interpretation, access and delivery of QoC-enriched context information, as well as

Table 5. QoC thresholds and its use in Healthcare systems

QoC threshold	General utility	Using in Healthcare systems
Sensor/context provider level	- Selecting context sources; - Identifying abnormal sensing patterns.	- Verifying the reliability of sensors/context provider that compose the gathering framework; - Investigating/correcting sensor-level problems and, if necessary, changing the defective/inaccurate context source.
System level	- Filtering context data, providing only context information that meet the minimum quality requirements; - Avoiding reasoning on low-quality raw context data in order derive/infer higher-level context information.	- Filtering context data before using that information to enforce inference rules; - Avoiding enforcing rules on raw context data that does not meet the quality requirements.
Decision-making level	- Verifying the quality of context used to make decisions.	- Verifying specific QoC requirements defined in each inference and decision rule.

other functionalities to efficiently handle QoC (e.g., delivering context with a minimum QoC).

CxtMF was defined to support context-aware applications, such as healthcare governance systems (Oliveira, et al., 2010). The main idea behind *CxtMF* is the quality management of health context information before their use by context-dependent healthcare services and applications (e.g., remote monitoring). This means, taking into account the quality of context information in all steps of context management operations.

The main entities of *CxtMF* are *Context Providers (CP)* and *Context Information Service (CIS)*. CP is an agent that sends *CxtObj* associated with some *QoCP* to the Context Information Service (CIS) belonging to the same domain, e.g., a U-Health smart home. Each CP is registered in a CIS, which is composed by various modules in charge of context management functions: *Context Collector (CC), Context Reasoner (CR), Context Obfuscator (CO), QoC Evaluator (QoCE)*, and *Context View Provider (CVP)*. The separation of *CxtMF* into two main entities (i.e., CP and CIS) is only functional, which means these entities may run together on a single processing unit (e.g., a server in a smart home running a CP and CIS) or on various distributed processing units (e.g., CP running on smartphones and CIS in a server). In the following, we give the definitions of some terms used in the remained of this chapter:

- *Health Context Information (HCI):* HCI represents the set of context information supported by the *CxtMF*. Each element of HCI, *hci*, has a domain of possible values, denoted as hci_{dv};
- *Entity (E):* E represents a set of real world entities that can be observed by the framework. For example, *e* could be a inhabitant of a smart home, a room, etc;
- *Sensor (S):* S represents a set of sensors that can be used to gather information about the observed entities E. A sensor can be classified as *physical* or *logical* (e.g., user-friendly interfaces, reasoning processes). Ex.: moving sensor, location sensor, door open sensor, smart home appliances;
- *Context Objects (SCxtObj):* SCxtObj is a set of context objects (*CxtObj*) that represents HCI and its values gathered by sensors S about entities E;
- *Quality of Context (QoC):* QoC is a set of information that describes the quality of a health context information *hci*. QoC can be classified as QoC parameter (QoCP) or QoC indicator (QoCI).

In this case, a *hci* ∈ *HCI* associated with a entity *e* ∈ *E* is sensed from the environment by using one sensor *s∈S*, which is represented in the framework by a *CxtObj∈SCxtObj*. Moreover, a

Figure 4. Architecture of our context management framework (CxtMF)

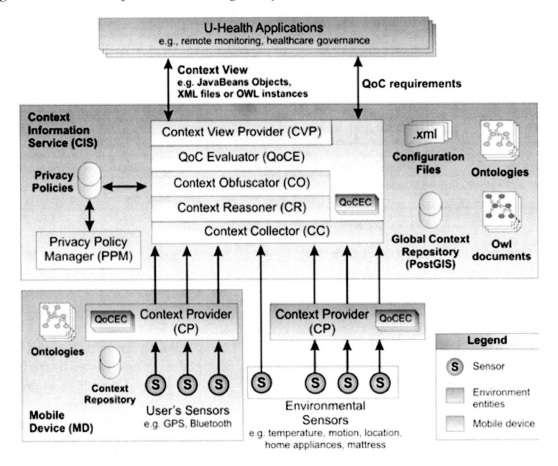

CxtObj can still be associated with some QoC information gathered and generated throughout the management process. Before describing in detail *CxtMF*, we present the Context, QoC, and QoC threshold models used as basis to represent semantically context, QoC, and QoC requirements in the *CxtMF*, respectively.

Modeling Context, QoC, and QoC Requirements

Various modeling approaches can be used to represent context and QoC information. Strang, (2004) presents a survey of existing context modeling solutions and provide taxonomy to classify the technologies to model a context: key-value models, markup scheme models, graphical models,

object-oriented models, logic-based models, and ontology-based models.

Our experience shows that ontology-based model is well suited for representing context information in U-Health systems. Indeed, ontologies are often used in order to achieve a shared semantic understanding of concepts and the relationships that hold among them. Besides that, ontologies allow semantic enrichment of context information through inference and/or derivation processes.

Therefore, we have defined three ontologies for modeling Context, QoC, QoC requirements in order to facilitate the context and QoC representation, sharing, and semantic interoperability in the CxtFM. We used the OWL Web Ontology Language to describe the proposed OWL-DL ontologies.

Figure 5. Health context model

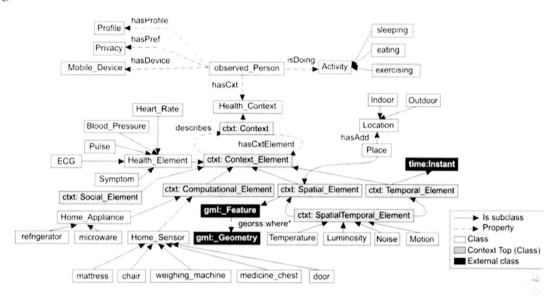

We proposed in (Viana, et al., 2008) a Context Top Ontology that classifies context information according to five different dimensions (see in Figure 5, the classes in gray represent the Context Top classes): *spatial* (e.g., location), *temporal* (e.g., date, instant, interval), *spatio-temporal* (e.g., temperature), *social* (e.g., nearby persons and friends), and *computational* (e.g., home appliances, home sensors). These dimensions are defined in the following:

- **Spatial dimension:** this contextual dimension characterizes the situation of observed entities from spatial point of view. For instance, whether the person is indoor or outdoor;
- **Temporal dimension:** a context element belongs to this dimension if it characterizes the situation from time aspects. For example, instant, period of day, month, year, day, etc;
- **Spatio-temporal dimension:** this dimension characterizes the situation of observed entities from both spatial and temporal aspects. Each piece of context information is associated with a particular location at a

particular time. For instance, temperature, noise, and luminosity in a particular room;

- **Social dimension:** this dimension characterizes the situation from social relationships. For example, a context management framework could identify the persons in the environment, such as relatives, friends and caregivers;
- **Computational dimension:** this dimension characterizes the situation from computational characteristics. We still classify this information in two different types: *invariable* and *variable*. Invariable context information is constant over the useful life of the sensor. For example, the capabilities of a smartphone are invariable context elements. Variable information is just the opposite, it may change during the useful life of the sensor. For example, the status of home appliances (on, off, in use) and home sensors (door open sensors, bed/chair occupancy sensors);

We are reusing the Context top Ontology that we defined (Viana, et al., 2008) as a basis to define the proposed ontologies. Moreover, we are reusing

Figure 6. QoC model

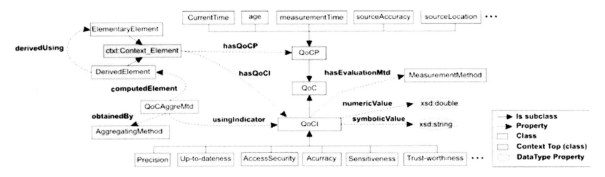

GeoRSS[12] concepts to describe GPS coordinates, OWLTime[13] ontology in order to express temporal information, and the RDF FOAF[14] ontology for describing social context dimensions.

Figure 5 illustrates the Context model, which is easily extensible to accommodate new concepts to represent the situation of an observed person. The main context concepts related to the observed person (class *observed_person*) are represented by the following classes: *Location* (Indoor and Outdoor), FOAF profile, *Activity* (e.g., sleeping, eating, and exercising), *Health_Element* (e.g., heart_Rate, blood_Pressure), *home_Appliance* (e.g., refrigerator, microwave), *Home_Sensor* (e.g., bed/chair occupancy sensors), and Time (Instant, period of day).

Health_Element represents the health situation of the observed person. In normal situation, this type of information is automatically obtained by sensors. Symptom information can be informed by users (e.g., observed person, relatives, caregivers, and doctors) or automatically inferred by the system. Context information from home appliance and sensors is used to derive the current activity of observed person (e.g., the activity sleeping is derived from the bed occupancy sensor and the door open/close sensor of the bedroom).

We are using IETF RFC 4119[15] as the basis to represent semantically indoor and outdoor locations. Indoor location can be described using any of the following formats: *building_name* (LMK); *building_name* and *floor* (LMK, FLR);

building_name, *floor*, and *room* (LMK, FLR, LOC). Outdoor location can be stated using four standard notations: *country* (country); *country, and city* (country, A3); *country, city, and street* (country, A3, A6-STS); *country, city, street, and house_number with suffix* (country, A3, A6-STS, HNO-HNS).

With regarding to the quality aspects, we proposed in (Filho, et al., 2010) a QoC ontology that offers a unified model able to represent QoC information. Figure 6 illustrates an extract of the proposed QoC ontology-based model, which extends our QoC model proposed in (Filho, et al., 2010) to accommodate new concepts, properties and relationships between the concepts.

QoC model is constructed around two main classes: QoCP and QoCI. The QoCP class has thirty-six pairwise disjoint sub-classes which define the set of QoCP that we are taking into account (see Table 2). *ElementaryElement* class represents the raw context data used to derive/infer a new higher-level context element, which is represented by *DerivedElement* class. The link between *ElementaryElement* concept (subclass of *the Context_Element* class defined in the Context Top ontology) and the QoCP and QoCI concepts is established using the object properties *hasQoCP* and *hasQoCI*, respectively.

New QoCP and QoCI can be defined if needed, as new specializations of the QoCP and QoCI class. A context element can be linked to every defined QoCP and to every defined QoCI. One

Figure 7. QoC threshold model

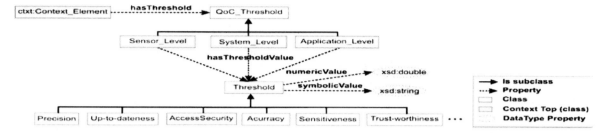

can also use QoC indicator classes defined in other ontologies by specifying alignments or correspondences with our QoC ontology. A derived context element, named DE (i.e., instance of the *DerivedElement* class), is calculated using one or several raw context information represented by *ElementaryElement* class, $E_1, \ldots, E_k$, designated by the *derivedUsing* object property. In order to calculate the QoCI attached to the derived context element DE, aggregating methods are applied to the defined QoCI for the elementary context elements, $E_1, \ldots, E_k$ (see in Section 2.4 these methods in detail).

We use rectification in order to specify the ternary relation (*QoCAggreMtd*) between the derived context element (*derivedElement*), the QoCI to be derived, and the aggregating method (AggregatingMethod) to be used. Each QoCI has two datatype properties to assign the measurement value: *numericValue, symbolicValue. numericValue* property represents the value obtained from the corresponding measurement method for evaluating the QoCI, which is a set in the range [0..1]. *symbolicValue* property describes the value of a QoCI using fuzzy terms, such as "low," "normal," and "high."

In order to represent QoC threshold values to be achieved at sensor, system, and application management level of U-Health systems, we defined the *QoC threshold* ontology illustrated in Figure 7. The *QoC_threshold* class has three sub-classes: *Sensor_level, System_level*, and *Application_level*. Each *Context_Element* may have one or various QoC threshold that should

be verified by the system, which is represented by the object property *hasThreshold*. As the QoCI class defined in the QoC ontology, each *threshold* has two datatype properties to assign the required level: *numericValue, symbolicValue*. The threshold could be defined on any QoCI defined in the QoC ontology.

Context Providers (CP)

Context Providers (CP) are the CxtMF entities in charge of gathering context information from the environment. CP is embedded in the environment (e.g., application server) or in smartphones. It role is to capture and transmit *CxtObj* to the *Context Information Service (CIS)*.

CP can be configured to run in one of these two operating modes: *push* and *pull*. In the push operating mode, CP sends automatically the gathered information to the Context Information Service (CIS) as alerts. However, in the pull mode the CIS should request the CP every time it needs a context element managed by that CP. A CP can manage one or more sensors, which can be of type *cxtSensors* (this sensor is in charge of gathering raw context data) and *QoCsensors* (this sensor is in charge of gathering QoC parameters when the QoC control is activated in the framework).

A CP keep a dynamic list of registered sensors S, controlling synchronous (push operating mode) and asynchronous (pull operating mode) notifications from them. Moreover, CP keeps a dynamic queue of receiving information from each registered sensor. A CP can have one or more registered

QoC Evaluating Components (QoCEC) in charge of gathering and evaluating QoC information associated with *CtxObj*. CP deploys dynamically the *QoC Evaluating Components (QoCEC)* in order to evaluate the quality of raw context data. Each QoCEC is in charge of evaluating a well-defined QoC dimension. For more detail about the QoCEC, see (Filho, et al., 2010). QoC-enriched CtxObj could be used to select sensors based on QoC thresholds (sensor level) defined by the context management administrator.

CP supports yet three sensing modes described below: *1) Default:* if a CP is configured to operate in this sensing mode, only raw context information will be gathered from the sensors controlled by it. In this case, the CxtFM will operate like a QoC-unaware context management system. *2) Sensing QoC:* by operating in this sensing mode, raw context information will be enriched with QoC parameters; *3) measurement QoC:* if a CP is configured to operate in this sensing model, raw context information *CtxObj* will be enriched with QoC Parameters and QoC Indicators. In this case, CP should call QoCE components in order to measure the QoCI values.

Context Information Service (CIS)

Context Information Service (CIS) is the main component of our context management framework. It is composed by the following sub-services: *Context Collector (CC), Context Reasoner (CR), Context Obfuscator (CO), QoC Evaluator (QoCE),* and *Context View Provider (CVP).* CxtMF is configurable, enabling the activation/ deactivation of the sub-services CR, CO, and QoCE. The deactivation of these services does not affect the core functionality of the context management framework, which makes the system very interesting.

Context Collector (CC) receives and aggregates context and QoC information sent by CP. Moreover, CC can collect context information sent directly by the sensors distributed in the environment. In this case, CC incorporates some features of CP. The collected context and QoC information is used to build the *health context* of the observed person. CC communicates directly with QoC Evaluator (QoCE) service in order to evaluate the QoC derived from raw context information. This process is performed only if the CC and the CxtMF are configured to support QoC control.

Health context is stored in the *Global Context Repository (GCR)* (i.e., a SGDB). Moreover, an instance of the health context associated with the observed person is generated with the most recent context information. This OWL-DL document will be used by the *Context Reasoner (CR)* and *Context Obfuscator (CO). Context Reasoner (CR)* runs inference operations on OWL-DL documents that describe the health context of observed entities, using Pellet[16] to evaluate SWRL rules predefined by the context management administrator.

Context Obfuscator (CO) enforces privacy policies on context information by running obfuscation and anonymization operations based on ontologies. Privacy policies are divided in two set of rules: personal privacy policies and global privacy policies. Personal privacy policies are defined with regard to the privacy requirements of a monitored person, while global privacy policies are applied to all people. Privacy policies are specified using SWRL rules, which are evaluated by the CO in order to limit and/ or to generalize the disclosure level of context information. As result, only the disclosed context concepts, properties, and datatype properties described in the health context document will be described in the resulting OWL document, named *Context View* (Context View ⊆ Health Context). Privacy policies are stored by the Privacy Policy Management (PPM), which provides a web interface to ease the writing of SWRL rules. After the enforcement of SWRL privacy rules, if the QoC support is activated in the framework the CO will call the QoCEC to re-evaluate the QoCI associated with the modified context in order to maintain the consistency.

QoC Evaluator (QoCE) is the core service for the QoC control. It allows dynamic deployment of QoC Evaluating Components (QoCEC) in order to evaluate QoC indicators supported by the *CxtMF*. There exists at least one QoCEC for each QoC indicator (e.g., precision, up-to-dateness). Let us note that *CxtMF* performs the QoC measurement methods in two steps: *i) step 1:* CxtMF evaluates QoC on raw sensed data, which is realized by CP/CC; *ii) step 2:* QoC of higher-level context information is re-evaluated by CR and CO.

Finally, the *Context View Provider (CVP)* answers the context information queries, providing *Context Views* to context consumers, such as U-health applications. They can operate in two modes: *push* and *pull*. Moreover, CVP supports two types of queries: *1) full query:* CVP answers the request by sending the full context view associated with a observed person; *2) personalized query:* CVP answers by sending the context view containing only the requested information. Before answering the request, CVP calls the *ContextObfuscator(CO)* in order to evaluate the privacy rules. If the QoC support is activated in the CxtMF, CVP is then able to provide context consumers *QoC-enriched context views*.

CASE STUDY

This section presents some case study describing the use of quality information to improve context-sensitive systems. Manzoor, et al. (2009) proposes the use of QoC to conflict resolving. Conflicts can take place at different context management layers, such as context acquisition, context processing, context distribution, and application level. Manzoor, et al. (2009) proposes the following set of QoC-based policies for conflict resolving: *1) Up-to-Dateness Based Policy:* this policy is used for resolving conflicts in the context objects that change their values very rapidly; *2) Trustworthiness Based Policy:* it is used for resolving the conflict between two or more sensors collecting the context of same entity or event; *3) Completeness Based Policy:* it is used to compose a complete picture of the current situation of the real world; *4) Significance Based Policy:* it is used to specify that the context objects with high values of significance should be reported on a priority basis. From this set of QoC fundamental policies, policies can also be defined based on two or more QoC indicators depending on the requirements of a particular application.

Muhlhauser, (2009) proposed the use of QoC information for improving context-aware user interfaces. QoC information is provided for cognitive user contexts: *1) correctness:* algorithms used to infer information from user's behavior usually return a confidence value along with the inferred information (i.e., probability of correctness); *2) trustworthiness:* it is derived in a similar way as for other context sources by measuring how often a context source returned data that proved to be useful; *3) resolution:* it reflects the population from which the information was derived (single user, users group, all potential users); *4) up-to-dateness:* it reflects the time of the last user model update.

Indeed, the probabilistic nature leads to inherent uncertainty of context information. Therefore, the uncertainty should be considered when using context to adapt UI. Muhlhauser (2009) proposes three meta-concepts to cope with uncertainty at UI: *1) Inform and mediate:* inform the user about uncertain context and let her confirm or correct the data; *2) Make multiple suggestions:* derive a weighted list of suggestions from context, not just a single one, and present them to the user for selection; *3) Adapt behavior:* consider the level of uncertainty for adjusting whether and how an action is executed and suggestions are made. The authors propose three ways to convey context quality at the UI: *1) Numerical:* a numeric value (number) is used to represent the certainty in a given action/suggestion; *2) Symbolic:* different icons represent different levels of uncertainty; *3) Gradual graphical attributes:* use a graphical attribute like color or line thickness to convey the certainty in the context quality.

Villalonga, et al. (2009) proposed the use of QoC for improving activity recognition system. User activity is a valuable piece of context and is worth to be made available to any application through context frameworks. By connecting to context frameworks the activity recognition systems could obtain additional data from environmental sensors and even incorporate them into the recognition chain. In the following we describe the mapping of QoC in activity recognition system: *1) Offline Performance Metrics:* accuracy as part of the QoC is one of the most relevant parameters as it gives an idea of the relation between the context value and reality. In wearable computing, the corresponding metrics are the offline performance metrics, i.e., accuracy, confusion matrix, precision, recall, and specificity. Even if accuracy is used in both domains, the concept is different since in activity recognition it is a statistical value saying how often the recognized class matches real class. The authors suggest the use of values on the diagonal of the confusion matrix as the quantification for the accuracy parameter in the QoC of the recognized class; *2) Online Performance Metrics:* Activity recognition systems usually operate online. The continuous recognition performance metrics are particularly important to quantify the errors of the classification for this system. The authors suggest extending QoC to include performance metrics (insertions, substitutions, deletion, merge, fragmentation, overfill, and underfill); *3) Cost of Context and Power Consumption:* context frameworks do not consider resource consumption when delivering or collecting context as the only goal is to deliver high quality context. In wearable computing, however, devices are running on batteries and only limited power is available. Thus, it is important to consider how much power is invested into the activity recognition. Power consumption can be traded-off for accuracy and can be used as performance metric of an activity

recognition system. However, it is not a QoC measure as it does not indicate how the context represents the real world, but only informs about the cost to calculate this context value. Cost of Context is therefore a new concept, which if defined as a parameter associated to the context that indicates the resource consumption used to measure or calculate the piece of context information; *4) Delay Time and Latency:* in a large scale framework, it is the time to find the appropriate context source. In wearable computing scenarios involving human assistance, the response time of an application is crucial for the acceptance by the user. In some cases, feedback must be delivered within milliseconds for meaningful interaction. Therefore, latency is another vital metric in human activity recognition and needs to be integrated into QoC. There is a clear matching between the latency and the delay time parameter of the QoC.

Filho, et al. (2010) deployed the CxtMF in a university building to simulate a u-health smart home, providing QoC-enriched context information to ubiquitous health services. In the current version of this system, there is a context-aware service to control heating and lighting according to the temperature and luminosity information provided by Sun Spots[17]. The main objective of this context-aware service is to provide comfortable life to old people. They installed in two different rooms two Sun Spots, in which was deployed a CP to gather context information. The gathered information is transferred to a Sun Spot base station connected to a server running a CIS (Intel Core Duo 2.GHz, 4 GB, Windows Vista 32 bits, MySql 5.0.45). In (Filho, et al., 2010), they describe an evaluation carried out during 24 hours, with intervals of 5 seconds between the sensor readings. The evaluation consisted of (1) a study of performance to verify the time overhead added by the quality support in the CxtMF and (2) and an analysis of the use of quality information for selecting context providers from redundant sources.

From the results, Filho, et al. (2010) observed that the time spent for sensing context information (temperature, luminosity) enriched with QoC remained almost constant in relation with the growing number of context providers (i.e., one, two, three, and four Sun Spots). Indeed, the execution time of the proposed QoC measuring methods for all QoCI supported by the framework is approximately 100 milliseconds, which is an acceptable impact on the performance of CxtMF.

Let CP_1 and CP_2 be two Sun Spots installed in the same room. To select a context provider from this redundant set of context sources, they compared two selection approaches of context providers: (1) FIFO and (2) QoC-aware approach. Using the FIFO approach, they observed that approximately 40% of cases the CIS has selected the information provided by the CP_2 and in the remaining 60% the CxtMF used the information from CP_1. This may have been caused by the different distances of the Sun Spots from the station base, or yet by the time synchronization problems. Using the QoC-aware approach, however, in 100% of cases the CIS selected the temperature provided by the CP_2. This occurred because the precision of the temperature provided by the CP_1 (0.67, which means that the temperature is described with only one decimal place) was lower than the precision of temperature provided by the CP_2. In this case, once the CIS identified that CP_2 offers information with higher global quality, it can select the CP_2 and put the CP_1 on its list of context providers that need to be checked in order to be able to provide context information in the future.

DISCUSSION

This chapter presented QoC definitions and existing approaches for modeling, measuring, and using QoC to improve context-aware systems, such as u-health smart homes. Table 6 presents a comparison between the existing solutions discussed in this chapter, according to the following criteria: 1) QoC indicators; 2) QoC parameters; 3)

measurement methods of QoC; 4) QoC model; 5) Context management framework; and 6) purpose.

Buchholz, et al. (2003), Kim (2006), Bu, et al. (2006), Manzoor, et al. (2008), Sheikh, et al. (2008), and Filho, et al. (2010) have proposed the most of QoC indicators described in the literature: probability of correctness, trust-worthiness, resolution, up-to-dateness, precision, freshness, spatial and temporal resolution, accuracy, completeness, representation-consistency, accessSecurity, delay time, and probability of Consistence. However, only the work described in (Filho, et al., 2010; Manzoor, et al., 2008) make the distinction between QoC indicators (i.e., high-level QoC information) and QoC parameters (i.e., raw quality data used to measure QoC indicators).

Despite the long list of proposed QoC indicators in the literature, few work proposes methods to evaluate them (Brgulja, 2010; Filho, et al., 2010; Grossmann, et al., 2009; Klein, 2010; Kim, 2006; Manzoor, et al., 2008). However, we observe yet the need to adapt the QoC measurement methods to each management layer. Moreover, context management frameworks should be able to represent quality indicator values as fuzzy sets.

With regard to the technology used to model QoC information, most work does not make an explicit choice. However, among those that explicitly propose QoC models, it is notorious the predominance of ontology-based approaches (Bu, et al., 2006; Filho, et al., 2010; Preuveneers, et al., 2006; Tang, et al., 2007). Indeed, there is a tendency in the use of ontologies to represent context and quality of context information in u-health smart homes.

Filho, et al. (2010), Manzoor, et al. (2009), Bu, et al. (2006), Tang, et al. (2007), and Krause, et al. (2005) proposed a context management framework that implements QoC control, while Sheikh, et al. (2008), Abid, et al. (2009), and Grossmann, et al. (2009) integrated QoC measurement methods with an existing context management framework.

The purpose of most work discussed in this chapter is general, proposing modeling and evaluating approaches that could be used by any

Table 6. Comparison between existing work

Approach	QoCI	QoCP	Measurement methods of QoC	QoC Model	Context Management Framework	Purpose
Buchholz, et al. (2003)	X	-	-	-	-	General
Krause (2005)	-	-	-	CMM	CoCo	General
Preuveneers, et al. (2006)	-	-	-	OWL-DL	-	Uncertainty handling
Tang, et al. (2007)	-	-	-	OWL-DL	X	File system
Manzoor, et al. (2008)	X	X	X	XML schema	X	Rescue situations
Sheikh, et al. (2008)	X	-	-	-	AWARENESS middleware	Privacy protection
Razzaque (2008)	-	-	-	QoC modeling process	-	General
Kim (2006)	X	-	X	-	-	General
Bu, et al. (2006)	X	-	-	OWL-DL	X	Inconsistency resolution
Abid, et al. (2009)	-	-	-	-	COSMOS	General
Grossmann, et al. (2009)	-	-	X	-	NEXUS	General
Manzoor, et al. (2009)	-	-	-	XML	X	Conflict resolving
Muhlhauser, et al. (2009)	-	-	-	-	-	UI improvement
Villalonga, et al. (2009)	-	-	-	-	-	Human Activity Recognition
Filho, et al. (2010)	X	X	X	OWL-DL	CxtMF	General
Brgulja (2010)	-	-	X	-	-	Inconsistency resolution
Klein (2010)	-	-	X	-	-	Temporal conflict

context-aware systems. However, we observe the use of QoC in some specific domains, such as uncertainty handling of context (Preuveneers, et al., 2006), rescue situations (Manzoor, et al., 2009), privacy protection of context (Sheikh, et al., 2008), inconsistency resolution (Brgulja, et al., 2010; Bu, et al., 2006; Klein, 2010), conflict resolving (Filho, et al., 2010; Manzoor, et al., 2009), and user-interface improvements (Muhlhauser, 2009). However, we observe yet the need to integrate QoC control in u-health smart homes to improve its management layers in specific healthcare application domains.

CONCLUSION

This chapter discussed the importance of controlling the quality of context information in order to improve U-health systems. We observe that although there are several studies proposing the use of QoC in pervasive and ubiquitous context-aware systems, it is still an incipient research. With this in mind, we presented and discussed the existing approaches for gathering, modeling, evaluating, and using QoC, which could be incorporated in U-Health systems to improve context-dependent decisions and reduce errors. In addition, this chapter presents how quality aspects of context information can be used to improve the main management layers of U-health systems.

Finally, we presented our semantic-based approach for gathering, modeling, providing, and using QoC, which was implemented in the ConteXT Management Framework (CxtMF). CxtMF was developed to support the deployment of U-Health systems, such as healthcare governance applications (Oliveira, et al., 2010). In order to maintain the interoperability of health context and quality information in all layers of context management, we defined three OWL-DL ontologies (health context ontology, QoC ontology, and QoC threshold ontology) for representing the health context, QoC information, and QoC thresholds, respectively. These ontologies can serve as basis for other further research from the community.

REFERENCES

Abid, Z., Chabridon, S., & Conan, D. (2009). A framework for quality of context management. In Proceedings of the 1st International Conference on Quality of Context, (pp. 120 – 131). Stuttgart, Germany: Springer.

Adami, A. M., Hayes, T. L., & Pavel, M. (2003). Unobtrusive monitoring of sleep patterns. In *Proceedings of the 25th Annual International Conference of the IEEE Engineering in Medicine and Biology Society*, (pp. 17 – 21). Cancun, Mexico: IEEE Press.

Arnrich, B., Mayora, O., Bardram, J., & Tröster, G. (2010). Pervasive healthcare: Paving the way for a pervasive, user-centered and preventive healthcare model. *Methods of Information in Medicine, 49*(1), 67–73.

Batini, C., Cappiello, C., Francalanci, C., & Maurino, A. (2009). Methodologies for data quality assessment and improvement. *ACM Computing Surveys, 41*(3), 1–52. doi:10.1145/1541880.1541883

Belbachir, A. N., Drobics, M., & Marschitz, W. (2010). Ambient assisted living for ageing well – An overview. *E&I Elektrotechnik und Informationstechnik, 127*(7-8), 200–205. doi:10.1007/s00502-010-0747-9

Bottazzi, D., Corradi, A., & Montanari, R. (2006). Context-aware middleware solutions for anytime and anywhere emergency assistance to elderly people. *IEEE Communications Magazine, 44*(4), 82–90. doi:10.1109/MCOM.2006.1632653

Brgulja, N., Kusber, R., David, K., & Baumgarten, M. (2009). Measuring the probability of correctness of contextual information in context aware systems. In *Proceedings of the IEEE International Symposium on Dependable, Autonomic and Secure Computing*, (pp. 246 – 253). Chengdu, China: IEEE Press.

Bu, Y., Gu, T., Tao, X., Li, J., Chen, S., & Lu, J. (2006). Managing quality of context in pervasive computing. In *Proceedings of the Sixth International Conference on Quality Software*, (pp. 193 – 200). IEEE Press.

Buchholz, T., Krause, M., Linnhoff-Popien, C., & Schiffers, M. (2004). CoCo: Dynamic composition of context information. In *Proceedings of the Annual International Conference on Mobile and Ubiquitous Systems*, (pp. 335 – 343). IEEE Press.

Buchholz, T., Küpper, A., & Schiffers, M. (2003). Quality of context: What it is and why we need it. In *Proceedings of the 10th International Workshop of the HP OpenView University Association (HPOVUA)*. Geneva, Switzerland: ACM Press.

Dengler, S., Awad, A., & Dressler, F. (2007). Sensor/actuator networks in smart homes for supporting elderly and handicapped people. In *Proceedings of the 21st International Conference on Advanced Information Networking and Applications Workshops*, (pp. 863 – 868). IEEE Press.

Dey, A. K., & Abowd, G. D. (1999). The context toolkit: Aiding the development of context-aware applications. In *Proceedings of the Workshop on Software Engineering for Wearable and Pervasive Computing*, (pp. 434 – 441). ACM Press.

Dongsoo, H., Sungjoon, P., & Minkyu, L. (2009). The-muss: Mobile u-health service system. *Communications in Computer and Information Science, 25*(4), 377–389.

Durresi, A., Durresi, M., & Barolli, L. (2008). Secure ubiquitous health monitoring system. *Lecture Notes in Computer Science, 5186*(1), 273–282. doi:10.1007/978-3-540-85693-1_29

Filho, J. B., Miron, A. D., Satoh, I., Gensel, J., & Martin, H. (2010). Modeling and measuring quality of context information in pervasive environments. In *Proceedings of the 24th IEEE International Conference on Advanced Information Networking and Applications*, (pp. 690–697). Perth, Australia: IEEE Press.

Fry, E. A., & Lenert, L. A. (2005). MASCAL: RFID tracking of patients, staff and equipment to enhance hospital response to mass casualty events. In *Proceedings of the AMIA Annual Symposium Proceedings*, (pp. 261 – 265). San Diego, CA: AMIA.

Gibbs, P., & Asada, H. H. (2005). Reducing motion artifact in wearable bio-sensors using MEMS accelerometers for active noise cancellation. *American Control Conference, 3*(1), 1581 – 1586.

Grossmann, M., Hönle, N., Lübbe, C., & Weinschrott, H. (2009). An abstract processing model for the quality of context data. In *Proceedings of the 1st International Conference on Quality of Context*, (pp. 132 – 143). Berlin, Germany: Springer.

Hagler, S., Austin, D., Hayes, T. L., Kaye, J., & Pavel, M. (2010). Unobtrusive and ubiquitous in-home monitoring: a methodology for continuous assessment of gait velocity in elders. *IEEE Transactions on Bio-Medical Engineering, 57*(4), 813–820. doi:10.1109/TBME.2009.2036732

Hansen, T. R., Bardram, J. E., & Soegaard, M. (2006). Moving out of the lab: Deploying pervasive technologies in a hospital. In *Proceedings of the IEEE Pervasive Computing*, (pp. 24 – 31). IEEE Press.

Henricksen, K., & Indulska, J. (2004). Modelling and using imperfect context information. In *Proceedings of the Conference on Pervasive Computing and Communications Workshops*, (pp. 33 – 37). IEEE.

Henricksen, K., Indulska, J., & Rakotonirainy, A. (2009). Modeling context information in pervasive computing systems. In *Proceedings of the First International Conference on Pervasive Computing*, (pp. 167 – 180). London, UK: IEEE Press.

Indulska, J., Robinson, R., Rakotonirainy, A., & Henricksen, K. (2003). Experiences in using CC/PP in context-aware systems. In *Proceedings of the 4th International Conference on Mobile Data Management*, (pp. 247 – 261). Springer.

Jantunen, I., Wang, X., Pekkola, M., & Korhonen, T. (2010). *Applying ethical guidelines to ubiquitous health care in China*. Paper presented at the 1st ETICA Conference. Tarragona, Spain.

Judd, G., & Steenkiste, P. (2003). Providing contextual information to pervasive computing applications. In *Proceedings of the 1st IEEE International Conference on Pervasive Computing and Communications*, (p. 133). IEEE Press.

Kim, J., Choi, H., Wang, H., Agoulmine, N., Deerv, M. J., & Hong, J. W. (2010). Postech's u-health smart home for elderly monitoring and support. In *Proceedings of the IEEE International Symposium on a World of Wireless, Mobile and Multimedia Networks*, (pp. 1 – 6). Montreal, Canada: IEEE Press.

Kim, Y., & Lee, K. (2006). A quality measurement method of context information in ubiquitous environments. In *Proceedings of the International Conference on Convergence and Hybrid Information Technology*, (pp. 576 - 581). Washington, DC: IEEE Press.

Klein, N., & David, K. (2010). Time locality: A novel parameter for quality of context. In *Proceedings of the Seventh International Conference on Networked Sensing Systems*, (pp. 277 – 280). IEEE Press.

Krause, M., & Hochstatter, I. (2005). Challenges in modelling and using quality of context (QoC). In *Proceedings of the Mobility Aware Technologies and Applications*, (pp. 324 - 333). Heidelberg, Germany: Springer.

Layouni, M., Verslype, K., Sandıkkaya, M. T., Decker, B., & Vangheluwe, H. (2009). Privacy-preserving telemonitoring for ehealth. *Lecture Notes in Computer Science, 5645*(1). doi:10.1007/978-3-642-03007-9_7

Lupu, E., Dulay, N., Sloman, M., Sventek, J., Heeps, S., & Strowes, S. (2008). AMUSE: Autonomic management of ubiquitous e-health systems. *Concurrency and Computation, 20*(3), 277–295. doi:10.1002/cpe.1194

Manzoor, A., Truong, H. L., & Dustdar, S. (2008). On the evaluation of quality of context. In *Proceedings of the Third European Conference in Smart Sensing and Context*, (pp. 140 – 153). Zurich, Switzerland: IEEE.

Manzoor, A., Truong, H. L., & Dustdar, S. (2009). Quality aware context information aggregation system for pervasive environments. In *Proceedings of the International Conference on Advanced Information Networking and Applications Workshops*, (pp. 266 – 271). Bradford, UK: IEEE Press.

Manzoor, A., Truong, H. L., & Dustdar, S. (2009). Using quality of context to resolve conflicts in context-aware systems. In *Proceedings of QuaCon* (pp. 144–155). Springer. doi:10.1007/978-3-642-04559-2_13

Matthews, R., McDonald, N. J., Hervieux, P., Turner, P. J., & Steindorf, M. A. (2007). A wearable physiological sensor suite for unobtrusive monitoring of physiological and cognitive state. In *Proceedings of the International Conference of IEEE Engineering in Medicine and Biology Society*, (pp. 5276 – 5281). IEEE Press.

Muhlsteff, J., & Such, O. (2004). Dry electrodes for monitoring of vital signs in functional textiles. In *Proceedings of the 26th Annual International Conference of the IEEE, Engineering in Medicine and Biology Society*, (pp. 2212 – 2215). San Francisco, CA: IEEE Press.

Neisse, R., Wegdam, M., & Van-Sinderen, M. (2008). Trustworthiness and quality of context information. In *Proceedings of the 9th International Conference for Young Computer Scientists, International Symposium on Trusted Computing*, (pp. 1925 – 1931). Zhang Jia Jie, China: IEEE.

Oliveira, M., Hairon, C., Andrade, O., Moura, R., Sicotte, C., & Denis, J.-L. … Martin, H. (2010). A context-aware framework for health care governance decision-making systems: A model based on the Brazilian digital TV. In *Proceedings of the IEEE International Symposium on a World of Wireless, Mobile and Multimedia Networks*, (pp. 1 – 6). Montreal, Canada: IEEE Press.

Orwat, C., Graefe, A., & Faulwasser, T. (2008). Towards pervasive computing in health care - A literature review. *BMC Medical Informatics and Decision Making, 8*(26).

Ottenbacher, J., Kirst, M., Jatoba, L., Großmann, U., & Stork, W. (2008). An approach to reliable motion artifact detection for mobile long-term ECG monitoring systems using dry electrodes. *Latin American Congress on Biomedical Engineering, 18*(3), 440 - 443.

Paoletti, M., & Marchesi, C. (2006). Discovering dangerous patterns in long-term ambulatory ECG recordings using a fast QRS detection algorithm and explorative data analysis. *Computer Methods and Programs in Biomedicine, 82*(1), 20–30. doi:10.1016/j.cmpb.2006.01.005

Preuveneers, D., Berbers, Y., Shvaiko, P., Euzenat, J., & Léger, A. (2006). Quality extensions and uncertainty handling for context ontologies. In *Proceedings of C&O,* (pp. 62 – 64). C&O.

Razzaque, M. A., Dobson, S., & Nixon, P. (2005). *Categorization and modelling of quality in context information.* Paper presented at the Workshop on AI and Autonomic Communications. New York, NY.

Schumm, J., Axmann, S., Arnrich, B., & Tröster, G. (2010). Automatic signal appraisal for unobtrusive ECG measurements. *International Journal of Bioelectromagnetism, 12*(4), 158–164.

Sheikh, K., Wegdam, M., & Van-Sinderen, M. (2007). Middleware support for quality of context in pervasive context-aware systems. In *Proceedings of the International Conference on Pervasive Computing and Communications Workshops,* (pp. 461 – 466). White Plains, NY: IEEE Press.

Sheikh, K., Wegdam, M., & Van-Sinderen, M. (2008). Quality-of-context and its use for protecting privacy in context aware systems. *Journal of Software, 3*(1), 83–93.

Sixsmith, A., & Johnson, N. (2004). A smart sensor to detect the falls of the elderly. In *Proceedings of the IEEE Pervasive Computing,* (pp. 42 – 47). IEEE Press.

Strang, T., & Linnhoff-Popien, C. (2004). A context modeling survey. In *Proceedings of the Workshop on Advanced Context Modelling Reasoning and Management as part of UbiComp,* (pp. 33 – 40). Nottingham, UK: IEEE.

Such, O., & Muehlsteff, J. (2006). The challenge of motion artifact suppression in wearable monitoring solutions. In *Proceedings of the 3rd IEEE/EMBS International Summer School on Medical Devices and Biosensors,* (pp. 49–52). Cambridge, MA: IEEE Press.

Szczepański, A., Saeed, H., & Ferscha, A. (2010). A new method for ECG signal feature extraction. In *Proceedings of the International Conference on Computer Vision and Graphics,* (pp. 334 – 341). IEEE.

Tang, S., Yang, J., & Wu, Z. (2007). A context quality model for ubiquitous applications. In *Proceedings of the IFIP International Conference on Network and Parallel Computing Workshops,* (pp. 282 – 287). IEEE Press.

Viana, W., Filho, J. B., Gensel, J., Villanova-Oliver, M., & Martin, H. (2008). PhotoMap: From location and time to context-aware photo annotations. *Journal of Location Based Services, 2*(1), 211–235. doi:10.1080/17489720802487956

Villalonga, C., Roggen, D., Lombriser, C., Zappi, P., & Tröster, G. (2009). Bringing quality of context into wearable human activity recognition systems quality of context. In *Proceedings of the First International Workshop on Quality of Context,* (pp. 164 – 173). Springer.

Wang, H., Choi, H., Agoulmine, N., Deen, M. J., & Hong, J. W. (2010). Information-based sensor tasking wireless body area networks in u-health systems. In *Proceedings of the 6th International Conference on Network and Service Management*, (pp. 517–522). Niagara Falls, Canada: IEEE Press.

Zadeh, L. A. (1965). Fuzzy sets. *Information and Control, 8*(3), 338–353. doi:10.1016/S0019-9958(65)90241-X

KEY TERMS AND DEFINITIONS

Context: context is any information that can be used to characterize the situation of an entity. An entity is a person, place, or object that is considered relevant to the interaction between a user and an application, including the user and applications themselves (Dey, 1999).

Health Context: it is any information that can be used to characterize the situation of monitored people and the environment around them, which is considered relevant for the decision-making support in U-Health systems (Oliveira, 2010).

Quality of Context (QoC): QoC is any information that describes the quality of information that is used as context information. Thus, QoC refers to information and not to the process or the hardware component that possibly provide the information (Buchholz, 2003).

QoC Indicator (QoCI): QoCI is any well-defined quality aspect that can be evaluated and used to describe the quality of context information (Filho, 2010).

QoC Parameter (QoCP): QoCP is as any information sensed from the environment that can be used to measure QoC indicators (Filho, 2010).

QoC control: QoC Control is a set of operations performed by context-aware systems and applications in order to provide means of evaluating and verifying the quality of context information used for context-sensitive decision-making.

OWL Language: The Web Ontology Language OWL is a semantic markup language for publishing and sharing ontologies on the World Wide Web. OWL is developed as a vocabulary extension of RDF (Resource Description Framework) and is derived from the DAML+OIL Web Ontology Language.

ENDNOTES

[1] http://www.un.org/esa/population/publications/worldageing19502050/.

[2] U.S. Department of Health & Human Services: http://www.aoa.gov/AoARoot/Aging_Statistics/index.aspx.

[3] Sensing t-shirt (Vital jacket). http://elite-choice.org/tag/heart.

[4] Pulse Oximetry

[5] Pulse CO-oximeter

[6] http://www.sensorcare.co.uk/products.aspx?page=24.

[7] http://www.netblue.co.kr/eng/html/sensor-technology.php.

[8] http://www.w3.org/Submission/SWRL/.

[9] http://www.w3.org/TR/owl-features/.

[10] http://www.math-interactive.com/Products/CalGraph/Help/Fit_Curve_to_Data/Root_Mean_Squared_Error.htm.

[11] OWL Web Ontology Language. http://www.w3.org/TR/owl-features/.

[12] http://www.georss.org/.

[13] http://www.w3.org/TR/owl-time.

[14] http://xmlns.com/foaf/spec/.

[15] http://www.ietf.org/rfc/rfc4119.txt?number=4119.

[16] http://clarkparsia.com/pellet.

[17] http://www.sunspotworld.com/.

Chapter 9
Designing the E–Health Message

Rupananda Misra
Drexel University, USA

Barbara C. Wallace
Columbia University, USA

ABSTRACT

The tremendous growth in the use of Web 2.0 technologies, interactive computer technologies, electronic records, and mobile devices for delivery of e-health necessitates attention to design. Designing e-health requires consideration of research, including best practices embodied in design principles. This chapter reviews key background information, including central definitions, concepts, and research, followed by a presentation of 9 key considerations that are recommended for guiding the design of e-health messages. An illustrative case example demonstrates how a typology that codifies design principles gave rise to a research tool that permits the evaluation of health care websites. The case example underscores the important role of findings from research evaluations in creating a feedback loop for designers, permitting research to inform refinements in design. Overall, the 9 key considerations suggest a new paradigm for design, while also giving rise to corresponding recommendations for future research to support evolution in the field of e-health.

INTRODUCTION

The design of health-related websites has emerged as critical for users (Misra & Wallace, 2011a), as is the design of a variety of electronic health information technologies. It is important to explore how design and presentation modalities incorporating user-centered design can contribute to the efficacy of health communication across health literacy levels—whether presenting health information via various large or small computer devices such as personal computers, mobile iPhones, interactive television, gaming consoles, or other technology. Thus, one may speak broadly of the critical importance of designing the e-health message.

DOI: 10.4018/978-1-4666-0888-7.ch009

There is also a role for the evaluation of designs, in order to obtain information that may guide improvements in design (Misra & Wallace, 2011b). The tremendous growth in electronic health information technology necessitates attention being paid to the task of designing the e-health message, and to evaluating what has been designed.

In this regard, Crilly et al. (2011) reported that the past decade "has experienced a rapid growth of electronic health information technology in hospital and health care provider systems to enhance access and quality for service recipients" (p. 1163). Progress has also been made toward the goal of having a "fully connected national health care system" within the present decade (p. 1163). Noteworthy developments are several, including how: the growth of the Internet has permitted wider access to health-related information and health promotion; online personal health records are accessible by patients, allowing them to control their own health data; and, broadband "Internet access and mobile wireless are available in all urban and most nonurban areas" in the United States, thereby "offering new opportunities to reach individuals outside health care networks" (p. 1164). Collectively, electronic health information technology holds out the hope for overcoming barriers to health care and health information, since it may reach geographically and socially isolated populations—especially with the use of wireless handheld devices. What is envisioned is the use of electronic health information technology both "to improve conventional health services" and "reduce health disparities"—while advancing public health goals, "without compromising privacy or security" (p. 1165).

There are those who dedicate their careers to informatics, "the science of information management in health care" (Adams & Leath, 2008, p. 297). Furthermore, one may identify the field of *Health Informatics and Information Technology* (HIIT) as one characterized by new advances that are constantly emerging. Adams and Leath (2008) explained how within the health care arena providers and consumers are facing a new challenge. This challenges involves the task of understanding what technologies are available, as well as learning how to use these tools for purposes of improving healthcare or self-management of one's own health.. The available range of effective HIIT tools support a variety of functions. These functions include the receipt, processing, transmission, retrieval, protection, and analysis of vast amounts of information and data. The breadth and scope of HIIT encompasses the global tracking of diseases, as well as reaching underserved populations, thereby impacting health disparities. Adams and Leath (2008) draw upon information disseminated by the World Health Organization in identifying potential outcomes from the use of information and communication technology, as follows:

- Health workers making better treatment decisions
- Hospitals providing higher quality and safer care
- People making informed choices about their own health
- Governments becoming more responsive to health needs
- National and local information systems supporting the development of effective, efficient and equitable health systems
- Policy makers and the public [being made] aware of health risks
- People having better access to the information and knowledge they need for better health (p. 302)

Clearly, HIIT can make vital contributions both nationally and globally. Those managing information in health care must also be concerned about the process of designing the e-health message. Information to be communicated to providers and consumers should reflect the use of designs that permit effective engagement and knowledge acquisition.

Others confirm the importance of the design of e-health messages. Woo (2008) has asserted the importance of websites being linguistically and culturally appropriate. In brief, Woo (2008) stressed the importance of the design of e-health effectively engaging users, providing information, and having interactive components—such as a chat room, question and answer service, e-mail service, and videos/films.

Within a pioneering approach, Moretti and Witte (2008) have also emphasized the importance of the process of design, including a role for research, while focusing on the interface of digital media technology and education. With regard to the design research process, they stressed how "the technology does not dictate its use, but we, its inventors" (p. 295). Yet, design is a complex and challenging process (Löwgren & Stolterman, 2004). Tools must be designed appropriately for effective use (Kreps & Neuhauser, 2010).

This chapter seeks to foster evolution in the field of e-health by focusing on the topic of designing the e-health message. More specifically, the objective of this chapter is to accomplish the following: 1) provide relevant background information, including a review of key concepts, issues, research findings, and recommendations for future research in light of gaps in current knowledge; 2) convey the importance of effectively and appropriately designing the e-health message, while offering recommendations in the form of 9 considerations that inform design—including an illustrative case example of the role of a typology and related research tool in fostering evolution in e-health message design; 3) discuss future and emerging trends, including recommendations for future research; and, 4) offer a final conclusion that highlights points deserving emphasis.

BACKGROUND DISCUSISON OF IMPORTANT CONCEPTS, ISSUES, AND RESEARCH

There is a need to ensure proper understanding of numerous key concepts, issues, and research find-

ings. This section provides important background information in this regard, while identifying gaps in knowledge and areas where more research needs to be conducted in the future.

E-Health as a Field, Services, and Information delivered via the Internet and Technologies

There is evidence that e-health should be defined ever so broadly. Eysenbach (2001) has defined e-health, while certain aspects of his definition deserve attention, as follows:

e-health is an emerging field..., referring to health services and information delivered or enhanced through the Internet and related technologies. In a broader sense, the term characterizes not only a technical development, but also a ....commitment for networked, global thinking, to improve health care locally, regionally, and worldwide by using information and communication technology. (Eysenbach, 2001, Introduction, para. 4)

The Potential Positive Impact of e-Health and Related Challenges

Both the potential positive impact of e-health and related challenges have been succinctly summarized in the literature. Toward this end, Eysenbach (2001) has asserted that there are 10 e's in "e-health," explaining each, as follows: 1) *efficiency*, as a key promise of e-health by decreasing costs from duplication of therapeutic interventions; 2) *enhancing quality* of care, including by directing patients to the providers of the best quality of care; 3) *evidence based*, as what e-health interventions should be—as an area needing much more work; 4) *empowerment*, as a positive outcome for consumers and patients, since they may access their electronic records and select evidence-based health care; 5) *encouragement* of new partnerships and the relationship between patients and health care providers, including shared decision-making; 6) *education* of medical doctors and consumers/patients via online information; 7) *enabling* of the exchange of information and communication across agencies; 8) *extending* the conventional geographic and other boundaries of conventional health care via access to global providers online; 9) *ethics*, as a challenge that arises when professionals provide online services, as well as when issues of informed consent, privacy and equity remain unresolved; and, 10) *equity* as an especially unresolved and challenging issue, since e-health can either make health care more equitable, or widen the gap between those who have versus those who do not have access to computers and Internet networks. Finally, Eysenbach (2001) concludes that e-health should be easy-to-use, entertaining, and exciting.

The Context for Prioritizing the Design of e-Health Messages

Data has validated priority being placed on the design of e-health messages. Data has revealed the widespread use of the Internet for accessing health care information. Of note, in research conducted by Pew, it was found that 61% of American adults have looked online for health information and about two-thirds talked to someone else about what they found online (Fox & Jones, 2009). In addition, about half of the respondents reported having read online other peoples' commentary or about their experiences with health issues. Reportedly, 60% of the people who access online health information report that the information had an impact on them, influencing their decision-making regarding the treatment of an illness or condition (Fox & Jones, 2009).

Research has also uncovered more details about Health Information-Seeking Behaviors (HISBs). According to Weaver, et al (2010), a sample (n=559) of adults living in the state of Washington were surveyed via e-mail about their HISBs—being mostly White (82.2%), women (51.9%), and college graduates (63.7%) with

most reporting household incomes of $75,000 or more (56.5%). Regarding their HISBs, 49.4% of the sample reported doing so in a typical week, as a behavior much more common among women (60.5%) relative to men (39.5%). Their online HISBs included the pursuit of illness information (14.1%), wellness information (15.2%), or both (20.1%). Also, the respondents seeking wellness information enjoyed the highest health status, engaged in more physical activities, and less prescription drug use.

Other relevant research was conducted with a sample (n=220) of primarily young African American and Hispanic women with a mean age of 32 years (Bacon, 2007). Data showed that the vast majority (72.5%) had been using the computer and Internet to access healthcare information for a period greater than 6 months—as a well-maintained behavior. In addition, the women reported high levels of self-efficacy or confidence in using the computer and Internet to access websites providing healthcare information. Also for a period greater than 6 months, the women reported a history of using the computer and Internet to access information about the following: prescription medications and other remedies and treatments (67.1%); to learn about their personal medical conditions and health concerns (69.8%); to share information with other family, friends, students, or clients (58.6%); and, to learn about sexual health issues (57.7%).

Noteworthy, is the manner in which this largely employed sample (82.9%) enjoyed high levels of education with the majority having obtained a college degree (34.2%), master's degree (26.2%), or doctorate degree (6.4%). Regarding income, 38.5% reported earning $50,000 to $99,000 a year, and 26.6% reported earning $30,000 to $49,000. Duly noted was how the sample of convenience may not be representative of those without such backgrounds (Bacon, 2007).

Yet, taken all together, this data suggests that accessing e-health messages is widespread in the United States, while also including diverse consumers. There are reasons why there is growth and expansion in accessing e-health messages, and a need to prioritize the design of e-health messages. Accessing such online health information gives individuals privacy, and helps people to make important decisions—whether for themselves or others.

One of the major challenges in consumer health informatics is to provide consumers with relevant information (that is contextualized and personalized), and to ensure that the information is presented is such a way that consumers can understand and act upon the information (Alpay, et al, 2009). Early applications in medical health informatics were focused solely on physicians and other care providers; but, now, patients and other lay people are also included in the equation (Eysenbach, 2000). One of the major challenges in developing comprehensive health-based applications involves figuring out how consumers interact with computer-based information, and how they digest and utilize the information (Eysenbach, 2000). An effective strategy involves first identifying the target audience, then assessing what they want, think, feel, and do when it comes to a particular health issue (Maibach & Parrott, 1995). This means conducting research. Having such information is important, because it can assist health message designers in selecting appropriate health message (stimuli) features which may prompt the target audience to attend to the message and trigger the motivation needed for action (Murray-Johnson & Witte, 2003).

There is an imperative to meet the needs of the growing number of consumers seeking out and accessing e-health. Both research and attention to the design of e-health messages emerge as vitally important.

Contemporary Trends in the Use of a Variety of Electronic Records: Promise and Challenges

Some of the considerations in designing e-health messages may apply to a variety of electronic records that contain health information. Adams and Leath (2008, p. 304) described the contemporary trends in the use of a variety of electronic records, below:

- EHR (electronic health record)—generic term for all electronic patient care systems
- CPR (computer-based patient record)—lifetime patient record that includes all information from all specialties (even dentist, psychiatrist) and requires full interoperability (potentially internationally); unlikely to be achieved in foreseeable future
- EMR (electronic medical record)—electronic record with full interoperability within an enterprise (hospital, clinic, practice)

Globally, many countries are using the Electronic Health Record (EHR)—as a record of patient health information that typically includes the patient's demographics, medications, progress notes, laboratory data, and other patient medical history. In countries such as the United States, the increasing use of EHRs is inevitable. In support of the growth in the use of the EHR, David Blumenthal, the US National Coordinator for Health Information Technology at the Department of Health and Human Services, asserted that EHRs "will improve caregivers' decisions and patients' outcomes" (Blumenthal & Tavenner, 2010). One implication is that considerations of design must also grow in importance to facilitate ease of access by varied medical personnel and patients.

In a similar vein, Crilly et al. (2011) reviewed Public Health Records (PHRs), summarizing contemporary trends in the use of this type of electronic record, as follows:

Recently, both Google (Google Health) and Microsoft (HealthVault) introduced publicly available, Internet-based PHRs at no cost... PHRs contain functions that can import data over the Internet directly from specific health devices (e.g. blood pressure monitors, weight scales, blood glucose tests) plugged into computers or handheld devices. Both Google and Microsoft products allow individuals to designate specific entities for data sharing... (p. 1165).

By way of an example, Odlum (2010) has described the use of Electronic Personal Health Management Tools (EPHMT) designed for use by patients with HIV/AIDS within an urban medical care system. The research on EPHMTs is important in seeking to improve, in particular, health care service delivery for the low-income, vulnerable, special population of underserved patients living with HIV/AIDS. From the perspective of the patients, focus group findings included recommended changes in design that would permit meeting practical needs, such as patient recall of appointment times. Ambivalence about the system was expressed; strengths included providers avoiding duplication of services and the repetitive asking of the same questions by varied providers, while concerns included issues of privacy, for example. Other findings on barriers to EPHMT from focus groups with providers uncovered concerns about patients' basic literacy, computer literacy, and health literacy.

Other studies have similarly suggested that patients with limited health literacy may require better designed communication mechanisms to support their self management strategies (Sarkar, et al., 2008). Fortunately, research is proceeding that may inform the ongoing design and re-design of e-health messages, as illustrated by the work of Odlum (2010).

Health Communication and Health Literacy

Meanwhile, what emerges as critical in e-health design is sufficient attention being paid to health communication and health literacy. Zarcadoolas et al. (2006, p. 5) define health communication as involving the use of "human and mass or multimedia and other communication skills and technologies to educate or inform an individual or public about a health issue"—meeting consumer demand for more and better health information.

Health communication must take into account the characteristics of consumers of health information. For example, level of health literacy is one especially relevant characteristic.

According to Zarcadoolas et al. (2006), health literacy involves the consumer's ability to understand and use health information, while defined as "the wide range of skills and competencies that people develop to seek out, comprehend, evaluate, and use health information and concepts to make informed choices, reduce health risks, and increase quality of life" (pp. 5-6). Level of health literacy must be considered, since low health literacy tends to be related to poorer health and early mortality on both the national and global scale (p. 21).

The Importance of Cultural Literacy, as well as Cultural and Linguistic Appropriateness

As another important characteristic of consumers of health information, Zarcadoolas et al. (2006) discuss how culture must be consistently considered in the design of all health communications; this suggests a role for "cultural literacy" (p. 260). Meanwhile, attention to culture means that e-health materials must be "linguistically appropriate," as when content must be presented in English and/or Spanish to meet the needs of particular communities (Perez-Rivera & Langston-Davis, 2008, p. 537). This is consistent with the call for e-health materials that are both culturally and linguistically appropriate (Woo, 2008).

Mobile Devices and e-Health: The Latest in m-Health

One blossoming area in e-health involves the use of mobile devices for accessing health information. Mobile health or m-health may be described as the use of wireless communication devices in support of public health and clinical practices. Mobile phones are increasingly used by people of all ages and literacy backgrounds. Mobile phones with internet connectivity (i.e., smart phones) are, indeed, much more than a phone. They are in fact a small computer with Internet access, along with a phone component. Designing e-health or m-health messages must take these devices into account, including their special features and the possibilities and opportunities that go along with them.

Mobile IT devices such as Personal Digital Assistants (PDAs) and cellular phones are increasingly being used in healthcare (Mitseva, et al., 2009). They are the most ubiquitous type of gadget in the world (Kahn, et al., 2010), suggesting promise for addressing global health needs.

According to a Pew study, the act of looking up health information using mobile devices, especially among young people, is on the rise; the study suggested that 29% of cell phone owners between the ages 18-29 have used their cell phones to look up health or medical information (Fox, 2010). Other Pew Internet Research indicated that, as of December 2009, 83% of adults owned a cell phone—whether a Blackberry, iPhone, or other similar device (Lenhart, et al., 2010).

Mobile phones empower and challenge patients to transition from the role of passive recipients of information to active participants and decision-makers (Mitseva, et al., 2009). These new "smart phones" can mimic what a personal computer can do with the transmission of a variety of forms of data, including permitting access to a multimedia learning environment that includes the use of text, graphics, audio and video (Patrick, et al., 2008).

Learning through mobile devices supports lifelong learning. This is because of both accessible formats, and the manner in which information is accessible at any time and from anyplace—permitting greater engagement with learning (Taylor, et al., 2010).

The technologies that underlie mobile phones are not only less expensive than they used to be, but they are also getting more powerful; this is being recognized in the delivery of healthcare services and the promotion of personal health (Patrick, et al, 2008). From an economic perspective, using mobile phones as a means of delivery of health care makes sense, given that the US expenditure on health care was projected to reach $4 trillion dollars per year (Patrick, et al., 2008). With these mobile technologies being widely available, there is an opportunity for this technology playing a critical role in health care at the regional, community, and individual level (Kahn, et al., 2010).

These devices are also permitting the remote capture of patient data, facilitating health assessments (Mitseva, et al., 2009). Also, the fact that mobile phone users can use text-based communication along with accessing the Internet makes such mobile technology a great resource that doctors and patients can use in order to communicate with each (Peirce & Bakke, 2010).

One study focused on patients diagnosed with Type 1 insulin dependent diabetes who managed their disease using mobile phones; findings indicated that the application was successful and the overall satisfaction level of patients was positive (Preuveneers & Berbers, 2008). Another study examined the feasibility of utilizing cell phone technology to assist with diabetes self-care in a clinic population; data showed that the intervention using cell phones had a positive impact on clinical outcome and self-efficacy (Faridi, et al., 2008). A recent systematic review of behavior change interventions delivered by a mobile telephone short message service indicated that in 13 out of 14 reviewed studies there were positive behavior change outcomes. The tailoring of SMS (Short Messaging Service), or text messaging, along with interactivity were found to be the key features supporting the successful use of these devices (Fjeldsoe, et al., 2009). Mobile phone intervention in healthcare has also been successfully implemented in varied parts of the world—such as Uganda (Chang, et al., 2008), again underscoring promise in addressing global health needs.

Though there are several commercial applications that run on mobile phones, a recent usability study on the design of mobile dietary and nutritional support for individuals living with diabetes was informative. Findings indicated that these commercial e-health applications still present opportunities for the enhancement of their design (Arsand, et al., 2008). Future research needs to evaluate users' preferences and needed improvements in design of mobile health applications.

Social Media, Web 2.0, and e-Health Blogging

"Web 2.0" refers to a collective group of tools that are in vogue. The "2.0" acknowledges the evolution of the Web into a medium that is known for its openness, vast sharing, and global nature; indeed, what it really does is provide a new way of socially constructing knowledge (Ravenscroft, 2009). The collective group of Web tools, or the contemporary family of technologies that the "2.0" refers to includes everything from social networking tools (e.g., Facebook), to media sharing tools (e.g., YouTube, Flickr), and virtual worlds (e.g., Second Life)—as noted elsewhere (Ravenscroft, 2009).

What distinguishes Web 1.0 from Web 2.0 involves how the content creators were few in Web 1.0, and most users were mere consumers of content (Miller & Pole, 2010). On the other hand, Miller and Pole (2010) explain what is new and distinct about Web 2.0, below:

User-generated content, the hallmark of Web 2.0, is responsible for the remarkable growth in health-related content on the Internet. This is reflected in tools ranging from Twitter to social networking sites to wikis. The blog (short for weblog) is the quintessential Web 2.0 application....

Data show that between 12.0 and 26.4 million Americans blog and 57.0 to 94.1 million are blog readers...Blogs that focus on health care (whose

exact number is unknown) have the potential to provide interactive support networks for caregivers and patients, generate real-time discussions about health news or policy, extend social and political mobilization efforts, and offer providers another forum in which to collaborate and consult. (p. 1514)

Chui et al (2009) have summarized how the new generation of contemporary Web tools assist users in numerous ways, as follows: supporting broad collaboration, such as via wikis which facilitate co-creation of content; permitting broad communication, such as via blogs; allowing collective estimation, as in the case of market predictions and polling; supporting meta data creation, such as tagging/RSS (Real Simple Syndication), which adds additional information to primary content; and, allowing social graphing, as in social networking, which leverages connections between people to offer new applications. As the popularity of Web 2.0 technologies has grown, so also has intense public engagement, collaboration and participation (Chui, et al., 2009).

The essence of the Web 2.0 is to harness a collective intelligence. It functions as a global brain (Oreilly, 2007).

Medical professionals also share information among themselves. This occurs, given Web 2.0 fosters an open and accessible resource from which ordinary people can learn—such as via blogs and Twitter.

The website, www.Twitter.com, invites others to "Follow your interests." And, it offers "Instant updates from your friends, industry experts, favorite celebrities, and what's happening around the world." The service is accessible globally via 12 different languages. Twitter is also described as permitting micro-blogging using text-based posts, or instant messaging, for example. And, as of the summer of 2011, Twitter announced access by all users to a new photograph sharing feature. This highlights the ongoing expansion and integration of technologies that may have implications for e-health or m-health design. Future research in e-health can explore ways to utilize the latest capabilities of Twitter now that photographic images may be shared.

Blogging is not only one of the most important features of Web 2.0, but also supports the social construction of knowledge. Some examples of health-related blogs are, as follows:

- http://www.webmd.com/dcfault.htm which claims to provide "Better information. Better health."
- http://www.medicalinsurance.org/52-blogs-run-by-doctors-or-nurses-offering-medical-advice-and-stories/ which provides links to "52 Blogs Run by Doctors or Nurses Offering Medical Advice and Stories"—beginning with a blog (#1) run by Dr. Kevin Poh, M.D. of New Hampshire in the United States, and ending with (#52) a collective blog that is interactive and socially driven (i.e., covering what happens in the emergency room from the perspective of the doctors, nurses, emergency medical technicians, and nurses).
- http://www.rntomsnprograms.net/52-excellent-twitter-accounts-every-medical-professional-should-follow.html which specifically identifies "52 Excellent Twitter Accounts Every Medical Professional Should Follow"—including that of Dr. Mehmet Oz (who began his television career on the Oprah Winfrey show and went on to have his own syndicated television show in the United States). Dr. Oz provides "interesting information on health and medicine, as well as the latest medical news." This website also provides access to the twitter accounts of nurses, surgeons, dentists, orthodontists, ophthalmologists, radiologists, medical assistants, and those practicing alternative medicine (i.e. homeopathy, naturopathic care).

As has been noted in the literature, people may even subscribe to blogs. They may also received notifications every time there is an update (Oreilly, 2007).

Social software such as blogs, wikis, and group forums are being used as healthcare tools. For example, there are blogs on topics such as dieting and weight loss, including access to experts offering advice. Blogging and micro-blogging are allowing individuals to provide social support to each other in dealing with a variety of diseases, while supporting learning about diseases. Examples of such social support being provided via the Web 2.0 appear below:

- http://www.experienceproject.com/groups/Want-To-Lose-Weight/984-here, the Experience Project allows individuals to access an Experience Group to "connect with others on common ground;" for example, the "I Want to Lose Weight" group. Here, subscribers can "Read true personal stories, chat & get advice, support, and help from a group of 11029 people who all say 'I Want to Lose Weight.'"
- http://www.dailystrength.org/support-groups—provides "Free, anonymous support from people just like you." Individuals are invited by Daily Strength to "Browse our +500 communities of people facing similar life challenges, medical conditions, and mental health issues and find people who understand exactly what you're going through." In addition to links to support groups, the Daily Strength website provides links to health blogs, expert answers to health questions, and information on treatments.

Another example of Web 2.0 technologies involves the use of AJAX for the creation of interactive web applications, including engagement with content. Some of the major weaknesses of this platform are the limited quality of interaction as well as the uncertainty of ownership of the content materials. One can argue that with the widespread use of some Web 2.0 software, there is a challenge to the quality management of health information technology resources.

All of these Web 2.0 technologies are blurring the lines between the traditional producers of healthcare information and consumers of that knowledge. The modern day consumers of that information are increasingly taking part in co-producing the healthcare information that they consume. Since the Web 2.0 environment is a very social space where the user generates content, it can provide patients and the general public with access to huge amounts of information about healthcare; and, at the same time, it provides a huge amount of data about the users. This data can be used in future research by healthcare researchers and researchers to understand consumers, their characteristics, and needs.

Yet, very "little systematic empirical research has documented the content and characteristics of health blogs and bloggers" (Miller & Pole, 2010, p. 1514). Using a sample of 951 health-related blogs, Miller and Pole (2010) found that 34.3% had a SiteMeter, 90.2% posted external links, 96% had a reader commentary section, 97.5% featured archives, 75% had a blogroll—while only 15.4% contained video, and only 5.5% featured audio; also, only 15% had sponsors, and 28.1% accepted commercial advertising. Regarding the characteristics of the category of health bloggers, most were women (56.8%) with an average age of 35.8 years, being highly educated, as two-thirds held a master's or doctoral degree. In addition, 49.8% worked in the health professions, including physicians (43.3%) with some being medical students (19.6%). The medical specialties represented were, as follows: internal medicine (14.9%), family practice and emergency medicine (9.8%), surgery (9.3%), psychiatry (5.2%), pediatrics (4.6%), obstetrics and gynecology (3.6%), oncology (2.1%), and other specialties (9.3%). Other professions represented included nursing (19.9%), health

counseling (8.7%), counseling (5.4%), research (4.7%), emergency response (3.1%), administration (2.0%), paraprofessionals (1.8%), medical journalism (1.3%), and other professions (8.2%). For those not in the health profession (50.2%), bloggers were journalists or writers (27.4%), professors (8.7%), information technology specialists (8.3%), students (7.3%), or lawyers (7.3%).

Regarding the perspective taken in their blog, findings reported by Miller and Pole (2010) revealed that most adopted a professional perspective (54.3%), while 37.7% took a patient-consumer perspective, and 8.0% took a caregiver perspective. Also, most blogs (42.6%) focused on bloggers' experiences with specific health conditions (e.g. mental health, reproduction, chronic disease, physical disability, HIV/AIDS, cancer). Miller and Pole (2010) concluded that because "most of these blogs were written from a patient-consumer or caregiver perspective" this "suggests that health blogs are being used, in part, to forge support networks among bloggers and their readers;" moreover, there appears to be the potential to create virtual support networks, given the presence of blogrolls, links, and comment sections—as interactive features (p. 1516). Also noteworthy was how the vast majority of health blogs did not feature audio or video. As a consequence, the health blogs were primarily text-based while also being more personal, highlighting "the journaling aspect of blogging" (p. 1516).

Although Eysenbach (2001) concluded that e-health should be easy-to-use, entertaining, and exciting, there are apparently categories of consumers with characteristics such as those which Miller and Pole (2010) identify. Thus, it is possible that the opportunity to journal and be a part of a social network in a largely text-based environment that is void of video and audio is sufficiently entertaining and exciting for some highly educated professionals who blog and journal. Yet, it is also possible that an entire audience of potential health bloggers is not being sufficiently engaged because blog sites are primarily text-based, lacking video and audio features; future research needs to investigate this, as findings will have implications for design.

Social Networking, Web 2.0 Technologies, and Biosurveillance

Others have focused on the uses of social networking and Web 2.0 technologies by groups of professionals for purpose of ensuring the general public health. As a case in point, Khan et al. (2010) asserted that the next public health revolution will involve the use of social networks by professionals and the fusion of information, using technologies such as those made available via Web 2.0. Valued applications include biosurveillance—the process of actively gathering, analyzing, and interpreting biosphere data for threats to life and disease activity; this includes early detection and warning systems. Khan et al (2010) noted how the events of September 11, 2001 in the United States in New York City have led to the creation of information-sharing environments or fusion centers. Fusion involves the integration of patient/individual level, community level, and inter-sectoral level information. Similarly, the Centers for Disease Control and Prevention (CDC) in the United States created and tested a public health fusion center; results may include public health alerts and control measures (Khan, et al., 2010), as in response to epidemics and natural/human-made disasters. Social networks are used for purposes of assessment of information, comparison of data, and dissemination of key information (Khan, et al., 2010). Khan et al. (2010) discussed recent developments, below:

... Tools such as the Global Public Health Information Network (GPHIN), HealthMap, EpiSpider, ARGUS, and Google.org Flu Trends mine low-cost unstructured data for event-based information. These data sources include news wire services, listserves, ProMED-mail, online newspapers, and search engines ....

...The response to the 2009 influenza pandemic (H1N1) showcased the power of Web 2.0 technologies for communications purposes because the CDC and other entities have used blogs, widgets, wikis, microblogs (e.g. Twitter), RSS (real Simple Syndication) feeds, and podcasts for communication with other public health officials, the health care industry, and the public.... (p. 1239)

The envisioned multidirectional information flow necessitates the design of electronic social networks that can support the management of information (Khan, et al., 2010). Designs need to be evaluated in future research.

Goals of Equity in Health for All: More Inclusive Care, Social Justice, and e-Health

The contemporary web and dissemination of well-designed e-health messages can play a potentially crucial role in achieving the equity goals elaborated upon by Wallace (2008), below:

Because of vast differences with regard to access to the resources associated with the pursuit and maintenance of health, there is a need for a global health transformation—one wherein we value and pursue equity in health for all as a global interdependent community with vast resources at our disposal for sharing and deployment to any group in need located on any part of the globe. To value and pursue equity in health means that we engage in fair play, act with impartiality, and allow a sense of social justice to guide us as we ensure that all human beings are free to enjoy the right to health and pursuit of physical, emotional, mental, and spiritual well-being—consistent with how any diverse groups may define it and elect to pursue it... (p. 2)

For example, in the case of natural disasters, or crises of drought and famine, or refugees (i.e., migrating to escape harsh conditions, violence or war), we have witnessed the power of Web 2.0 technologies to achieve Wallace's (2008) equity goals. Technology has played a role in mobilizing and organizing assistance, humanitarian aid, and fund-raising for the sake of preserving life and ensuring access to health. Thus, new social media tools are facilitating organized responses to the needs of vulnerable populations. Web 2.0 technologies can play an important role in promoting the goals of equity in health, social justice, and access for all. The achievement of these goals depends on effectively designing e-health messages.

By way of example, Prochaska (2008) pioneered the design of innovative interactive computer-based approaches to "that can enhance health, reduce health care costs, and provide more inclusive care" (p. 61). Prochaska (2008) described the results of interactive computer-based interventions delivered at home via programmed algorithms; findings on interventions for cigarette smoking cessation revealed how interactive computers alone produced a 24% abstinence rate; this was relative to the 18% abstinence rate obtained by counselors plus computers. And, the computers produced an abstinence rate that was twice that of the manuals provided by the American Lung Association.

Of note, these advances are reminiscent of an approach that combines the work of professional social workers with the use of computers. Moretti and Witte (2008) described the successful transformation of the first couples-based, HIV/Sexually Transmitted Infections (STI) prevention intervention developed by El-Bassel et al (2008) into a multi-media intervention accessible online. The El-Bassel et al (2008) model is important in being evidence-based and targeting for HIV/AIDS prevention interventions those heterosexual women at highest risk in the United States, specifically, African American and Latina women.

Moretti and Witte (2008) detailed their design research structure, while the end product was called Multimedia Connect. Multimedia Connect was used as a new tool for training social workers in how to work with couples, as well as

deployed by professionals working with couples in community-based settings. Multimedia Connect also has international applications.

The Multimedia Connect intervention promotes equity in health and the elimination of regional, national, and global health disparities for vulnerable stigmatized populations with HIV/AIDS. Providing such populations with access to an evidence-based intervention also constitutes social justice. Hence, there are a variety of contemporary pioneering approaches involving interactive computer-based intervention and treatment—possessing tremendous value.

Regarding the rationale for the pioneering interactive computer-based approaches of Prochaska (2008), he explained how "most behavioral treatments are action-oriented and are designed for people who are prepared to take action in the immediate future;" or, designed based on the assumption that people do not have co-morbidities or more than one problem (p. 64). Yet, some people are just contemplating taking action, for example, while having multiple problems (e.g., cigarette smoking, anxiety, and depression). And, interactive computer-based interventions can also be designed to reach entire populations with chronic conditions (i.e., versus the typical paradigm where the focus is on acute conditions among patients in clinics); this population approach via the use of home-based computers permits much greater impacts on behavioral health, relative to a patient-level approach followed by clinicians in clinics. The result is an alternative to health care systems designed primarily for the delivery of diagnoses and drugs; furthermore, this new alternative approach promotes scientific and practice paradigms that are designed to treat some of the highest risk and highest cost behaviors. The result is a "more inclusive" approach to care, as "social justice" (p. 75).

In support of the assertion that Prochaska's (2008) pioneering approach produces a more inclusive approach to treatment, as social justice, consider the following evidence:

...Across our population trials, we found that African American smokers and Hispanic-American smokers had somewhat higher quit rates than non-Hispanic Whites. The oldest smokers had the highest quit rates....Treatment stereotypes have suggested that certain populations, like younger, older, minority, or impaired individuals do not have the same ability to change. These results indicate that the problem is not inability to change: the problem is inaccessibility to quality change programs. (p. 72)

Looking forward, Prochaska (2008) suggested a viable future. This is one wherein the emerging paradigms need to rely much more "on proactive approaches to reaching entire populations;" the goal is to maximize impacts on "multiple behaviors treated by tailored communications delivered primarily by patients using technologies at home" (p. 75).

The results are likely to assist in achieving the goals of equity in health, social justice, and access for all. This is the possible, in particular, when applications include the newer, less expensive mobile smart phone technology; and, when the digital divide is being closed by making smart phones, computers, and the Internet widely accessible to those of all socioeconomic statuses.

The Internet can also be used to make materials typically purchased or downloaded for a fee available for free—in order to foster equity in health, social justice, and access for all. For example, the HIV/AIDS prevention peer education training manual created by Wallace (2005) has been made freely available on the Web at the Global HELP-Health Education and Leadership Program website as part of a recommended toolkit for global use (i.e. https://sites.google.com/a/globalhelp.columbia.edu/globalhelp/toolkit) by communities in need.

In all cases, design factors remain critical. Research needs to investigate the effectiveness of design in meeting the needs of vulnerable and stigmatized populations, as well as the global community, in an attempt to promote equity in health, social justice, and access for all.

DESIGNING e-HEALTH MESSAGES: KEY CONSIDERATIONS

This section of the chapter introduces 9 key considerations in e-health design; also offered in this section is an illustrative case example of a typology and research tool created to permit the evaluation of e-health design, thereby fostering evolution in design. Figure 1, displays the 9 key considerations in e-health design, as part of recommended movement from the old paradigm (i.e. wherein designers considered the technology at hand, the people and the content for e-health) to a new paradigm; within the new paradigm, it is recommended that designers engage in the recommended 9 key considerations elaborated upon in this section, thereby expanding the factors impacting design.

Consideration of Categories of Consumers in Design

This first key consideration emerged from the background information and review of research. The background review revealed many *categories of consumers,* or varied target audiences. The emergent categories of consumers included the following: patients seeking health information; patients interacting with electronic records or mobile devices for purposes of self-management; medical personnel across various hospital, clinic, and government surveillance systems accessing a variety of electronic records, while also engaging in patient care, as well as communicating with patients; ordinary people seeking wellness information or illness information, whether for themselves or others; patients, family members and caregivers seeking and sharing information, as well as social support, while forming social networks; varied members of the medical profession,

Figure 1. Movement from the old paradigm to the new paradigm guiding design: introducing the nine key considerations for designing e-health

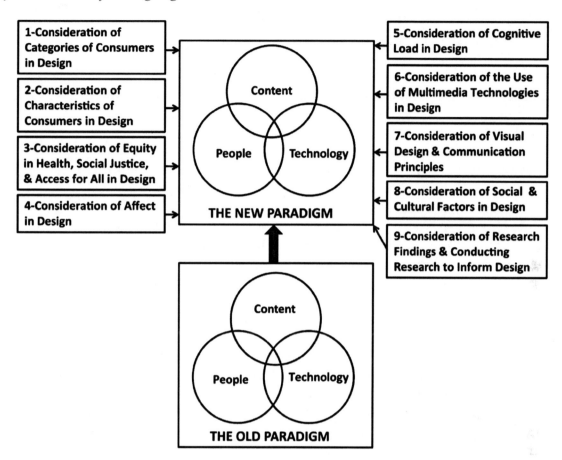

other health professionals, journalists/writers, and others participating in blogs and forming social support networks; professional social networks seeking to ensure the public health through biosurveillance and the integration and management of multiple streams of data; professionals working with clients, while using computers and interacting in virtual environments in order to deliver tailored interventions and treatment; a variety of special, vulnerable, and historically stigmatized populations (e.g., adolescents, minorities, the elderly, disabled, those with HIV/AIDS), frequently assumed to lack the ability to change, while suffering health disparities, and in need of exposure to evidence-based interventions in order to attain equity in health, social justice, and access; and, people with multiple problem behaviors, both mental and physical in nature, seeking access to interventions –such as via computers at home that can deliver tailored interventions that are driven by algorithms. Most importantly, the background review was not comprehensive, only being suggestive of the vast diversity in categories of consumers of e-health.

Consideration of Characteristics of Consumers in Design

The second key consideration also arose from the background and review of research, revealing how many *characteristics of consumers* must be considered when designing the e-health messages. Examples of important characteristics included levels of basic literacy, computer literacy, and health literacy. What also emerged from the background review were issues of cultural literacy, including the goal of ensuring that messages are appropriate, both linguistically and culturally; cultural characteristics must, therefore, be considered.

Other key characteristics may include stage of change/readiness to take action on health information, chronic disease conditions, the presence of multiple problem behaviors, or being a member of a special, vulnerable, or stigmatized population. As with data on bloggers, other key characteristics may include a level of education and comfort with primarily text-based information.

Consideration of Equity in Health, Social Justice, and Access for All in Design

The background review and research also revealed how the latest developments in e-health hold the promise of helping to foster *equity in health, social justice, and access for all*. However, only effectively and appropriately designed e-health messages can permit meeting the needs and addressing the characteristics of diverse consumers around the globe. This also means paying attention to special populations of the most vulnerable and stigmatized, seeking to meet their needs in design. Considerations of equity in health, social justice, and access for all emerge as important in e-health design.

Consideration of Effect in Design

There is a mandate for interface design to include considerations of *affect* (Kalbach, 2006), including users' reactions of frustration or satisfaction. Research supports a focus on that which elicits feeling. Many e-health activities require what Pink (2005) would describe as L-Directed Thinking; i.e. focusing on engaging the left hemisphere of the brain, which is where the logical and analytic part of the brain makes the computer programmer triumph. But, there is also a need for utilizing R-Directed Thinking; i.e., focusing on the right hemisphere of the brain, which is underemphasized in the information age. The right side of the brain helps us to see the whole, as well as focus on aesthetics, creativity and feeling—or affect (Pink, 2005)

Consideration of Cognitive Load in Design

Research in Cognitive Load Theory (CLT) contributed significantly towards understanding engagement during learning and problem solving. *Cognitive load* is said to be the mental load in performing a task, having two aspects: mental load, as the task-based dimension; and, the mental effort, as the learner based dimension—while both of these impact performance (Sweller, 1994). The effective design of health materials should be geared towards effective patient learning and recall of health information (Wilson & Wolf, 2009). Working memory provides limited capacity in the representation of information (Repovs & Baddeley, 2006). This means that designers should understand the limitations of the working memory.

Working memory load can be affected by the intrinsic nature of the material (i.e., intrinsic cognitive load), as well as how the material is presented (i.e., extraneous cognitive load) or the activities required by the users. The third type of cognitive load involves processes relevant to schema construction (i.e., germane cognitive load). Intrinsic cognitive load is determined by interaction between the material to be learned, given the complexity of the information, and the expertise of the learner. Extraneous cognitive load is determined by the format of the material—which is determined by design. The combination of high intrinsic cognitive load (i.e., level of complexity in the material) and high extraneous cognitive load (i.e., level of complexity in the format presenta-

Table 1. Design principles arising from cognitive load theory and research

Cognitive Load Design Principles	Explanation of the Principle
1-Extraneous cognitive load demands	It is important for e-health message designers to keep in mind the extraneous cognitive load demands (Sweller, 1994) placed on consumers/patients; it is better to free up mental resources for the processing of relevant health information. (Sweller, 1994).
2-Limited processing capacity of working memory	Working memory provides limited capacity in the representation of information (Repovs & Baddeley, 2006). Design e-health material that does not overload the working memory of the user.
3-Animation segmentation and the expertise reversal effect	Presenting animations in segments (i.e., as a means to reduce cognitive load) has a positive effect on cognitive load and learning for students with lower levels of prior knowledge; yet, this segmentation impact may be reversed in some cases, thereby not being effective for students with higher levels of prior knowledge or expertise (Spanjers, et al., 2011).

tion or design of material) would be detrimental to learning; this is because of too much load is placed on working memory (Sweller, 1994).

Though intrinsic load cannot be directly influenced by the designers, it is something to be considered by the designers. However, the extraneous cognitive load of the health material is directly under the control of the designer. Therefore, it is important to design e-health material that does not overload the working memory of the user.

Research shows that presenting animations in segments (i.e., to reduce cognitive load) has a positive effect on cognitive load and learning for students with lower levels of prior knowledge; yet, this might not be effective for students with higher levels of prior knowledge (Spanjers, et al., 2011). Designers should consider such cognitive variables in an effort to create health information materials that can be processed and understood by the users, especially those with limited literacy skills or declining cognitive abilities (Wilson & Wolf, 2009).

Three design principles that emerge from cognitive load theory and research are presented in Table 1. These should be considered in design and research studies.

Consideration of the Use of Multimedia Technologies in Design

From the learner-centered perspective, research studies show that the use of *multimedia technolo-gies* in design are consistent with the way the human mind works; they put less cognitive load on the learner and foster greater learning relative to those designs not using multimedia systems (Mayer, 2001). On the other hand, multimedia instructional presentations that are designed ineffectively—e.g., duplication of the same information using different modes of presentation—can potentially increase the risk of overloading working memory and negatively impact learning (Kalyuga, et al., 2000).

Mayer and Moreno (2003) define multimedia instruction as the use of words and pictures with the intent to foster learning, while cognitively organizing material so that it is coherent and emphasizes importance. Studies suggest that multimedia educational aids have been successful in education and healthcare (Jeste, et al., 2008). Multimedia educational aids hold promise for improving the provision of complex medical information to patients and caregivers (Jeste, et al., 2008). The design of multimedia educational tools may be very important to harness the power of this new media (Strecher, et al., 1999). Interactive multimedia communication tools have the potential to help learners acquire a deeper understanding of subject matter (Lajoie, 2000). Acquiring a deeper understanding of material holds the potential for users retaining information longer and applying it to new situations (Mayer & Moreno, 2003).

Table 2. Multimedia design principles arising from Mayer and Moreno's (2002) work

Multimedia Design Principles	Explanation of the Principle
1-Multimedia principle	Users learn more deeply from animation and narration than they do from the use of narration alone (Mayer & Moreno, 2002).
2-Spatial continuity principle	Users learn more deeply when on-screen text is presented next to the animation that it describes, versus instances when text is presented at a distance from the animation (Mayer & Moreno, 2002).
3-Temporal contiguity principle	Users learn more deeply when corresponding portions of the narration and animation are presented at the same time, versus instances when they are separated in time (Mayer & Moreno, 2002).
4-Coherence principle	Users learn more deeply from animation and narration when extraneous words, sounds (including music), and video are excluded rather than included (Mayer & Moreno, 2002).
5-Redundancy principle	Users learn more deeply from the combination of animation and narration, versus the use of animation, narration, and on screen text (Mayer & Moreno, 2002).
6-Personalization principle	Users learn more deeply from animation and narration when the narration is in a conversational mode rather than a formal style (Mayer & Moreno, 2002).

Best practice recommendations by Fox (2009) for interactive computer-based programs included the following: (1) multimedia capabilities should be deployed effectively in order to engage patients and hold interest; (2) programs should incorporate voice-over and script messaging written for patients with low literacy levels and visual deficits; (3) programs should be web-based to allow for ease of access and providing updates; (4) programs should incorporate questions and answers to reinforce important constructs and promote interaction; and (5) programs should allow for user control over program presentation sequence.

A number of multimedia design principles arise from the work of Mayer and Moreno (2002) that may be considered in design and research. See Table 2, including explanations.

Consideration of Visual Design and Communication Principles

In designing e-health messages, *visual design and communication principles* are very important. These can be especially important in representing how reality is defined by a particular social group (Kress & Van Leeuwen, 1996, pp. 161-162). Visual images can powerfully communicate meaning (Lester, 2003). Pye (1995) argues that appearance and value are intertwined. Along with

color, which carries an abundance of psychological and emotional meaning, concepts such as visual hierarchy and legibility, for example, are important in visual communication (Samara, 2007). Gestalt psychology is particularly helpful in explaining human perception and tendencies to group things together (Graham, 2008). Kress and Van Leeuwen (1996) stressed the meaning of the horizontal position of images in order to suggest involvement, how "power over" relationships may be created by vertical angels, and how images at eye level suggest equality or no power difference; also, narrative visual structures can suggest action and convey meaning.

Table 3 offers a compilation of visual design principles that designers should keep in mind when designing e-health materials and conducting research.

Consideration of Social and Cultural Factors in Design

It is important for designers to keep in mind *social and cultural factors* that inform design. Misra (2007) relied upon the prior work of others (i.e., Papanek, 1984) in making the case that one should consider the telesic content of a design, in order to ensure that designs accurately reflect the current social times and conditions in which

Table 3. Visual design and communications principles

Visual Design and Communication Principles	Explanation of the Principle
1-Have a concept	No matter how amazing something looks, without a clear message it is an empty though beautiful shell (Samara, 2007).
2-Communicate - don't decorate	Form carries meaning no matter how simple or abstract, therefore communicate meaning and avoid merely decorating (Samara, 2007).
3-Treat the type as image, being as important as everything else	Type is visual material— made up of lines, dots, shapes and textures— that needs to relate compositionally to everything else in the design (Samara, 2007).
4-Select colors with purpose	Color carries an abundance of psychological and emotional meaning. It also affects visual hierarchy, legibility and how people make connections between disparate items (Samara, 2007)
5-Restraint	Limit the content and elements in the design to what your audience needs (Lipton, 2004).
6-Proximity	Using space, move the elements together or apart (Lipton, 2004).
7-Similarity, Consistency, and Repetition	Use style— the size, face, style, color and color of elements—in order to show their relationships with other elements (Lipton, 2004).
8-Visual hierarchy and Emphasis	Emphasize what is most important to the least (Lipton, 2007).
9-Alignment, unity and balance	Align elements with others to assist the audience with navigation through the material, and to create unity as well as balance (Lipton, 2004).
10-Figure/Ground	Make the content stand out clearly from the background, emphasizing figure-ground relationships (Lipton, 2004).
11-Clarity	Use clear and legible images (Lipton, 2004).
12-Size of frame and social distance	The interactive meaning of images is related to the size of the frame; this involves the selection of either the close-up shot, medium shot, or long shot (Kress & Van Leeuwen, 1996).
13-The image and the gazer	Images serve different communicative functions, such as to create an imaginary relationship between the represented participant and the viewer/gazer (Kress & Van Leeuwen, 1996)
14-Involvement and the horizontal angle	The use of the horizontal angle serves to represent the involvement between the image-producer and represented participants (Kress & Van Leeuwen, 1996)
15-Power and vertical angle	The use of the vertical angle serves to represent the power relationship between the image-producer and the represented participants (Kress & Van Leeuwen, 1996)
16-Split-attention effect	All elements and their relations must be learned. For example, integrating diagrams with explanatory text was found to be far superior to the conventional split-source format of having diagrams and separate text (Sweller, 1994).
17-Narrative structures	Narrative structures are represented by the presence of a line (vector) that goes across or connects the participants in the picture. For example, the outstretching of arms to hold another person. The vector expresses a relationship and action (Lipton, 2007).

prospective users live. Misra (2007) surmised that telesic content can permit an evaluation of the extent to which the design content matches the cultural context, and is appropriate for that cultural context. Thus, the consideration and evaluation of telesic content in the design process emerges as a very important dimension; this can serve to determine whether or not designs are sufficiently user-oriented, thereby meeting the client where they are in their own cultural context; the alternative involves failing to do so, or even alienating or failing to engage those of a particular culture (Misra, 2007). Results may mean that content is not culturally appropriate (Woo, 2008).

Consideration of Research Findings and Conducting Research to Inform Design: An Illustrative Case Example

The design of e-health messages should reflect a *consideration of research findings* during the design process. Once e-health messages have been designed, also important is *conducting research to inform design*—toward the goal of using findings to improve and refine the e-health messages.

As an illustrative case example, first, Misra's (2007) consideration of research findings informed the creation of a *Typology for Evaluating Healthcare Websites Arising from a Systematic Review and Analysis of Design Research and Scholarship: 13 Principles of Design.* The typology embodies standards and principles that should guide the design and creation of healthcare websites, as well their evaluation. Second, Misra's (2007) typology gave rise to a measure co-created by the authors that is of value in conducting research to inform design: the *Evaluating and Rating Healthcare Websites (ERHCW-20)* scale. The ERHCW contains 20 items that permit research subjects to evaluate and rate websites against the 13 design principles within the typology. The ERHCW-20 is actually a sub-scale of a larger tool co-created by the authors, entitled the *Rating and Evaluating Healthcare Websites Survey (REHWS-74),* having 74 items (including other sub-scales). Together, the typology and the ERHCW-20, respectively permit consideration of research findings and conducting research to inform design. See Tables 4 and 5.

Findings with both ERHCW-20 sub-scale and the other scales of the REHWS-74 have been presented and discussed elsewhere (i.e. Misra, 2007; Misra & Wallace, 2011a, 2011b). Findings for the ERHCW-20 have provided evidence of excellent internal consistency (Misra & Wallace, 2011a, 2011b). The scales have been used in numerous research studies where the authors served as webmaster/design consultant and research sponsor/content consultant, respectively. For example, Bacon (2007) conducted a study, reporting excellent Cronbach's Alpha (.966) for the ERHCW-20 sub-scale with a sample (n=220) of largely African American and Hispanic women who evaluated a sexual healthcare information website (i.e. www.DIVAhealth.org).

Consider what Bacon (2007) reported as the most highly rated website features (1=extremely poor to 10 = excellent), using the ERHCW-20, as follows: for health literacy (i.e. easy for me to understand the information in the website's written material), the mean rating was 8.77 (SD=1.36); for reflecting the current times and real life conditions of people with health problems, or being culturally appropriate, the mean rating was 8.66 (SD=1.51); for the feature of the website being pleasing to the eye and having some beauty to it, while also providing information that had a real impact, so women thought about changing beliefs or behavior, or wanted to learn more, the mean rating was 8.55 (SD=1.66). Aside from these three top rated design features, the overall rating of the website (i.e. given everything the women knew about websites and their personal preferences and needs) was also high (mean = 8.44, SD=1.55). A relevant finding revealed in the open-ended response (i.e., qualitative data) component was how women appreciated the website being tailored primarily for Black women, culturally appropriate, easy to navigate, incorporating emotional issues in a way that was not cold, promoting justice, while also being colorful, attractive and beautiful. However, the website was criticized for lacking photographs or images of overweight or obese women by at least a small minority of consumers.

Findings are noteworthy for illustrating the value of the ERHCW-20 tool in assessing the design of e-health messages, and creating a feedback loop for designers—who can use the data to further improve and refine e-health messages. In this manner, the illustrative case example (i.e., provided by the typology and the ERHCW-20 research tool the typology gave rise to) serves to demonstrate the importance of designers engaging in consideration of research findings and conducting research to inform design.

Table 4. Typology for evaluating healthcare websites arising from a systematic review and analysis of design research and scholarship: 13 principles of design

1. Level of Health Literacy of the Written Material
2. Degree to Which Dual Channels Are Being Used: Verbal and Pictorial
3. Six Principles of Design in Advertising: Application to the Design of Web-Based Messages (a) Method: The interaction among tools, processes, and materials. (i.e., if visual materials do a better job of explaining the content, then the designer should use pictorial elements rather than textual content. (b) Use: Does it work? (c) Need: Is the designer ignoring the needs of the consumers? (d) Telesic: This involves the purposeful utilization of resources to reach one's goal, reflecting the times and conditions, while fitting in with the general human and socioeconomic order, or being culturally appropriate. (e) Association: It is the psychological conditioning influencing whether to like or dislike a certain product, being based on memories associated with similar things. (f) Aesthetics: Beauty is one of the elements of good design, but not everything. So, consider content versus interface design (visual design), while the results are most important (i.e., Does it impact you enough to change beliefs, behaviors, or compel you to want to interact with the website?)
4) Ensuring the Website is Not a Mono-modality: Is There Too Much Text?
5) To What Degree is the Website Multimodal, Multimedia, and Multisensory?
6) To What Degree is the Learning of New Information Occurring via the Website?
7) To What Degree is the Presentation and Structure of the Website Favorable, Supporting the User's Interactive Behavior? (a) Presenting one idea per paragraph and using the inverted pyramid style of writing—presenting the conclusion first. (b) Using half the word count to present information found in standard writing. (c) Laying text out in bullets, using spacing and indenting, using bolding, varying size and type of fonts.
8) How Do Users Rate the Presentation and Structure of Text So It Supports Their Interactive Behavior? (a) Supporting scanning versus reading word for word
9) Following Other Emergent Textual Design Suggestions (i.e., using the following: bullet-points; spacing, indenting, and white space; bulleted lists; text that looks good and is colorful, using bold and differentiation in size and font of text; good spatial positioning of images and texts; structure as well as detail; word headings that are 3-4 words; brief descriptions that are 10-20 words; meaningful headings and subheadings, as users are likely to read text that has a good subheading; interactive areas that are clear and practical; words, pictures and icons so they are harmonized; the power of interactivity with hypertext links; writings that are kept short so users do not have to scroll both vertically and horizontally).
10) Placement of Pictorial Images to the Left and Textual Content to the Right: What Do Users Prefer?
11) Maximizing the Interactive Meaning of Images (a) Using a frontal angle that says that the producer/viewer is involved with the represented objects (b) Using pictures at eye level, so the point of view is one of equality and there is no power difference involved (c) Good use of modality and color (d) Good use of narrative structures–such as when the presence of a line (vector) goes across or connects participants in the picture, expressing desired relationships and action.
12) Are There Practical Relationships between Multi-modal Messages and the Goal of Behavior Change?
13) To What Extent Are Messages Diffused as a Social or Interactive Process?: Use of Videos, Chat Rooms, Peer Feedback, and Interaction as Valuable Features in Websites

FUTURE AND EMERGING TRENDS: DIRECTIONS IN E-HEALTH AND RECOMMENDATIONS FOR FUTURE RESEARCH

The 9 key considerations for e-health design within a new paradigm—which were introduced in the prior section—served to suggest emerging and future trends in e-health design. These 9 key considerations give rise to corresponding new directions in e-health and recommendations for future research, as follows:

1. Designers of e-health must strive to identify and consider *categories of consumers*. As technology expands, new categories

Table 5: The 20 items on the evaluating and rating healthcare websites (ERHCW-20) measure

1. For level of health literacy (i.e., how easy it was for me to understand the information in the website's written materials), I rate this website as...
2. For the degree to which my two main (dual) channels (i.e., both my verbal/language and mental/visual systems) for processing information were used, I rate this website as...
3. In terms of the kind of design elements I think are used in billboard and magazine advertising (i.e., using pictures and images, and written text when it seems needed), I rate this website as...
4. In terms of the kind of design elements I think are used in billboard and magazine advertising, and whether the overall website design was *useful* for me and *"worked"* for me, I rate this website as...
5. In terms of considering the needs of people like me who are browsing this website, and *meeting my needs*, I rate this website as...
6. In terms of this website reflecting the current times and real life conditions of people with health problems, being what I consider culturally appropriate, I rate this website as...
7. In terms of this website using the technique of attempting to trigger memories or associations in me (i.e., stimulating me to associate the information with similar images and information that I already had), I rate this website as...
8. In terms of this website being pleasing to the eye and having some beauty to it, while *also* providing information that had a real impact on me (i.e., so I thought about changing my beliefs or behavior, or wanted to learn more from the website), I rate this website as...
9. In terms of the amount of written text this website had, and a suggested standard where the best websites *avoid having a majority of written material to convey information*, I rate this website as...
10. In terms of the *mix* of written text, visual images, pictures, moving videos/images, and music/sound, and a suggested standard where the best websites use *some mixture* of these, I rate this website as...
11. In terms of the amount of learning of new information that occurred for me, I rate this website as...
12. Given the overall presentation of information/structure of the website, and how *favorable* my experience was and how *supported I felt* when interacting with the website, I rate this website as...
13. In terms of presentation of information (i.e., stating key conclusions up front or at the beginning, avoiding use of too many words; and, good use of bullets, spacing, bolding, and lettering format/font size), I rate this website as...
14. Given the overall presentation/structure of written text, how easy it was for me to *interact* with the website, and to *scan for information* (versus having to read every single word to find the information I wanted), I rate this website as...
15. In terms of the use of: meaningful headings and sub-headings; spatial placement of images, text, pictures, and icons; support for my interacting with the website via hypertext links; and, avoidance of too much left/right or up/down scrolling—I rate this website as...
16. Given placement of pictorial images (e.g. a suggested standard where it is better to put images on the left and written textual content to the right), I rate this website as...
17. In terms of arrangement of pictorial images, and the feeling one sometimes gets from looking at billboards and magazine advertisements—like the people in the pictures are involved with you as the viewer or equal to you in power, creating a connection—I rate this website as...
18. In terms of using multiple modalities to convey messages (i.e., written text, pictures, sounds, movement, videos, etc...), and whether they served the practical purpose of promoting healthy behavior change, I rate this website as...
19. In terms of having messages conveyed as a social or interactive process (i.e., use of videos, "chat rooms," and access to peer feedback and interaction, etc...), I rate this website as...
20. Given everything I know about websites and my personal preferences and needs, *overall*, I rate this website as...

Note: *All items are rated on the following scale:*
Extremely Poor 1 2 3 4 5 6 7 8 9 10 Excellent
Not Applicable (this did not seem to apply to the website)

of consumers may arise. This necessitates future research which expands the base of knowledge about categories of consumers. This information may then be used in designing e-health messages for specific categories of consumers.

2. *Consumer characteristics,* in general, need to be a focus of research—both determining what they are, and investigating the relationship between those characteristics and how various e-health messages are rated and evaluated (e.g., using tools such as the

ERHCW-20 developed by the authors). Results of such research can lead to better tailoring of e-health messages so they are well-suited for and accepted by consumers with specific characteristics.

3. Designers should strive to ensure that e-health has been designed with considerations of *equity in health, social justice, and access for all* being held in mind—including from the perspective of various categories of consumers with varied characteristics. Experts in diversity, multiculturalism, equity, and justice should be consulted in the design process, as well as in research evaluation. Research should also investigate diverse and underrepresented consumers' responses to that which has been embodied in the design of e-health messages. Research also needs to investigate the extent to which the digital divide is being closed, and whether consumers that have historically lacked access to computers and the Internet are gaining greater access, including via the use of smart phones.

4. As a result of prioritizing attention to considerations of *affect*, research and evaluation within the design process can determine users' affective reactions, including experiences of frustration, preferences, and level of satisfaction with e-health messages.

5. It is important to design e-health material and conduct research from the perspective of *cognitive load*—as in exploring the relationship between the extent of cognitive load demanded of consumers by certain designs, and their characteristics (e.g., levels of knowledge, education and expertise).

6. The use of *multimedia technologies*, and interactive computer-based designs need to be evaluated through research that determines how design features are rated and evaluated by various categories of consumers (e.g., professionals versus patients) with certain characteristics (e.g., level of education, literacy, health literacy, cultural characteristics).

7. Research needs to analyze the use of various *visual design and communication principles,* in terms of the extent to which e-health designers are following them; and, research can explore how various categories of consumers with various characteristics respond to various e-health messages from the perspective of the degree to which e-health designs adhere to varied visual design and communication principles.

8. Regarding *social and cultural factors*, research needs to evaluate the extent to which e-health messages are linguistically and culturally appropriate, or the extent to which they reflect the current social times and conditions in which consumers live. There is a role for formative evaluation research, using interviews and focus groups—allowing either multiculturalism experts or members of cultural groups to identify important socio-cultural characteristics, and what is culturally appropriate—which then informs design and factors to be studied in research.

9. Designing e-health messages should involve consideration of *research on design, and research needs to be conducted to evaluate and inform refinements in design.* The large, varied and growing body of e-health messages supported by Web 2.0 technologies all need to incorporate a research process that includes both consideration of research in design, as well as the evaluation of e-health messages.

Thus, the 9 key considerations introduced in this chapter have demonstrated their effectiveness in suggesting future directions in research. A focus on the design of e-health holds the potential to drive evolution in the field in ways that can significantly benefit individuals, communities, health-care systems, professionals, the public health, and the global community—including the most vulnerable, underrepresented, and stigmatized populations.

Given this book's focus on telemedicine and e-health services, including policies and applications, this chapter contributes understanding of the importance of design. When it comes to e-health services broadly conceived, formal policies need to include directing attention to the importance of design. No matter the advancements in e-health applications, if they are poorly designed, then they will not have the desired impact; the health of communities on the local, national, and global levels are at stake and may be compromised by poor design features. Policies must direct researchers to include assessments of elements of design in their e-health studies. Toward realization of these goals, the authors have contributed the *ERHCW-20* research measure to facilitate such research, while the larger survey of which the ERHCW-20 is a part (i.e., the *REHWS-74)* can support research exploring relationships between ERHCW-20 findings on design features and data on various categories of consumers and their characteristics (See Misra & Wallace, 2011a, for more details).

CONCLUSION

This chapter has covered the topic of designing e-health messages. More specifically, the chapter first provided relevant background information and a review of research. Next, the chapter focused on the importance of designing e-health messages, providing 9 key considerations that may serve to move the field toward a new paradigm. Discussion of the 9 key considerations that inform design included an illustrative case example of the role of a typology and related research tool (i.e. ERHCW-20) in fostering evolution in e-health message design. Discussion in the chapter also covered future and emerging trends, including recommendations for future research in the field of e-health that corresponded to each of the 9 key considerations.

The chapter demonstrated how the 9 key considerations are important, while the chapter sought to make a valuable contribution to advancements and developments in the field of e-health; this was done by highlighting how, among the elements considered important to advancements in e-health, design must be identified as a vital element. Indeed, designing the e-health message in light of the principles, typology, and key considerations identified in this chapter holds the promise for creating e-health services with the potential to have great impact around the globe. Substantial evolution in the field of e-health may follow from what has been offered through this chapter's discussion.

REFERENCES

Adams, D. L., & Leath, B. A. (2008). A role for health informatics and information technology (HIIT): Shaping a global research agenda to eliminate health disparities. In Wallace, B. C. (Ed.), *Toward Equity in Health: A New Global Approach to Health Disparities* (pp. 297–321). New York, NY: Springer Publications.

Alpay, L., Verhoef, J., Xie, B., Te'eni, D., & Zwetsloot-Schonk, J. (2009). Current challenge in consumer health informatics: Bridging the gap between access to information and information understanding. *Biomedical informatics insights, 2*(1), 1.

Arsand, E., Tufano, J., Ralston, J., & Hjortdahl, P. (2008). Designing mobile dietary management support technologies for people with diabetes. *Journal of Telemedicine and Telecare, 14*(7), 329. doi:10.1258/jtt.2008.007001

Bacon, D. T. (2007). *An internet evaluation of "DIVAS": A website designed to prevent human immunodeficiency virus and other sexually transmitted infections (STIs) among young black women.* Unpublished Doctoral Dissertation. New York, NY: Columbia University.

Blumenthal, D., & Tavenner, M. (2010). The "meaningful use" regulation for electronic health records. *The New England Journal of Medicine, 363*(6), 501–504. doi:10.1056/NEJMp1006114

Chang, L., Kagaayi, J., Nakigozi, G., Packer, A., Serwadda, D., & Quinn, T. (2008). Responding to the human resource crisis: Peer health workers, mobile phones, and HIV care in Rakai, Uganda. *AIDS Patient Care and STDs, 22*(3), 173. doi:10.1089/apc.2007.0234

Chui, M., Miller, A., & Roberts, R. (2009). Six ways to make web 2.0 work. *The McKinsey Quarterly, n.d.,* 1–7.

Crilly, J. F., Keefe, R. H., & Volpe, F. (2011). Use of electronic technologies to promote community and personal health for individuals unconnected to health care systems. *American Journal of Public Health, 101*(7), 1163–1167. doi:10.2105/AJPH.2010.300003

El-Bassel, N., Witte, S. S., & Gilbert, L. (2008). HIV/AIDS risk reduction with couples: Implications for reducing health disparities in HIV/AIDS prevention. In Wallace, B. C. (Ed.), *Toward Equity in Health: A New Global Approach to Health Disparities* (pp. 253–274). New York, NY: Springer Publications.

Eysenbach, G. (2000). Recent advances: Consumer health informatics. *British Medical Journal, 320*(7251), 1713. doi:10.1136/bmj.320.7251.1713

Eysenbach, G. (2001). What is e-health? *Journal of Medical Internet Research, 3*(2), 20. Retrieved from http://www.jmir.org/2001/2/e20/; doi:10.2196/jmir.3.2.e20; PMID, 11720962.

Faridi, Z., Liberti, L., Shuval, K., Northrup, V., Ali, A., & Katz, D. (2008). Evaluating the impact of mobile telephone technology on type 2 diabetic patients' self-management: The NICHE pilot study. *Journal of Evaluation in Clinical Practice, 14*(3), 465–469. doi:10.1111/j.1365-2753.2007.00881.x

Fjeldsoe, B., Marshall, A., & Miller, Y. (2009). Behavior change interventions delivered by mobile telephone short-message service. *American Journal of Preventive Medicine, 36*(2), 165–173. doi:10.1016/j.amepre.2008.09.040

Fox, M. (2009). A systematic review of the literature reporting on studies that examined the impact of interactive, computer-based patient education programs. *Patient Education and Counseling, 77*(1), 6–13. doi:10.1016/j.pec.2009.02.011

Fox, S. (2010). Mobile health 2010. *Pew Internet and American Life Project.* Retrieved November, 2010 from http://pewinternet.org/~/media//Files/Reports/2010/PIP_Mobile_Health_2010.pdf.

Fox, S., & Jones, S. (2009). The social life of health information. *Pew Internet and American Life Project.* Retrieved November, 2010 from http://www.pewinternet.org/~/media//Files/Reports/2009/PIP_Health_2009.pdf.

Graham, L. (2008). Gestalt theory in interactive media design. *Gestalt Theory, 2*(1).

Jeste, D. V., Dunn, L. B., Folsom, D. P., & Zisook, D. (2008). Multimedia educational aids for improving consumer knowledge about illness management and treatment decisions: A review of randomized controlled trials. *Journal of Psychiatric Research, 42*(1), 1–21. doi:10.1016/j.jpsychires.2006.10.004

Kahn, J., Yang, J., & Kahn, J. (2010). 'Mobile' health needs and opportunities in developing countries. *Health Affairs, 29*(2), 252. doi:10.1377/hlthaff.2009.0965

Kalbach, J. (2006). "I'm feeling lucky": The role of emotions in seeking information on the web. *Journal of the American Society for Information Science and Technology, 57*(6), 813–818. doi:10.1002/asi.20299

Kalyuga, S., Chandler, P., & Sweller, J. (2000). Incorporating learner experience into the design of multimedia instruction. *Journal of Educational Psychology, 92*(1), 126–136. doi:10.1037/0022-0663.92.1.126

Khan, A. S., Fleischauer, , Casani, J., & Groseclose, S. L. (2010). The next public health revolution: Public health information fusion and social networks. *American Journal of Public Health, 100*(7), 1237–1242. doi:10.2105/AJPH.2009.180489

Kreps, G. L., & Neuhauser, L. (2010). New directions in ehealth communication: Opportunities and challenges. *Patient Education and Counseling, 78*(3), 329–336. doi:10.1016/j.pec.2010.01.013

Kress, G., & Van Leeuwen, T. (2001). *Multimodal discourse: The modes and media of contemporary communication*. New York, NY: Hodder Arnold.

Kress, G. R. (2003). *Literacy in the new media age literacies*. London, UK: Taylor & Francis. doi:10.4324/9780203164754

Kress, G. R., & Van Leeuwen, T. (1996). *Reading images: The grammar of visual design*. London, UK: Routledge.

Kress, G. R., & NetLibrary Inc. (2003). Literacy in the new media age. *Literaciespp, 13*, 186. Retrieved from http://www.columbia.edu/cgi-bin/cul/resolve?clio4255051.

Lajoie, S. (Ed.). (2000). *Computers as cognitive tools: No more walls (Vol. 2)*. Mahwah, NJ: Lawrence Erlbaum.

Lenhart, A., Purcell, K., Smith, A., & Zickuhr, K. (2010). Social media & mobile internet use among teens and young adults. *Pew Internet and American Life Project*. Retrieved February, 6, 2010 from http://www.pewinternet.org.

Lester, P. M. (2003). *Visual communication: Images with messages* (3rd ed.). Belmont, CA: Thomson/Wadsworth.

Lipton, R. (2004). *Information graphics and visual clues*. Gloucester, MA: Rockport Publishers.

Lipton, R. (2007). *The practical guide to information design*. Hoboken, NJ: Wiley.

Löwgren, J., & Stolterman, E. (2004). *Thoughtful interaction design: A design perspective on information technology*. Cambridge, MA: MIT Press.

Maibach, E., & Parrott, R. (1995). *Designing health messages: Approaches from communication theory and public health practice*. Thousand Oaks, CA: Sage Publications.

Mayer, R. E. (2001). *Multimedia learning*. Cambridge, UK: Cambridge University Press.

Mayer, R. E., & Moreno, R. (2002). Animation as an aid to multimedia learning. *Educational Psychology Review, 14*(1), 87–99. doi:10.1023/A:1013184611077

Mayer, R. E., & Moreno, R. (2003). Nine ways to reduce cognitive load in multimedia learning. *Educational Psychologist, 38*(1), 43–52. doi:10.1207/S15326985EP3801_6

Miller, E. A., & Pole, A. (2010). Diagnosis blog: Checking up on health blogs in the blogosphere. *American Journal of Public Health, 100*(8), 1514–1519. doi:10.2105/AJPH.2009.175125

Misra, R. (2007). *The significance of design: A multimodal analysis of government and non-government websites*. Unpublished Doctoral Dissertation. New York, NY: Columbia University.

Misra, R., & Wallace, B. C. (2011a). Improving the design of health information websites: A study of users' expectations. *Design Principles and Practices: An International Journal, 5*. Retrieved from http://www.Design-Journal.com.

Misra, R., & Wallace, B. C. (2011b). Evaluating the design of two government and two non-government HIV/AIDS websites. *The International Journal of Health, Wellness and Society, 1*. Retrieved from http://www.HealthandSocietyJournal.com/.

Mitseva, A., Kyriazakos, S., Litke, A., Papadakis, N., & Prasad, N. (2009). ISISEMD: Intelligent system for independent living and self-care of seniors with mild cognitive impairment or mild dementia. *The Journal on Information Technology in Healthcare, 7*(6), 383–399.

Moretti, F., & Witte, S. S. (2008). Using new media to improve learning: Multimedia connect for HIV/AIDS reduction and the triangle initiative. In Wallace, B. C. (Ed.), *Toward Equity in Health: A New Global Approach to Health Disparities* (pp. 277–296). New York, NY: Springer Publications.

Murray-Johnson, L., & Witte, K. (2003). Looking toward the future: Health message design strategies. In *Handbook of Health Communication* (pp. 473–495). Mahwah, NJ: Lawrence Erlbaum.

Odlum, M. (2010). *An exploratory analysis of factors associated with use and comprehension of the internet and a continuity of care document for persons living with HIV in New York City.* Unpublished Doctoral Dissertation. New York, NY: Columbia University.

Oreilly, T. (2007). *What is web 2.0: Design patterns and business models for the next generation of software.* Retrieved from http://oreilly.com/web2/archive/what-is-web-20.html.

Papanek, V. (1984). *Design for the real world: Human ecology and social change.* Chicago, IL: Academy Chicago Publishers.

Patrick, K., Griswold, W., Raab, F., & Intille, S. (2008). Health and the mobile phone. *American Journal of Preventive Medicine, 35*(2), 177. doi:10.1016/j.amepre.2008.05.001

Peirce, L., & Bakke, E. (2010). *Healthcare perceptions and mobile phone use: A predictive model of text-based health communication.* Paper presented at the Annual Meeting of the International Communication Association. Suntec City, Singapore. Retrieved from http://www.allacademic.com/meta/p404783_index.

Perez-Rivera, B., & Langston-Davis, N. (2008). A model for comprehensive community-wide asthma education using partnerships and the public school curriculum. In Wallace, B. C. (Ed.), *Toward Equity in Health: A New Global Approach to Health Disparities* (pp. 529–545). New York, NY: Springer Publications.

Pink, D. H. (2005). *A whole new mind: Moving from the information age to the conceptual age.* New York, NY: Riverhead Books.

Preuveneers, D., & Berbers, Y. (2008). Mobile phones assisting with health self-care: A diabetes case study. In *Proceedings of the 10th international Conference on Human Computer interaction with Mobile Devices and Services.* Amsterdam, The Netherlands: ACM.

Prochaska, J. O. (2008). New paradigms for inclusive health care: Toward individual patient and population health. In Wallace, B. C. (Ed.), *Toward Equity in Health: A New Global Approach to Health Disparities* (pp. 61–78). New York, NY: Springer Publications.

Pye, D. (1995). *The nature and aesthetics of design.* New York, NY: Cambium Press.

Ravenscroft, A. (2009). Social software, Web 2.0 and learning: Status and implications of an evolving paradigm. *Journal of Computer Assisted Learning, 25*(1), 1–5. doi:10.1111/j.1365-2729.2008.00308.x

Repovs, G., & Baddeley, A. (2006). The multicomponent model of working memory: Explorations in experimental cognitive psychology. *Neuroscience, 139*(1), 5–21. doi:10.1016/j.neuroscience.2005.12.061

Samara, T. (2007). *Design elements: A graphic style manual: Understanding the rules and knowing when to break them.* Gloucester, MA: Rockport Publishers.

Sarkar, U., Piette, J. D., Gonzales, R., Lessler, D., Chew, L. D., & Reilly, B. (2008). Preferences for self-management support: Findings from a survey of diabetes patients in safety-net health systems. *Patient Education and Counseling, 70*(1), 102–110. doi:10.1016/j.pec.2007.09.008

Spanjers, I. A. E., Wouters, P., van Gog, T., & van Merriënboer, J. J. G. (2011). An expertise reversal effect of segmentation in learning from animated worked-out examples. *Computers in Human Behavior, 27*(1), 46–52. doi:10.1016/j.chb.2010.05.011

Strecher, V. J., Greenwood, T., Wang, C., & Dumont, D. (1999). Interactive multimedia and risk communication. *Journal of the National Cancer Institute. Monographs, 25*, 134–139.

Sweller, J. (1994). Cognitive load theory, learning difficulty, and instructional design. *Learning and Instruction, 4*(4), 295–312. doi:10.1016/0959-4752(94)90003-5

Taylor, J., Dearnley, C., Laxton, J., Coates, C., Treasure-Jones, T., & Campbell, R. (2010). Developing a mobile learning solution for health and social care practice. *Distance Education, 31*(2), 175–192. doi:10.1080/01587919.2010.503343

Wallace, B. C. (2005). *HIV/AIDS peer education training manual: Combining African healing wisdom and evidence-based behavior change strategies.* Philadelphia, PA: StarSpirit Press.

Wallace, B. C. (2008). Introduction: The forces driving and embodied within a new field of equity in health. In Wallace, B. C. (Ed.), *Toward Equity in Health: A New Global Approach to Health Disparities.* New York, NY: Springer Publications.

Weaver, J. B., Mays, D., Weaver, S. S., Hopkins, G. L., Eroglu, D., & Bernhardt, J. M. (2010). Health information-seeking behaviors, health indicators, and health risks. *American Journal of Public Health, 100*(8), 1520–1525. doi:10.2105/AJPH.2009.180521

Wilson, E. A. H., & Wolf, M. S. (2009). Working memory and the design of health materials: A cognitive factors perspective. *Patient Education and Counseling, 74*(3), 318–322. doi:10.1016/j.pec.2008.11.005

Zarcadoolas, C., Pleasant, A. F., & Greer, D. S. (2006). *Advancing health literacy: A framework for understanding and action.* San Francisco, CA: Josey-Bass.

ADDITIONAL READING

Ballard, B. (2007). *Designing the mobile user experience.* West Sussex, UK: John Wiley & Sons, Ltd. doi:10.1002/9780470060575

Beaird, J. (2010). *The principles of beautiful web design* (2nd ed.). Canada: Sitepoint.

Cheng, Q., Qu, H., Wang, Y., & Tan, J. (2005). Mobile health networks case: Unconfined mobile Bluetooth technology for e-medical services. In Tan, J. (Ed.), *E-Health Care Information Systems: An Introduction for Students and Professionals* (pp. 190–200). San Francisco, CA: Jossey-Bass.

Cheong, P. H., Wilkin, H. A., & Ball-Rokeach, S. (2004). Diagnosing the communication infrastructure in order to reach target audiences: A study of Hispanic communities in Los Angeles. In Whitten, P., & Cook, D. (Eds.), *Understanding Health Communication Technologies* (pp. 101–110). San Francisco, CA: Jossey-Bass.

Clemens, C. M., Sypher, B. D., & Doolittle, G. C. (2004). The role of telehospice in end-of-life care. In Whitten, P., & Cook, D. (Eds.), *Understanding Health Communication Technologies* (pp. 111–117). San Francisco, CA: Jossey-Bass.

Effertz, G., Beffort, S., Preston, A., Pullara, F. D., & Alverson, D. C. (2004). A model for persuading decision makers and findings new partners. In Whitten, P., & Cook, D. (Eds.), *Understanding Health Communication Technologies* (pp. 46–58). San Francisco, CA: Jossey-Bass.

Fling, B. (2009). *Mobile design and development: Practical concepts and techniques for creating mobile sites and web apps*. Sebastopol, CA: O'Reilly Media, Inc.

Forducey, P., & Kaur, K. Scheidman-Miller, & Tan, J. (2005). E-health domains: Surveying the e-health landscape—Cases and Applications. In J. Tan (Ed.), *E-Health Care Information Systems: An Introduction for Students and Professionals*, (pp. 203-223). San Francisco, CA: Jossey-Bass.

Golombisky, K., & Hagen, R. (2010). *White space is not your enemy: A beginner's guide to communicating visually through graphic, web and multimedia design*. Burlington, MA: Focal Press.

Harris, L. M., Kobb, R., Ryan, P., Darkins, A., & Kreps, G. L. (2004). Research as dialogue: Health communication and behavior change in patients' natural habitat. In Whitten, P., & Cook, D. (Eds.), *Understanding Health Communication Technologies* (pp. 91–101). San Francisco, CA: Jossey-Bass.

Maheu, M. M., & McMenamin, J. P. (2004). Successful web site construction and management: Harness the skill and enthusiasm of volunteers. In Whitten, P., & Cook, D. (Eds.), *Understanding Health Communication Technologies* (pp. 187–201). San Francisco, CA: Jossey-Bass.

McNeil, P. (2008). *The web designer's idea book: The ultimate guide to themes, trends and styles in website designs*. Cincinatti, OH: F&W Publications.

McNeil, P. (2010). The web designer's idea book: *Vol. 2. More of the best themes, trends and styles in website design*. Cincinatti, OH: F&W Media, Inc.

Patterson, J., & Shulman, G. M. (2004). Leadership issues facing an e-start-up management team. In Whitten, P., & Cook, D. (Eds.), *Understanding Health Communication Technologies* (pp. 59–68). San Francisco, CA: Jossey-Bass.

Rice, R. E. (2004). Social aspects of implementing a medical information system: Cure or symptom. In Whitten, P., & Cook, D. (Eds.), *Understanding Health Communication Technologies* (pp. 19–29). San Francisco, CA: Jossey-Bass.

Tan, J. (Ed.). (2005). *E-health care information systems: An introduction for students and professionals*. San Francisco, CA: Jossey-Bass.

Tan, J. (2005). E-health: The next health care frontier. In Tan, J. (Ed.), *E-Health Care Information Systems: An Introduction for Students and Professionals* (pp. 3–26). San Francisco, CA: Jossey-Bass.

Tan, J. (2005). E-health vision: Drivers of and barriers to e-health care. In Tan, J. (Ed.), *E-Health Care Information Systems: An Introduction for Students and Professionals* (pp. 37–51). San Francisco, CA: Jossey-Bass.

Tan, J. (2005). E-health perspectives: General systems concepts, chaos and string theories, and social science thinking. In Tan, J. (Ed.), *E-Health Care Information Systems: An Introduction for Students and Professionals* (pp. 59–81). San Francisco, CA: Jossey-Bass.

Tan, J. (2005). E-health records: The lifeblood of e-health care. In Tan, J. (Ed.), *E-Health Care Information Systems: An Introduction for Students and Professionals* (pp. 91–115). San Francisco, CA: Jossey-Bass.

Tan, J., & Cheng, W. (2005). E-networking: The backbone of e-health care. In Tan, J. (Ed.), *E-Health Care Information Systems: An Introduction for Students and Professionals* (pp. 163–189). San Francisco, CA: Jossey-Bass.

Tan, J., Soto Mas, F. G., & Hsu, C. E. (2005). E-public health information systems: E-technologies for public health preparedness and surveillance. In Tan, J. (Ed.), *E-Health Care Information Systems: An Introduction for Students and Professionals* (pp. 127–154). San Francisco, CA: Jossey-Bass.

Wallace, B. C. (2008a). *Toward equity in health: A new global approach to health disparities*. New York, NY: Springer Publications.

Wallace, P. (2004). The United Kingdom virtual outreach project. In Whitten, P., & Cook, D. (Eds.), *Understanding Health Communication Technologies* (pp. 160–170). San Francisco, CA: Jossey-Bass.

Whitten, P., & Cook, D. (Eds.). (2004). *Understanding health communication technologies*. San Francisco, CA: Jossey-Bass.

Wooten, R., & Tahir, M. S. M. (2004). Challenges in launching a Malaysian teleconsulting network. In Whitten, P., & Cook, D. (Eds.), *Understanding Health Communication Technologies* (pp. 11–18). San Francisco, CA: Jossey-Bass.

KEY TERMS AND DEFINITIONS

Culturally appropriate: A description for content, research, or interventions that reflect an appreciation of the cultural background and history of the consumers, research subjects, or clients—being designed in accordance with the characteristics and needs of the target audience or population, based on prior information, data, or experiences.

E-Health Messages: This term includes all of the forms of communication that convey health information or health data, being broadly conceived---including the written and multimedia content associated with electronic records, web sites, blogs, micro-blogs, e-mails, and texts.

Health Equity: First, equity is a desired state and goal involving fairness, fair play, and the experience of enjoying impartiality with regard to access to opportunities. Thus, one may speak of health equity, or the state or goal of enjoying equal access to the opportunity to experience health and all associated with attaining and maintaining health.

Health Disparities: Those gaps in health or differences on indicators of health status that may be found when comparing groups across various categories—whether, for example, race, ethnicity, socioeconomic status, or geographic region. These gaps or differences in health status are also known as health inequities.

Linguistically Appropriate: A description for content that is in a language that may be comprehended by the target audience.

M-Health: The health information content that is shared via mobile phone technology, or "smart phones"—as devices combining telephone and computer components with Internet access.

Paradigm: A model that reflects an era or generation of thinking and standards with regard to how to conceptualize and approach an endeavor, including a field of study or discipline.

Typically, the guiding or dominant paradigms within fields of study and disciplines change across time, given natural processes of evolution. Thus, old paradigms tend to be replaced by new paradigms.

Social Justice: The manner in which human beings, as social beings, may experience equity when interacting within all societal institutions, including gaining equal access to all opportunities, and rectifying all past instances when such equality did not prevail within communities. Hence, for many historically marginalized, underrepresented, or oppressed groups, social justice remains an important goal.

Chapter 10

Health Systems for Syndromic and Epidemiological Surveillance

Débora Helena Job
National Laboratory for Scientific Computing (LNCC), Brazil

Antônio Tadeu Azevedo Gomes
National Laboratory for Scientific Computing (LNCC), Brazil & National Institute of Science and Technology on Medicine Assisted by Scientific Computing (INCT-MACC), Brazil

Artur Ziviani
National Laboratory for Scientific Computing (LNCC), Brazil & National Institute of Science and Technology on Medicine Assisted by Scientific Computing (INCT-MACC), Brazil

ABSTRACT

Health surveillance practices date back to decades ago. Traditionally, such practices to gather health data have been manual; more recently, however, computerized health information systems have been applied to enhance and facilitate health information acquisition for surveillance. The so-called health surveillance systems put in practice the systematic acquisition of health data, which is stored and processed for expert analysis. This chapter makes a survey of health surveillance systems dedicated to syndromic and epidemiological surveillance, identifying the different design and technological strategies adopted in the development of such systems. The aims of such a survey are: (1) to provide practitioners with some information about the collective expertise of health information system architects in the design and implementation of syndromic and epidemiological surveillance systems; and (2) to pave the way for the establishment of software product lines dedicated to such systems.

INTRODUCTION

Surveillance practices date back to decades ago. They aim at monitoring outbreaks, emerging infectious diseases and the like, as well as their impacts on population health, according to national or international targets for disease control and eradication (WHO, 1999). Traditionally, such practices have been manual, using standardized diagnostic laboratory testing, and health notification reports (Forslund, et al., 2004). More recently, however, computerized Health Information Systems (HIS) have been also applied to enhance and facilitate

DOI: 10.4018/978-1-4666-0888-7.ch010

health information acquisition for surveillance (Chen, Zeng, & Yan, 2010). The so-called *health surveillance systems* put in practice the systematic acquisition of health data, which are stored and processed for expert analysis. Such systems are usually composed of typical software artifacts such as graphical user interfaces and databases, but also employ somewhat sophisticated analysis techniques such as data (typically text) mining, ontologies, and mathematical disease spreading models. A particularly important aspect of such systems is the process of health information transmission, which relies on health protocol standards that aim at ensuring reliability, security, and interoperability on data acquisition.

For the sake of this chapter, we divide health surveillance systems into two groups: *epidemiological* and *syndromic* surveillance systems. Epidemiological surveillance systems collect and monitor data related to specific diseases and other health problems. Syndromic surveillance systems are wider in scope, relying on algorithms that are able to categorize health information in general and detect specific syndromes that, for example, might suggest the possibility of an underlying disease. The categorization into these two groups is blurry, though, and systems that implement both epidemiological and syndromic surveillance are more common than not. There are certainly other definitions and forms of classification related to health surveillance systems. One example is that of *sentinel surveillance systems*, in which a set of pre-arranged samples of reporting sources (e.g. hospitals)—usually distributed over a wide region—agree to report all cases of one or more notifiable health conditions. In this chapter, we try to collapse these alternative classifications into the ones of epidemiological and syndromic surveillance.

This chapter makes a survey of HISes dedicated to syndromic and epidemiological surveillance, identifying the different design and technological strategies adopted in the development of such systems. The aims of such a survey are: (1)

to provide practitioners with some information about the collective expertise of HIS architects in the design and implementation of syndromic and epidemiological surveillance systems; and (2) to pave the way for the establishment of software product lines better aligned with the requirements imposed by such systems. The adopted methodology for structuring this survey comprises the definition of a set of criteria (data collection, data storage, data analysis, and data visualization) for comparative analysis of the discussed HISes as well as the presentation and comparison of such HISes in the light of the defined criteria.

The remainder of this chapter is organized as follows. Next section brings background information that provides the main definitions adopted along the chapter involving health surveillance systems. The considered criteria for comparative analysis of health surveillance systems are then introduced. There is then a section that reports a survey of epidemiological and syndromic surveillance systems. Another section compares the main characteristics of the surveyed systems. Finally, in the latest two sections we present the future trends and conclusions, respectively.

BACKGROUND

The last years have witnessed an increasing amount of work dedicated to the study and development of Health Information Systems (HISes) in general, and surveillance systems in particular. Thacker, Stroup, and Dicker (2003) define surveillance systems as HISes that allow the

"Ongoing, systematic collection, analysis, and interpretation of health data essential to the planning, implementation, and evaluation of public health practice, closely integrated with the timely dissemination of these data to those who need to know" (p. 225).

Crucially, such systems aim at providing decision makers with access to information of adequate quality when they need. Wilkins, Nsubuga, Mendlein, Mercer, and Pappaioanou (2008) report some surveillance system types, such as: systems for notification of potentially epidemic diseases; systems that collect periodic information from mortality reports; systems for prevention and control of specific diseases or groups of diseases; sentinel reporting systems; and periodic surveys. Such system types differ in scope and functionality, but all of them are based on epidemiological and/or syndromic surveillance concepts.

Epidemiological surveillance has its definition rooted on the epidemiology topic definition from the World Health Organization (WHO)[1]:

"Epidemiology is the study of the distribution and determinants of health-related states or events (including disease), and the application of this study to the control of diseases and other health problems. Various methods can be used to carry out epidemiological investigations: surveillance and descriptive studies can be used to study distribution; analytical studies are used to study determinants."

Nevertheless, the term *epidemiological surveillance* is also commonly used to refer to the processes of collection, analysis, and dissemination of health data, as well as the actions related to the prevention and the control of diseases. As put by Frerichs (1991):

"The final link in the surveillance chain is the application of [health] data to prevention and control. A surveillance system includes a functional capacity for data collection, analysis, and dissemination to linked public health programs" (p. 258).

Syndromic surveillance is concerned with the continuous monitoring of public health-related information sources and the early detection of public health aberrations such as outbreaks. As Chen et al. (2010) explain:

"In practice, syndromic surveillance systems are being increasingly adopted to meet the critical needs of effective prevention, detection, and management of infectious disease outbreaks, either naturally-occurring or caused by bioterrorism attacks" (p. 3).

A broader view of surveillance systems is described by Castillo-Salgado (2010), which enumerates the following key functions for both epidemiological and syndromic systems: (1) detecting cases of disease in specific populations and reporting the information; (2) analyzing and confirming reported cases' information to detect outbreaks; (3) providing timely and appropriate responses at the national and international level to prevent and control disease outbreaks; and (4) providing epidemiologic intelligence information to assist in long-term management of public health.

As can be inferred from the above, a common point in surveillance systems is that they must allow for health-related alerts and corresponding responses *in a highly distributed fashion*, so as to ensure that decision makers adequately accomplish the committed healthcare policies and programs. This commonality has led to the informal transmission of architectural idioms between such systems, which share as a result much about their structure and underlying functional model, as discussed in the following section. Nevertheless, the outstanding technological development in mobile computing and networking in the last decade has been a key enabler to the production of a new family of HISes, which we collectively call in this chapter *ubiquitous HISes*. For instance, as a recent contribution to this trend, platforms such as EpiCollect (Aanensen, Huntley, Feil, al-Own, & Spratt, 2009) are targeted at providing a basic framework to collect data using mobile devices in the field and synchronize the gathered data offering a centralized view through web applications for further data analysis. The existence of such recent alternatives eases the implementation and deployment of ubiquitous HISes.

Ubiquitous HISes expose a new set of non-functional requirements to be addressed—see Gomes, Ziviani, Souza e Silva, and Feijóo (2006) for an example in the area of emergency healthcare. For health surveillance systems, in particular, such wireless communication technologies are instrumental in providing the necessary timeliness of alerts and responses. Such timeliness, however, will mostly depend on the specific scenario for application of the intended surveillance practices. Each scenario may differ in one or more of the following characteristics, as described in WHO (1999):

- the specific case detection method used (active *vs* passive);
- the speed at which data need to flow through the system (immediate *vs* routine);
- the rapidity of response required (immediate investigation of cases or clusters of cases *vs* analysis of data on a regular basis with subsequent adjustments to a control policy).

As an example, for a surveillance system to provide early warnings, the involved steps of reporting, confirmation, decision-making, and response must be taken fast. On the other hand, for more endemic diseases, the aim may be to carefully consider data collected in widespread areas in order to adjust or target the control policy of public healthcare services. This leads to differences in the specific non-functional requirements that must be addressed not only by the systems themselves, but also by the computational and communication infrastructure that underlies them.

In the following, we comment on the overall design space for health surveillance systems and how the existing systems fit in with such space, emphasizing the structural and functional commonalities and the non-functional differences between such systems.

CRITERIA FOR COMPARATIVE ANALYSIS

In this section, we will present some criteria for the comparative analysis of epidemiological and syndromic surveillance information systems, including a discussion about architectural styles, technologies, and standards specifications employed in such systems. For the sake of such a presentation, we adopt a common vocabulary of design elements that cover the main functions expected from such systems: data collection, data analysis (which includes outbreak detection on syndromic surveillance systems), data visualization, and data storage/sharing. Figure 1 depicts the main relationships between such design elements. This vocabulary is based on guidelines from WHO (2001).

Data Collection

The first goal of a surveillance system is to efficiently collect information about a population's health. Data collection is therefore a key element in such systems, and usually one of the most complex to implement as well. The main challenge is to collect such data in a standardized way. Many countries' surveillance systems have been developed in an uneven way, leading to field workers participating in multiple systems and using different surveillance methods, terminology, reporting forms, and frequency (WHO, 2001). This scenario may result in extra costs and de-motivation for the health workers.

Data collection is usually accomplished from multiple data sources, including emergency rooms, ambulatory records, hospital admissions, medication prescriptions, national reference laboratories, and health departments (Chen, et al., 2010). Epidemiological surveillance systems collect data in all places where there are epidemiological case notifications, whereas syndromic surveillance systems collect data from regular electronic records providing timely health information. Chief

Figure 1. Typical design elements in a surveillance system

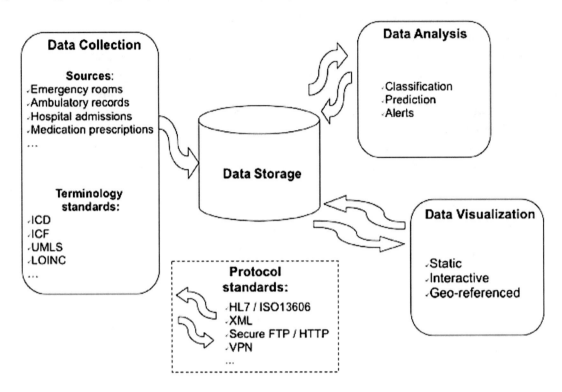

Complaint (CC) records, in particular, are widely used in syndromic surveillance systems, as they report the most common symptoms and conditions of medical interest—e.g. abdominal pain is a very common CC in emergency rooms (Graff & Robinson, 2001). CCes are usually reported in textual format, which makes the processing of such information rather complex, as they often have misspells and abbreviations (Chen, et al., 2010).

Primary data acquisition can be conducted is several different ways, including paper, Web or PDA forms, or directly from other HIS databases. Such data is ultimately published in a data storage so that it can be more easily made accessible to data analysis and visualization tools. This publication process typically involves the transmission of such data over shared networking resources—Internet being the common choice nowadays. Such data transmission over the Internet brings out technical issues such as the messaging protocol and the security procedures being adopted.

In this context, researchers and international bodies have been working to standardize data collection in HISes (Mandl, et al., 2004). The standard specifications related to surveillance systems have been mainly issued by WHO and the Centers for Disease Control and Prevention (CDC), a major operating component of the U.S. Department of Health and Human Services (HHS). Such specifications encompass terminology, communications, and security standardization:

- ICD (The International Classification of Diseases) is a WHO standard providing indexing codes to the diagnostic classification for all general epidemiological, many health management purposes and clinical use (ICD, 2011);
- ICF (The International Classification of Functioning, Disability, and Health) is a WHO standard that offers a framework for

measuring health and disability at both individual and population levels (ICF, 2011);

- UMLS (The Unified Medical Language System) is a development from HHS providing databases and associated software tools and programs for use by system developers in building or enhancing electronic information systems that create, process, retrieve, integrate, and/or aggregate biomedical and health data and information (Lindberg, Humphreys, & McCray, 1993);

- LOINC (The Logical Observation Identifiers Names and Codes) is a database and universal standard for identifying laboratory and clinical observations developed by the Regenstrief Institute, which is closely affiliated with the Indiana University School of Medicine and the Health and Hospital Corporation of Marion County, Indiana, U.S. (McDonald, Huff, Mercer, Hernandez, & Vreeman, 2010).

- *open*EHR (Open Electronic Health Records) is an open standard specification in health informatics that describes the management and storage of health data in Electronic Health Records (EHRs). In openEHR, all health data for a person is stored in a vendor-independent, person-centered EHR (Beale, 2002). The security and communications standardization covers both technical and regulatory aspects of health information storage and dissemination:

- The Standards for Privacy of Individually Identifiable Health Information from HHS is a regulation based on the HIPAA (Health Insurance Portability and Accountability Act) Privacy Rule enacted by the U.S. Congress in 1996 (Thacker, 2003). This regulation aims at giving patients more control over the sharing and availability of their health information, setting boundaries on the use and release of health records and holding violators accountable both civilly and criminally. It establishes appropriate safeguards that must be achieved to protect the privacy of health information, but also strikes a balance when public responsibility requires disclosure of some forms of personal data—for example, to protect public health.

- Health Level Seven (HL7) is a non-profit organization headquartered in Ann Arbor, Michigan, U.S., accredited by the American National Standards Institute (ANSI). HL7 is involved in the development of international standards for the exchange, integration, sharing, and retrieval of electronic health information. Such standards range from conceptual and documentation standardization, to messaging standardization. Currently in its third version, the HL7 messaging standard defines XML as the required encoding syntax to support all healthcare data and work flows (HL7, 2011).

- The International Organization for Standardization (ISO) has published the 13606 Recommendations Series as an international standard that specifies the communication of part or all of the EHR of a single identified subject of care between EHR systems, or between EHR systems and a centralized EHR data repository. ISO 13606 aims at supporting either the direct care given to identifiable individuals or surveillance systems (ISO, 2008).

Despite the many standardization efforts mentioned above, it remains unclear how they cope with the challenges the current network environment may impose on surveillance systems. For instance, if a 3G network is available during a data collection, one could expect a minimum data rate of 2 Mbps for stationary or walking users, and 384 kbps in a moving vehicle, whereas for an ordinary cellular network the maximum transmission rate is 64 kbps. If we are referring to countries characterized by large territorial areas, some of which lacking advanced—if not any—telecommunications capability[2], 64 kbps may be the only available data transmission rate for both wireless and wired communications. We comment more on this issue later in this chapter.

Data Storage

Another common element in all surveillance systems is data storage. It is responsible for providing efficient data update and retrieval mechanisms. This element can be implemented based on a variety of technologies. Nevertheless, Relational Database Management Systems (RDBMSes), such as Oracle and PostgreSQL, are the common choice for HISes in general, and for surveillance systems, this is not different. In a nutshell, such systems store data as relational tables row-by-row and use sophisticated data structures—e.g. B-trees—for indexing. RDBMSes are particularly fit to online transaction processing, as they fill all the ACID (atomicity, consistency, isolation, durability) properties. RDBMSes offer the Structured Query Language (SQL) as a standard way for transactionally updating and retrieving information on data storages.

Nonetheless, RDBMSes have been used to support many data-centric applications with widely varying characteristics and requirements that not necessarily fit well with such systems. Surveillance systems are arguably an example of application that does not fit well with RDBMSes. We comment more on this issue later in this chapter.

Data Analysis

Data analysis is the element responsible for extracting relevant information from health data. It accomplishes its task by synthesizing data from multiple data sources, detecting and identifying inconsistencies, contradictions, and anomalies to produce consistent assessments (HMN, 2008).

Data analysis is of particular importance to syndromic surveillance systems. Outbreak detection is a main feature of data analysis in such systems, and prediction algorithms are usually employed for implementing it. Data standardization (e.g. as the one provided by ICD) is crucial for such a feature, as it allows the classification of data into syndromes, which may reveal either known or novel diseases (Chen, et al., 2010).

Data analysis may raise alerts whenever a new outbreak is detected. Many different alerts are employed in syndromic surveillance systems, ranging from e-mail and short messages (SMS) to direct phone and fax calls.

Data Visualization

All surveillance systems provide visualization facilities. Chen et al. (2010) divide data visualization facilities into two types: static and interactive visual information. The first type shows both raw data and results from data analysis by means of tables, graphs, and maps. The second type provides navigational features, which allow users to access information in a dynamic and exploratory way.

The coupling of data visualization facilities with Geographic Information Systems (GISes) is increasingly common in health surveillance systems. Such coupling renders geo-referenced data visualization features, which are a powerful tool especially for syndromic surveillance, as they allow understanding the dynamics of syndromes' propagation. Nevertheless, such features can be only available if GPS-enabled equipment is used for data collection.

SURVEY

There are several HISes for epidemiological and syndromic surveillance. This study will mainly survey systems that are currently in operation, including their origins, goals, and architecture. Each system will be described in terms of the criteria described in the preceding section. Other development efforts (most of them from academia) are pointed out in the following section. In the end of this section, we provide a summary and comparison of such systems in tabular form.

NEDSS

The National Electronic Disease Surveillance System (NEDSS) is a public health project that aims at providing a standards-based, integrated approach to disease surveillance. NEDSS is a component system that integrates and replaces various surveillance systems and its primary goal is the ongoing, automatic capture and analysis of electronic data. The NEDSS Base System is a main part of NEDSS, offering a secure, standards-based environment over which other surveillance systems can be developed (Velikina, Dato, & Wagner, 2006).

The NEDSS base system architecture includes Web-based modules, a Web application server and an integrated database to store data shared between the modules. The system has a messaging tool and provides authentication and data security functions (NEDSS, 2001). The system defines various standard data types for collection. Data are collected from several sources, for example, diseases reports, healthcare systems, and health department documents. NEDSS employs the HL7 standard and XML documents conveyed in HTTP or HTTPS messages as its data transmission mechanisms. The database uses standard RDBMSes such as Oracle and SQL Servers by default, but supports other RDBMSes through ODBC, JDBC, and ANSI standard SQL.

ESSENCE

The Electronic Surveillance System for the Early Notification of Community-Based Epidemics (ESSENCE) is a syndromic surveillance system that integrates both military and civilian health data. It was created in 1999 and was jointly developed by

the Applied Physics Laboratory at Johns Hopkins University, Maryland Department of Health and Mental Hygiene, the District of Columbia Department of Health, and the Virginia Department of Health under the sponsorship of the Defense Advanced Research Projects Agency (DARPA) (Chen, et al., 2010). ESSENCE was developed in phases and the current version is ESSENCE IV, which is maintained by the Defense Health Service Systems (DHSS) of the Military Health System.

ESSENCE collects data from military clinical sources, including outpatient clinical visits, pharmacy transactions, and laboratory orders, and clusters them into disease syndrome groupings intended to promote early detection of disease outbreaks. The data acquisition may occur electronically or manually. The standards employed in ESSENCE include HL-7 and XML for message formatting and Secure FTP and VPN for data transmission. The system uses the syndrome classification defined by the 9th edition of ICD (ICD-9) to process the data by employing either a natural language processing algorithm or a weighted keyword matching-based parser. ESSENCE then runs on the processed data an analysis method composed of a set of algorithms that employ Exponentially Weighted Moving Average (EWMA) and Early Aberration Reporting System (EARS) as basic statistic tools for outbreak detection. The analysis results are made available on a web page through maps and tables to health and governmental entities. The system also provides alerts via e-mail, pagers, and mobile phones based on such analysis results.

RODS

The Real-time Outbreak and Disease Surveillance (RODS) system was created in 1999 in the Department of Biomedical Informatics at University of Pittsburgh. RODS is an open source project developed in Java and under the GNU license aiming at accelerating the software development process for surveillance systems and to stimulate the creation of a community-based outbreak and disease surveillance system (Szczepaniak, 2011).

RODS is a syndromic surveillance information system. It is a data-driven system and the data acquisition is regarded as its most important stage. Data are collected as CC records from emergency departments, emergency room clinicians, results of laboratory tests, and others (Tsui, et al., 2002). The data collection may occur in real time or at predefined times using HL7 as the messaging protocol between computer systems. The CC records (typically encoded as free text) are analyzed and classified according to a syndromes dataset stored in an Oracle RDBMS. The system uses Recursive Least Squares (RLS) and Cumulative Sum (CUSUM) algorithms together to help detect the presence of a disease outbreak. The RODS system includes information from a GIS, thus allowing the geo-referenced visualization of the data from different time series plots views (Wong, 2005).

SSIC

The Syndromic Surveillance Information Collection (SSIC) system was developed by the Clinical Informatics Research Group (CIRG) at the University of Washington and the Public Health-Seattle and King County (PHSKC) and its aim is at the early detection of disease outbreaks.

SSIC periodically collects data from a variety of sources, such as CC records or discharge summaries[3] from emergency departments. After the data are collected, they are "normalized" in a standard format and stored in a cluster of servers. The data storage format is based on XML. The data are then analyzed by aberration detection algorithms and made available to epidemiologists (Lober, et al., 2003).

CheSS

The Country Health Systems Surveillance (CheSS) is a project from WHO that provides a common platform for global partners and countries to implement harmonized, surveillance-related monitoring and evaluation systems. The platform aims to improve availability, quality, and use of data needed to monitor health progress and inform governmental health sectors at the regional, national, and global levels. A key feature of CheSS is the health "observatories" in which data from all relevant sources are publicly accessible and synthesized to monitor a population's health condition (Boerma, et al., 2010).

BioPortal

BioPortal is a project to develop infectious-disease surveillance systems. The project started in 2003 and was developed by the University of Arizona Artificial Intelligence Laboratory and sponsored by NSF, DHS, DoD, the Arizona Department of Health Services, and the Kansas State University's BioSecurity Center, under the guidance of a federal inter-agency working group (the Infectious Disease Informatics Working Committee—IDIWC) (Chen, et al., 2010).

The BioPortal architecture follows the traditional three-tiered architecture style. The data store tier is implemented using a SQL Server. The business-logic tier is responsible for information sharing, and is composed of a set of web services that support data search and query, data analysis, visualization, and alerting functionalities. These services are made available to the end user through a web-based presentation tier. BioPortal uses the Public Health Information Network Messaging System and HL7 with SSL connections as its data transmission mechanisms (Chen & Zeng, 2009).

BioPortal features advanced spatial-temporal data analysis methods that include industry standard hotspot analysis algorithms and in-house developed innovative clustering-based techniques for retrospective and prospective data analysis. The analysis results can be displayed via a Spatio-Temporal Visualizer (STV). BioPortal also has a social network analysis module that can be used to aid in the understanding of infectious disease transmission processes.

The BioPortal project has originally focused on two infectious diseases—the West Nile Virus (WNV) and Botulism (BOT)—but since its launching it has been continuously extended to cater for other diseases and syndromes. Two particularly interesting extensions of BioPortal have been the Food-and-Mouth Disease (FMD) BioPortal system and the BioPortal Syndromic Surveillance (SS) system.

The FMD-BioPortal system is a customization of BioPortal for the monitoring of the Food-and-Mouth Disease (FMD), a highly infectious disease that can affect all cloven-hoofed animals. It uses functionalities such as (near) real-time epidemiological data collection, gene sequence analysis, and news related to FMD to provide web-based situation awareness and crisis management facilities.

The BioPortal-SS system uses a data store built in batch mode using as sources the Arizona Department of Health Services and several hospitals. It implements the automatic classification of syndromes from CC records in free-text format using a concept ontology derived from UMLS. Various methods for detecting unusual and spatial clusters are used for disease outbreak detection.

WHOIS/GHO Databases

Surveillance is a data-intensive method of epidemiological investigation. As such, global databases play a crucial role in surveillance practices. Because of that, in spite of not being fully-fledged surveillance systems in their own right, WHOIS, and GHO are also presented here.

The WHO Statistical Information System (WHOIS) is the official WHO guide to health and health-related epidemiological and statistical information, which has recently been incorporated into the Global Health Observatory (GHO). GHO is a database that stores the main health statistics, such as: mortality, burden of diseases, infectious diseases, risk factors, and health expenditure. It is made available by WHO through a web interface that provides the meta-data codes currently in use for disease/syndrome classification, as well as several health statistical measurements, all of which can be downloaded as XML documents (WHOIS, GHO).

Comparison between Surveyed Systems

Table 1 summarizes the main characteristics of the systems surveyed in this section.

Table 1. Review of surveyed systems

System	Data Collection and Sources	Data Standards	Messaging Standards	Protocol Standards
NEDSS	Diseases reports, healthcare systems, health departments	N/A	HL7, XML, ODBC, JDBC	HTTP, HTTPS, SSL
ESSENCE	Military clinical, pharmacy, laboratory	ICD-9	Real time, HL7, XML	VPN, FTP
RODS	Emergency departments, emergency room clinicians, results from laboratory tests, CCes in free-text format	ICD-9	HL7, ODBC, XML	SSH
SSIC	Emergency departments	ICD-9	XML	SSL, HTTP
CheSS		IDC, ICF		
BioPortal	Hospital, health departments, CCes in free-text format	N/A	HL7	SSL
WHOIS / GHO		IDC, ICF		

As can be inferred from the table, the surveyed systems share a lot of similarities. The data collection element is implemented in different ways in each system, but all of such systems gather data of interest from heterogeneous data sources, so they must somehow deal with data interoperability issues. Data transmission using HL7 as the messaging standard is commonplace, and it is usually associated with secure protocols such as HTTPS and SSH. Data storage is typically based either on RDBMSes deployed "in-house" or on third-party data warehouses. Data analysis strategies vary a lot among such systems, but most of them use the ICD-9 standard to classify and categorize data for analysis.

An open issue observed in the analyzed systems is how much they are flexible to changes. Despite a huge effort to develop health surveillance systems for complying with healthcare standards, there seems to be little concern in developing "future-proof" systems. This issue can be observed in emergency situations where there is a need for rapidly adapting existing systems. For instance, during the Swine-flu outbreak in Japan in 2009, the national surveillance systems faced several problems because they were not flexible enough to support the changes in the surveillance policies caused by the phase transitions of a previously unknown disease. The outcome of this situation was the development of a whole new system. Even though agile development methods were employed at the time, the issues of standardization, interoperability, and cost of development were not taken into consideration appropriately (Murota, Kato, & Okumura, 2010). Specifications such as *open*EHR aim at tackling this issue from a data-modeling standpoint, but broader model-centric approaches in the development of HISes are still to be employed in wider scope. We come back to this issue in the following section when discussing future trends.

Another point to be considered is the relationship between the set of development initiatives of national surveillance systems and the corresponding country's welfare. On the one hand, several efforts

in U.S. have been launched to develop systems for the monitoring of bioterrorism threats and public health emergencies. Castillo-Salgado (2010) reports that after the anthrax threat, nearly US$32 billion were made available in the U.S. for the development of such systems. There is also an increasing number of health surveillance systems being developed and deployed both in European and Asian countries—and to some extent in Pan-American countries as well (Castillo-Salgado, 2010). Most of such systems are for syndromic surveillance.

On the other hand, in the majority of African countries the surveillance practices are still manual, with health data being collected almost exclusively from medical visits. When HISes are available, such data are entered on these systems and eventually published to a global surveillance database, e.g. GHO (Burnham & Gospodinov, 2008; Haux, 2006).

Despite the historical gap presented above, this situation is bound to change due to the role the Internet has started to play in providing a global mobilization about—mainly syndromic—surveillance practices (WHO, 1999; Ginsberg, et al., 2009; Castillo-Salgado, 2010).

FUTURE TRENDS

Our general overview of current surveillance systems naturally leads to a reference architecture pretty much aligned with the elements depicted in Figure 1. Moreover, we can observe from such an overview that there is a lot of possibilities for further technological improvements on the landscape of surveillance systems. We comment on some possibilities for such improvements in the following.

Communications Infrastructure and Protocols

Current surveillance systems take the omnipresence of network environments for granted. Nevertheless, there are some situations in which a communications infrastructure is scarce or even absent. As one example, disaster scenarios in urban areas (e.g. the ones caused by the Indian Ocean tsunami in Dec. 2004, the hurricane Katrina in Aug. 2005, or the Japanese earthquake and tsunami in Mar. 2011) ask for the seamless integration of on-site mobile devices—following the concept of *hastly formed networks* (Denning, 2006)—so that they can collect and automatically process information about groups of injured people (e.g. for triage) and thus better allocate medical resources. As another example, health data gathering on isolated areas—such as the large semi-arid region in the Northeastern Brazil—is not economically feasible to be conducted online due to the lack of a terrestrial communications infrastructure.

Adapting existing surveillance systems to operate in intermittent network environments such as the ones depicted above is likely to be challenging. Such systems are unable to gracefully handle disconnection conditions, forcing users to retry connections manually. Using intermittent connectivity requires new techniques to detect when a network connection has come and gone, new approaches to data routing to dynamically deal with the disconnected network, and new mechanisms to temporarily store in-transit data.

In this context, there has been considerable research work in the areas of Challenged/Opportunistic Networks (Chen, Yu, Sun, Chen, & Chu, 2006) and Delay-/Disruption-Tolerant Networks (DTNs) (Demmer, et al., 2004). Crucially, such approaches address the technical issues in networks of devices that may lack continuous connectivity among themselves and the Internet. Nevertheless, there is yet a lot of work to be done to make such technologies available to the surveillance systems development community, which seems yet rather unaware of the possibilities of such technologies.

Database Management Systems

As mentioned earlier in this chapter, RDBMSes do not necessarily fit well with health surveillance

systems. First, RDBMSes require that a data model (the database *schema*) be defined prior to any operation on the data storage, and any redefinition of such model implies a complete change in the data storage structure. Nevertheless, as a HIS takes form, it is far from uncommon that the members of the medical staff—who are in general beset by articulating their knowledge in layman's terms—require continuous data modeling changes in the system. This is one of the reasons for the creation of specifications such as *open*EHR. Second, ad hoc and associative queries (e.g. "select *everything* related with H1N1") are difficult (if not impossible) to define in SQL. Third, stream-processing applications—syndromic surveillance systems being a clear example—must be capable of dealing with sophisticated alerting and historical queries. As put by Stonebraker and Cetintemel (2005), there is a widespread speculation that RDBMSes do not perform well on this class of stream-processing applications. In this sense, other database approaches have come into play and should be better considered during the development of surveillance systems. Among such approaches, we can mention:

- Correlation Database Management Systems (CDBMSes), which employ key-value pairs as the unit of storage, and are particularly amenable to analytic processing. Examples include Amazon's SimpleDB and Apache's CouchDB;
- Column-Oriented Database Management Systems, which allows aggregates to be computed over large numbers of similar data items. Examples include Google's Bigtable and Apache's Cassandra;
- Data Streaming Management Systems (DSMSes), for continuous querying against data streams. Stanford University's SHARE is the most well known example of DSMS (Arasu et al., 2004).

Model-Centric Software Design

Despite the large number of surveillance systems already developed, we can observe that none of them has systematically departed from a concrete representation of a reference architecture (e.g. the one illustrated in Figure 1), such as an application framework or set of domain-specific software components. This approach is, however, crucial for such systems to rapidly respond to changing requirements.

In this context, some development efforts have emerged, mostly from academia. The AL-PHA Project (Turner, Bishay, Peng, & Merifield, 2006) is a Canadian initiative with the purpose of developing a software architecture based on the philosophy of configuring and reusing common components to produce services that would be used to enable faster development of robust, maintainable surveillance systems. The goal is to reduce the amount of new development work required for each new application, in order to reduce its time-to-market. Inline with this trend, EpiCollect (Aanensen, Huntley, Feil, al-Own, & Spratt, 2009) provides a framework to facilitate the development of applications, such as health surveillance systems, that need data collection from mobile devices and further analysis of such data on a centralized repository. In these projects, new components or services that have to be built are designed in such a way that other applications can use them, and contribute to the architecture. Consequently, software becomes more maintainable, since applications share many of their components.

More recently, attention has been drawn to the potential of Model-Driven Engineering (MDE) in general, and OMG's Model-Driven Architecture (MDA) approach (Miller & Mukerji, 2003) in particular, for overcoming inhibitor factors to the deployment of maintainable HISes. Exploratory papers like (Raghupathi & Umar, 2008; Tuomainen, Mykkänen, Luostarinen, Pöyhölä, and Paakkanen, 2007) have set an initial basis in terms

of the potential MDE could offer, as previously mentioned, for the systematic engineering of HIS. Nevertheless, despite reporting an increase in the use of model-centric approaches in healthcare, these papers are also critical about the difficulties in reaching rationale for general design decisions. According to their analysis, a non-trivial effort is often required for localized tuning.

Lopez and Blobel (2009) discuss several software engineering methodologies (e.g., RUP), modeling languages (e.g., UML), architectural frameworks (e.g., MDA, RM-ODP), and health-care standards (e.g., HL7, *open*EHR) in the pursuit of a feasible configuration for enabling semantic interoperability in healthcare. The main assumption behind this initiative seems to be a need for integrating methodologies and standards from software engineering in general to those born in health informatics in particular. It is worth highlighting in this sense the difficulty in integrating and evolving proprietary artifacts such as RUP and HL7. On a different path, Janamanchi, Katsamakas, Raghupathi, & Gao (2009) discuss the potential of dissemination of open artifacts such as the Eclipse Modeling Framework (EMF) (EMF, 2010) and the *open*EHR specifications. The authors conclude there exists an active and thriving open-source software development community that is focusing on health and medical informatics.

From this brief review on the literature, we highlight that the application of MDE in healthcare is in progress, and the existing initiatives are in general still restricted to the standard MDA approach.

The MDA approach lies in the use of (semi-) automatic transformation rules for translating a Platform-Independent Model (PIM) into different Platform-Specific Models (PSMs) and then generating code from the latter. This allows one to manage, say, functional changes, directly in the PIM to then regenerate PSM and code, rather than (at worst) handling changes as bug fixes in the code. This means a better management of the so-called roundtrip problem (Hailpern &

Tarr, 2006), i.e., handling multiple artifacts that represent different levels of abstraction in the development workflow in such a way to avoid redundancy and inconsistency. This feature constitutes an important step to reduce the high development cost of HIS.

The MDA approach itself can be a valuable resource for developing HIS with separation between healthcare processes and technology. Nevertheless, we understand it should be augmented in order to improve reuse in terms of application-independent modeling. In the case of healthcare, particularly, modeling clinical data as well as software architecture in an application-by-application basis may well not be worth it.

On the one hand, it is our experience with the development of a teleconsultation system for prehospital delivery of thrombolysis for infarction patients (Gomes, et al., 2006) that clinical data modeling takes much of the attention of the development team. In fact, it is not new for the medical informatics community that clinical data modeling turns out to be a tough job for either clinicians or computing professionals, if both are not committed to working together (Schulz, Suntisrivaraporn, Baader, & Boeker, 2009).

On the other hand, the architectural modeling of the sought-after HIS—e.g., to provide users with easy interaction to permanently available clinical systems—is far from a trivial task. Therefore, either by being model-driven or not, for those systems to be "future-proof," a careful architectural design is important, if not indispensable. In this sense, MDA is able to ease the reuse of a good architecture, but it still cannot systematically help one to come up with new good architectures. Nonetheless, one can envision within the HIS domain typical communication and control patterns that are fit to specific system families. For instance, the near real-time requirements in syndromic surveillance systems do not necessarily bother in epidemiological surveillance systems. In the latter, however, the robustness and reliability of the available information is of foremost importance.

Along these lines, the established principles of software architecture in general, and of architectural styles (Garlan, Allen, & Ockerbloom, 1994) in particular, make up a clear synergy within the model-driven philosophy.

To summarize, we believe the development of HISes in general, and surveillance systems in particular, can capitalize on the following set of principles, which are yet to be attained by a single, unified approach:

- Transversalization of data and architecture models, so that health domain specialists do not care about *how* data is to be conveyed, whereas software architects do not bother with *what* data is to be conveyed.
- Dualization of information and clinical data models, to lessen the development team's effort on HIS maintenance and evolution.
- Stylization of architecture models, to capture commonalities within families of HIS as reusable design artifacts.

CONCLUSION

In this chapter, we survey a set of representative syndromic and epidemiological surveillance systems currently in operation either regionally, nationally, or globally, identifying not only the different design and technological strategies adopted in their development, but also the many similarities shared between them. With this survey, we expect to have provided practitioners with some information about the collective expertise of HIS architects in the design and implementation of such systems.

We have also tried in this chapter to present some of the design space yet to be properly addressed by the groups somehow involved with the development of health surveillance systems. More specifically, we showed some possibilities for further developments in communications infrastructure and protocols, database management systems, and model-centric software design. This way, we hope to have contributed in paving the way for the establishment of software product lines better aligned with the requirements imposed by such systems.

ACKNOWLEDGMENT

This work has been funded by the Brazilian Ministry of Science and Technology (MCT), the Brazilian National Council for Scientific and Technological Development (CNPq), and the Brazilian National Institute of Science and Technology on Medicine Assisted by Scientific Computing (INCT-MACC).

REFERENCES

Aanensen, D. M., Huntley, D. M., Feil, E. J., al-Own, F., & Spratt, B. G. (2009). EpiCollect: Linking smartphones to web applications for epidemiology, ecology and community data collection. *PLoS ONE*, *4*(9), 6968. doi:10.1371/journal.pone.0006968

Arasu, A., Babcock, B., Babu, S., Cieslewicz, J., Datar, M., & Ito, K. (2004). *STREAM: The Stanford data stream management system. Technical Report*. Palo Alto, CA: Stanford InfoLab.

Beale, T. (2002). *Archetypes: Constraint-based domain models for future-proof information systems*. Paper presented at the Eleventh OOPSLA Workshop on Behavioral Semantics: Serving the Customer. Seattle, WA.

Boerma, T., Zahr, C. A., Bos, E., Hansen, P., Addai, E., & Beer, D. L. (2010). *Monitoring and evaluation of health systems strengthening: An operational framework*. Retrieved October 20, 2011, from http://www.who.int/entity/healthinfo/HSS_MandE_framework_Oct_2010.pdf.

Che, S. S. (2011). *Country health systems surveillance: Improving data availability, quality and use for better performance*. Retrieved February 11, 2011, from http://www.internationalhealthpartnership.net/en/working_groups/monitoring_and_evaluation.

Chen, H., & Zeng, D. (2009). AI for global disease surveillance: Trends & controversies. *IEEE Intelligent Systems*, *24*(6), 66–69. doi:10.1109/MIS.2009.126

Chen, H., Zeng, D., & Yan, P. (2010). *Infectious disease informatics: Syndromic surveillance for public health and BioDefense*. New York, NY: Springer Science+Business Media, LLC.

Chen, L., Yu, C., Sun, T., Chen, Y., & Chu, H. (2006). Hybrid routing approach for opportunistic networks. In *Proceedings of the ACM SIGCOMM Workshop on Challenged Networks (CHANTS)*, (pp. 213-220). ACM Press.

Demmer, M., Brewer, E., Fall, K., Jain, S., Ho, M., & Patra, R. (2004). *Implementing delay tolerant networking*. IRB-TR-04-020. Retrieved from http://www.dtnrg.org/docs/papers/demmer-irb-tr-04-020.pdf.

Denning, P. J. (2006). Hastily formed networks. *Communications of the ACM*, *49*(4), 15–20. doi:10.1145/1121949.1121966

EMF. (2010). *Eclipse modeling framework project*. Retrieved Mach 05, 2011, from http://www.eclipse.org/modeling/emf/.

FCC. (2010). *Federal communications commission – FCC - 10-129*. Retrieved March 05, 2011, from http://www.fcc.gov/Daily_Releases/Daily_Business/2010/db0720/FCC-10-129A1.pdf.

Forslund, D. W., Joyce, E. L., Burr, T., Picard, R., Wokoun, D., & Umland, E. (2004). Setting standards for improved syndromic surveillance: The importance of using standard, distributed components for medical surveillance for discovering and managing a public health threat. *IEEE Engineering in Medicine and Biology Magazine*, *24*(1), 65–70. doi:10.1109/MEMB.2004.1297176

Frerichs, R. R. (1991). *Epidemiologic surveillance in developing countries. Annual Revision Public Health* (pp. 257–280). Los Angeles, CA: University of California.

Garlan, D., Allen, R., & Ockerbloom, J. (1994). Exploiting style in architectural design environments. In *Proceedings of the SIGSOFT 1994 Symposium on the Foundations of Software Engineering*, (pp. 175 – 188). SIGSOFT.

GHO. (2011). *Global health observatory*. Retrieved February 11, 2011, from http://apps.who.int/ghodata/.

Ginsberg, J., Mohebbi, M. H., Patel, R. S., Brammer, L., Smolinski, M. S., & Brilliant, L. (2009). Detecting influenza epidemics using search engine query data. *Nature, n.d.*, 457.

Gomes, A. T. A., Ziviani, A., Souza e Silva, N. A., & Feijóo, R. A. (2006). Towards a ubiquitous healthcare system for acute myocardial infarction patients in Brazil. In *Proceedings of the IEEE International Workshop on Pervasive and Ubiquitous Health Care – UbiCare 2006*, (pp. 585-589). IEEE Press.

Graff, L. G., & Robinson, D. (2001). Abdominal pain and emergency department evaluation. *Emergency Medicine Clinics of North America*, *19*(1), 123–136. doi:10.1016/S0733-8627(05)70171-1

HL7. (2011). *Health level seven international*. Retrieved January 28, 2011, from http://www.HL7.org.

Hailpern, B., & Tarr, P. (2006). Model-driven development: The good, the bad, and the ugly. *IBM Systems Journal*, *45*(3), 451–461. doi:10.1147/sj.453.0451

Haux, R. (2006). Health information systems - Past, present, future. *International Journal of Medical Informatics*, *75*, 268–281. doi:10.1016/j.ijmedinf.2005.08.002

HMN. (2008). *Framework and standards for country health information systems - Health metrics network*. Geneva, Switzerland: World Health Organization.

ICD. (2011). *International classification of diseases*. Retrieved January 20, 2011, from http://www.who.int/classifications/icd/en/.

ICF. (2011). *International classification of functioning, disability and health*. Retrieved January 20, 2011, from http://www.who.int/classifications/icf/en/.

ISO. (2008). *ISO 13606 - Health informatics - Electronic health record communication*. Geneva, Switzerland: International Organization for Standardization (ISO).

Janamanchi, B., Katsamakas, E., Raghupathi, W., & Gao, W. (2009). The state and profile of open source software projects in health and medical informatics. *International Journal of Medical Informatics*, *78*(7), 457–472. doi:10.1016/j.ijmedinf.2009.02.006

Lindberg, D. A. B., Humphreys, B. L., & McCray, A. T. (1993). The unified medical language system. *Methods of Information in Medicine*, *32*, 281–291.

Lober, W. B., Trigg, L. J., Karras, B. T., Bliss, D., Ciliberti, J., Stewart, L., & Duchin, J. S. (2003). Syndromic surveillance using automated collection of computerized discharge diagnoses. *Journal of Urban Health: Bulletin of the New York Academy of Medicine*, *80*(2), 97–106.

Lopez, D. M., & Blobel, B. (2009). A development framework for semantically interoperable health information systems. *International Journal of Medical Informatics, 78*(2), 83–103. doi:10.1016/j.ijmedinf.2008.05.009

Mandl, K. D., Overhage, J. M., Wagner, M. M., Lober, W. B., Sebastiani, P., & Mostashari, F. (2004). Implementing syndromic surveillance: A practical guide informed by the early experience. *Journal of the American Medical Informatics Association, 11*(2), 141–150. doi:10.1197/jamia. M1356

McDonald, C., Huff, S., Mercer, K., Hernandez, J. A., & Vreeman, D. J. (Eds.). (2010). *Logical observation identifiers names and codes (LOINC®): Users' guide.* Indianapolis, IN: Regenstrief Institutes, Inc.

Miller, J., & Mukerji, J. (2003). *MDA guide version 1.0.1.* Tech. Rep. No. omg/2003-06-01. New York, NY: Object Management Group (OMG).

Murota, T., Kato, A., & Okumura, T. (2010). Emergency management for information systems in public health: A case study of the 2009 pandemic-flu response in Japan. In *Proceedings of the Pervasive Computing and Communications Workshops (PERCOM Workshops), 8th IEEE International Conference,* (pp. 394 – 399). IEEE Press.

Raghupathi, W., & Umar, A. (2008). Exploring a model-driven architecture (MDA) approach to health care information systems development. *International Journal of Medical Informatics, 77*(5), 305–414. doi:10.1016/j.ijmedinf.2007.04.009

Castillo-Salgado, C. (2010). Trends and directions of global public health surveillance. *Epidemiologic Reviews, 32,* 93–109. doi:10.1093/epirev/mxq008

Schulz, S., Suntisrivaraporn, B., Baader, F., & Boeker, M. (2009). SNOMED reaching its adolescence: Ontologists' and logicians' health check. *International Journal of Medical Informatics, 78*(1), 86–94. doi:10.1016/j.ijmedinf.2008.06.004

Stonebraker, M., & Cetintemel, U. (2005). One size fits all: An idea whose time has come and gone. In *Proceedings of the 2005 International Conference on Data Engineering.* IEEE.

Systems Architecture, N. E. D. S. S. (2001). *Centers for disease control and prevention.* Retrieved by January 15, 2011, from http://www.cdc.gov/nedss/BaseSystem/NEDSSsysarch2.0.pdf.

Szczepaniak, M. C. (2011). *Real-time outbreak and disease surveillance laboratory.* Retrieved January 11, 2011, from https://www.rods.pitt.edu/site/content/view/14/77/.

Thacker, S. B. (2003). *HIPAA privacy rule and public healthL Guidance from CDC and the U.S. Department of Health and Human Services.* Retrieved Mach 05, 2011, from http://www.cdc.gov/mmwr/preview/mmwrhtml/m2e411a1.htm.

Thacker, S. B., Stroup, D. F., & Dicker, R. C. (2003). Health data management for public health. In F. D. Scutchfield & C. W. KecK (Eds.), *Principles of Public Health Practices,* (p. 225). New York, NY: Thomson Delmar Learning.

Tsui, F. C., Espino, J. U., Wagner, M. M., Gesteland, P., Ivanov, O., & Olszewski, R. T. … Moore, A. (2002). *Data, network, and application: Technical description of the Utah RODS winter olympic biosurveillance system.* Retrieved January 05, 2011, from http://rods.health.pitt.edu/LIBRARY/AMIA02-TsuiJue-Final.pdf.

Tuomainen, M., Mykkänen, J., Luostarinen, H., Pöyhölä, A., & Paakkanen, E. (2007). Model-centric approaches for the development of health information systems. *Studies in Health Technology and Informatics, 129*(1), 28–32.

Turner, C., Bishay, H., Peng, B., & Merifield, A. (2006). The ALPHA project: An architecture for leveraging public health applications. *International Journal of Medical Informatics, 75*(10-11), 741–754. doi:10.1016/j.ijmedinf.2005.10.006

Velikina, R., Dato, V., & Wagner, M. M. (2006). Governmental public health. In Wagner, M. M., Moore, A. W., & Aryel, R. M. (Eds.), *Handbook of Biossurveilance* (pp. 67–87). Burlington, MA: Elsevier Academic Press. doi:10.1016/B978-012369378-5/50007-7

Wagner, M. M., Moore, A. W., & Aryel, R. M. (Eds.). (2006). *Handbook of biosurveillance*. Burlington, MA: Elsevier Academic Press.

WHO. (1999). *Recommended surveillance standards*. Retrieved February 05, 2011, from http://www.who.int/csr/resources/publications/surveillance/whocdscsrisr992.pdf.

WHO. (2001). *Protocol for the assessment of national communicable disease surveillance and response systems*. Retrieved February 05, 2011, from http://www.who.int/csr/resources/publications/surveillance/whocdscsrisr20012.pdf.

WHO-CheSS. (2011). *Country health systems surveillance: Health statistics and health information systems*. Retrieved October 20, 2011, from http://www.who.int/healthinfo/country_monitoring_evaluation/en/index.html.

WHOSIS. (2011). *Statistical information system*. Retrieved February 11, 2011, from http://www.who.int/whosis/en/.

Wilkins, K., Nsubuga, P., Mendlein, J., Mercer, D., & Pappaioanou, M. (2008). The data for decision making project: Assessment of surveillance systems in developing countries to improve access to public health information. *The Journal of the Royal Institute of Public Health and Hygiene, 122*, 914–922.

Wong, R. (2005). *Early CBRN attack detection by computerized record surveillance (ECADS) project: RODS user manual*. Retrieved February 05, 2011, from http://openrods.sourceforge.net/contrib/AMITA_RODS3_documentation.zip.

ENDNOTES

[1] http://www.who.int/topics/epidemiology/en/.

[2] For an overview of the current situation of U.S., for instance, the reader may refer to the 7th 706 report from the Federal Communications Commission (FCC) (FCC, 2010).

[3] A doctor may dictate a discharge summary on the release of a patient from a course of care.

Chapter 11
Distributed Monitoring and Supervising System for E-Health Applications

Silviu Folea
Technical University of Cluj-Napoca, Romania

Mihai Hulea
Technical University of Cluj-Napoca, Romania

Camelia Avram
Technical University of Cluj-Napoca, Romania

Adina Aştilean
Technical University of Cluj-Napoca, Romania

ABSTRACT

The system presented in this chapter is mainly destined to offer support and to monitor chronic and elderly patients. In accordance with the new tendencies in the field, it integrates innovative components for data acquisition systems, Web-based virtual instrumentation, personalized user interfaces, and relational data in a complex, modular, flexible, and opened structure. Compared with other similar integrated communication systems, which are based on Wi-Fi technology, the presented one has as distinctive features: small dimensions, low power consumption, and a considerable autonomy. A large set of experiments and the corresponding results illustrates the functionality of the configurable virtual web instrument principle materialized in the E-Health Monitoring and Supervising System (EMSS) that has many possible applications. As an example, a cheap, easy to use, and personalized support destined to improve the quality of life for subjects suffering from chronic diseases or elderly patients was chosen. The implementation of the complete application included a model for gesture recognition, which allows the classification and assessment of the characteristics of the subject's movement, highlighting even small progresses of the monitored patients.

DOI: 10.4018/978-1-4666-0888-7.ch011

INTRODUCTION

Following the new requests, resulted from the complex social and medical necessities of the present moment and some specific problems of chronic patients, the chapter presents a Web based monitoring and supervising system, which integrates many innovative characteristics. The main design concepts included in the presented experimental system aim to offer a cheaper, easier to use, and personalized support destined to improve the quality of life of the subjects suffering from chronic diseases or of the elderly patients. The flexible and modular structure of the system offers reliable solutions for an adequate and permanently updated treatment, adaptable to a long-term evolution of the disease. In order to enrich the practice of medical staff besides the borders resulted from each individual experience, suggestions, case studies, and especially long-term observations and obtained results will be stored in common, accessible data bases. So, even though it was not the main priority in the presented context, the system can bring a considerable contribution to the improvement of the defective relationship among groups of researches involved in similar or close area of interest.

Using adequate, performing, and promising technologies, the presented virtual monitoring system integrates innovative components for data acquisition systems, WEB based virtual instrumentation, personalized user interfaces, and relational data in a complex and open structure. Compared with other similar integrated communication systems which are based on the Wi-Fi technology, the presented one has as distinctive features small dimensions, low power consumption and a considerable autonomy. Consequently, the resulting assembly is easy to wear and to use. Furthermore, neither specialty knowledge, nor prior special training of the users is required. It is not necessary to install a dedicated soft on the users' computers, wired connections are eliminated, the freedom of movement in the working space is preserved and the effectuation of routine, daily activities is possible without restrictions or drawbacks.

Resuming the above considerations, the main objectives of our presented research were:

1. To offer to clinicians, doctors and therapists, not only new conceptual but also implemented technical solutions regarding the supervising and adapting of the rehabilitation process for many categories of subjects affected by neuromotor disorders. stage is at the level of "proof of concept," being possible many improvements and developments;

2. Based on repetitive practice, to offer to the subjects, the solutions are based on two core elements: a new, Wi-Fi based, performing acquisition system and the concept of web virtual instrument. It is important to mention that the implementation the possibility to perform compensatory tasks and to re-learn the main steps involved in complex activities;

3. To complete the significant statistical information regarding the evolution and treatment results for many categories of chronic diseases.

The content of the chapter is organized as follows:

The first two sections focus on the necessity to assess the human movement in a close relationship with the health status as a consequent of the increasing number of patients having motor impairments and their special rehabilitation necessities.

A brief overview of the technical solutions applied to measure and quantify the human motion, a special emphasize being given to configurations containing accelerometers is presented in the third section of the chapter.

Recent techniques for the signal processing such as Fast Fourier and Wavelets Transformation are presented, as are the key elements which can generate innovative features. The main advantages of LabVIEW are considered to be the implementation facilities, a superior optimization from the point of view of runtime and needed CPU resources and more important, the support offered for built-in libraries and virtual instruments. This part ends with an overview and some considerations regarding the Virtual WEB Instruments concept and the possible, new corresponding applications.

The main part of the chapter is dedicated to the presentation of the E-Health Monitoring and Supervising System. After the description of the multilevel, distributed architecture of the system, details about E-Health PostgresSQL Database and the functionalities of E-health EMSS Middleware and about the components responsible for handling biomedical sensors are given.

A particular interest represents the introducing of the concept of configurable virtual web instruments, the configuration being defined by the users in accordance with their own necessities. The designed interfaces allow a selection from a list containing the WiFiSmartDAQ devices.

A considerable space was allocated to WiFiSmartDAQ Biomedical Device, the core element around which the system was developed. It is characterized as a special Wi-Fi module having low power consumption and reduced dimensions, many of the technical solutions, which lead to the obtained performances being mentioned in the associated explanations and descriptions.

Later, a large set of experiments and the corresponding results illustrates the functionality of the configurable virtual web instrument principle materialized in EMSS system and having a lot of possible applications.

First, different configurations were chosen, the measured values were preprocessed and the signal evolutions were stored and visualized. A complete application which highlights the possible progress of the monitored patients is presented. After the chosen of the configuration for the WiFiSmartDAQ device, the signals preprocessing and the signal analysis, based on the wavelet transformation, a model for gesture recognition based on hidden Markov chain is used to classify

and to assess the characteristics of the patient's movement.

The final section presents the conclusions. Several directions of future research are suggested.

THE PHYSICAL IMPAIRMENTS AND THE HEALTH STATUS

Some Aspects Related to Incidence, Characteristics, Causes, and Some Manifestations of Chronic Diseases

In a close connection with some aspects of technical progress, chronic diseases have a distribution depending on economical conditions, age, and geographical zone. Consequently, the quality of life of the affected population is directly and permanently influenced by the presence of the specific symptoms. On the other hand, the constant rising number of patients belonging to this category leads to huge health care costs. Seventy percent of health-care costs in the United States are for chronic diseases.

Over the past three decades, chronic kidney disease, diabetes, cardiovascular, and chronic respiratory diseases, cancers, and Alzheimer' disease are the most important causes of death among older patients. From a medical point of view, the leading causes of death vary among different age, sex, and origin groups (race) and can be classified taking into account several criteria. Medical statistics for many years show that cancer accounted for about one-fifth of all deaths in the elderly patient group and nearly one-third of all deaths among older persons were due to heart diseases (heart attacks and chronic ischemic heart disease). Europe averages approximately 650,000 stroke deaths each year. More, ischemic stroke is one of the most frequent causes of long-term deficiencies or even severe disabilities in Western Europe. Worldwide, according to some recent statistics of World Health Organization, 15 million people suffer a stroke each year. Of these, 5 million die and another 5 million are disabled for the rest of their lives. It is important to mention that there are certain, important risk factors for stroke, such as: high blood pressure (the most important), age (the risk factor is double for each decade after the age of 55), smoking, stress due to working conditions, atrial fibrillation (independent risk factor).

Other important factors which contribute to the increasing of the morbidity rate of the old persons are unintentional injuries. The most frequent are, falls, burns, accidental ingestion of toxic substances, other home accidents, road accidents, suffocation. These remain an important cause of death and disabilities for all the rest of life into this category.

There is a strong interdependency between health status and physical activity, which is also progressively accentuated with the age. A declining physical activity level represents a major factor in multiple illnesses and symptoms related to functional impairment (Steele, et al., 2000). Human movements and their relationship to health status were studied especially in the area of cardiovascular diseases, diabetes mellitus, and obesity (Yang & Hsu, 2010). A lot of similarities among the physical impairments caused by chronic diseases and that developed in the case of elderly persons lead to the possibility to use many common monitoring, treatment, and support.

Rehabilitation

In a large sense, rehabilitation means the recovery of the lost functions with the main purpose to live independently in the community. Many causes such as surgical interventions (amputations), accidents, falls and fractures (due to age), cardiac and neurologic disorders, other impairments related to age and chronic diseases involve long periods of physical and occupational therapy. In this context, two categories of patients need a particularly attention, their rehabilitation being carefully personalized: elderly persons and post-stroke patients. The result of the recovery process depends on multiple factors, the most important being the gravity of illness, the patient's motivation, and the correctness of initial and long-term evaluation, and of prescribed therapy. Patients' initial condition expressed by muscle strength, coordination, joint mobility, and agility also play an important role.

The assessment of patients that suffered a cerebrovascular accident in order to maximize their functional recovery is a difficult process, which can begin in an acute care hospital and continues periodically, long after their discharge. The recovery potential of the patients is determinant for the manner in which is initiated and established the formal rehabilitation therapy. The used evaluation methods, the reliability and validity of measures, the sensitivity of assessment tools to changes are crucial factors, which determine the relevance of the assembly result. In most of the cases, an interdisciplinary approach is necessary. Frequently, the patients present cognitive, sensory, and motor impairments. The manifestations of the last are reflected in mobility, flexibility, postural control, and balance and lead to difficulties and even to the impossibility to be independent during the performance of daily activities that often includes taking care of oneself. The increased risk of falls can have a negative impact on the possible progress of the subject.

Multiple tests were developed and adopted to measure motor performances in many areas, being helpful in determining appropriate placement of persons with disabilities. These tests includes perceptual motor function, object control, loco-motors skills, and have as results scores giving the possibility to quantify low levels of performance and to determine even a small progress. The rehabilitation techniques aim to improve motor malfunctions, gait instability, difficulties to maintain the postures and to perform stable motion trajectories.

The most known, accepted, and utilized scales, which asses physical and cognitive disabilities adopted in many countries from many continents

(Europe, Asia, and America) are Functional Independence Measure (FIM) and Functional Assessment Measure (FAM) which includes the first. The 13 items of FIM scale which refers to physical domains and are based on Barthel index were used widely in rehabilitation settings (e.g. for stroke and multiple sclerosis). Currently, FIM is considered the most robust global outcome measure of disability (Mackintosh, 2009).

More recently, new methods were developed in order to establish causal relationships between the activities of some selected muscles and movement kinematics and to obtain quantitative evaluation of neurological disorders using EMG signals captured from different many muscles. (Lee, et al., 2009) developed a new method to identify causal muscles activities for movement disorders.

Beyond all doubt, regular screening can reduce morbidity and mortality of patients belonging to many groups of chronic diseases. Clinical preventive services play also a very important role to prevent and delay the complications of cardiovascular diseases.

In these conditions, beside the periodical screening and in hospitals evaluations for diagnosis and establishment of disease and/or disability status (severity), the close monitoring of old persons for surveillance purposes, and for the registration of relevant data resulted from long term observations becomes important and poses special problems.

It is important to mention that the difficulties in diagnosis and in defining differences in the levels of illness are partially due to the heterogeneous nature of diseases patterns.

SYSTEMS, DEVICES, AND TECHNIQUES USED FOR THE EVALUATION, MONITORING, AND SUPPORT OF HUMAN PHYSICAL ACTIVITY

Many systems were designed for the quantitative evaluations of mobility and flexibility, to asses balance stability or to detect the fall risk. Human motion was measured and quantified using objective techniques based on image systems and/or inertial measurements, wearable, or body-fixed motion sensors, which range from switches, pedometers, actometers, goniometers, accelerometers, and gyroscopes (Steele, et al., 2000). While the systems including vision are cost expensive, more efficiency have proved that are based on accelerometers, gyroscopes, magnetometers and more recently, EMG sensors.

Often, accelerometers measures include all accelerations (because of the gravitational field), while the gyroscopes based results have to take into consideration that these are affected by sensing errors, manifesting as bias drift. In applications where the integration is necessary, the resulted errors are also integrated, leading to the increasing of error (Painter & Shkel, 2001). A solution to obtain complete information regarding full position and rate sensing is given by (on a chip) integrated devices including many accelerometers and gyroscopes. More, inertial measurements systems (tri-axes) accelerometers and gyroscopes are often combined with others types of sensors and widely used to assess the human motion and to interpret it. In Shi et al. (2009) a method of human motion recognition based on MEMS inertial sensors data is presented. A unit, consisting of three dimensional MEMS accelerometers, gyroscopes, a Bluetooth module, and a MCU (Micro Controller Unit), can record and transfer inertial data to a computer via wireless technology. Five categories of human motion were analyzed including walking, running, going upstairs, falling, and standing. Fourier series analysis was used to extract the feature from the measured data and categorize the human motions through HMM (Hidden Markov Model) process.

Miniature acceleration sensors are extensively used for ambulatory monitoring, allowing the measurement of important gait parameters, to identify postures, to measure balance during walking (Lindemann, et al., 2005; Mathies, et al., 2008). Intelligent and wearable devices integrate accelerometers in different ways. Many accelerometers have to be attached to a single segment to solve its complete Kinematics (Aminian, et al., 1998). Some suggestive examples are given below.

The design and evaluation of a miniature kinematic sensor based three dimensional (3D) joint angle measurement technique is presented in O'Donovan et al. (2007). The technique uses a combination of rate gyroscope, accelerometer and magnetometer sensor signals. The solution based on a 3D inter-segment joint angle measurement can be useful in a variety of applications, which require monitoring of joint angles.

An alternative method for measuring human motion, by placing small acceleration sensors on the body is presented in Takeda et al. (2009).

Joint angle and segment inclination measurement techniques have been developed for gait analysis which use accelerometers on their own (de Vries, et al., 1994; Willemsen, et al., 1990) or combined with rate gyroscopes (Williamson & Andrews, 2001; Luinge & Veltink, 2005; Mayagoitia, et al., 2002). These techniques measure the inclination of a segment with respect to a common reference axis (the gravity vector) and hence determine a two-dimensional (2D) joint angle between two segments (O'Donovan, et al., 2007).

The based sensor fusion approaches, using information obtained from various sensors, allow the characterization of oscillations, which have significance for diagnostic purposes.

Common methods of gait analysis include using cameras to track the position of body-mounted reflective markers, from which information on joint and limb segment motion can be derived (Liu, et al., 2010). However, such systems are large, expensive, and complex. Accurate three-dimensional (3D) inter-segment joint angle measurement is an important biomechanical measure for a variety of applications. Such a measure, when applied to ankle joint measurement, could be used for the monitoring of lower leg activity in the case of persons with limited mobility that presents the risk of remaining inactive for prolonged periods.

It could also be used for the measure of balanced dorsiflexion (rotation about the medio-lateral axis of the joint, which does not also involve rotation about the other axes of the joint) in drop foot correction applications or for the monitoring of foot rotation in clinical trials (O'Donovan, et al., 2007).

The monitoring of elderly and extern patients supposes less an accurate assessment of physical activity and more the identification of changes in movement patterns followed by the quantification of the corresponding disorders and deficits. Different devices, methods, and algorithms, depending on the patient's specific needs are used in this purpose.

A special attention was given to the integration of accelerometers and gyroscopes, data processing algorithms known as filters being used in this purpose. Accelerometers on two or three axis and gyroscopes can be used in difference combination being integrated through Kalman Filters. Other versions of more simple algorithms, inspired by Kalman Filter included ideas were also introduced and implemented on embedded devices.

Signal Analysis

The main purpose of the analysis of a measured signal is to obtain supplementary information on the *hidden features* of an interest element.

Signal processing methods are used to reduce (eliminate) the noise, to extract the characteristics changes in the signal and to characterize these changes. The denoising process (signal filtering) precede the signal analysis, Discrete Wavelet Transform (DWT), conventional filtering or statistical denoising being currently utilized. In order to give the best interpretation to the measured values, appropriate chosen of the analysis approaches is crucial (Giurgiutiu & Yu, 2003).

A special place in the analysis of motion for chronic patients and elderly persons is occupied by frequency-based techniques. Since the introduction of the Discrete Fourier Transform and especially the Fast Fourier Transform (FFT), spectral analysis has been applied extensively to physiological signals (Jain, et al., 1996). The FFT is the most popular method to perform transformation in the frequency domain, being computationally simple and fast (Grimaldi & Manto, 2010).

The analysis techniques based on Fourier transform are not suitable for non-stationary signals analysis because perform poorly in that case and cannot given relevant information about the evolution of frequencies over time and if the sample window on which the FT is calculated is not large enough.

The wavelet analysis is considered the most recent solution to overcome the shortcomings of the Fourier transform (Mallat & Zhong, 1992; Mallat, 1989; Bidargaddi, et al., 2007), providing an alternative to classical Fourier methods and providing access to information that can be obscured by applying other time frequency methods. The main advantages are both its ability to perform local analysis and to preserve time information (Deligianni, et al., 2004). Having this double advantage, Wavelet-based methods are suitable to characterize signals having transitory and non-stationary characteristics.

Wavelets transforms are classified in two main categories: continuous (CWTs) and discrete (DWTs).

The Continuous Wavelet Transform (CWT) is a transformation into a wavelet basis space. To apply this transformation, first, the signal must be projected onto different shifted and scaled versions of a so called 'mother wavelet,' an oscillating signal that only exists over a finite period of time and considered as a prototype for the windows of the process (Martinez-Ramirez, et al., 2010). The CWT implies a high computational cost. This is the reason why the Discrete Wavelet Transform (DWT) is the most popular approach applied.

The DWT implementation can be performed by repeatedly filtering the signal with a pair of filters. Specifically, the DWT decomposes a signal into an approximate signal, the result being subsequently divided into new approximation and detail signals (Martinez-Ramirez, et al., 2010). This process is carried out iteratively producing a set of approximate signals at different detail levels (scales) and a final gross approximation of the signal (Murugappan, Rizon, Nagarajan, Yaacob, Hazry, Zunaidi, 2008).

The Importance of Medical Data Recording

Generally, the existing databases belonging to different care units or even to more complex administrative structures are incomplete from the medical, management, and patient diseases history points of view. For these reasons, a major interest presents the creation of a network of databases in which are stored, at the individual patients level, multiple information referring to the observed evolution of the chronic disease, short and long term treatments and their efficiency, recurrences, co morbidities, costs collected for each hospital-treatment of the patient, case fatality. Data can be measured several times each day allowing comparisons and the observation of new trends in patient's evolution. These data represent more consistent information for at least two reasons:

- Their volume is considerably increased (collected during several days, or even months) comparative to those obtained by sporadic medical appointments and the measurements can be done (made) in the daily environment conditions, at work or patient's home, without creating discomfort, or adding new stress elements;
- The access of the implied factors to these interconnected databases could facility the access to a more rich medical experience, a more complete vision on recent and traditional interest fields.

New Concepts and Technologies Used to Improve the Actual Monitoring and Assisting Capabilities

Taking into account all the reasons and facts described above, it is desirable to combine the surveillance methods with the support offered to patients. A designing concept, having in view multiple possible objectives, presents the advantage to be at the same time efficient and cost effective. Following this idea, a system could integrate, in an embedded modular structure, some capabilities for the monitoring of persons' activities and status, means to support the rehabilitations and could be also used in prevention strategies. A system based on technologies which are also usually used for others services and activities, (internet, mobile telephony etc.), being familiar to patients, presented in a way that doesn't imply new knowledge and learning efforts, has increased chances to be accepted and utilized.

LabVIEW Instruments

In the context of the application presented above, LabVIEW has major advantages especially due to some specific, characteristic features. It is a graphical programming, which utilizes graphical interconnected icons (functions, structures connected by wires), resembling with a flowchart, and being more intuitive. Taking into account different objectives, LabVIEW can be considered as an equivalent or an alternative of the classic programming languages. It is important to mention that the implementation time for a software application is reduced in comparison with other software environments.

Built-in libraries and virtual instruments examples (based on VIs), as well as the software drivers for almost all data acquisition devices, including industrial instruments, oscilloscopes, multimeters, and signal generators, produced by more than fifties companies, could have support in

LabVIEW and are ready to be used. More, presenting implementation facilities, it was increasingly adopted in various fields such as engineering, chemistry, physics, and medicine.

The LabVIEW platform is scalable across multiple targets (devices) and operating systems like Windows 7 or Mobile, or Real Time Operating Systems (RTOSs): Phar Lap, VxWorks, etc. Programming in LabVIEW involves the creation of the graphical code (G), developed on a PC where it is compiled. Specific tools for the different targets such as industrial computers with RTOSs (PXI), programmable automation controller (Compact RIO), PDAs, microcontrollers, or Field-Programmable Gate Arrays (FPGAs) are used and the compiled code is downloaded to the target.

Due to the graphical programming approach, a major benefit for different categories of users is the ability to scale applications for multiple cores, often with no additional programming effort or advanced programming knowledge. The programs written in LabVIEW could be more optimized to use less CPU resources and to have a shorter runtime comparative with other programming environments. Based on FPGAs target, the applications can run in a hard real time mode with a low jitter value (less than 500 picoseconds).

The LabVIEW platform includes many modules dedicated for programming: FPGA module, real time, signal processing etc. or remotely monitor and control measurement and automation systems, which can be integrated with LabVIEW based web browsers to create "virtual web instruments."

Web Instruments Concept

Web instruments concept has been adopted as a solution in many applications. There is not a standard generally applied solution for all types of applications. This depends on the characteristics of the application.

Ursutiu et al. (2010) present the WEB instruments as web applications which are implemented using WEB technologies (web pages, server side and client side programming technologies). The sensors are connected using a Wi-Fi link to a main Data Acquisition Service (DAS) to which data are sent. The DAS is seen as gateway through which sensors data are accessible through internet in web pages and widgets that reside at remote locations all over the world.

"WEB Instruments move the concept of virtual instrumentation beyond computer based, beyond LabVIEW and into the Internet space where instruments are built, and shared across the world using web pages. WEB Instruments are built on the power of the Internet network" (Ursutiu, et al., 2010).

The Sensor Web concept is presented in Delin and Jackson (2001), which consists of a system of wireless, intercommunicating, spatially distributed sensor pods that can be easily deployed in new environments for monitoring and exploring purpose.

The macros-instrument concept has been introduced in Delin (2002) that allows for the spatial discovery of an environment using distributed sensing platforms which communicate using a series of wireless network communication services. The sensing platforms are heterogeneous, including both orbital and terrestrial and both fixed and mobile.

The evolution of technologies, including increased communication bandwidth, increasing processing power and miniaturization, has accelerated development in the field of mobile telemedicine has been remarked in Xin et al. (2007). Integration of wireless transmission technologies in the area of telemedicine systems makes development of such systems more practical and convenient. It has become possible to monitor patient's biomedical parameters from any computer in any part of the world if that computer is connected to the internet.

The increasing internet bandwidth provides a fast way method to transmit multimedia information. Virtual medical instrument accessible over the Internet through a terminal is a new concept with application in telemedicine. These instruments are used to enable remote monitoring and patient care based on the physiological parameters that have been sent over computer networks to the remote physician. For the communication of the physiological signals, the Internet is used as a transport vehicle (Natesan, 2001).

In Bai and Lu (2005) it is proposed a Web-based remote digital stethoscope. The functions provided by the digital stethoscope are: local data storage, data transmission and processing for both breathing and heartbeat sounds. The solution incorporates the following components: microphone, amplifier, analog to digital conversion, PC interfaces, PC software, and power line communication software and hardware. The system uses low cost modules. In the same time the usage PC based systems for running monitoring applications provides high capacity of storage and a good processing power at an accessible price. As in other systems of the same type, the internet is used for sending medical data to remote locations.

The concept of "cloud instrument" presented in Figure 1 implies the integration of sensor devices into an infrastructure network providing them communication capabilities in order to exchange data with other peer devices or with application localized in Internet (Ursutiu, 2010). The Tag4M system has been implemented in order to take advantage of the presented concept. The device can be connected to an 802.11 b/g wireless network trough, which it communicates with the so called "cloud." One of the supporters of this idea is Pachube whose website offer utilities for such kind of devices. Therefore using the device internal features one can display trends of measurements, view logs, and even send SMS on threshold value triggers.

The screenshot presented in Figure 2 is a Java applet, which implements the concept of web

Figure 1. Generic cloud instrument (Ghercioiu, 2011)

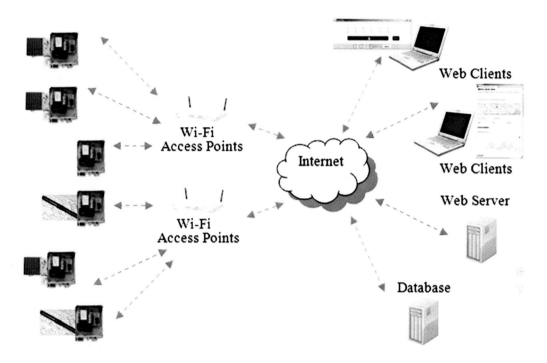

instrument. The application communicates with a data server from where gets sensors data and display them to the user. At the same time, the instrument provides a mechanism for device configuration by sending to it a package containing new parameters when the user changes them (Zapartan, 2010).

In Figure 3, a web instrument used for monitoring data sent by a Tag4M device through Internet to the Pachube data server is presented (Folea, et al., 2010). All the informa-

tion is being plotted on a graphic web instrument in real time (Emmerich, 2000). The instrument can be displayed in web pages and can also be accessed from mobile devices. The data are sent through a channel called data feed. There are two methods for sending the data. In the first method, the Pachube server is requesting the data with a frequency configured in advance and in the second one the device has the initiative of sending the data when new set of data are available.

Figure 2. Web instrument example, using Java applet

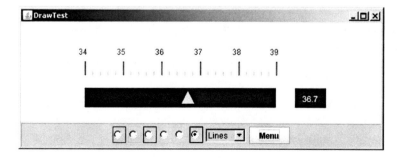

Figure 3. Pachube panel on WSN-Tech.net site

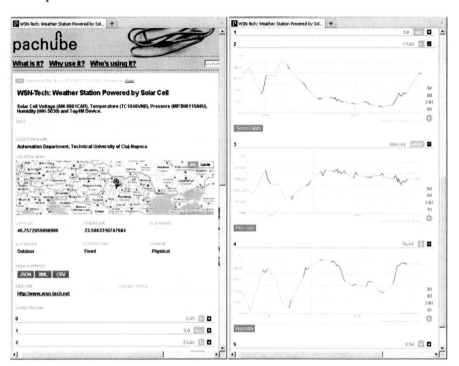

E-HEALTH MONITORING AND SUPERVISING SYSTEM OVERVIEW

The E-Health Monitoring and Supervising System (EMSS) presented here illustrates a complete medical solution comprised of software components and hardware equipments which implements services which can be equally accessed by the persons benefiting of medical monitoring and supervision and by the medical staff, increasing the efficiency of the last category. It must be emphasized that the system does not replace the role of the doctor, but it is a useful tool, which offers support and facilitates the mentioned activities. The most important features of EMSS is the possibility to create dynamic web instruments which are accessible from a web page. So, the concept of configurable virtual web instruments, in which the user has a finer control over the data displayed in the web interfaces, is introduced. Using a Virtual Web Instruments Configurator, the user can define its own virtual instrument by selecting from a list

of available physical devices, the ones that are of interest for him. The virtual instrument can be customized more by selecting from each device only signals of some specific sensors.

Part of the EMSS system has been also developed the WiFiSmartDAQ equipment, which is a low-cost, flexible solution, used for biomedical signal data acquisition. This device has been developed starting from the Tag4M hardware to which extension modules has been added and a new firmware has been developed. Details about this device are presented later in this chapter.

EMSS System Architecture

A multilevel, distributed architecture has been proposed for the EMSS system. Figure 4 presents the hardware components and how they are interconnected.

The system is composed of the following main components: WiFiSmartDAQ devices for biomedical data acquisition, Wi-Fi Access Points for

Figure 4. The general hardware architecture

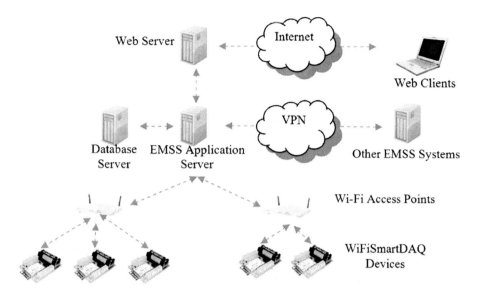

providing wireless communication services for the mobile devices (including WiFiSmartDAQ modules), Database Server where applications data are stored, and Application Server, which is the PC where the core engine components of the EMSS are installed. The services are accessible by users through a Web Server. Using Virtual Private Network (VPN) technologies is also possible that distributed EMSS systems to communicate in a secure manner. The software components of the EMSS system are presented bellow in the Figure 5.

The core engine of the EMSS application is the E-Health EMSS Middleware. A middleware is software that connects other software components or some people and their applications. "A middleware consists of a set of services that allows multiple processes running on one or more machines to interact. This technology evolved to provide for interoperability in support of the move to coherent distributed architectures, which are most often used to support and simplify complex distributed applications" [Wikipedia]. A middleware resides between the applications and the underlying operating systems, network protocol stacks, and hardware.

As stated in (Hadim & Mohamed, 2006), a middleware application can used as a support layer for Wireless Sensor Network (WSN) applications in order to meet challenges associated with this type of applications.

The E-Health EMSS Middleware (EHM) implements the main functionalities of the system, including real-time data processing, data integration and aggregation and alarm and notification handling. The components, part of the EHM, responsible for handling biomedical sensors data are:

- LabVIEW Instruments (LVI) implements the data communication protocol with the WiFiSmartDAQ devices. The LabVIEW instruments receive messages from biomedical devices, apply a set of processing and conversion operations and then forward the messages to the DSS component;
- Data Storage Service (DSS) component is responsible for storing the data in the relational database;
- Time Synchronization Function (TSF) is used for clock synchronization of the sensor devices;

Figure 5. Software architecture of the EMSS system

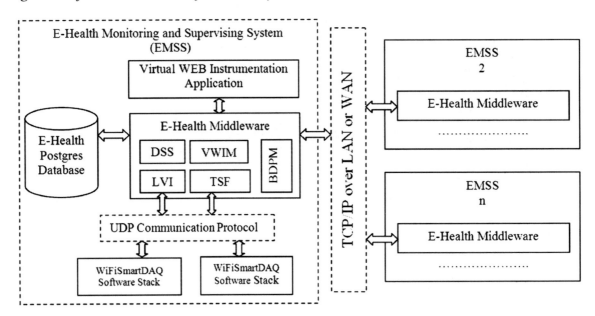

- Virtual Web Instruments Manager (VWIM) is responsible for managing the virtual instruments (creation, deletion and modification);
- Biomedical Data Processing Module (BDPM) implements the medical data processing and interpretation functions. The results of the interpretations are stored back into database and are accessible by user with the help of the virtual web instruments.

The EMSS middleware is implementing using J2EE technologies and deployed on a Glassfish J2EE application server. J2EE provides a reusable component model for building distributed applications. Also, it provides automatic load-balancing, scaling, fault-tolerance, and fail-over. Components deployed in J2EE environment automatically inherit these facilities, and there is no deliberate coding effort required.

The implemented middleware provides the following services:

- Guarantees the exchange of data between distributed EMSS nodes. Therefore, fa-

cilitating transparent access to patient data from remote EMSS nodes;
- Real-time WiFiSmartDAQ sensor data acquisition and processing;
- Alarms and notification services for users or other applications;
- Provides authentication mechanisms, cryptography services, and electronic signing functions in order to protect patient data for unauthorized access;
- Provides functions for activation, deactivation of services;
- Network layer bellow the middleware ensure that communication errors and fault of the network are transparently recovered, but EHM need to handle errors which arise in the usual activities of the system;

The EHM must have the ability to manage growing load with the addition of new EMSS nodes. The typical mechanism to accomplish this issue is transparency. Of particular interest is location transparency on which detailed discussions can be found in Emmerich (2000).

The WiFiSmartDAQ Software Stack represents the software components installed on the biomedical data acquisition device responsible for implementing the sensor measurements and data transmission protocol.

PostgresSQL E-Health Database is used for storing persistent data in a PostgreSQL relational database. At this level biomedical sensor configurations, collected sensors data and virtual instruments configurations are stored.

E-Health WEB Virtual Instrumentation Application (WebVI) is the web application through which users have access to patient monitored data.

The proposed architecture directly offers the following benefits:

1. *Lower cost of hardware* – The existing WiFi infrastructure can serve the purpose for communication between WiFiSmartDAQ and application server, thereby reducing the overall cost;
2. *Scalability* – The system is designed from ground-up to handle large number of sensor devices without imposing software restrictions. Server based processing ensures minimal network communication;
3. *Better performance* – Core processing is done by the server, which has the capability to handle huge loads, unlike the microcontroller devices. This ensures better performance.

High quality industry proven open source and free software libraries, database and framework are used for the EMSS system. *C++* is used as the programming language for developing the WiFiSmartDAQ software stack. *Java* is used as the programming language for developing the application server backend and user interfaces. *Java 2 Platform Standard Edition 5.0 (J2SE)* and *Java 2 Platform Enterprise Edition 5.0 (J2EE)* are used for development of the user interface and backend software. J2SE and J2EE provide additional capability to develop highly functional user interface and provides mature and robust set of technologies for backend software development. *PostgresSQL* is used as relational database to store persistent data.

E-Health PostgresSQL Database

The EMSS uses PostgresSQL as the database engine for storing persistent data. PostgreSQL is a powerful, open source relational database system. It is a reliable, scalable and a proven architecture with a strong reputation. It provides versions for most of the operating systems, including Windows, Linux, and Unix. Integration with the other components of the EMSS application is easy since it provides native programming interfaces in Java. The Data Acquisition Service is responsible for feeding the database with data received from WiFiSmartDAQ devices or from other sources—for example is possible to receive biomedical signals from a remote EMSS application using the middleware communication capabilities.

In Figure 6, the proposed database structure for storing received sensors data and virtual instruments configuration where the main tables for storing received sensors data and virtual instruments configurations are presented. The database has a flexible and scalable structure capable of handling an unlimited number of physical device types and sensor types. For storing device configurations the tables *WiFiSmartDAQDevices*, *ChannelConfiguration* and *ChannelsConfiguration* are used. The received data are stored in *DAQDeviceData*, *Package* and *ChannelData* tables. The effective values are stored in the *ChannelData* table, while the information regarding the channels, which are part of the same device, are stored in the *ChannelConfiguration* table. Virtual instruments configurations are stored in *VirtualInstrument* and *VirtualInstrumentConfiguration* table.

We define a read cycle as the set of operations executed at WiFiSmartDAQ level for reading each attached sensor value. All values from a read cycle are added in a package and are sent to over

Figure 6. Database tables structure

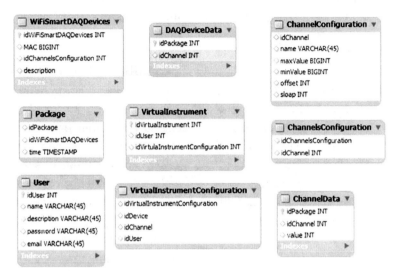

the Wi-Fi to the processing module (LVI component).

In order to identify the packages and therefore knowing each stored value from which package belongs the *packagecounter* and *tagpacket* tables are used. For each received package a unique ID is generated. This ID is generated in a sequential order so that based on this value can be determined also the order in which package arrived, therefore being possible to reconstitute the signal in a function of time.

Data Storage Service

Data Storage Service (DSS) is used by external devices or by other EMSS components to feed sensors data into the system. The received data are stored into the EMSS E-Health Database. In the current implementation, this service is used by LVI components, which receive data from WiFiSmartDAQ modules, convert them into a specific format, and forward them to the DSS. It is also possible that some devices to report data directly to the DSS component bypassing the LVI component.

DSS is implemented as a Web Service (WS) using Java Technology APIs and tools provided by

the integrated Web Service Stack of the Glassfish application server. Because access to WS uses standard Internet technologies, the client of a WS can utilize any platform without knowing any details of the WS implementation. These characteristics are important since the LVI components are implemented in LabVIEW.

In order to provide interoperability with applications and components written in other languages the description of the DSS is implemented using WSDL (Web Service Description Language). WSDL represents a common language for describing services and a platform for integrating Web Services. In the following paragraph a small part of the WSDL file is presented, where the operation for inserting sensors data is defined.

Where the following parameters were defined:

- *mac* – unique identifier of the WiFiSmartDAQ device;
- *mask* – identify the data types sent in this package;
- *data_count* – number of data samples;
- *data* – sensors data;
- *package_count* – the package counter;
- *status* – the status of the insert action;

Table 1. A part of the WSDL definition file

```
...
<wsdl:message name="insertDataRequest">
        <wsdl:part name="mac" type="xsd:string"></wsdl:part>
        <wsdl:part name="mask" type="xsd:string"></wsdl:part>
        <wsdl:part name="data_count" type="xsd:string"></wsdl:part>
        <wsdl:part name="data" type="xsd:string"></wsdl:part>
        <wsdl:part name="package_count" type="xsd:string"></wsdl:part>
</wsdl:message>
<wsdl:message name="insertDataResponse">
        <wsdl:part name="status" type="xsd:string"></wsdl:part>
</wsdl:message>
...
<wsdl:operation name="insertData">
        <wsdl:input message="tns:insertDataRequest"></wsdl:input>
        <wsdl:output message="tns:insertDataResponse"></wsdl:output>
</wsdl:operation>
...
```

The DSS is accessible through Hypertext Transfer Protocol (HTTP). For security reasons, the DSS service is exposed only internally in the LAN for LVI modules and is not accessible from Internet.

In order to reduce the database load, the LVI components are buffering the messages received from the device sensors and send the data as a single package (containing values resulting from 1000 read cycles) to the DSS service. This is particularly useful for devices, which are configured to read sensors with a high sampling rate.

EMSS Web Instruments Application

One of the Java technologies, which made Java one of the most used technologies for Internet, is the Java Applet, which enables Java application to be executed in a Web browser or in other environments, which have support for this technology. In this context, applets can be used to develop powerful J2EE client applications. Browser based applets provides reach GUIs that can be managed from a single location but are hard to deploy in heterogeneous network because of the diversity of the Java virtual machines installed on the client browser.

The applet based J2EE clients are more suitable to be deployed in intranet controlled environments.

In the Virtual Web Instrumentation (VWI) application, part of the EMSS system, the Java Applet technology is used for creating dynamic web instruments. The instruments are accessible from a web page.

The VWI Application (VWIA) introduces the concept of configurable virtual web instruments, in which the user has a finer control over the data displayed in the web interfaces. Using a Virtual Web Instruments Configurator (VWIC), the user can define its own virtual instrument by selecting from a list of available physical WiFiSmartDAQ devices, the ones which are of interest for him. The virtual instrument can be customized more by selecting from each device only signals of some specific sensors. In Figure 7 and 8, the main interface of the VWIC Applet is presented.

A virtual instrument configuration contains the available devices, which will be aggregated in the corresponding defined instrument. As it can be seen in the previous figures, the user can select only a subset of the available data types from each physical device to be aggregated in the virtual instrument, providing in this way a high level of flexibility.

Figure 7. VWIC applet user interface – first instrument added

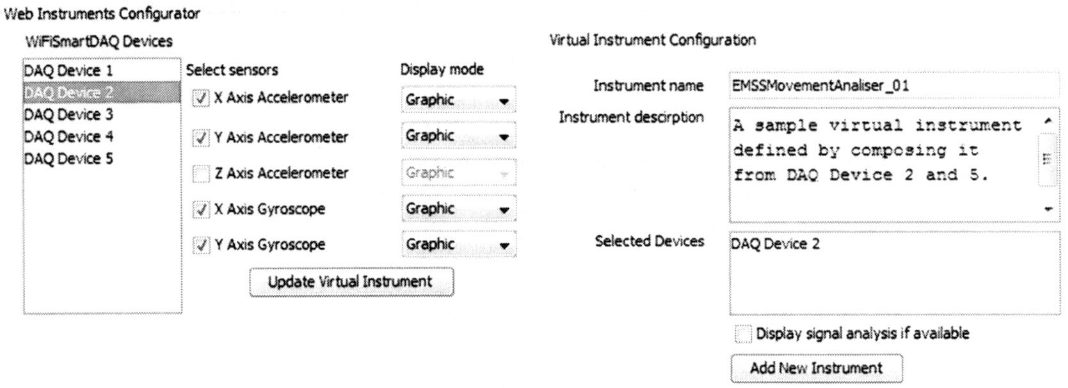

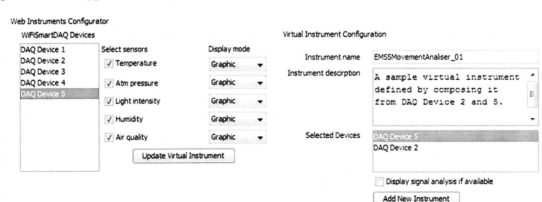

The request for creating a new instrument is managed by VWIM component which receive the instrument creation request and will save the virtual instrument configuration in the E-Health EMSS database.

In Figure 9, it is presented the user interface corresponding to Virtual Web Instrument Signal Analyzer (VWISA) Applet, which is used for comparing two signals. Two signals can be selected in "Signal analysis configuration" area and the analysis results are displayed depending on the analysis objectives selected.

Another component developed part of the VWIA is the Virtual Web Instruments Viewer (VWIW) applet which is responsible for display-

ing the virtual instruments. When a user will select one of the previously created instruments, the user interface will be dynamically generated based on the previously stored configuration. Usually that will imply the creation of a panel containing graphical display zones and/ or table display zones for the selected sensor values.

In Figure 10, the main user interface of the VWIW application is presented, where a virtual instrument has been created. In the presented figure, a virtual device called *EMSSAcelGyroTest* is selected. This virtual device has been configured to displays acceleration and gyroscope on axis X and Y.

Figure 8. VWIC applet user interface – second instrument added

Figure 9. VWISA applet user interface

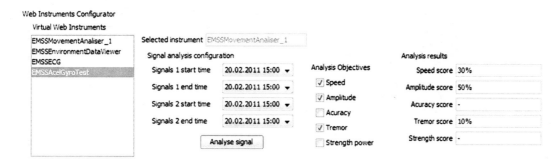

WiFiSmartDAQ Biomedical Device

WiFiSmartDAQ System

Tag4M on which is based the modular structure of the proposed system is presented in Figure 11 (scale 1:1). This is a Wi-Fi RFID active device with measurement capabilities. By attaching sensors to its I/O terminal blocks, in a similar manner as for a data acquisition device, the user can build wireless proof-of-concept sensor solutions for a wide range of applications. The system has the advantage of reduced dimensions (4.7 cm x 7.0 cm) and the weight of 50 g, reducible to 2.0 x 3.0

cm and runs on battery power, being portable. It is a complete Wi-Fi and networking solution, incorporating a 32-bit CPU, a memory unit, an eCos real-time operating system and UDP stack. Other included components are the analog sensor interface, power management unit, hardware cryptographic accelerator and real time clock (G2 Microsystems, 2009).

The General Architecture of the Based WiFiSmartDAQ System

The hardware architecture of the acquisition system is presented in Figure 12. In this version,

Figure 10. VWIW applet user interface

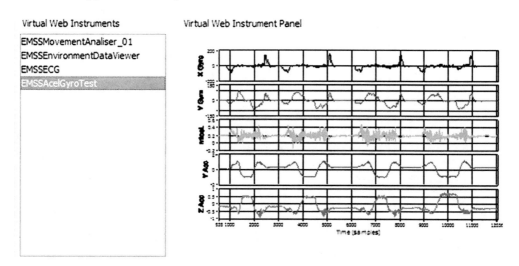

Figure 11. Tag4M data acquisition system

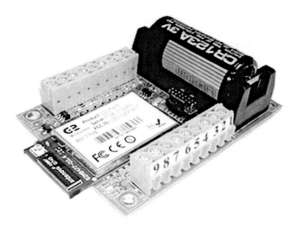

8 analogic channels, 10 digital channels, and 2 serial ports are available. A general interface was implemented to fit the acquisitions from more sources like: 3-axis accelerations, 3-axis gyroscopes, 2-channels ECG, 2-channels myoelectric, temperatures, humidity, light intensity, atmospheric pressure, dust air, sound, tilt, magnetic sensor and more others parameters, which can be combined in many configurations.

Because the UDP protocol does not guarantee the integrity of data transmission, many transmission tests were accomplished and the results were analyzed. Supposing the transmission implies many tags and a considerable number of connections per second (about 1000) to an Access Point (AP), it leads to losing data of up to 5-10%. A detection method of lost points was implemented. The specified maximum number of connections to an AP is less than 20.000. Another important aspect, which was solved, is the synchronizations of transmissions in the case of multiple tags utilization.

The correct interpretation of data received from many tags, which transmit simultaneously, is conditioned by a corresponding synchronization of data acquisition processes. Recently, several power saving protocols have been proposed for IEEE 802.11 wireless LANs. The presented

Figure 12. The hardware architecture of the WiFiSmartDAQ system

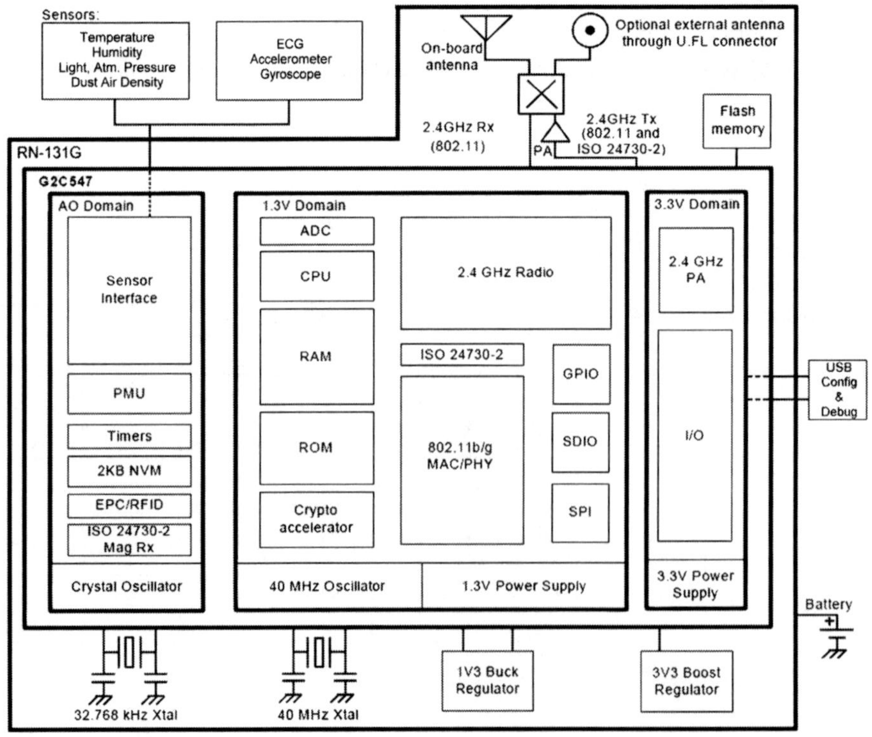

system uses for synchronization purposes, Time Synchronization Function (TSF).

The main steeps of IEEE 802.11 TSF are:

- Each node randomly generates a beacon-generation timer in millisecond (ms); when the timer times out, the node will send a beacon with a 32-bit timestamp;
- If a node receives a beacon before its beacon-generation timer times out, it will cancel the timer and keeps quite in this beacon interval;
- A node will update its clock to synchronize with a faster timestamp it has received; and it will ignore slower timestamps; each node has the same probability to contend sending a beacon.

WiFiSmartDAQ System Power Consumption

The battery of the WiFiSmartDAQ system has the needed capacity to provide the peak power required for all tasks, including data transmission. Obviously, the battery cannot supply energy for a Tag4M system, which operates in its high-power state indefinitely (Folea, et al., 2010).

The Wi-Fi radio module was designed for three separate power domains in order to have a flexible power management and lower power consumption. Therefore, when the module is *asleep*, only the "The Always On" domain is powered; in *awake* mode the 1.3V rail is powered; the 3.3V domain is enabled only in the *awake* state.

In *asleep* mode, the average power consumption is 10 microwatts; CPU and almost all components being unavailable and a limited number of functions, specified below, are utilised in this case:

- Decrementing timers and detecting expiry;
- Detecting state change of the switch sensors;
- Monitoring the sampled comparator and detecting when external parameters pass preset thresholds;

- Responding to battery brownout (low voltage) etc.

The specific functions in *awake* mode are: loading and executing programs from flash memory, communication based on Wi-Fi radio, measurements using the sensor interface, utilization of GPIO, SPI, SDIO, and UART interfaces, reading and writing flash memory or NVM (Non Volatile Memory).

In *doze* mode the 1.3V domain remains powered but the CPU is not clocked. The module uses less power than in the case of *awake* state, and responds very quickly to interrupt source (45ns). The transition from *asleep* to *awake* mode is triggered by an awake event, a subset of specific interrupts.

The overall bi-directional communication time is about 35...120ms, corresponding to a wake-up period. A wake-up event has five distinct periods of power consumption (Tag4M, 2009), Figure 13, where:

1. Boot-up period: is a short-term period during which the Tag4M system reads the application from flash and starts execution. The sensors system consumes 10mA in this state.
2. Transmit Data period: is a very short period, the system consuming up to 210mA while it transmits the 802.11b frames.

Figure 13. Power consumption periods during a wake-up event

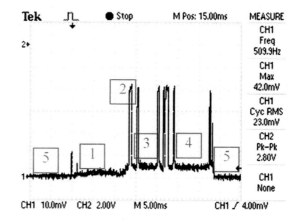

3. Measurement period: is a period during which the Tag4M system consumes on average 20mA, while it performs measurements and executes programs with the CPU.
4. Receive Data period: is a "dead" period, where the Tag4M system consumes up to 30mA while it waits to receive 802.11b data from AP or computer with the new configuration if needed. This period always succeeds the last transmission period (G2 Microsystems, 2008).
5. Sleep period: happens during the most part of life time of the Tag4M system; during it, the current consume is in the 4-10uA range.

The power-management implemented at the hardware level is enhanced at the software level, giving a continuous action time of the sensors of about 1-5 years. This long action time is possible, taking into account that the wake-up time represents only 0.1%-0.6% of the sleep time.

A prediction table for the lifetime of the Tag4M system is given in Table 2.

In order to predict the battery lifetime, some choices have to be made for an entire range of parameters; these affect the consumed power when the sensors are sending reports.

The based WiFiSmartDAQ system was specially developed for a low power consumption benefiting from a new hardware and software technology offered by WSN–Tech Cluj-Napoca a small team from Automation Department, Technical University of Cluj-Napoca, using a hardware developed by Tag4M Company, Austin, Texas, USA.

Table 2. Battery lifetime

Length of Sleep period	Battery life time
1 s	90 hours
10 s	37 days
100 s	1 year
500 s	5 years

The maximum values of data transmission rate and acquisition speed are 54 Mbps and respectively, 33 kSPS at 16-bits. At more reduced acquisition rates, the average of power consumption has a lower value (e.g.: 150 mW for about 1 kSPS), allowing a continuous functioning for 36 hours when a usual CR 123A battery (1.5A and 3V) is used. An important feature is that the power consumption can be drastically reduced by combining the acquisition, processing, and transmission periods with sleeps periods. An important reduction of the power consumption was obtained by specific improvement (Table 2). So, the resulted, average power consumption will attain only 18 mW at a rate of 10 SPS. In these conditions, the life expectation of a continuously utilized lithium battery spectacularly increases at 11 days. Taking into account the above rate, 11 days of continuous functionality represents a true performance for the acquisition, processing, and Wi-Fi based communication system.

The low power consumption performance at this moment is a tag that functions without any external power supply using only solar energy, gold capacitor and a special hardware designed. The results were presented in *International Journal of Online Engineering (iJOE)* and more online journals.

Sensors and Equipment Used for Bio Parameters Monitoring

From the point of view of this specific application, an important measure component is the ECG units. The Figure 14 presents a photo of the ECG device, in order to see the real small dimensions of the device implemented. Our target is to reduce more of the system dimensions up to that of a simple ECG electrode.

The simplified hardware scheme for ECG monitoring device is presented in Figure 9. A differential amplifier and a low pass filter followed by a high pass filter are used. The simplified scheme is presented at the principle level. The value of

Figure 14. Photos with the ECG device, real dimensions

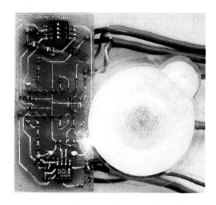 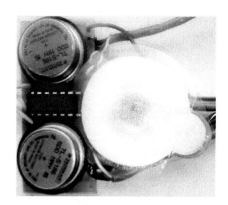

the total gain necessary to acquire an ECG or myoelectric signal is equal by ten, because the analogic inputs range for Tag4M system is -200 mV to +600 mV and the value of the resolution is 12.20 uV. This value of the resolution corresponds to an analog to digital converter with 16-bits.

The signal to noise ratio of the entire system has high value. The performances obtained due to the wireless system used being superior to that reported in the case of similar wired devices. The ECG circuit is used in this situation to determine the heart rate, but a similar scheme is used to measure the myoelectric signal. The circuits used for ECG are presented in the Figure 15.

3-Axis Acceleration Sensor

The acceleration sensor (Figure 16) allows the measurement on three axes, of static or dynamic

acceleration (in ±3g range). It was chosen to be included on the extensions, ADXL330 of iMEMS type, from Analog Devices.

External components are used to establish the period of the output signal between 2 and 1000 ms, the frequency band being limited between 0.5 Hz and 1.6 kHz. The typical noise level is 280 $\mu g/\sqrt{Hz}$ rms and allows the acquisition of signals under 5 mg level. (Analog Devices, 2007).

2-Axis Gyroscope Sensor

The chosen gyroscope (LPR530AL) is the combination of one actuator and one accelerometer integrated in a single micro machined structure. It is based on the Coriolis principle and is able to react when an angular rate is applied on the sensing element which is kept in continuous oscillating movement (ST Microelectronics, 2009). The

Figure 15. ECG basic scheme and the output signal

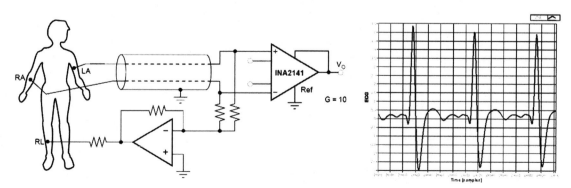

Figure 16. Acceleration sensor scheme

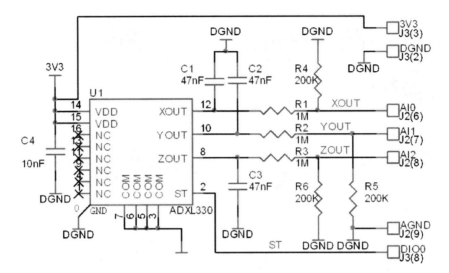

electric scheme is presented in Figure 17 and has a full scale of ±300 °/s and is capable of detecting rates with a -3 dB bandwidth up to 140 Hz.

Environment Parameters Monitoring

The WiFiSmartDAQ system monitors the following parameters which are considered to have a variable influence on the patients' health conditions:

- temperature, using the TC1046VNB sensor that is connected to tag line AI2 (Microchip, 2004);
- humidity, using the HIH-5030/5031 sensor that is connected to tag line AI0 (Honeywell, 2010);
- light intensity or solar radiation, using the LX1792 sensor that is connected to the AI0 line of the tag (Microsemi, 2005);

Figure 17. Gyroscope sensor scheme

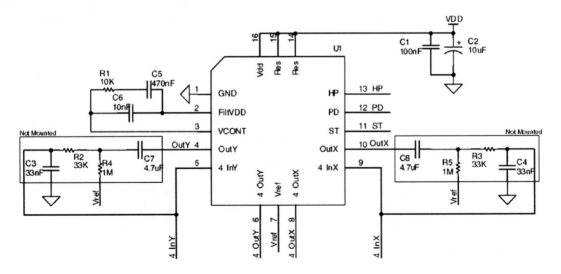

- atmospheric pressure, using the MP3H6115A6U sensor connected to tag line AI1 (Freescale Semiconductor, 2009);
- the dust air density, using the GP2Y1010AU0F sensor connected to tag line AI2 (Sharp, 2006).

The temperature and humidity sensors (if it is necessary to extend the number of measured parameters) are presented in Figures 18 and 19. A sample corresponding to a registration of over 700 hours of the two parameters, observing their changes according with alternation of day and night, is given in Figure 18 and 19.

The TC1046 can accurately measure temperature in the range -40°C to +125°C having linear output with a 6.25mV/°C voltage slope (Microchip, 2004).

The HIH-5030 is an analog sensor (voltage) which means it is faster (Honeywell, 2010). The reading time of the values sent by sensors is a very important factor in terms of power con-

sumption. It must be mentioned that the tag reads the values given by analogical sensors at higher speed compared with that of read values sent by digital sensors.

The light sensor (LX1972) extension presented in Figure 20 is used to measure ambient light in the WiFiSmartDAQ system vicinity. The light measured intensity can highlight the alternation of day and night through the voltage generated by a photocell. The photocell is able to distinguish different degrees of light intensity (darkness and the time of day). The LX1972 is a low cost silicon light sensor which emulates the human eye producing a spectral response. The response is produced at 520nm, with IR response less than 5%, of the peak response, above 900nm. According to Microsemi (2005) it is usable at ambient light from 1 to more than 5000 Lux.

The pressure sensor (MP3H6115A6U) is usually used to measure atmospheric pressure in weather forecasting applications, and the corre-

Figure 18. Temperature sensor and output signal

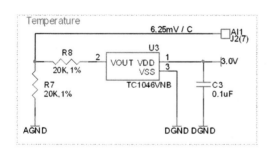 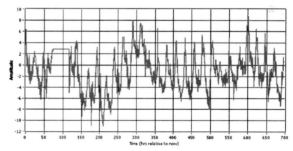

Figure 19. Humidity sensor and output signal

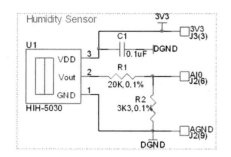 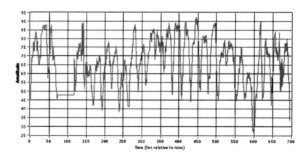

Figure 20. Light sensor and output signal

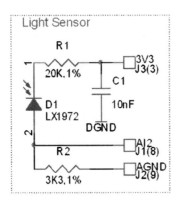 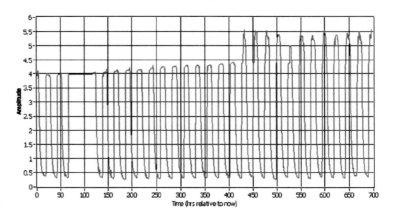

sponding signal conditioning circuitry are shown in Figure 21 (Freescale Semiconductor, 2009). An example of a measured atmospheric pressure for a period of 700 hours is also given.

Dust air density detector module is implemented with the GP2Y1010AU0F device, a dust sensor based on an optical sensing system, presented in Figure 22. The basic principle on which the sensor detects the dust air density is to quantify the reflected light of dust in air. An Infrared Emitting Diode (IRED) and a phototransistor are diagonally arranged into this device (Sharp, 2006). The high sensitivity in detecting even very small dust particles (like the ones contained in the cigarette smoke) and the possibility to distinguish the house dust and smoke, contributed to the inclusion of this type of sensor in the WiFiSmartDAQ configuration.

WiFiSmartDAQ Software Stack

In this section, the software stack installed on the WiFiSmartDAQ is described. The device is powered by a G2C547 module from G2 Microsystem. It has an eCos real-time operating system installed on ROM, which boots when the system is powered on.

The eCos operating system runtime provides full preemtability, low latency, synchronization primitives, and scheduling policies and interrupt handling mechanisms which are applicable in real-time applications. The embedded applications also can take advantage of the eCos functionalities such as device drivers, memory management mechanisms, exception handling, math libraries and many more. Is also includes all necessary tools for developers like: build tools, compilers,

Figure 21. Pressure sensor and output signal

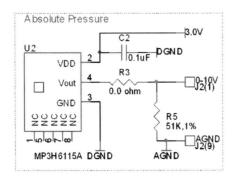 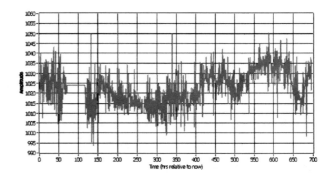

Figure 22. Dust sensors and output signal

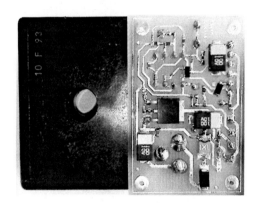
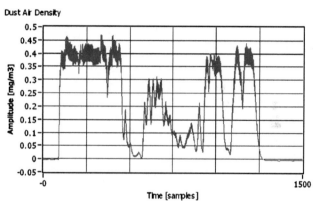

assemblers, linkers, assemblers, debugger, and simulators.

Programming for microcontroller devices presents unique set of challenges. Firstly there are several points of failure. The WiFiSmartDAQ device itself may fail. There can be transient or permanent communication errors between connected devices and microcontroller device like overlapping signals, accidental disconnection etc. The C Application on WiFiSmartDAQ itself may fail, however unlikely. Then there could be communication failure between the WiFiSmartDAQ

device and the application server. The application needs to handle these multiple points of failure and hide the complexity from the end user.

Secondly programming for devices requires much more debugging and testing iterations than normal application development because of direct low-level interaction with underlying hardware.

The application need to provide robust error handling capability. Automatic error correction code must be incorporated to correct several types of transient errors. This will minimize maintenance requirements and manual intervention.

As shown in the Figure 23, the The WiFiSmart-DAQ software stack is composed from an eCos operating systems, eCos libraries for accessing low level services, G2 library for accessing sensors and measurements services and two user applications (Main DAQ App and Config App) which are stored in the Nonvolatile Memory (NVM). At any given moment, only one user application can be in execution. The applications are designed to minimize memory and processor requirements on the WiFiSmartDAQ devices.

The Main DAQ application is used for performing the sensors measuring activities and sending data to the remote LabVIEW instruments. When the device is powered one, after the system boots, this main application is launched.

The second application is the Config application, which is used for configuring the main measuring application through a serial RS232 interface.

The DAQ application is responsible for executing the measuring and communication activities. It has an event-driven architecture (Hanson, 2005) and the loop for handling events which, executed in the main application thread, is presented in Table 3:

When the application starts, the digital and analog lines are initialized. After that, the DHCP procedure is started. The events handled by the application for connecting to a Wi-Fi access point are:

Figure 23. WiFiSmartDAQ software stack

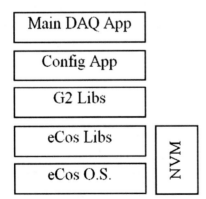

Table 3. Events executed in the main application thread

```
activateAnalogDigitalLines();
startDHCP();
whiel(1){
        evntID = getNextEvent();
        case RESET_EVENT:
                startConfigurationApplication();
                break;
        case MEASURE_EVENT:
                measure();
                postEvent(REPORTING_EVENT);
                break;
        case REPORTING_EVENT:
                sendData();
                break;
        case FIND_ACCESSPOINT_EVENT:
                associate();
                break;
        case DHCP_COMPLEAT:
                dhcpConfigure();
                initializeMeasureTimer(frequency);
        case DHCP_RENEW:
                dhcpConfigure();
                break;
        case WATCHDOG_RESET:
                restartApplication();
}
```

- FIND_ACCESSPOINT_EVENT – is triggered after the startDHCP() function is executed. The application receives a list of available access points. The *associate()* implements the operations needed for the device to connect to an access point. The operations involve association, authentication and obtaining IP address.;
- DHCP_COMPLEAT – is generated when the application obtains a valid IP address and is ready for communication. After the IP address is obtained the main thread can initialize the data acquisition process;
- DHCP_RENEW – is generated when the device IP address has been renewed by the access point.

The application uses eCos timers for generating the application events. A custom MeasureTimer periodic timer has been defined for controlling the measuring frequency. The timer period can be configured depending on the application characteristics. Supposing a high number of samples are needed, the timer period can be decreased to 1 millisecond which will provide a maximum number of 1000 readings in a second. The MEASURE_EVENT is generated each time when measure timer expires.

The *measure()* function performs the reading of the analog and digital sensors connected to the device. The measurements are added in a data buffer and then REPORTING_EVENT is generated.

The handler for REPORTING_EVENT is implemented by the *sendData()* functions read the data buffer containing the sensor values and send it to the reporting server.

The communication is done via UDP protocol, which provides several advantages over TCP, like an increased transmission speed, low latency, smaller packages and no need to maintain a connection between client and server.

The configuration application is started when the device reset button is pressed which generates a RESET_EVENT event. This will cause the measuring application to be shut down and the configuration application to be started. The user can configure over RS232 the following device parameters: active sensors, reporting server IP (in this case the IP is where LVI modules are installed), reporting port, secured access points to which the device is allowed to connect, WEP or WAP password for the access points and reporting frequency. All configuration parameters are stored in the device NVM and are not lost in case of a battery change. After the parameters are configured the system can be restarted by pressing again the reset button and the measuring application will be automatically restarted.

This mechanism provides an easy way for a user to configure the devices, but has a drawback because there is need to have direct access to the device and to connect to it using a wired link (RS232 connection). A second mechanism by using UDP packages can be used for configura-

tion. This second mechanism does not make it necessary to restart the device and to enter in configuration mode, but it is necessary for the main DAQ application to stay in a receive mode, which will decrease the acquisition rate. Therefore, this second mechanism has been disabled.

EXPERIMENTAL RESULTS

WiFiSmartDAQ Signal Acquisitions Test

The functioning of different configurations of the acquisition system and sensors was tested, some results being presented below. Specific configurations are needed depending on the therapeutic and rehabilitation profile.

The Figure 24 presents the placement of the sensors and a capture with the signals for the first test. A correlation between the signals from 3-axis accelerometer, 2-axis gyroscope and myoelectric signals are realized.

The 2-axis gyroscope, 3-axis accelerometer and the WiFiSmartDAQ system are placed on the leg and the ECG circuit is placed right on the heart. The signals are from a normal subject and are used only for the reference to compare with a patient presented in the figure 24 and to calibrate the system.

The Figure 25 presents the placement of the sensors and the signals capture for the second test. The 2-axis gyroscope, 3-axis accelerometer and the WiFiSmartDAQ System are placed on the hand and the myoelectric circuit is placed on the forearm.

The Figure 26 presents a zoom on the figure 25, for the signals captured to see the detailed for a single motion.

The Figure 27 presents the placement of the sensors and the signals capture for the third test. The movement corresponds to the squeeze. The acceleration sensors and the gyroscope are placed

Figure 24. First test, sensors placement and signals

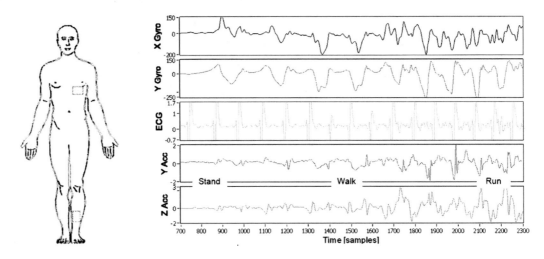

Figure 25. The second test, sensors placement and signals

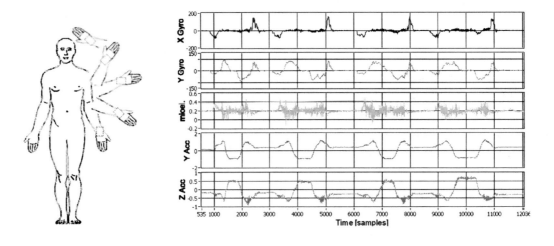

Figure 26. The second test, zoom for a single motion

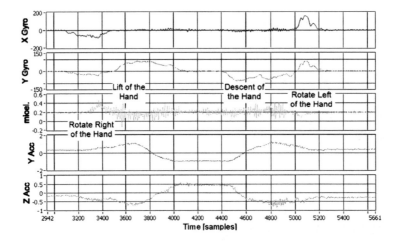

on a finger and the electrodes of the myoelectric sensor are positioned on the forearm.

Details of the signal, which correspond to the movement registered in Figure 27, are presented (zoomed) in Figure 28 ZOOM.

The Figure 29 presents the placement of the sensors and the signals capture for the fourth test. This movement corresponds to the right leg; the acceleration sensor is positioned below the knee while the gyroscope sensor and the electrodes of the myoelectric sensor are positioned on the muscle above the knee. Figure 29 illustrates the signal corresponding to the normal movement of the leg for the first part of the registration and a corresponding signal to the drag of the leg, in the second half.

The next two figures illustrate details (by zoom) for the two movement types described above, Figure 30.

Wi-Fi Biomedical Sensors Signal Analysis

Several experimental trials were designed to evaluate the forearm and leg mobility and tremor measurement technique.

A method for leg and arm movement's analysis using wearable acceleration sensors, gyro sensors and a myoelectric sensor was implemented.

The volunteers wired the WiFi sensors unit, which included a tri-axis acceleration sensor, a two-axis gyro sensor and myoelectric sensor. The signals received from the sensors are pre filtered and interpreted for movement type and intensity detection.

A LabVIEW application was used for the signal acquisition, the pre-processing, and the sending to the database of the measure data. The signal and the representation of the instrument panel are given in Figure 31.

The signals acquired by the accelerometer, gyroscope myoelectric sensors were filtered implementing a Butterworth filter - which has as essential characteristic a smooth and monotonically decreasing frequency response (National Instruments, 2009). LabVIEW application allows an operative and rapid change of filter parameters or the using of other types of filters.

After the calling of the corresponding function *Butterworth Coefficients VI* (Virtual Instrument), the *Butterworth Filter VI* function calls the *IIR Cascade Filter VI* in order to obtain the final filtered sequence. Obviously, the values for high cutoff frequency (f_H) and low cutoff frequency (f_L) must observe the relationship:

$$0 < f_L < f_H < 0.5f_S$$

where $f_S = 200$Hz is the sampling frequency.

A part of the bloc diagram for the above application, with a graphical programming example, is shown in Figure 32.

Data analysis was performed on-line using the WiFiSmartDAQ system, containing 2 or 3-axis acceleration sensors, 2-axis gyroscope sensors, 1 or 2 myoelectric channels and LabVIEW graphical programming. From the time origin of each separate axis where the measured values are represented (on five channels) were taken 200 sps for trial periods from 100 to 300 seconds.

The angular velocity data measured by the gyro sensor is used for signal movement analysis. The acceleration sensor measurements are processed and the orientation of analyzed body segments is obtained. Experiments were carried out on the normal movements and predefined scenarios of several healthy volunteers.

It is difficult to observe detailed movement, such as twisting arms or rising arm on different degree. In order to observe these detailed motions of the forearm in a predefined repetitive scenarios a tri-axis acceleration sensor and a two-axis gyro sensor are used by a data logger and analyzed. The myoelectric sensor is placed on forearm to determine the contraction or tremor muscle.

An example of arm movement with slow speed is presented in Figure 33. The myoelectric signals

Figure 27. The third test, sensors placement and signals

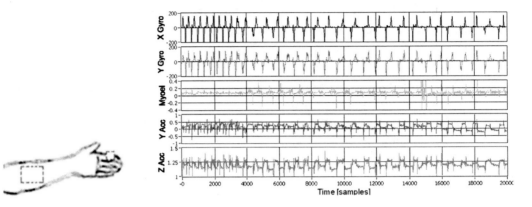

Figure 28. The third test, sensors placement and signals (zoom)

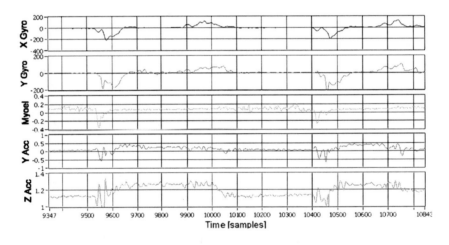

Figure 29. The fourth test, sensors placement and signals

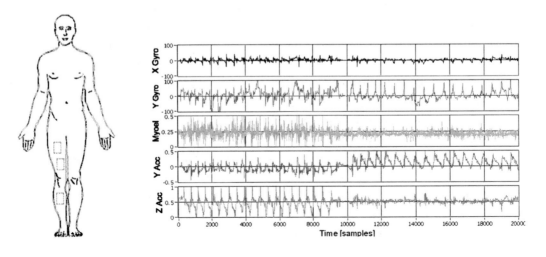

Figure 30. The fourth test, sensors placement and signals (zoom)

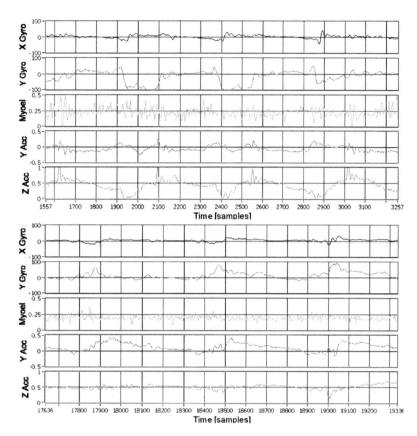

Figure 31. Application panel

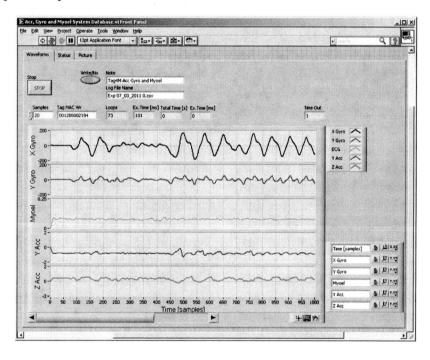

Figure 32. Application bloc diagram

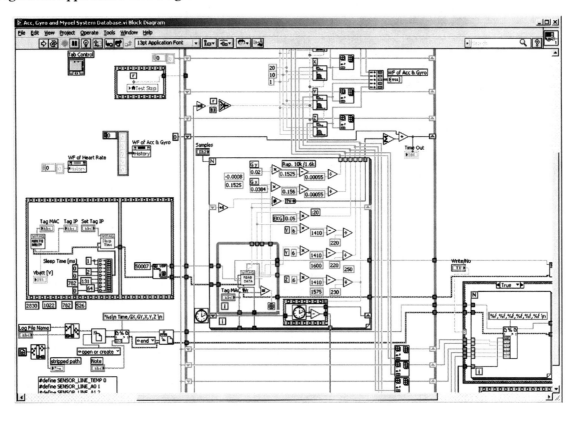

presented in Figures 33-36 are not very evident without a signal zoom.

In Figure 33 the five signals (first two are corresponding to gyro sensor on two axes, third correspond to myoelectric sensor and the last two are corresponding to accelerometer with two axes) of DAQ representing four, slow speed, movements of the subject arm to 45°, 90 °, 135°, and 180° are presented.

In Figure 34 the five signals (first two are corresponding to gyro sensor on two axes, third correspond to myoelectric sensor and the last two are corresponding to accelerometer with two axes) of DAQ representing four, high speed, movements of the subject arm to 45°, 90 °, 135°, 180°, and 230° are presented.

In Figure 35 the five signals (first two are corresponding to gyro sensor on two axes, third correspond to myoelectric sensor and the last two

are corresponding to accelerometer with two axes) of DAQ representing three, normal speed with tremor, movements of the subject arm to 45°, 90°, and 135° are presented.

In Figure 36 the five signals (first two are corresponding to gyro sensor on two axes, third correspond to myoelectric sensor and the last two are corresponding to accelerometer with two axes) of DAQ representing four, normal speed with rhythmic contraction, movements of the subject arm to 45°, 90°, and 135° are presented.

The interdecadal fluctuations have the effect of modulating the amplitude and frequency of occurrence of specific movement. The simplest method for analyzing non-stationary of a time series would be to compute statistics such as the mean and variance for different time periods and see if they are significantly different.

Figure 33. Arm movement – slow speed

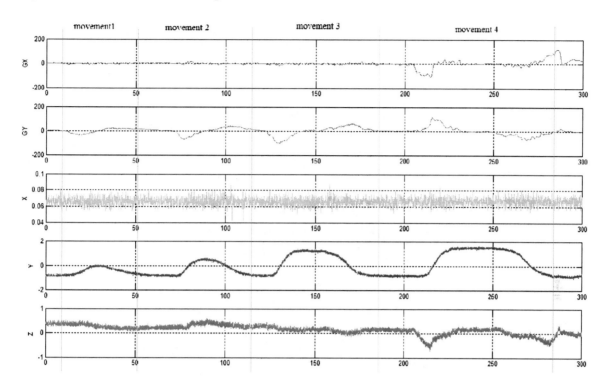

Figure 34. Arm movement – high speed

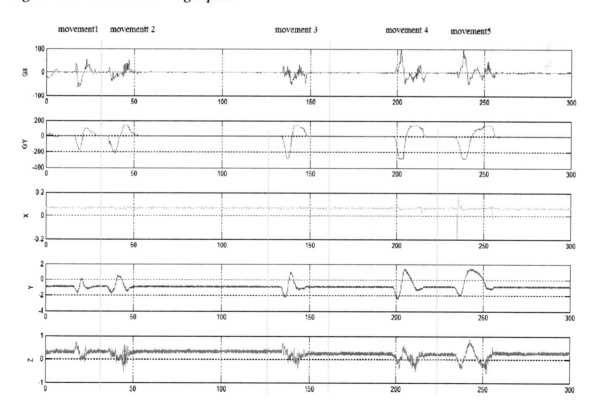

Figure 35. Arm movement – normal speed with tremor

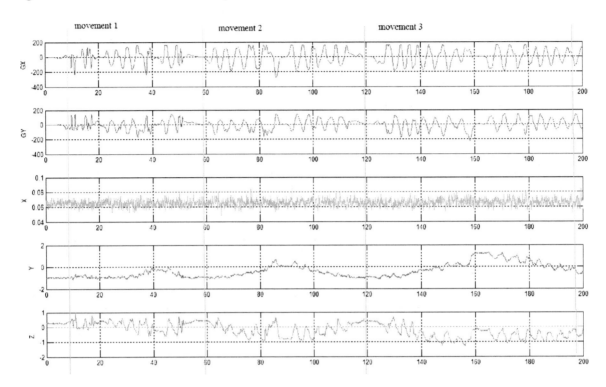

Figure 36. Arm movement – normal speed with rhythmic contraction

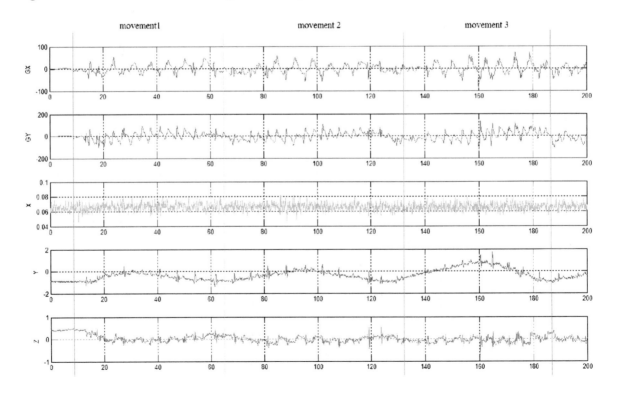

While the running variance tells us what the overall strength of the signal was at certain times, it suffers from two major defects:

- Time Localization. The shape of the result processed signal is dependent on the length of the window used. A method to overcome this problem is to apply different window sizes depending on the scales.
- Frequency Localization. The analyze signal contains no information about the frequency, only its amplitude.

One possible solution is to apply Windowed Fourier Transform (WFT), using a predefined window size and to slide along it during the time interval, computing the FFT at each time using only the data within the window. This approach would solve the frequency localization, but would still be dependent on the window size used. The major problem while WFT is applied is that at low frequencies, the frequency localization is lost because of few oscillations and high frequencies cause many oscillations the time localization is lost.

Wavelet method tries to solve these problems by decomposing a time series into time/frequency space simultaneously, by getting information on amplitude of a periodic signals and how this amplitude varies with time.

The total width of the analyzed wavelets is about 3 – 5 minutes and a movement a few seconds. This value gives a measure of how much (amplitude) the period for a movement resemble a Sine wave of this width (frequency). Sliding the calculated wavelet, along the time series we can construct a new time series of the projection amplitude versus time. Changing the width has the result of varying the "scale" of the wavelet, which brings a real advantage over a moving Fourier spectrum.

Appling the wavelet transform for a time series imply the following steps:

1. Choose a mother wavelet,
2. Find the Fourier transform of the mother wavelet,
3. Find the Fourier transform of the time series,
4. Choose a minimum scale s_0, and all other scales,
5. For each scale the mother wavelet is processed.

For this experiments the Morlet mother wavelet was selected but several other mother wavelets could be chosen and several.

$$W_n\left(s\right) = \sum_{k=0}^{n-1} \hat{x}_k \, \hat{\varphi}^*\left(sw_k\right)e^{iw_k ndt}; \qquad (1)$$

Wn – wavelet transform in Fourier domain;
Several parameters must be chosen for wavelet implementation:

$$\varphi_0\left(n\right) = \pi^{-1/4}e^{iw_0 n}e^{-n^2/2}; \qquad (2)$$

w_0 – is wave number; (represent the number of oscillations)

$$s_j = s_0 2^{j\delta_j}, j = 0 \div J; \qquad (3)$$

$$J = \delta_j^{-1}log_2\left(\frac{N\delta_t}{s_0}\right) \qquad (4)$$

s – scaling parameter;
dt – time resolution;
The largest scale chosen is less than 1/2 the length of the entire time series.
The Fourier transform of the time series is given by:

$$\hat{x}_k = \frac{1}{N}\sum_{n=0}^{N-1}x_n e^{-2\pi ikn/N}; \qquad (5)$$

To normalize the wavelet:

$$\varphi(\hat{sw}_k) = \left(\frac{2\pi s}{dt}\right)^{1/2} \hat{\varphi}_0\left(sw_k\right) \qquad (6)$$

The wavelet transform in Fourier space brings a problem because this method starts with the assumption that the time series is periodic. A method to avoid this is to pad with enough zeroes to make the length of the time series equal to a power of two, and also will speed up the FFT.

Sensors signal are processed and the results of wavelet transform are presented in Figure 37 – 41 (gyro on axes x and y, myoelectric and accelerometer on axes y and z).

The *x*-axis is the wavelet location in time. The *y*-axis is the wavelet period in years. The black contours are the 10% significance regions, using a red-noise background spectrum. The red areas indicate that a movement occurred. The lower line is the theoretical mean white noise spectrum. The top line is the 95% confidence level.

The confidence interval is defined as the probability that the true wavelet power at a certain time and scale lies within a certain interval about the estimated wavelet power (Tirtom, et al., 2008).

From the signal of the Oy axe accelerometer sensor the occurrence of arm movement can be determined. Synchronizing the scaled signals of all sensors the type, intensity, and trajectory of a movement can be obtained.

A model for gesture recognition was design based on Hidden Markov Model (HMM).

The HMM is a finite set of *states*, each of which is associated with a (generally multidimensional) probability distribution. Transitions among the states are governed by a set of probabilities called *transition probabilities*. In a particular state an outcome or *observation* can be generated, according to the associated probability distribution. It is only the outcome, not the state visible to an external observer and therefore states are „hidden" to the outside; hence the name Hidden Markov Model (Narada, et al., 1996).

A discrete-time HMM, can be viewed as a Markov model whose states cannot be explicitly observed (each state has an associated probability

Figure 37. Wavelet transform power spectrum and average variance of distribution for gyro sensor on ox axe

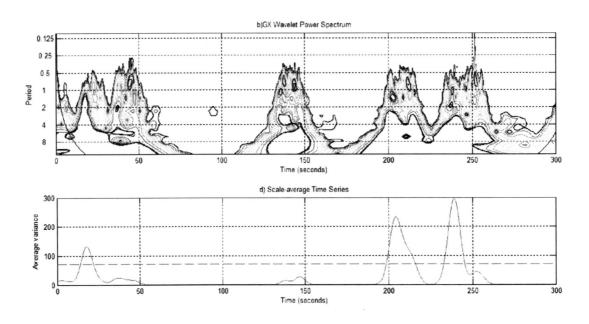

Figure 38. Wavelet transform power spectrum and average variance of distribution for gyro sensor on oy axe

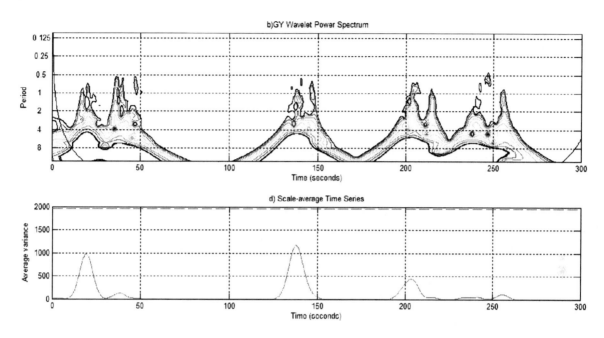

Figure 39. Wavelet transform power spectrum and average variance of distribution for myoelectric sensor placed on forearm

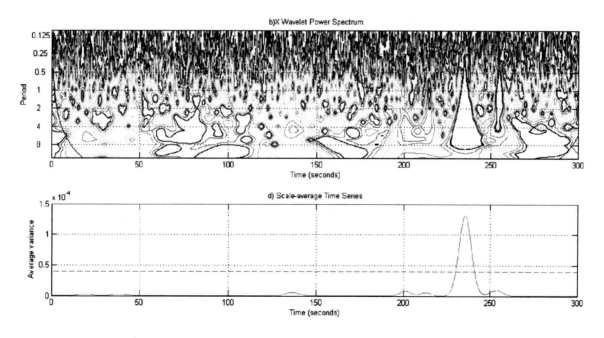

Figure 40. Wavelet transform power spectrum and average variance of distribution for accelerometer sensor on oy axe

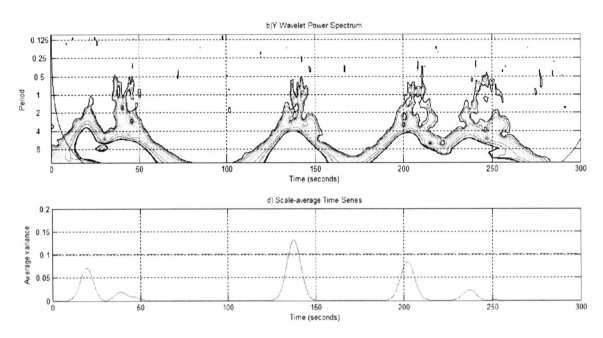

Figure 41. Wavelet transform power spectrum and average variance of distribution for accelerometer sensor on oz axe

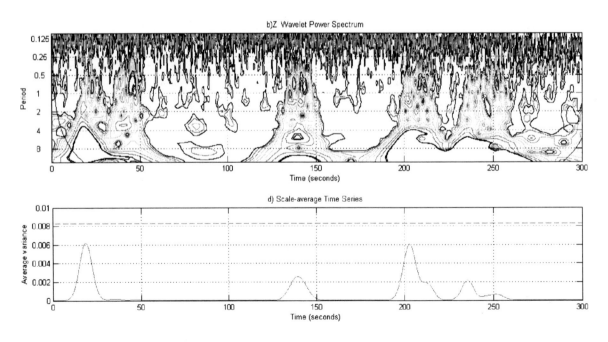

distribution function, modeling the probability of emitting symbols from that state). More formally, a HMM is de□ned by the following entities (Salah, et al., 2007):

Set of hidden states;

$$S = \{S_1, S_2, ..., S_n\}; \quad (7)$$

S – is a finite set of hidden states;

Probabilities of going from one state to another;

$$A = \{a_{ij}, 1 \leq j \leq N\}$$

$$a_{ij} = P[q_{t+1} = S_j | q_t = S_i] \ 1 \leq i, j \leq N;$$

Where:

$$a_{ij} \geq 0 \ \& \ \sum_{j=1}^{N} a_{ij} = 1; \quad (8)$$

Emission parameters,

$$B = \{b(o | S_j)\} \quad (9)$$

Indicating the probability of emission of the symbol o when the system state is S_j and b is different based on the chosen distribution. In our experiments $b\{o|S_j\}$ is a Chi–square distribution.

$$b(o | S_j) = N(o | k_j, 2k_j);$$

Where:

N(o|k, 2k)- is the Chi – square density of mean k and covariance 2k, evaluated at o. (10)

Initial state probability distribution

$$\pi_i = P[q_i = S_i]; 1 \leq i \leq N$$

Where:

$$\pi_i \geq 0; \sum_{i=1}^{N} \pi_i = 1 \quad (11)$$

Based on average values from Wavelet analysis the probabilities for HMM model are determined (see Tables 4 and 5).

In Figure 42 the HMM of the analysing system is presented.

$S = \{S\_0°, S\_45°, S\_90°, S\_135°, S\_180°\}$ – states set;

$$A = \begin{bmatrix} a_{11} & \cdots & a_{15} \\ \vdots & \ddots & \vdots \\ a_{51} & \cdots & a_{55} \end{bmatrix}; - \text{probability matrix;}$$

Table 4. Average values from wavelet analysis of the gyro sensors signal

	45°	90°	135°	180°
Gx	0.6	0.1	0.4	0.9
Gy	0.4	0.9	0.6	0.1

Table 5. Average values from wavelet analysis of the accelerometer sensors signal

	45°	90°	135°	180°
Axe Y	0.2	0.9	0.2	0.9
Axe Z	0.8	0.2	0.8	0.9

Figure 42. The HMM of the analyze system

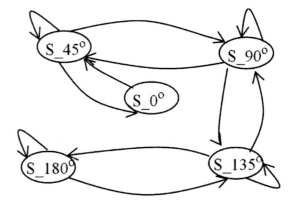

$a_{11} = P[q_{t+1} = S_1 \mid q_t = S_1] \neq 0;$

$a_{12} = P[q_{t+1} = S_1 \mid q_t = S_2] \neq 0;$

$a_{13} = P[q_{t+1} = S_1 \mid q_t = S_3] = 0;$

$a_{14} = P[q_{t+1} = S_1 \mid q_t = S_4] = 0;$

$a_{15} = P[q_{t+1} = S_1 \mid q_t = S_5] = 0;$

$a_{21} = P[q_{t+1} = S_2 \mid q_t = S_1] \neq 0;$

$a_{22} = P[q_{t+1} = S_2 \mid q_t = S_2] \neq 0;$

$a_{23} = P[q_{t+1} = S_2 \mid q_t = S_3] \neq 0;$

$a_{24} = P[q_{t+1} = S_2 \mid q_t = S_4] = 0;$

$a_{25} = P[q_{t+1} = S_2 \mid q_t = S_5] = 0;$

...

$a_{51} = P[q_{t+1} = S_5 \mid q_t = S_1] = 0;$

$a_{52} = P[q_{t+1} = S_5 \mid q_t = S_2] = 0;$

$a_{53} = P[q_{t+1} = S_5 \mid q_t = S_3] = 0;$

$a_{54} = P[q_{t+1} = S_5 \mid q_t = S_4] \neq 0;$

$a_{55} = P[q_{t+1} = S_5 \mid q_t = S_5] \neq 0;$

Interpreting and analyzing the Figures 33 – 42:

- $t = 200$ the $a_{45} = 0.8$ and $a_{55} = 0.2$.
- ...
- $t = 205$ the $a_{45} = 0.9$ and $a_{55} = 0.1$.

Movements presented and analyzed in figures 33 – 42 are correctly executed and can be chosen as etalon. The experiments were concentrated also to determine the intensity and trajectory, not only the speed movements. In figures 43 – 46 the sensors signal for movements with slow speed rhythmic contractions or slow speed and tremor.

Where: a) the gyro on Ox axe sensor signal; b) the wavelet power spectrum, using the Morlet wavelet. The x-axis is the wavelet location in time. The y-axis is the wavelet period in years. The black contours are the 10% significance regions, using a red-noise background spectrum. The red areas indicate that a movement occurred; d) the lower line is the theoretical mean white noise spectrum. The top line is the 95% confidence level.

In case of a subject with difficulties to perform a correct movement, it is important to use all the sensor signals and to realize a correlation between interpretations.

If only one of the signals from Figure 46 or Figure 49 is considered, we cannot decide which kind of movement is realized. A correlation of the wavelets interpretation is necessary to form a conclusion.

FUTURE RESEARCH DIRECTIONS

Virtual Web Instruments technology can provide users a convenient way to have remote access to their physical equipments from Internet using a mobile or fix web client. A high-level communication protocol can be developed in order to provide hardware devices with a standardized way to advertise their capabilities on Internet. This information can be used by application servers in order to generate and expose on internet web components allowing user to access devices functionalities.

Another challenge is to reduce the system dimensions up to that of a simple ECG electrode using on the shell electronic components. The further reducing of power consumption is possible using software methods and remains a priority. Multiple tags synchronization at higher data acquisition rate with reduced data lost is another future work proposal.

Figure 43. Wavelet transform power spectrum and average variance of distribution for gyro sensor on ox axe – slow speed with rhythmic contraction

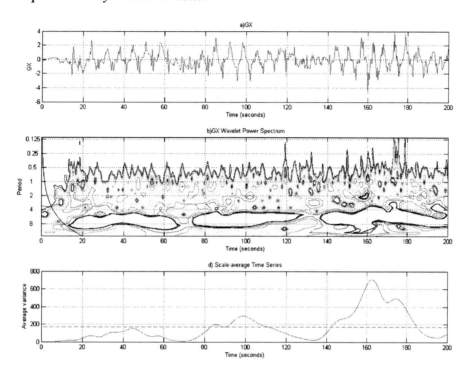

Figure 44. Wavelet transform power spectrum and average variance of distribution for giro sensor on Oy axe – slow speed with rhythmic contraction

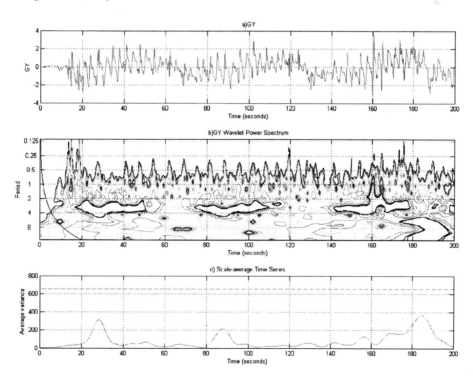

Figure 45. Wavelet transform power spectrum and average variance of distribution for accelerometer sensor on Oz axe – slow speed with rhythmic contraction

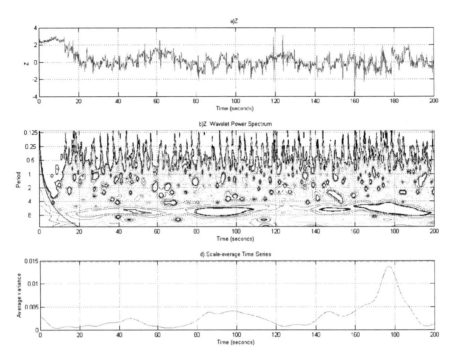

Figure 46. Wavelet transform power spectrum and average variance of distribution for mioelectric sensor – slow speed with rhythmic contraction

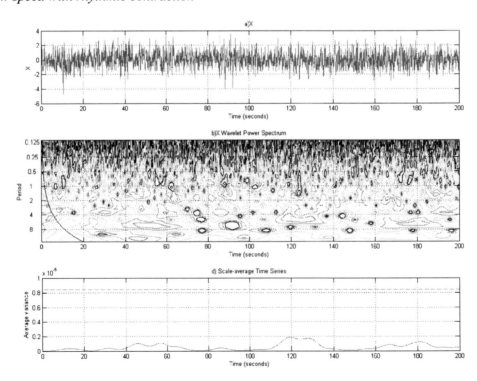

Figure 47. Wavelet transform power spectrum and average variance of distribution for gyro sensor on Ox axe – slow speed with tremor

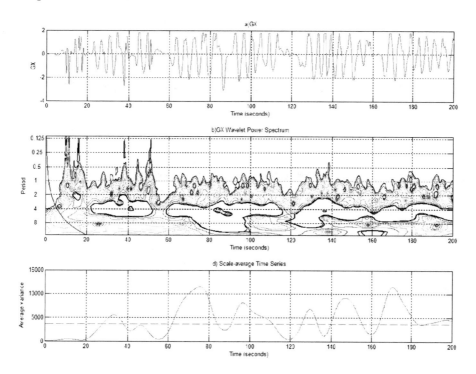

Figure 48. Wavelet transform power spectrum and average variance of distribution for accelerometer sensor on Oy axe – slow speed with tremor

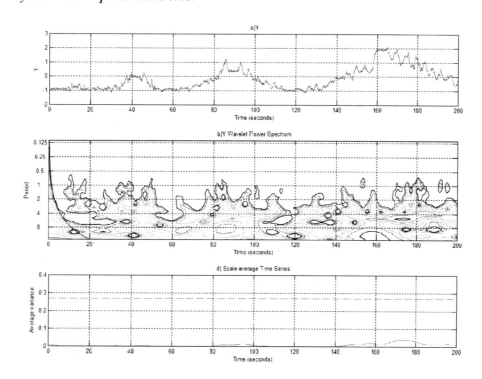

Figure 49. Wavelet transform power spectrum and average variance of distribution for mioelectric sensor – slow speed with tremor

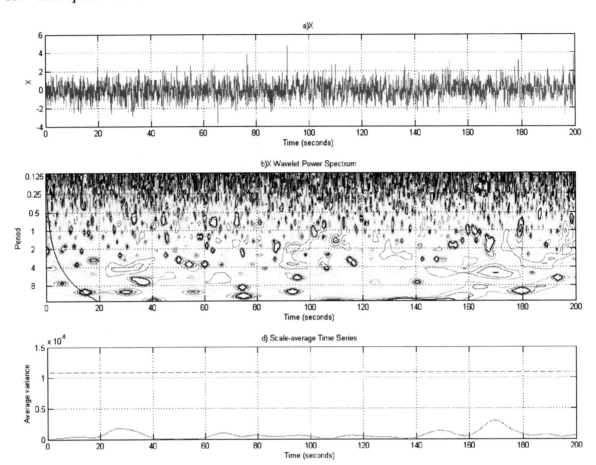

CONCLUSION

Compared with other similar systems a main advantage of the presented one consists of the possibility to choose different configuration of the hardware and software components using a web browser. A proof of concept was implemented, including hardware, software application, and firmware.

The presented system is in a development stage, the main modules and functionalities being implemented and tested. Many aspects regarding the integration and information exchange among the components of the system have to be completed.

Specific solutions were applied to measure and asses the human motion. A special emphasis was given to different configurations of the wireless sensors network.

The proposed system presents many new characteristics, one of the most important consisting of the embedding of ultra-low power, performing, Wi-Fi transmission capabilities in a very small package. The system is running on a battery having characteristic life time of years and offering a platform for sensor measurements. Thus, unlike other proposed systems dedicated to distance surveillance of main chronic diseases, this one offers a reliable, low cost and low power consuming solution for distance data acquisition, during long periods of times and assuring a flexible, simultaneous monitoring of many body parts. The functions of all components of the proposed system were tested.

Although the device presents the corresponding sensitivity and measurement range required to detect all interest signals, more clinical supervised tests are necessary. These must be oriented to evaluate and detect the distinguished feature specific of different patients' mobility and flexibility. A considerable volume of work is necessary to increase the system performances and capabilities oriented to real necessities.

REFERENCES

G2 Microsystems. (2008). *G2C547 SoC data sheet*. Technical Report. Retrieved from www.g2microsystems.com.

G2 Microsystems. (2008). *G2C547 software, example application*. Technical Report. Retrieved from www.g2microsystems.com.

G2 Microsystems. (2008). *G2M5477 wi-fi module data sheet*. Technical Report. Retrieved from www.g2microsystems.com.

Abhaya, G. (2008). *Measurement scales used in elderly care*. New York, NY: Radclife Publishing.

Aminian, K., De Andres, E., Rezakhanlou, K., Fritch, C., Schutz, Y., & Depairon, M. … Robert, P. (1998). *Motion analysis in clinical practice using ambulatory accelerometry, modelling and motion capture techniques for virtual environments*. Berlin, Germany: Springer.

Analog Devices. (2007). *Small, low power, 3-axis 3g MEMS accelerometer*. Technical Report. Retrieved from www.analog.com.

Bai, Y., & Lu, C. (2005). Web-based remote digital stethoscope. In *Proceedings EuroIMSA, (423-428)*. Springer.

Bidargaddi, N., Klingbeil, L., Sarela, A., Boyle, J., Cheung, V., & Yelland, C. … Gray, L. (2007). Wavelet based approach for posture transition estimation using a waist worn accelerometer. In *Proceedings,* (pp. 1884-1887). IEEE Press.

Burr-Brown. (1996). *Dual, low power, G-10, 100 instrumentation amplifier*. Technical Report. Retrieved from http://focus.ti.com.cn.

de Vries, W., Veltink, P. H., Koper, M. P., & Koopman, B. F. J. M. (1994). Calculation of segment and joint angles of the lower extremities during gait using accelerometers. In *Proceedings of the Second World Congress of Biomechanics on Dynamic Analysis Using Body Fixed Sensors*. Amsterdam, The Netherlands: McRoberts.

Deligianni, F., Chung, A., & Yang, G. (2004). Decoupling of respiratory motion with wavelet and principal component analysis. In *Proceedings of Medical Image Understanding and Analysis (MIUA04)* (pp. 13–16). London, UK: Springer.

Delin, K. A. (2002). The sensor web: A macro-instrument for coordinated sensing. *Sensors Journal, 2*(7), 270–285. doi:10.3390/s20700270

Delin, K. A., & Jackson, S. P. (2001). *The sensor web: A new instrument concept*. Paper presented at SPIE's Symposium on Integrated Optics. San Jose, CA.

Emmerich, W. (2000). *Engineering distributed objects*. New York, NY: John Wiley & Sons.

Folea, S., Avram, C., Vidican, S., & Astilean, A. (2010). Telemonitoring system of neurological signs in a health telematique network. *International Journal of E-Health and Medical Communications, 1*(4), 14–33. doi:10.4018/jehmc.2010100102

Folea, S., & Ghercioiu, M. (2010). Tag4M, a Wi-Fi RFID active tag optimized for sensor measurements. In Turcu, C. (Ed.), *Radio Frequency Identification Fundamentals and Applications Design Methods and Solutions* (pp. 287–310). PA, Austria: InTech Education and Publishing.

Folea, S., Ghercioiu, M., & Ursuțiu, D. (2010). cloud instrument powered by solar cell sends data to pachube. *International Journal of Online Engineering, 6*(4), 20–25.

Freescale Semiconductor. (2009). *High temperature accuracy integrated silicon pressure sensor for measuring absolute pressure, on-chip signal conditioned, temperature compensated and calibrated.* Technical Report. Retrieved from www.freescale.com.

Ganti, R. K., Jayachandran, P., Abdelzaher, T. F., & Stankovic, J. A. (2006). SATIRE: A software architecture for smart attire. In *Proceedings of MobiSys 2006*. Uppsala, Sweden: ACM Press.

Giurgiutiu, V., & Yu, L. (2003). *Comparison of short-time Fourier transform and wavelet transform of transient and tone burst wave propagation signals for structural health monitoring.* Paper presented at the 4th International Workshop on Structural Health Monitoring. Palo Alto, CA.

Grimaldi, G., & Manto, M. (2010). Neurological tremor: Sensors, signal processing and emerging applications. *Sensors (Basel, Switzerland), 10*, 1399–1422. doi:10.3390/s100201399

Hadim, S., & Mohamed, N. (2006). Middleware challenges and approaches for wireless sensor networks. *IEEE Distributed Systems Online, 7*(3).

Hanson, J. (2005). *Event-driven services in SOA.* Javaworld.

Honeywell. (2010). *HIH 5030/5031 series, low voltage humidity sensors.* Technical Report. Retrieved from http://sensing.honeywell.com.

Ito, S., & Okuno, K. (2010). Visualization and motion analysis of swimming. In *Proceedings of the 8th Conference of the International Sports Engineering Association (ISEA)*. London, UK: Elsevier.

Jain, A., Wim, L., Martens, J., Mutz, G., Weiss, R. K., & Stephan, E. (1996). Towards a comprehensive technology for recording and analysis of multiple physiological parameters within their behavioral and environmental context. *Journal of Psychophysiology, 13*(13).

Jongho, L. (2009). Yasuhiro Kagamihara and Shinji Kakei: A new method for quantitative evaluation of neurological disorders based on eMG signals. In Naik, G. R. (Ed.), *Recent Advances in Biomedical Engineering.* Philadelphia, PA: InTech.

Lindemann, U., Hock, A., Stuber, M., Keck, W., & Becker, C. (2005). Evaluation of a fall detector based on accelerometers: A pilot study. *Medical & Biological Engineering & Computing, 43*, 548–551. doi:10.1007/BF02351026

Liu, K., Liu, T., Shibata, K., & Inoue, Y. (2010). Visual estimation of lower limb motion using physical and virtual sensors. In *Proceedings of IEEE International Conference on Information and Automation (ICIA)*, (pp. 179 – 184). IEEE Press.

Luinge, H. J., & Veltink, P. H. (2005). Measuring orientation of human body segments using miniature gyroscopes and accelerometers. *Medical & Biological Engineering & Computing, 43*, 273–282. doi:10.1007/BF02345966

Mallat, S., & Zhong, S. (1992). Characterization of signals from multiscale edges. *IEEE Transactions on Pattern Analysis and Machine Intelligence, 14*(7), 710–732. doi:10.1109/34.142909

Mallat, S. G. (1989). Theory for multiresolution signal decomposition: The wavelet representation. *IEEE Transactions on Pattern Analysis and Machine Intelligence, 11*(7), 674–693. doi:10.1109/34.192463

Martinez-Ramirez, A., Lecumberri, P., Gomez, M., & Izquierdo, M. (2010). *Tri-axial inertial magnetic tracking in quiet standing analysis using wavelet transform*. Paper presented at the International Multi-Conference on Engineering and Technological Innovation, IMETI. Miami, FL.

Mathies, M., Coster, A., Lovell, N., & Celle, B. (2008). Accelerometry: Providing an integrated, practical method for long-term, ambulatory monitoring of human movement. *Journal Physiological Measurement, 25*(2).

Mayagoitia, R. E., Nene, A. V., & Veltink, P. H. (2002). Accelerometer and rate gyroscope measurement of kinematics: An inexpensive alternative to optical motion analysis systems. *Journal of Biomechanics, 35*, 537–542. doi:10.1016/S0021-9290(01)00231-7

Menz, H. B., Lord, S. R., & Fitzpatrick, R. C. (2003). Acceleration patterns of the head and pelvis when walking are associated with risk of falling in community-dwelling older people. *Journal of Gerontology, 58*, 446–452.

Microchip. (2004). *High precision temperature-to-voltage converter*. Technical Report. Retrieved from http://ww1.microchip.com.

Microsemi. (2005). *Ambient light detector, LX1972*. Technical Report. Retrieved from www.microsemi.com.

Murugappan, M., Rizon, M., Nagarajan, R., Yaacob, S., Hazry, D., & Zunaidi, I. (2008). Time-frequency analysis of EEG signals for human emotion detection. In *Proceedings of the 4th Kuala Lumpur International Conference on Biomedical Engineering*. Kuala Lampur, India: IEEE.

Natesan, T. R. (2001). Web based multi-functional virtual instrument for telemedicine. *Medindia Networking for Health*. Retrieved from http://www.medindia.net/articles/webmedicine.htm

National Instruments. (2009). Working with LabVIEW filtering VIs and the LabVIEW. *Digital Filter Design Toolkit VIs*. Retrieved from www.ni.com.

O'Donovan, K. J., Kamnik, R., O'Keeffe, D. T., & Lyons, G. M. (2007). An inertial and magnetic sensor based technique for joint angle measurement. *Journal of Biomechanics, 40*, 2604–2611. doi:10.1016/j.jbiomech.2006.12.010

Painter, C. C., & Shkel, A. M. (2001). Structural and thermal analysis of a MEMS angular gyroscope. In *Proceedings of Smart Structures and Materials 2001: Smart Electronics and MEMS*, (pp. 86-94). IEEE.

Salah, A. A., Bicego, M., Akarun, L., Grosso, E., & Tistarelli, M. (2007). *Hidden Markov model-based face recognition using selective attention*. Paper presented at the Human Vision and Electronic Imaging XII. San Jose, CA.

Sharp. (2006). *GP2Y1010AU0F compact optical dust sensor*. Technical Report. Retrieved from www.sharp-world.com.

Shi, G., Zou, Y., Jin, Y., Cui, X., & Li, W. J. (2009). Towards HMM based human motion recognition using MEMS inertial sensors. In *Proceedings of the 2008 IEEE International Conference on Robotics and Biomimetics*. Bangkok, Thailand: IEEE Press.

Shylie, M. (2009). Functional independence measure. *The Australian Journal of Physiotherapy, n.d.*, 55.

Steele, B. G., Holt, R. N. L., Belza, B., Ferris, S., Lakshminaryan, S., & Buchner, D. M. (2000). Quantitating physical activity in COPD using a triaxial accelerometer. *Chest, 117*, 1359–1367. doi:10.1378/chest.117.5.1359

STMicroelectronics. (2009). *LPR530AP MEMS motion sensor: dual axis pitch and roll 300/s analog gyroscope*. Technical Report. Retrieved from www.nex-robotics.com.

Takeda, R., Tadano, S., Natorigawa, A., Todoh, M., & Yoshinari, S. (2009). Gait posture estimation using wearable acceleration and gyro sensors. *Journal of Biomechanics, 42*, 2486–2494. doi:10.1016/j.jbiomech.2009.07.016

Tan, X., Guo, X. M., Cheng, M., & Yan, Y. (2007). Wireless telemedicine physiological monitoring center based on virtual instruments. In *Proceedings of the Bioinformatics and Biomedical Engineering*, (pp. 1157 – 1160). Wuhan, China: IEEE Press.

Tirtom, H., Mehmet, E., & Erkan, Z. E. (2008). Enhancement of time-frequency properties of ECG for detecting micropotentials by wavelet transform based method. *Expert Systems with Applications, 34*(1), 746–753. doi:10.1016/j.eswa.2006.10.009

Ursutiu, D. (2010). Wireless sensor networks and cloud instruments for web based measurements, guest editorial. *International Journal of Online Engineering, 6*(4), 4–5.

Ursutiu, D., Cotfas, D. T., Ghercioiu, M., Samoila, C., Cotfas, P. A., & Auer, M. (2010). WEB instruments. In *Proceedings of the Education Engineering (EDUCON) – The Future of Global Learning Engineering Education*, (pp. 585 - 590). Madrid, Spain: IEEE Press.

Warakagoda, N. D., & Hogskole, N. T. (1996). *A hybrid ANN-HMM ASR system with NN based adaptive preprocessing*. Retrieved from http://jedlik.phy.bme.hu/~gerjanos/HMM/hoved.html.

Willemsen, A. T., van Alste, J. A., & Boom, H. B. (1990). Real-time gait assessment utilizing a new way of accelerometry. *Journal of Biomechanics, 23*, 859–863. doi:10.1016/0021-9290(90)90033-Y

Williamson, R., & Andrews, B. J. (2001). Detecting absolute human knee angle and angular velocity using accelerometers and rate gyroscopes. *Medical & Biological Engineering & Computing, 39*, 294–302. doi:10.1007/BF02345283

Yang, C. C., & Hsu, Y. L. (2010). A review of accelerometry-based wearable motion detectors for physical activity monitoring sensors. *Sensors in Biomechanics and Biomedicine, 10*.

Zapartan, A. (2010). *Tag4 applet - The cloud instrument*. Unpublished Master's Thesis. Cluj-Napoca, Romania: Technical University of Cluj-Napoca. Retrieved from http://www.scribd.com/doc/46245362/Alin-Zapartan-Tag4Applet.

ADDITIONAL READING

Ayrulu-Erdem, B., & Barshan, B. (2011). Leg motion classification with artificial neural networks using wavelet-based features of gyroscope signals. *Sensors (Basel, Switzerland), 11*, 1721–1743. doi:10.3390/s110201721

Darpe, A. K. (2010). *Wavelet transforms and its application to fault detection*. Retrieved from http://www.scribd.com/doc/36571471/Wavelet.

Davis, R. I. A., & Lovell, B. C. (2003). Comparing and evaluating HMM ensemble training algorithms using train and test and condition number criteria. *Pattern Analysis & Applications, 6*, 327–336.

Hua, W., Wang, A., & Tung, C. L. (2007). Dynamic gesture recognition based on dynamic Bayesian networks. *WSEAS Transactions on Business and Economics, 4*(11), 1109–9526.

Hussain, S., Erdogen, S. Z., & Park, J. H. (2009). *Monitoring user activities in smart home environments*. Hingham, MA: Kluwer Academic Publishers.

Iso, T., & Yamazaki, K. (2006). Gait analyzer based on a cell phone with a single three-axis accelerometer. In *Proceedings of the 8th Conference on Human-Computer Interaction with Mobile Devices and Services*, (pp. 141–144). New York, NY: ACM.

Jamil, M., Zain, M. F. M., Krishnamurthy, V., & Sazonov, E. (2009). Scientific data acquisition for structural health monitoring by using wireless intelligent sensor. *European Journal of Scientific Research, 33*(4), 585–593.

Jin, G. H., Lee, S. B., & Lee, T. S. (2008). Context awareness of human motion states using accelerometer. *Journal of Medical Systems, 32*, 93–100. doi:10.1007/s10916-007-9111-y

Karantonis, D. M., Narayanan, M. R., Mathie, M., Lovell, N. H., & Celler, B. G. (2006). Implementation of a real-time human movement classifier using a triaxial accelerometer for ambulatory monitoring. *IEEE Transactions on Information Technology in Biomedicine, 10*, 156–167. doi:10.1109/TITB.2005.856864

Li, Q., Stankovic, J. A., Hanson, M., Barth, A., & Lach, J. (2009). Accurate, fast fall detection using gyroscopes and accelerometer-derived posture information. In *Proceedings of the Sixth International Workshop on Wearable and Implantable Body Sensor Networks*. IEEE.

Long, X., Yin, B., & Aarts, R. M. (2009). Single-accelerometer-based daily physical activity classification. In *Proceedings of the 31st Annual International Conference of the IEEE EMBS*, (pp. 6107-6110). Minneapolis, MN: IEEE Press.

Lu, G., & Krishnamachari, B. (2007). Minimum latency joint scheduling and routing in wireless sensor networks. *Science Direct, 5*, 832–843.

Luinge, H. J., & Veltink, P. H. (2004). Inclination measurement of human movement using a 3-D accelerometer with autocalibration. *IEEE Transactions on Neural Systems and Rehabilitation Engineering, 12*(1). doi:10.1109/TNSRE.2003.822759

Lyons, G. M., Culhane, K. M., Hilton, D., Grace, P. A., & Lyons, D. (2005). A description of an accelerometer-based mobility monitoring technique. *Medical Engineering & Physics, 27*, 497–504. doi:10.1016/j.medengphy.2004.11.006

Mannini, A., & Sabatini, A. M. (n.d.). (2019). Machine learning methods for classifying human physical activity from on-body accelerometers. *Sensors (Basel, Switzerland), 10*, 1154–1175. doi:10.3390/s100201154

Najafi, B., Aminian, K., Loew, F., Blanc, Y., & Robert, P. A. (2002). Measurement of stand-sit and sit-stand transitions using a miniature gyroscope and its application in fall risk evaluation in the elderly. *IEEE Transactions on Bio-Medical Engineering, 49*, 843–851. doi:10.1109/TBME.2002.800763

Niezen, G. (2008). *The optimization of gesture recognition techniques for resource-Constrained devices*. Master Thesis. Pretoria, South Africa: University of Pretoria.

Pober, D. M., Staudenmayer, J., Raphael, C., & Freedson, P. S. (2006). Development of novel techniques to classify physical activity mode using accelerometers. *Medicine and Science in Sports and Exercise, 38*, 1626–1634. doi:10.1249/01.mss.0000227542.43669.45

Ren, Y. F., & Ke, X. Z. (2010). Selection of wavelet decomposition level in multi-scale sensor data fusion of MEMS gyroscope. *International Journal of Digital Content Technology and its Applications, 4*(8).

Schlömer, T., Poppinga, B., Henze, N., & Boll, S. (2008). Gesture recognition with a Wii controller. In *Proceedings of Tangible and Embedded Interaction*. IEEE. doi:10.1145/1347390.1347395

Stankovic, J. A. (2008). When sensor and actuator networks cover the world. *ETRI Journal, 30*(5).

Stojmenovic, I. (2005). *Handbook of sensor networks, algorithms and architectures*. New York, NY: Wiley Interscience. doi:10.1002/047174414X

Xiaoli, M., Zhiqiang, Z., Gang, L., & Jiankang, W. (2009). Human motion capture and personal localization system using micro sensors. In *Proceedings of the IEEE International Conference on Computer Science and Information Technology*. IEEE Press.

Xie, Y., & Wiltgen, B. (2010). Adaptive feature based dynamic time warping. *International Journal of Computer Science and Network Security, 10*(1).

KEY TERMS AND DEFINITIONS

Cloud Instrument: A sensor becomes a Cloud Instrument when it is connected to a wireless tag such as a Wi-Fi tag. The tag digitizes the data to send it on to an access point, where the data is routed to the Internet and a server IP. Here a customized engine is collecting data to feed into applications like metering, charting, control, analysis, modeling, data mining and so forth, with display on Web page and Web widget instruments.

E-Health: Is a complex field based on medical data, public health and information delivered through Internet and other related technologies.

Gesture Recognition: Software applications and mathematical algorithms used to interpret the human gestures.

Signal Processing: Is a merge area of electrical devices and applied mathematical operations used to analyze signals to perform useful operations.

Tag4M: a Wi-Fi Data Acquisition System manufactured by Tag4M Company, Austin, Texas, USA.

Web Instrument: the concept of virtual instrumentation beyond computer based, beyond LabVIEW, Java, C# and into the Internet space where instruments are built, and shared across the world using web pages. WEB Instruments are built on the power of the Internet network.

WiFiSmartDAQ: a Tag4M device with dedicated firmware and external hardware developed special for E-health applications.

Chapter 12
Overview of the Most Important Open Source Software:
Analysis of the Benefits of OpenMRS, OpenEMR, and VistA

Beatriz Sainz de Abajo
University of Valladolid, Spain

Agustín Llamas Ballestero
University of Valladolid, Spain

ABSTRACT

In this chapter, the authors review software that enables the proper management of EHR. The different types of software share the feature of being open source and offer the best opportunity in health care to developing countries—an overall integrated approach. The authors analyze the main free software programs (technical features, programming languages, places for introduction, etc.). Then they focus on the description and the comparison of the three most important open source software programs EHR (OpenMRS, OpenVistA, and OpenEMR) that are installed on two operating systems (Linux Ubuntu and Windows). Finally, the authors show the results of the various parameters measured in these systems after using different Web browsers. The results show us how the three main EHR applications work depending on which operating system is installed and which web browser is used.

INTRODUCTION

Computer applications are an effective tool to solve many problems, most notably the fast management of medical records. The use of computres for this kind of documents provides a faster search and organization of patient data (Sainz, et al., 2010).

DOI: 10.4018/978-1-4666-0888-7.ch012

New technology plays a relevant role in areas where pandemics are a major problem. In undeveloped countries, where economic resources are often slender, the budget for health issues is not enough and therefore the right management of such financial resources might save a large number of lives (Fraser, et al., 2006; Noor, et al., 2004; Stansfield, 2005; Tomasi, et al., 2004). From the binomial "lack of financial resources versus epidemics" comes the idea and the implementation of Electronic Health Record (EHR) as it solves the problems related to the information management in a fast, efficient way while the deployment budget is not too high (Diero, et al., 2006; Mamlin & Biondich, 2005). The advantages are to save work and to gain faster access to the information about a patient. Far from the disadvantages of deploying a system of medical records management with proprietary software (Biondich, et al., 2003; Fraser, et al., 2005), free software systems avoid the payment for expensive proprietary software licenses for installation, but the services provided by the program are not reduced in any case (Fraser, et al., 2004; Mamlin & Biondich, 2005).

Open source software provides effective support to the research that is carried out in underdeveloped countries, and allows the assessment of new diagnostic procedures, measures to prevent diseases, pandemics, as well as epidemiological and statistical analysis of public health by regions (Häyrinen, et al., 2008; Murray, et al., 2004; Siika, et al., 2005).

This chapter is organized as follows:

In section 2 we review a set of applications, which are all open sources as a common characteristic and enable the proper management of EHR. We briefly analysis the most prominent free software on the market by services (number of managed patients, number of sites that are used and heterogeneity of the clinics, higher level software development, functionalities) or by technical characteristics (technology of the core, programming language that implements the application interface, language of interaction with database).

In sections 3, 4, and 5, we focus on the description of the three most important applications of open source worldwide: OpenMRS, OpenEMR, and VistA. Their importance lies mainly in technological development, rapid evolution, and efficient implementation. Regarding the medical improvements that are introduced, we may highlight the number of modules that allows functionalities both

specific and general, the large number of patients they manage, etc. These applications are mostly used in hospitals and clinics around the world and their current development process suggests that this trend will continue in the foreseeable future.

In section 6, we compare OpenMRS, Vista, and OpenEMR systems according to their historical and technological development and the current state of software.

In section 7, we make a comparison among these three main types of EHR software solution (OpenMRS, OpenVistA, and OpenEMR) installed on two operating systems (Linux Ubuntu and Windows).

Finally, in section 8, we show the conclusions of the chapter.

CHARACTERISTICS OF SOME OPEN SOURCE SOFTWARE

Electronic Health Records (EHR) are applications that came from the use of computing for medical records. There is no universal, compatible format to date. The large amount of technological, cultural—or even philosophical—variants stopped the imposition of a standard so far. In order to support this type of EHR, integrated systems should be considered. These systems must be stable, modular, configurable, versatile, safe, and comprehensive. This second section shows some of the most important Open Source Software and their characteristics.

CHITS

Community Health Information Tracking System (CHITS) is prestigious open source software for medical records management designed for local health centers in the Philippines. It has been developed and managed by the National Telehealth Centre in Manila.

This application generates reports in a standard format weekly and monthly. It can store patient information digitally to recover it quickly as well. It allows also the collecting of data routinely and its use for statistical analyses, in order to open an interesting area of study on the prediction of outbreaks and to assure adequate medicaments supply.

CHITS can be configured to work with cabled or wireless connections. In order to use a wireless setup, you can use a wireless router instead of the network switch or hub. In any case, you will need to configure your wireless router or network hub to provide private IP addresses (chits.ph/web, 2011).

ClearHealth

ClearHealth is an open source application where the used EHR are compliant with the General Public License (GNU), which has emerged as a possible open source option for the use of electronic health records. Currently, it is used in approximately 600 places all over the world including marketing support. There are a great number of facilities in non-profit health settings.

Fred Trotter and David Uhlman were the developers of this application. Fred Trotter and David Uhlman were also involved in the creation and review of FreeBE invoicing system that was the first open source program to apply the HIPAA X12 procedure for electronic invoicing. In the U.S.A., a medical invoicing system available under a GPL license has motivated the creation of other open source systems such as FreeMed, OpenEMR, ClearHealth, and MirrorMed. Clear-Health released its first version in 2003, allowing many different possibilities to be programmed. Version 1.0 was released in October 2005 and included important additions to the original programming capabilities, including support for patient registration and demographics, though it also had electronic invoicing. In July 2007, the 2.0 version added the implementation of electronic medical records due to their release and the ability to use SQL databases.

In 2006, the Tides Foundation granted monetary assistance that financed the development of a wide set of new characteristics to support the specialized needs of health centers, which gave a boost to open source systems for medical applications. This program is written in PHP language and it is possible to execute it on the majority of the server configurations such as Windows, Linux, or Mac OS X. ClearHealth, like Apache and MySQL, follows the rules of most web-based open source systems.

Between the different open source solutions for the California HealthCare Foundation health industry, ClearHealth application can be identified as a viable solution based on the idea of using open source software creation, which can be used in medicine (en.wikipedia.org/wiki/ClearHealth, 2011).

elementalClinic

elementalClinic is an application based on web technology for the management of mentally handicapped patients. This program executes the following tasks: programming, assessment, objectives definition, group treatment, and electronic invoicing. This open source software was released in 2002. In 2005, Randall Hansen joined the company OpenSourcery of open source software in Portland (Oregon), which now supports and develops this application. They have dedicated thousands of hours developing the program with the objective of helping mental health clinics to have an EHR system. Randall Hansen assumed the leadership of the base-source project in 2004. Due to a strong belief in the power of open source software, Randall and others have made significant personal sacrifices to keep the project going. As a result, this application allows physicians and patients to enjoy very useful software. Security and community development that implements electronic medical records applications as well as free licenses concessions of EHR are the main characteristics of elementalClinic.

elemcntalClinic application is made in the Perl programming language using the PostgreSQL database that has excellent performance for that programming language. All these are under the open source philosophy (directory.fsf.org/project/elemental_clinc, 2011).

FreeMedForms

FreeMedForms (FMF) is a multi-platform software (available in MacOS, Linux, FreeBSD, and Windows), multilingual, and open source, released under the new BSD license and basically programmed in C++. This application is developed by physicians and it is intended mainly for health professionals. The main objective of FreeMedForms is the management of EHR based on his medical practice or based on the practice of clinical research groups. Their records can be totally customizable by the use of plugins. Some parts of the software are already working and they are being used in the medical practice such as the FreeDiams application (before DrugsInteractions).

FreeDiams is a prescription FreeMedForms plugin integrated into an independent application. This software is a multi-platform (MacOS, Linux, FreeBSD, and Windows) and it is an open source application released under the new BSD license. It is being developed by physicians and it is assigned for the use of these same professionals. It is used only to prescribe medicaments. This plugin can be linked to any application, thanks to its command line parameters input.

FreeMedForms is a multi-user application used to manage EHR. It is open source and based on open source electronic medical records. The main objective of the application is to create a powerful highly dynamic EHR manager and manage the patient data by a set of XML files. Interoperability and internationalization are the objectives to be achieved. The authors have made the software install the simpler possible for each operating system. The general steps are downloading, unzipping, and installing. FreeMedForms has a wizard that helps you in all configuration phases. The application can be quickly improved thanks to the easy installation of the many supplements

in the form of plugins. The main idea behind the project is that any physician can create their own "forms" to their patients without any tedious setup.

This multi-platform software, free and open source is addressed for health professionals. When the project is finished, FreeMedForms submits a full version that will allow the correct management of medical records. The application has an intuitive interface and it is very modular. Its characteristics are totally customizable through the plugins listed above. The program also allows the management of medical records (freemedforms.com/en/start, 2011).

FreeMED

It is an application for managing open source electronic medical records, based on Linux, Apache, MySQL, and PHP. The FreeMED project was officially started in 1999 by Jeffrey Buchbinder in the U.S.A. Since then it has become an international effort, with thousands of downloads and several translations. It is a direct descendant of the AMOS application, that was a program implemented in Pascal and was created in 1983 before the widespread use of relational databases and object-oriented programming. Now it comes to the ninth revision. When we started this review there have been changes in medicine and medical assistance, and therefore in this review we intend to adapt the application to the new requirements.

FreeMED is mainly written in PHP and makes intensive use of SQL, which favours the MySQL database engine. It also uses bash, Perl, and small modules written in other languages. Its interface is mainly based on the web, but web service interfaces such as XML-RPC are also available. It is an application designed for Linux. If you want to use it in any other operating system like Windows or Mac OSX, then you must use a virtual machine to proceed to the installation of FreeMED application for VMware. The installation of FreeMED on Windows is known to be unstable and dangerous, hence it is not recommended.

Once the installation has been done, in order to access the application, you should check the EHR FreeMed system homepage, which contains some useful information. The username (administrator) is in the lower right corner of the screen. There are four general fields (Freemed main menu) in the center of the header bar: System, main, users, patients. The Help button is next to the tab. The Help menu related to the context provides information about the page in use. Each of these tabs contains sub menu items with different options.

The FreeMED application shows the medical data as a group of "modules," which consists of a database model and user interfaces. Modules are virtually connected between each other by the relation fields of the reference table to another modules and patients database. This gives FreeMED the possibility to add and delete functionalities in the central database by installing or deleting modules without re-programming the interface.

FreeMED uses an external invoicing program called Electronic Medical Record Information Translation and Transmission (REMITT). Is communicates with REMITT XML by an authenticated RPC connection. This connection, once established, allows the transmission of medical invoicing data as a monolithic block of XML. This information is converted into a meta-model by XSLT, which is transferred to the final destination once converted into the final form. This methodology allows many output formats that are created from the same database (freemedsoftware. org, 2011).

GNUmed

GNUmed is an open source program designed mainly for the management of EHR and can be installed on Unix-like systems (BSD, Linux, and UNIX), Microsoft Windows, Mac OS X and other platforms. GNUmed community is developing a medical software package that will be open source, free, secure, and respectful of patient privacy, open standards-based, flexible, and fully equipped. For use on the network (client-server architecture) the characteristics are: easy to use, multi-platform, and multilingual. It is based on open source tools such as PostgreSQL and it is mainly written in Python. It relies on a Graphical User Interface (GUI) based on wxPython. The first version was created by Horst GNUmed Herb. When Herb stopped his active development, the work was led by Karsten Hilbert who assumed the role of project manager.

Karsten Hilbert was not alone in his efforts. Several developers around the world joined the team and helped at one time or another: Syan Tan, Ian Haywood, Hilmar Berger, Sebastian Hilbert, Carlos Moro, Michael Bonert, Richard Terry, Tony Lembke, and more. While some were concentrated on programming the code, many more contributed enormously by the creation of an excellent documentation (Jim Busser).

The name was initially chosen to give credit to the GNU project and the connection to the medical profession. The logo represents a gnu as a reference to the GNU project accompanied by a python as a reference to the programming language in which the application develops, as well as the medical profession.

Technical Data

GNUmed supports a variety of characteristics, many of them executed as plugins that extend the basic functionality. Some of the uses of this application are:

- Use of different applications associated with GNUmed.
- Manage waiting lists.
- Control of allergies in patients.
- Documents management.

FFEHR

FFEHR is an application developed using the Mozilla programming framework. This program can execute independently or within the Firefox browser. It was chosen because of its network data exchange security and multi-platform capability. This software can be executed as an extension of Firefox, Mozilla, or other browsers. It can also work as an independent local application by Xulrunner.

The initial objective of the project is to design a common user interface that is effective, efficient, and acceptable for medical professionals in the Philippines and, in the future, in the entire world. FFEHR has license under the GNU GPLv3 and therefore it is available for free download and use, including source code.

Design Objectives of FFEHR

- To develop a Firefox extension that serves as an electronic medical record, the main objective is to generate standard reports, such as clinical summaries.
- Must be able to save files in XML format.
- The XML file must check whit HL7 scheme (scheme local copy).
- To simplify the implementation, specific XML format will be provided to developers (these are simple implementations of HL7 scheme).
- FORMS: will try to avoid the problems associated with SOAP (Subjective, Objective, Assessment, Plan diagnostics, Plan therapeutics).
- Add new patient.
- Add a new SOAP for the patient.

In short, the application must be like a notepad with ability to present structured forms, save data as XML and generate reports (XML files) in a structured format.

HealthForge

This application has been designed for deployment in different hospitals to support the needs of the health community. The main objective is to provide a flexible solution for managing medical records, medical center, and connecting to the healthcare community. The entire application has been developed in open source using the most robust tools and can be installed on any Microsoft server with MS SQL. Once installed, the physicians and their patients can be in touch with many telematic tools that make it possible to monitor the evolution of a patient.

The application contains EHR; Practice Management System (PMS); Patient-physician tools; Tools for the management of contents; Tools for user access.

It is a totally interoperable platform that allows you to connect to the healthcare community to which it belongs. This allows the patients to be in contact with other healthcare organizations that connect their services to a wider network.

The development of the all application is realized under the open source philosophy using the concept of modularity that helps the integration of the program in all types of systems used by hospitals. The adaptation will consist of the installation of the appropriate module and, if it does not exist, there is always the possibility of realizing the implementation of the module thanks to open source.

Every day new modules that can be used appear. They can be downloaded installed free of charge since they are open source, which is an important characteristic that helps its spread. The software can be easily modified to meet the needs of the hospital where it is deployed. For example, you can personalize different characteristics such as: changing page layouts, adding users, and personalizing the appearance. Everything is available within the solution presented in this open source software.

You can also say that the application is a secure solution for hospitals and health centers. The software is totally compatible and easily integrated within a network environment with LDAP (Lightweight Directory Access Protocol) (healthforge.codeplex.com, 2011).

Hospital OS

Hospital OS is a research and development project of a health management software to support small hospitals. The Thailand Research Fund (TRF) finances it.

The project efforts are focused on facilitating the work to hospitals in remote areas where the technology seems to have difficulties. An information system for the hospital, called "Hospital OS," has been developed. This software is an open source program directed at providing efficient medical services and hospital management. Despite the lack of budget and technological advancement in rural communities, the task of developers is to create an effective information system, along with competent people in order to promote a sustainable development for all communities in Thailand. Hospital OS program has been used in 80 hospitals and 60 government health centers throughout Thailand so far.

Hospital OS is a system for management of hospital information that focuses on the organization of tasks and resources. This is a client-server model in which the server works as a central unit that stores all the information, and the clients are software units that access the server remotely to look up, add, or modify different data.

The application uses the Linux operating system and PostgreSQL as database. Linux and PostgreSQL are open source software available for download. The software used by the client is developed using the Java programming language and can execute under Windows 98, ME, 2000, XP, Linux, and other operating systems that offer the possibility of installing the virtual machine Java.

The developed software helps to support the digital database, providing reduction in processing time. In the beginning of the project, it was observed that people had to wait a long time to obtain medical services in hospitals. Therefore, the idea of a system that can help patients to improve services has emerged.

The application helps the hospitals to do the transition to electronic systems. It is estimated that the program Hospital OS can reduce waiting time for outpatients in clinics by 20 per cent.

Hospital OS comes with support modules for the Outpatient Department (OPD) and Inpatient Department (IPD). The modules include workflow management, registration, diagnosis, medical history and patient service order, pharmacy, invoicing, laboratory, and radiology reports, helping to put all these medical services in the electronic database.

Since the registration process to identify the patient or the numbers used in the hospital, health personnel can quickly access the records through the system and send patients to the medical specialist immediately.

Doctors can also add new medical information very easily about a patient of the system. In addiction, they can also send prescriptions electronically to pharmacists through the application. Instead of reading the writing of a doctor, the pharmacist can read the prescription directly from the computer and this helps to reduce the mistakes.

On the other hand, once a great number of public hospitals and clinics install the Hospital OS software, its systems can be connected. The public provincial health office can use the health information to do a correct planning. The application can also link to Google Maps and keep the public health civil servants informed about the general health situation and thus they are able to manage the epidemics quicker. The health information is available in the form of image, text and maps. When the hospitals are connected, the civil health servant will be able to test how the health in each area is and find the people infected with an illness and they will be able to concentrate to the area that seems to have an outbreak. (hospital-os.com/en, 2011).

HOSxP

HOSxP is a system for the management of information in hospitals, including the EHR. Nowadays it is in use in more than 70 hospitals of the whole Thailand. The program has as objectives to facilitate the workflow in health centers and central hospitals.

Before becoming HOSxP, the software was called KSK-HDBMS. They sought a friendly name, so the development team has chosen the name HOSxP, which comes from Hospital and experience. The name also reflects the graphical user interface software that it imitates the Windows XP theme. Distributed under the GNU General Public License (GPL), HOSxP is a free software.

Its development began in 1999. It came up a solitary project of Suratemekul Chaiyaporn, a pharmacist. The main developers of the software are the staff of Bangkok Medical Software Co., Ltd., a company managed by Chaiyaporn. The development of the application infrastructure, including source code repository, is hosted at SourceForge.net (hosxp.net, 2011).

Indivo

Indivo is a system used to save medical records with the possibility of personal control. This application allows an individual to have and to manage a complete and secure digital copy of your medical record where you can see your health state. Indivo is free and open source. It is actively used in various places, particularly at the Hospital of Boston and the Consorcio de Dossia. It is designed to be expanded and customized: users can connect their registration to third party applications that improve the management and analysis of health information.

Indivo system is essentially a future project for the management of medical records, in which the patients granted permission for the management of clinical data to institutions, doctors, researchers, and other users of medical information. Indivo is a distribution based on web technology and available under open source license.

This project has had its origin in the project "Guardian Angel," a collaboration between Harvard University and MIT, which provides a web-based automated with a manager to organize health information and decisions. Indivo model has inspired a number of commercial efforts along its evolution. More recently, it has promoted a shift to a platform model, so that other applications can connect to extend its basic functionality.

In order to share the concept of "personally controlled health record," and promote their adoption, two conferences on PCHR infrastructure in the Harvard Medical School have been promoted. 100 participants came each year, including government leaders (CDC, NIH, FDA, SSA, CMS, VA) information technology (Google, Microsoft, Intuit), business (Wal-Mart, Intel, AT & T), and the teaching staff.

In 2006, a broad agreement was established about the model of personal control. In 2007, a broad consensus has been reached about the structure of the platform, where innovation and variation live side by side, as if they formed an ecosystem.

A few months after the conference, Google, Microsoft and Dossia started to work in projects related to medical records. Microsoft HealthVault launched with Indivo is an open source product. Dossia signed a contract with children's hospitals to adapt Indivo like its informatics program in order to be used by millions of employees in the field of medicine. Later Google announced Google Health. Indivo (formerly PING) has been financed by the National Library of Medicine from 1998 to 2004 when it began to be financed by the Centers for Disease Control and Prevention until 2008, in which the financing is produced by the Boston Children's Hospital (indivohealth.org, 2011).

Medical

The Medical software offers the functionality of an EHR, a Hospital, and Health Information System for the implementation OpenERP. The main objective is to provide an open source universal hospital and Health Information System, in which doctors and institutions around the world, especially in developing countries, will benefit of a scalable, centralized, and free system to improve quality of life for its inhabitants.

The data model is designed to centralize information so that no duplication occurs. On the other hand, Medical optimizes collaboration and communication among health professionals. For example, when a doctor order specific lab tests to a patient, it is processed by the pathologist, and the results are fed to the system. The doctor now has all the patient related information in the record. Medical allows you to attach documents (X-rays, biopsy results, etc.) to the patient registry.

Information generated and gathered in Medical uses industry standards. ICD-10 is used for pathologies/diagnoses and ICD-10-PCS for medical procedures. For example, instead of typing an arbitrary name, the doctor can choose from over 14,000 unique disease variables. This is very important for epidemiological and statistical studies as well as interoperability between institutions in other countries. Thus, the history of the patient will be in a format that medical centers around the world would be able to process. Medical software is effective, saving paper, and providing a quick way to practice medicine.

This software uses genetic information of the "National Center for Biotechnology Information" (NCBI) and "GeneCards" to link genetic disorders with diseases. This information is important to assess the patient risks of contracting a specific disease and probably transmit it on to future generations. Medical also saves the patients' medical records.

The main language is English, but it can be easily translated into other languages using the translation module OpenERP 5.0. The Spanish version coexists with English (medical.sourceforge.net, 2011).

Open Healthcare

The group responsible for the development of the Open Healthcare project is an organization dedicated to the promotion and the distribution of an open source application used to manage medical records. It is implemented with XML technology and it has been developed to help automate and improve the practice of medicine. Also, it is developed in open-source and can also be developed and customized to your preferences by creating your own templates.

Like other open source software, this application for health records allows everyone to use and modify it for free.

The group developing this project wants to create a community of people who share the goal of improving medical care. This community will be able to freely use the Open Healthcare application. This maximizes the universal access to the health technology Open Group.

The commercialization of health care and software has often led to the development of "business secrets." This has stifled cooperation and progress in both industries. The members of the Open Healthcare project believe that we can work together to create a health record that will significantly improve the practice of medicine.

The application is developed in native XML. The aim is to create a long-lived universal tool for the search of electronic health records. Because the information is stored as native XML is independent of the operating system and the application of software. A system to enable the processing of XML-based XML is under development.

Techniques have been developed to interoperate with traditional technologies used by databases such as SQL, which was used in the initial deployment. Currently, this system is being transformed to a fully native XML and techniques have been developed to edit XML files as if they were SQL tables.

The servlet application uses the XMTP transformation technique to request a MIME originated from an XML representation (SAX really), which is introduced in a chain of SAX processing. The TRAX interface makes the work easier by using the transformation engines of Xalan like SAX filters.

323

This software building process of medical records is based in XML as a sequence of individual packets allows the study of medical research, medical test results, and reports of medical errors. Their authors strongly believe that this approach will provide great benefits to the health system, although there is clearly more research and work to do. This is a start and seems to be in the right direction (openhealth.org, 2011).

OSCAR McMaster

OSCAR McMaster is an application for EHR managing based on web technology. The system was initially developed for university hospitals primary care. It has become a global application also used as a billing system used by many private doctors and clinics primarily in Canada but in other parts of the world as well. The name is derived from where it was created—OSCAR stands for "Open Source Clinical Application and Resource" and McMaster refers to McMaster University, where it was developed.

On December 1, 2005, the group of the project announced that OSCAR had been certified as part of medical applications. Notably, OSCAR is the only open source application (from a list of 19 certified products from 15 suppliers) to meet or exceed the requirements to ensure that the product is compatible with the standards defined by the clinical management software.

OSCAR basically works as a web server, which must be installed on a Linux machine. We recommend the use of Ubuntu (one of the many Linux distributions) which is really easy to install and use, as there is much information online about this distribution that can be downloaded for free. It is important to install the English language in the operating system of the server. Once the server is installed, the program is accessed like a web page through a browser on a machine with any operating system.

In order to access OSCAR, simply fill in your username and password. This measure, known as authentication ensures that only you can access your account. Therefore, you should never reveal your password to anyone. Your password is stored in an encrypted format so that even the system administrator cannot know what it is. If you have forgotten your username and or password, the administrator can reset the initial password.

Depending on the privacy information of your account, the settings can be a key to access the second level. This is typically a code that the OSCAR administrator has provided the user with and it is typically required when connecting from outside the office or local network (for example, from home or hospital). This is a security feature. It is unlikely that a hacker will be able to guess your password in both the access codes of the second level.

If you enter the wrong password three times, the computer you are using OSCAR at will be prevented from accessing the system for a period of time. If this happens, you may wait a set time to access the application or tell your administrator that proceed to unlock the computer (he can do it remotely). This security feature helps to prevent hackers may have from trying to hack more than three times. After working with the application, exit by pressing the button at the top right corner of the screen. Closing the session will ensure that no unauthorized person can access the account OSCAR (en.wikipedia.org/wiki/OSCAR_McMaster, 2011).

SmartCare

The SmartCare application is a system for the management of medical records to ensure the continuity of medical care that has been developed and deployed by the Ministry of Health of Zambia, in collaboration with the Centers for Disease Control and Prevention and other many development partners.

Given the resource constraints in developing countries like Zambia, where electricity is not yet available in some parts of the country, Internet access throughout the country will take long to be widely deployed. The data management is carried out at each health center in a distributed design, unlike the designs of most centralized systems.

The SmartCare client is used with flash drives so you have a connectivity solution and high technology that works today. Information on the health of an individual is stored in a single compressed file.

The Data capture may be the most difficult part of the designing of an application for medical records. SmartCare extends an idea of success, the touch screen for data entry. The software works well with a touch screen that allows the doctor to view and record patient data. This tool, combined with customer specific data, can provide decision support for diagnosis.

The data stored in the health facilities can be displayed on GIS maps. This includes live patient data and static data from health surveys.

SmartCare is an application written in C#. The database was implemented in Microsoft MSDE (which is a free version of SQL Server 2000) and has been migrated to SQL Server 2005 Express (the free version of SQL Server 2000). The application is installed on computers with Windows XP operating system that will be the only licensed software is used for system implementation (smartcare.org.zm, 2011).

Functionality

- Each resident of Zambia receives confidential health care when and where needed and he or she also has an electronic medical record.
- Each point of clinical service can access and update this record.
- Each doctor understands the value of this record and promises to keep it secret.
- Each medical center, municipal, provincial, and national sends the data to the Ministry of Health where they systematically monitor and evaluate the reports. This informa-

tion is used to optimally allocate human resources and others to achieve a continuous and systematic improvement in health services.

Tolven Healthcare

Released early in 2009, Tolven RC1 allows new and innovative solutions. The solution proposed by the application Tolven ensures to the medical staff the ownership of all the most recent information and guide them in their decision-making. An electronic records system like this offers to the consumer an intuitive way to surf the patient information based in Web applications with the objective to create, view, store and share health information. With the purpose of communicating with service providers and allow the necessary access to health information located on servers situated far from their Local Area Network (LAN) using Internet, although simply performing routine tasks such as re-checking a recipe.

The electronic records are not simply a static record, but allow the medical personnel to selectively include the information that a doctor has collected in an initial assessment of a patient, it allows that the medical personnel can easily and safely take partial or complete medical information that is available to other doctors who may treat the patient. One of the main advantages of using electronic records is the speed that doctors have to know the ailments of a patient because all the necessary information is available online and can be checked without having to search in huge paper forms. The emergency doctors are among the big beneficed for the use of electronic records since this can avoid unnecessary risks and delays in treating patients.

The use of the Tolven open source application extends beyond the United States in regions such as Europe and the Pacific coast of Asia. The rapid use of Tolven software is a direct reflection of the quality and breadth of the products and services that have been introduced in the last three years.

The Tolven platform and the framework of the application provide a complete set of technical services that can be used to easily deploy tools based on health standards.

At the application level, Tolven supports a number of new features, including "favorites lists" for accounts and the individual users, like this as Tolven Plug-Ins to add various extra features to the platform.

In the upcoming months, Tolven will release a set of healthcare applications that can be used on phones and mobile devices.

The last version of the Tolven platform, Tolven Plug-Ins, has been the result of 3.5 years of work to apply to medicine, especially electronic records, the available technology in order to create a secure and scalable architecture with the objective of occupying the worldwide market for which international applicability tests have been run for Tolven solutions. The latest version uses resource bundles to provide a translation of the application in many languages, including the ability to support Traditional Chinese and Arabic character sets.

In short, the Tolven applications are web-based solutions that can be accessed using the latest versions of Internet Explorer or Firefox. The system administrator will provide users with a Web address (e.g. URL) so they can securely access Tolven applications. Tolven provides a demo environment that can be used for training purposes (tolven.org, 2011).

TORCH

The application Trusted Open source Records for Care and Health (TORCH) is developed in Python language, which is allowed to be executed in different platforms with the unique requirement of having the Python interpreter installed.

One of the main features of the application is the use of templates in order to complete the patient information more quickly. Using a well-designed set of templates makes the health care professional quick and accurate, producing a patient history while asking their ailments.

Operation

Before you create your own templates, it is advisable to know the full operation of the program and of the different templates generated by default, which are installed with the program. To begin the manipulation of the program the first step will be look the selection of patient records that appear in the main screen of TORCH. Then you can make a list of all patient records or search a patient if you have several already saved. To open in a window the history of a patient, simply click on the link of the surname.

The main templates are created from other defined templates. A template can be as simple as "if" selection or as complicated as a selection of multiple items in a list of many items.

If you create a circular reference, referring to a template that points to the current template, the system constantly try to put the data in the two fields and the template will be useless. In case of circular reference, it can be repaired by editing the template.

All templates are created and edited using the FreePM template generator. The screen template generator has three frames. The upper frame contains the menu. The box right under the new template is where the data is entered or where you edit existing templates. The left frame contains a list of all templates or a list of only the main templates.

Server Connection

The first thing to do is access your server using the user ID. To do this, put the URL in a browser http://:9080/manage where the TORCH network name server is installed. By doing this you should get a login box HTTP. From here, you must enter your user ID and password.

The user "admin" is created during the installation where you need to set the startup password.

In case that you do not remember this key can be changed to the user you want by clicking on the username. The user "admin" is basically a user of emergency and can not be the owner of any object.

The user "torch_admin" comes with a very simple and basic password "abc123." Each copy of the application TORCH has the same username and password. Therefore, it should change the password for this user immediately. It must click the user name and fill out both password fields. Then click the Change button. Then, you must close the browser and then log in using your user ID and password new user "torch_admin." You MUST NOT delete this user. This user owns all objects of the TORCH program. It can ruin all the installation work if you delete it (launchpad. net/trusted, 2011).

ZEPRS

At the beginning of 2001, a medical team of Alabama University in Birmingham conceived the idea to the implementation of an application of EHR, which will begin to be used in Zambia.

The team of Alabama University requested the proposal for technical design and the application of the system to several private companies of the information sector before awarding a contract. Once decided the company in charge of the implementation, they agreed the basis of the project whose most important feature more was its non-profit development. Other partners of the project have been the Center for Infectious Disease Research in Zambia (CIDRZ) and the health district of Lusaka.

Since the implementation (in February 2006) ZEPRS has been continuously revised and improved in many aspects due to the contributions of doctors and the changing needs. In 2008 an interface has implemented, letting you see the results of laboratory tests. Nowadays testing a version of the software can be installed locally, so it can be used in a facility in the absence of network connectivity and it is also possible to

automatically synchronize the records when it detects connectivity (ictedge.org/zeprs, 2011).

ZEPRS was designed to improve motherly and perinatal results for improve the perinatal attention for the women and the postnatal attention for the newborn baby in order to promote the practice of care, identify and document the potentials health problems so that the effective treatment could be administrated, improve the communication between the suppliers and the references and improve the supervision and the assessment of the results. It also improves the efficient, integrity, exactness of the documentation and show of reports.

ZEPRS has been developed used the Java programming language. Other technologies used are AJAX, Quartz, MySQL and others. ZEPRS has its own content management system called DynaSite, which presents easier add shapes, different fields and some more characteristics without the need for programming. Also, it has developed a local installable version of the software with the integrate database. This last version uses the open source platform and open zcore, which uses an application to transmit data over intermittent networks such as mobile phone networks.

The Main Components

ZEPRS achieve these objectives by means of the following contributions:

- An EHR system with a database that contains the medical records and that is shared between different health centers.
- A system that guides the doctor through the standard attention of Zambia.
- An electronic system used for the first time by the doctor during the attention of the patient.
- An electronic remission system to improve the efficient and the efficacy of the references.

OpenMRS

In section 3, 4, and 5, we focus on the description of the three most important applications of open source worldwide: OpenMRS, OpenEMR, and VistA. Each of these sections are subdivided into a brief introduction, technical specifications and development projects.

Introduction

OpenMRS was designed as a generic system for the management of medical records that may assist on patient healthcare, collection of observations, visits to specialists, explanatory notes on individual patients, and other necessary data for diagnosis. The purpose of the application is to facilitate the processing of information about patients to doctors. Consequently, diagnosis might be done by spending less time and decreasing the waiting time between patients.

It has proved to be highly effective in the management of medical data of patients with HIV (Human Immunodeficiency Virus) and tuberculosis, mainly in Kenya, but later in Rwanda and South Africa. Once verified the good performance, it was installed in other countries such as Malawi, Mozambique, Lesotho, Tanzania, Uganda, and Haiti (Allen, et al., 2006.) At the moment, OpenMRS is being used in more hospitals and medical management centers, and it is important to stress its high functionality and low installation cost. A clear example is the OpenMRS version created by the World Health Organization (WHO), known as OpenMRS Express, which is able to adapt the software to the requirements demanded by a large managing institution.

All basic concepts used in the system are defined in OpenMRS. By using combinations of questions and answers, the observations (important data to be taken into account) can be defined, as well as the forms to collect multiple observations. The first systems were built by converting paper forms into an electronic format, and were based on the documentation of all forms and the cataloguing of such forms into a hierarchy.

OpenMRS is an application developed in Java and its utility is the management of EHR records through a Web interface. The initial approach was a simple data model that obtained the proper operation by using an Application Programming Interface (API). Then the developers built a Web-based application that uses the API to make the proper function (Mamlin, et al., 2006). OpenMRS API works as a "black box," that is to say by hiding the complexity of the data model, and ensures that applications and modules are working properly.

Although there was a small development team and a slow implementation at the beginning, OpenMRS development project organizers have made use of weekly conferences, mailing lists, Wikis, a version code and the project tracking software in order to manage the collaboration of people interested in working on the project in an altruistic way (Allen, et al., 2007).

Technical Specifications

The application has been implemented with an architecture defined at different levels. The layers are clearly separated, as shown in Figure 1.

Each and every one of the layers that form the OpenMRS application architecture is explained below.

- **MySQL** database is very fast in reading, but can cause problems in high concurrency environments. Regarding Web applications, there is a low turnout in the modification of data, while the environment is intensive in data reading, what makes MySQL perfect for this kind of OpenMRS applications (mysql.com, 2010).
- **SQL** (Structured Query Language) is a language to access relational databases. It allows you to make queries to recover, in a simple way, interesting information from a database, as well as to make changes to

Figure 1. OpenMRS technical architecture

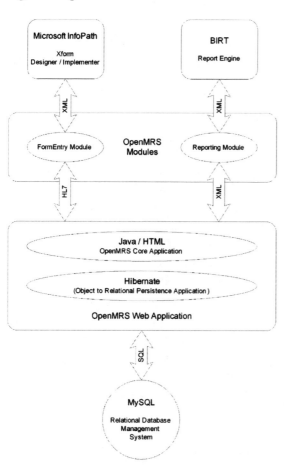

the database. It is a "high level" or "not applicable," declarative computer language of fourth generation, that allows encoding and object orientation thanks to its high productivity. A single statement may amount to one or more programs to be used in a low-level language aimed at making more efficient records (sql.org, 2010).

- **Hibernate** is an object-relational mapping tool used for Java Platform (also available for .NET under the name of NHibernate). It facilitates the mapping of attributes between a traditional relational database and the objects model of an application by declarative files of type eXtensible Markup Language (XML) or by annota-

tions in the beans of the entities that establish these relationships. Hibernate is a free software, distributed under the terms of GNU (GNU is Not Unix) LGPL (Lesser General Public License). Basically, this tool seeks to solve the problem of the difference between the two data models co-existing in an application: the one used in the computer memory (object oriented) and the one used in the database (relational model). To achieve this purpose, it allows the developer to fully detail how the data model is, what kind of relationships exist and how their shape is. Thanks to all this information, Hibernate allows the application to manipulate the information in the database to operate on objects, with all the features of Object Oriented Programming (OOP). Hibernate will convert information between the data types used by Java and those defined by SQL. This tool generates SQL statements and releases the developer from manual handling of data resulting from the enforcement of such awards, while maintaining portability across all database engines with a slight increase in execution time that compensates for the amount of work done. Regarding the schedule of tables that is used, it is a very flexible tool, able to get adapted to the use on an existing database. It has also the ability to create the database from the information available at any given time. Moreover, Hibernate tool provides a data query language called Hibernate Query Language (HQL), as well as an API for building queries. In case of using the described tool for Java, it can be used in Java independent applications or in Java Enterprise Edition (Java EE), by the Hibernate Annotations component that implements the Java Persistence API (JPA), which is part of this platform (hibernate.org, 2010).

- **Java** is an object-oriented programming language. Most of the syntax is similar to C and C++, but it has a simpler object model and cancels low-level tools, which often leads to many errors, such as direct manipulation of pointers or memory, thus facilitating the work to the developer. The software programmed in Java is compiled into bytecode, although compilation to native machine code is also possible. At runtime, bytecode is usually either interpreted or compiled into machine code for execution, although direct hardware execution of bytecode by a Java processor is also possible, but generally less used (java.com/es, 2010).

- **HTML** (HyperText Markup Language) is the predominant markup language, mainly used for Web page development. It is used to describe the structure and the content as a text, as well as to complement the text with objects such as images. HTML is written in the form of tags, surrounded by angle brackets (<,>). This language also describes the appearance of a document and can include a script (e.g. Javascript), which can affect the behavior of Web browsers and other HTML code interpreters (w3.org/html, 2010).

- **XML** (eXtensible Markup Language) is an extensible, tagging metalanguage developed by the World Wide Web Consortium (W3C). It simplifies and adapts the Standard Generalized Markup Language (SGML), which defines the grammar of specific languages. Therefore, XML is not actually a particular language, but a way of defining languages for different needs that might appear. XML is not only used for the Internet, as it is proposed as a standard for the exchange of structured information between different platforms. It can be used in databases, text editors, spreadsheets, etc. XML is a simple technology surrounded by

other technologies in order to get complemented and to increase the chances of use. Nowadays it plays a very important role, as it allows compatibility between systems to share information in a safe, reliable, and easy way (w3.org/XML, 2010).

- **HL7** (Health Level 7) is a system created for the exchange of information in medical-related environments and provides an integrated environment to manage medical data more easily. To carry out the implementation of the standard, it was designed the HL7 (Health Message Server [HMS]) message server—as an interface installed in each medical institution—, and the HL7 Message Archiver (HMA)—as an interface for the central database. Both interfaces communicate with each other through the use of HL7 messages. Thanks to its efficiency in data exchange, it has been proposed as a communication standard for transactions of medical information (hl7.org, 2010).

- **Microsoft InfoPath** is an application used to develop data entry forms based on XML. It was initially called "Xdocs." The main feature of InfoPath is the possibility of creating and viewing XML documents with support for XML schemata. InfoPath can connect to external systems by using XML Web services through Microsoft XML Core Services (MSXML) and Simple Object Access Protocol (SOAP) Toolkit, back-end and middle-tier systems. Communication may be set up communication by using Web services standards like SOAP, UDDI (Universal Description, Discovery, and Integration), and Web Services Description Language (WSDL). By using the InfoPath client, users fill forms on their computers while working offline. The form fields can also be checked for validation. Users can also attach a digital signature for security (office.microsoft.com/en-us/infopath, 2010).

- **BIRT** (Business Intelligence and Reporting Tools) is an open source project that provides the client and the Web applications—especially those based on Java and Java EE—with information and business intelligence abilities. It was designed to work with business intelligence processes in organizations. It is specifically made of tools that assist the analysis and presentation of data. Although some business intelligence tools include ETL functionality (Extraction, Transformation, and Load), they are not generally considered as business intelligence tools. The main aim is to address a wide range of information needs within an application (eclipse.org/birt/phoenix, 2010).

In Figure 1, there is a layer that shows the possibility of implementing different modules in the application. This is a very important feature. Thanks to modularity, the program can significantly change functions with little need for major changes in the software. Almost all installations of OpenMRS application use FormEntry module to capture data and login. The current version of the FormEntry module uses InfoPath, which is an application software package of Microsoft Office Professional. Even if it is not free, InfoPath is preferred since it uses XML and is a model that allows you to easily distinguish the data in the form from the data entered by the user. InfoPath is also used to fill out forms, providing an environment similar to a word processor, what helps people with limited IT knowledge to change the form fields. Although there is a project to create an alternative open source tool to InfoPath, its functionality is lower for the moment. For the right operation of OpenMRS application on a client-server model, distributed applications and other systems without interoperability problems, data and forms are represented in XML and XForms (XML Forms), respectively. Data may be communicated between the FormEntry module and

the application layer by using the HL7 system. Information is stored in the database according to an open relationship model that could be both manipulated and queried by using SQL language (Seebregts, et al., 2009).

The main feature of the program lies in a sturdy, flexible OpenMRS data model. From the initial design, the application kept its technical architecture, specially modularity. Implementing an API layer allows developers to work more easily, as they do not need full disclosure of the data model, but only the java objects to be used. The API layer is the backbone of the application, with methods for all major functions. The main types to be used within the API are PatientService, ConceptService, EncounterService, and ObsService. The context is a static class used to allow the application to store data in the memory. The context of services is divided into two categories: methods of the Services and methods for the users. The services are held at the class ServiceContext. On the other hand, the UserContext contains methods to influence users: authentication and authorization, login, logout, etc. For each new user who joins the system there is a new class UserContext instance and the current class UserContext is stored in the current thread. Every time you access the system, it is defined in a "work unit." This unit is bordered by calls to Context.openSession() and Context.closeSession(), which are made in Openmrs-Filter in a Web application, so most developers do not have to worry about making those calls. This procedure facilitates the fast deployment of OpenMRS modules and allows the application to be developed in quickly. As noted above, whether to stress something in the specifications, the API would be the main highlight (openmrs.org, 2011).

OpenMRS Projects in Development

During 2009 the OpenMRS project experienced significant progress in developing new tools that completed the proper running of the application and added new options that allowed doctors to manage medical records better, especially in patients with HIV and tuberculosis. In Rwanda, tools for primary care and chronic disease management, such as heart failure, were also developed, and therefore the time management in these systems was improved.

The module MDR-TB, developed in Rwanda in collaboration with the government, permits the continuation of the treatment of patients taking many medicines, as tuberculosis or other diseases. It is currently being used in Haiti and Pakistan with efficient results. Other countries, such as Peru, have also developed new tools for OpenMRS that improve information management.

With the support from the Government of Canada—the International Development Research Centre (IDRC)—, the OpenMRS project organization released a training course aimed at joining staff to the team in charge of the computer application development in Rwanda. The course is focused on teaching the techniques of Java programming language and various practical skills in health informatics. Nowadays, qualified programmers in Rwanda are interested in joining the development of the application, thanks to the Rwandan Government's plan to implement OpenMRS at a national level.

It is also important to consider that the Partners In Health (PIH) organization is working with the Rwandan Government on an ambitious plan to integrate OpenMRS into 250 clinics across the country. The application is mainly addressed to the management of medical records for patients on HIV treatment, primary care and other medical problems.

After the catastrophic earthquake in Haiti on 12th January 2010, it was considered to extend OpenMRS into 12 clinics and hospitals in Zanmi Lasante (Haiti), what meant a greater emphasis on primary care and women's health, as well as the creation of a surgical EHR system, which allowed health professionals to work more effectively in such a chaotic situation. The team in charge of implementing the software in different hospitals and clinics worked in Haiti with other key organizations that have implemented health information systems to improve care assistance for all victims (pih.org/pages/electronic-medical-records, 2010).

VistA

Introduction

Veterans Health Information Systems and Technology Architecture (VistA) is mainly aimed at creating an electronic health record application. This application was developed for the U.S.A. medical system and it is known as the Veterans Health Administration (VHA). In 2003, the VHA was the largest health care system in U.S.A. and paid attention to more than 4 million potential patients, employed 180,000 doctors in 163 hospitals and more than 800 clinics, regarding 135 nursing homes. Currently, half of all hospitals in U.S.A. use VistA.

Due to the large amount of data needed for the proper running of the VHA health system, several departments were started to be computerized from 1985 in order to manage data in a better way. It was initially called Decentralized Hospital Computer Program (DHCP) and it became so successful that it was awarded with the Computerworld Smithsonian Award for best use of IT applied to medicine in 1995.

VistA application is compatible with both small outpatient and large inpatient centers, and it includes several improvements to the original DHCP system. The most significant change is a graphical user interface for hospitals known as the Computerized Patient Record System (CPRS), which was released in 1997. In addition, VistA includes computerized order entry, bar code medication administration, electronic prescribing and clinical guidelines. It was also proved that the application improves the efficient work of a doctor by 6% per year.

CPRS provides a client-server interface that allows healthcare providers to review and update the medical record of a patient. This includes the ability to place orders and medicines, special procedures, X-rays, nursing interventions, diets and laboratory tests. CPRS provides flexibility in a wide variety of settings so that it is guided to events, it has a Windows style interface, and consequently presents a broad spectrum of workers in the health field.

VistA program is a free software application that consists of a collection of about 100 integrated software modules. VistA was developed by using the M language or MUMPS (Massachusetts General Hospital Utility Multi-Programming System) for the use of databases. Most VistA systems are now running on InterSystems proprietary version, even if it was developed a free version using the open source engine MUMPS for interaction with the database. The free version is basically planned for Linux and Unix computers. There is a free open source M module/Gateway, called MGWSI, that was developed to act as a gateway between GT.M (free version to manage the database) and Cache (proprietary version to manage database) by using programming tools like PHP, ASP, .NET, or Java, to create a Web-based interface.

VHA partnership is running a pilot project, known as HealtheVet (HEV), which is planning the next generation of VistA to upgrade the capacity of databases and interfaces.

The development is continuous, as necessary updates are performed illimitably (500-600 patches per year) and offered as public domain software. This was implemented by the U.S.A. Government to make VistA available at low cost for non-governmental hospitals and other healthcare centers. Universities, such as California and Texas, as well as nonprofit organizations such as WorldVistA, have worked to expand and improve the VistA application.

Technical Specifications

Implementing VistA Imaging is a coordinated system for communicating with radiology images and other types of images such as electrocardiograms, pathology slides, and scanned documents that are added to the VistA medical records system. This kind of integration of information on a medical history is basic for an efficient use. VistA imaging has become open source and it is available in the public domain to be used by both private and public hospitals. It may be used independently or integrated into the electronic medical records of VistA.

VistAWeb module is a web application used to review the patient information that is placed in the Vista medical records management system. To a certain extent, VistAWeb is the module that reflects the medical reports. There are three ways to access VistAWeb, but the main one is available by adding to the Tools menu and may be selected as the default method of data recovery. VistAWeb is compatible with the standard HL7, used in most healthcare software.

VistAWeb design is based on n-tier architecture and VistAWeb represents the level of presentation. The business process layer is represented by several components that VistAWeb uses to gain access to the data tier. The business process components include items such as code-behind pages (a function of Microsoft.NET programming language), Medical Domain Objects (MDO) and a collection of other reusable components. The data tier has multiple data sources, such as VistA, XML and many relational databases with SQL (e.g., Oracle, Microsoft SQL Server and Microsoft Access). Although some code-behind pages do not interact with a database with SQL and XML, the rest of the data level interactions take place in reusable components, such as MDO. Figure 2 shows the interaction of different levels of implementation in high level (va.gov/vista_monograph, 2011).

VistA Projects in Development

Since VistA is an open source application, it has been implemented in many health centers

Figure 2. VistAWeb application tiers interaction

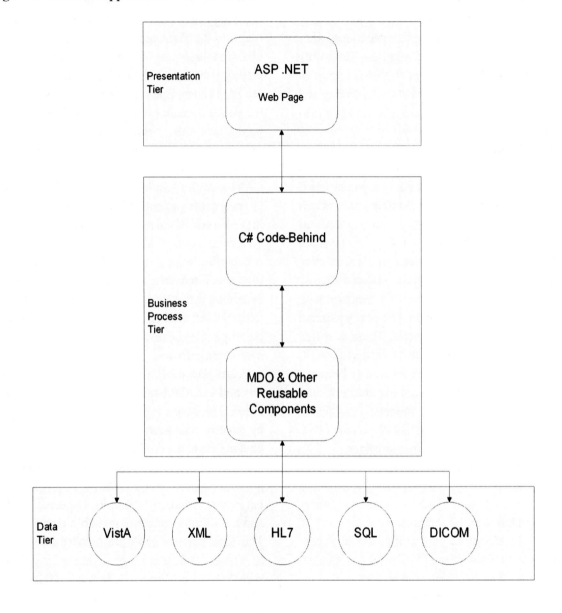

in Texas, Arizona, Florida, Hawaii, Oklahoma, West Virginia, California, New York, and Washington.

A piece of research confirmed that the budget assigned to a hospital for EHR VistA-based was a tenth of the cost of a retail version of the application used in a hospital of the same State ($9 million versus $90 million of the retail version). Both VistA and the retail system used MUMPS for the use of databases.

The VistA software modules have been installed or are being evaluated for installation in health institutions like WHO and countries such as Mexico, Finland, Jordan, Germany, Kenya, Nigeria, Egypt, Malaysia, India, Brazil, and Pakistan.

The project OpenVista came up to make good use of funds and effort invested in VistA and to extend it around the world. Therefore, starting from an initial development by VistA, some things have been changed in the application, but compatibility between both systems is total for the use of different modules, as well as in the field of communications. Then, from a technical point of view we can state that it is the same software. The main difference lies in who is the use of the application addressed to. In the case of VistA, it was firstly addressed to veterans, but later it was extended to many hospitals in U.S.A. due to the smooth operation, while OpenVista is addressed to all types of users, especially to places where economic resources are very limited (worldvista. sourceforge.net/openvista/index.html, 2011).

OpenEMR

Introduction

As all applications for medical records, this software was developed in order to facilitate access and management of medical records with a minimum cost. The development in a Web environment and the transparency allow many users to enter data simultaneously from different locations. The first implementation of the software dates from June 2001. In a nutshell, the application allows users to gain access to patient data from any computer on the Internet or Intranet. In July, 2002, a new version of the application with major improvements in security came up. Currently, all improvements are thoroughly reviewed by the OpenEMR community, which is mainly constituted by software developers and doctors and keeps the status of the application as a free software solution. They all work to make OpenEMR application better than other alternatives released by proprietary software.

Technical Specifications

The technical architecture of OpenEMR can be considered as a "LAMP" (Linux, Apache, MySQL, Perl, PHP, or Python). It is a different type of Web-based software that uses a Web server such as Apache, MySQL database and PHP program-

ming language. As most architectures such as "LAMP," OpenEMR can run on Linux, Unix, BSD (Berkeley Software Distribution), Mac OS X, and Microsoft architectures.

The patient data on OpenEMR can be transferred over the Internet by using the technology of Wide Area Network (WAN) or in an Intranet by a Local Area Network (LAN). OpenEMR is based on the use of Transmission Control Protocol/Internet Protocol (TCP/IP) for the exchange of data over the network. TCP/IP is a set of communication protocols commonly used in Internet or in different Intranet private networks. The application layer includes the Hyper-Text Transfer Protocol (HTTP), which supports the implementation of the World Wide Web and is represented by the browser window in OpenEMR. TCP ensures the transmission of accurate, reliable data across the network. The normal way to ensure OpenEMR is to enable Secure Socket Layer (SSL) Web server. In case of accessing through the Internet, the SSL certificate might be installed in your Web browser, so the client authenticates himself in the server to avoid intrusions.

OpenEMR can export some of their data to other systems—such as names, addresses, phone numbers, insurance information, etc. This kind of data cannot be transferred directly, but it requires a filter in the receiving system to know what is the meaning of the different fields. The easiest way to transfer information is output in a standard format such as HL7. Other data are stored in the database only as a series of yes/no check boxes. It would be very difficult to interpret this information without the information of associated Web pages. This is a common feature in the medical visit forms, where medical professionals do prefer to point and click instead of typing. These actions are stored in the database of Boolean information (yes/no, true/false), which will be more difficult to transfer as it will require an interpretation.

It works as follows: the Web server receives a browser request, which uses the PHP interpreter to assess the request and acts on incoming packets to finally pass the queries to the database engine as needed. Then, the engine performs database queries on the database server (MySQL). After running the query, the result is returned to the Web server through the PHP engine, which is an http page with the suitable format. The Web server returns the http to the requesting browser. The Web server could be any PHP-compatible, although Apache is commonly used for Open-EMR. The database server could be, in theory, any SQL database. MySQL is the database that uses OpenEMR. MS SQL Server or Oracle have not been tested yet as databases for this application.

Another feature of OpenEMR is that it might run as a distributed (client/server) or as a centralized computer system, depending on the settings made by the administrator. Taking into account that this operation is a set of autonomous computers connected through a distribution network, middleware to enable teams to coordinate activities and share system resources, in the case of a distributed model all components of OpenEMR—database servers, billing servers, etc.—can be distributed transparently over a heterogeneous computer network and they would be still seen as a computer center. This distributed architecture increases the OpenEMR configuration flexibility in a hospital, where major changes are made in a machine and replicated to all computers on the same network. In addition, data transmission costs are lower and the capacity of information processing is higher. However, compared to centralized computing, costs of end-user equipment and network management increase in a distributed computing environment, making it perfect for large hospitals.

In small clinics, small private hospitals, and outpatient care centers, which do not need the processing power provided by distributed computing systems, OpenEMR is flexible enough to allow centralized computing to reduce costs. In a centralized computing environment all critical data and programs are stored on a host computer, known as the central computer. Centralized computing environment has low costs of end-user devices and reduces network management costs, even though the performance is closely tied to the hardware and software, which have been normally used for a long time.

OpenEMR Projects in Development

There are professionals who are currently developing or testing the software in countries such as U.S.A., Puerto Rico, Australia, Sweden, etc. The application is being expanded throughout the world and has been translated into languages like Spanish, Dutch, Greek, Portuguese, etc., and partially translated into other languages like Swedish, Norwegian, or Chinese. OpenEMR receives more than $815,000 through grants (oemr.org, 2011).

COMPARISON OF OpenMRS, VistA, AND OpenEMR SYSTEMS

Taking into account that the main advantage of using free software has no economic cost in terms of copyright and evaluated applications are a common feature, this section is going to evaluate the features of the three programs described previously. The fields of the software to be analyzed are: evolution of the application, technical details and current status of the program.

- Evolution of the application

Within this term of comparison, it is necessary make a distinction between historical evolution and current evolution.

OpenMRS is the least developed. However, if we consider the evolution of applications, OpenMRS is currently the most noteworthy because of the large projects in which it is being installed.

VistA is the project that has evolved the most, thanks to more than 40 years of development with a great work during all this time. To complete its many functions, it is equipped with 500 to 600 new modules every year.

OpenEMR has been worked on for 10 years continuously with a large budget and its development is remarkable thanks to several grants.

• Technical details

OpenMRS is the most efficient application, as it was recently created and there was a firm commitment to the latest technology at that time by using Java and HTML for the core and MySQL to interact with the database.

In contrast, VistA, which is the oldest project, uses M or MUMPS language for interaction with the database while its core is developed in PHP, ASP, .NET and Java.

OpenEMR is also relatively modern and uses PHP for core application and MySQL to interact with the database.

• Current status of software

OpenMRS is being used in major projects such as the management of patients in Rwanda, Kenya, and Haiti, where the effectiveness of the application has been widely proved. The great work made on the OpenMRS project makes it able to live up high expectations.

VistA has also demonstrated its efficiency to be the software managing the largest number of patients in USA.

OpenEMR is the most universal software because it has been translated into many languages and also installed in a large number of countries throughout the world (see Table 1).

OpenMRS surpasses VistA as it is the software developed with the latest technology. Its modular design gives it the ability to modify system behavior to meet local, medical needs without requiring big, global changes. The modules have full access to the system, so you can add tables in the database, modify the behavior of the API and add or change the Web page of the application

as needed. Another advantage of OpenMRS is the use of HL7 as the primary mode of transmission of data between external applications and the repository, which promotes reuse and interoperability. This software is compatible with existing standards such as Logical Observation Identifiers Names and Codes (LOINC), ICD-10 (International Statistical Classification of Diseases and Related Health Problems), SNOMED (Systematized Nomenclature of Medicine) and CPT (The Current Procedural Terminology) (Mamlin, et al., 2006). Another great advantage is the use of OpenMRS to boost the development of outstanding projects.

Regarding the disadvantages, OpenMRS had a short life so far, so it is much less developed and evolved than VistA. Another drawback against OpenEMR is that it was translated into a shorter number of languages, hence the more limited use.

RESULTS

In this section, we compare three main types of EHR software solution (OpenMRS, OpenEMR, and OpenVistA) installed on two operating systems (Linux Ubuntu and Windows). Firstly, we explain the hardware server. The hardware server is used for installation on Linux Ubuntu and Windows. Secondly, we talk about software installed on the server. Finally, we show the results of the various parameters measured on Linux Ubuntu and Windows using five web browsers such as Firefox, Chrome, Internet Explorer, Opera, and Safari. All results obtained are shown in the data Tables 2-9. The results help us see how the three main EHR applications work depending on which operating system is installed and which web browser used.

Hardware Server

AMD Athlon (tm) Processor, Socket-A, 1150 MHz, 32 bits, 1024 MB RAM memory and 320 GB hard disc.

Table 1. Characteristics of the three applications

Terms of comparative	OpenMRS	VistA	OpenEMR
Start Date	2006	1970	June 2001
Core Technology	Java / HTML	PHP, ASP, .NET, Java.	PHP
Interaction with the database	MySQL	M o MUMPS	MySQL
Interface type	Web based.	Web based.	Web based.
Operating systems to be used in	Linux and Microsoft architectures.	Linux, Unix and Microsoft architectures.	Linux, Unix, BSD, Mac OS X and Microsoft architectures.
Level of development	Low due mainly to the short time from the beginning of the project	Very high because of high budget and long-lived project (between 500-600 modules are generated per year at the moment)	Medium since it is aided by important grants and has 10 years of continuous development
Languages of the application	English, Spanish, French, Italian and Portuguese.	English.	English, Spanish, Dutch, Greek and Portuguese. Some Swedish, Norwegian and Chinese.
Countries in use	Kenya, Rwanda, South Africa, Malawi, Mozambique, Lesotho, Tanzania, Uganda and Haiti.	United States, Mexico, Finland, Jordan, Germany, Kenya, Nigeria, Egypt, Malaysia, India, Brazil and Pakistan.	U.S.A., Puerto Rico, Australia, Sweden, Holland, Israel, India, Malaysia, Nepal, Indonesia, Bermuda, Armenia and Kenya.
Steps to obtain the software	Through an easy Web download.	Through an easy Web download.	Through an easy Web download.
Previous computer skills	Basic user level.	Basic user level.	Basic user level.
Easy to use?	Yes, because of its Web interface.	Yes, because of its Web interface.	Yes, because of its Web interface.
Current Status	Management of very important international projects (Kenya, Rwanda, HIV management and earthquake disaster in Haiti.)	Mainly management of many U.S.A. hospitals.	Management of different hospitals around the world.
Current development	Very high because of the important projects being developed	Not very high as it has been distributed by many hospitals in U.S.A. previously.	High because of the financial resources from grants

Table 2. Measurement parameters

Parameters	Time (seconds)	Percentage CPU use
Initial CPU use	*	14%
The reboot time of the server	100,8	**
The startup time of tomcat	0,043	90%
The shutdown time of tomcat	1,653	30%
The reboot time of the apache	2,024	70%
The reboot time of MySQL	5,974	100%

*In the initial CPU use the time is irrelevant.

** In the reboot time of the server, the percentage CPU use varies between 0% & 100%.

Software Server

- Ubuntu 11.04 natty
- Apache – tomcat 6.0.29
- MySQL 5.1.54-lubuntu4 (Ubuntu)
- PHP 5.3.5-lubuntu7.2
- Apache 2.2.17 (Ubuntu)
- OpenMRS 1.7.1
- OpenEMR 4.0.0
- OpenVistA release 6
- Firefox 4.0.1 with firebug 1.7.1

- Chrome 11.0.696.71
- Internet Explorer 8.0.6001.18702
- Opera 11.50
- Safari 5.1(7534.50)

Table 2 shows data related to installed software components for correct operation of OpenMRS, OpenVista and OpenEMR. These measurements offer us a temporary efficiency reference Linux Ubuntu operating system with the EHR.

Table 3 presents delays that are considered most relevant for operation of OpenMRS. The delays have been measured with five different browsers (Firefox, Chrome, Internet Explorer, Opera, and Safari). Also, we have realized a measurement of CPU use for each of the delays assessed. All data shown together with the previous table we do see the efficiency of work of the server and the efficiency in connecting through a browser or another.

Table 4 presents delays that are considered most relevant for operation of OpenEMR. The delays have been measured with five different browsers (Firefox, Chrome, Internet Explorer, Opera, and Safari). Also, we have realized a measurement of CPU use for each of the delays assessed. All data shown together with the Table 2 we do see the efficiency of work of the server and the efficiency in connecting through a browser or another.

Table 5 presents delays that are considered most relevant for operation of OpenVistA. (http://www.worldvista.org; http://www.medsphere.org; http://www.astronautvista.com http://www.vistapedia.net). The delays have been measured with the client application. Also we have realized a measurement of CPU use for each of the delays assessed. All data shown we do see the efficiency of work of the server.

Software Server

- Microsoft Windows XP Professional Version 2002 with Servi Pack 2
- Apache Tomcat 6.0.32 Server
- XAMP for Windows Version 1.7.2
- MySQL Server 5.5
- PHP 5.3.1
- Apache 2.2.12
- OpenMRS 1.7.1
- OpenEMR 4.0.0
- OpenVistA release 6
- Firefox 4.0.1 with firebug 1.7.1
- Chrome 11.0.696.71
- Internet Explorer 8.0.6001.18702
- Opera 11.50
- Safari 5.1(7534.50)

Table 6, with the same parameters of Table 2 shows results for the Windows operating system. Measurements show the behavior of the software components necessary for the operation of the EHR evaluated. With these measurements, you can see the CPU usage and delay obtained at the start, restart, or shutdown of a program. These measurements give us a temporary efficiency reference Windows operating system with the EHR.

In Table 7, we are measuring the same parameters as in Table 3 for the Windows operating system. The results are different by the characteristics and singularities of the Windows operating system. The data in the Table 7 allow us to know the CPU utilization, delay times, etc. and therefore the operation of the records evaluated.

Table 8 presents delays that are considered most relevant for operation of OpenEMR. The delays have been measured with five different browsers (Firefox, Chrome, Internet Explorer, Opera, and Safari). Also, we have realized a measurement of CPU use for each of the delays assessed. All data shown together with the Table 6 we do see the efficiency of work of the server

Table 3. OpenMRS on Linux operating systems

Parameters	OpenMRS				
	Firefox	Chrome	Internet Explorer	Opera	Safari
Request Web time	3,24	4,07	11,6	0,725	2,9
CPU use	65%	70%	100%	70%	80%
Log in time	3,41	2,66	3,4	1,125	4,9
CPU use	90%	90%	90%	50%	90%
Patient search time	0,528	0,726	0,630	0,341	1,2
CPU use	60%	60%	90%	80%	90%
Time for create new patient	21	5,44	6,2	3,720	7,1
CPU use	80%	80%	90%	90%	90%
Time for change of patient	20,53	11,31	15,27	7,14	10,87
CPU use	80%	80%	90%	80%	90%
The average time navigating for the main menu	0,703	0,343	0,617	0,107	0,343
CPU use	70%	70%	80%	50%	50%
Log out time	2,86	1,93	2,6	0,934	1,225
CPU use	85%	80%	90%	60%	90%

Note: time is in seconds.

Table 4. OpenEMR on Linux operating systems

Parameters	OpenEMR				
	Firefox	Chrome	Internet Explorer	Opera	Safari
Request Web time	4,04	2,53	4,01	1,4	3,5
CPU use	60%	60%	80%	80%	80%
Log in time	13,75	7,81	7,9	4,4	8,3
CPU use	80%	80%	100%	100%	100%
Patient search time	8,06	7,10	4,4	1,6	3,4
CPU use	50%	50%	80%	80%	80%
Time for create new patient	12,08	10,86	9,308	4,18	5,8
CPU use	60%	60%	80%	80%	80%
Time for change of patient	5,96	4,28	4,57	3,14	3,72
CPU use	70%	70%	70%	60%	70%
The average time navigating for the main menu	3,11	2,19	2,31	1,02	1,972
CPU use	60%	60%	60%	60%	60%
Log out time	4,26	2,26	3,3	1,6	2,982
CPU use	60%	60%	100%	100%	100%

Note: time is in seconds.

Table 5. OpenVistA on Linux operating systems

Parameters	OpenVistA
	OpenVistA CIS
Request Web time	Not based on Web
CPU use	Not based on Web
Log in time	16,6
CPU use	100%
Patient search time	3,7
CPU use	100%
Time for create new patient	9,76
CPU use	100%
Time for change of patient	11,8
CPU use	100%
The average time navigating for the main menu	2,8
CPU use	100%
Log out time	5,2
CPU use	100%

Note: time is in seconds.

and the efficiency in connecting through a browser or another.

Table 9 presents delays that are considered most relevant for operation of OpenVistA on Windows operating systems. The delays have been measured with the client application. Also, we have realized a measurement of CPU use for each of the delays assessed. All data shown we do see the efficiency of work of the server.

There is nothing most objective that the numbers. Tables show how behave the main EHR in two operating systems using five different browsers. OpenMRS application has less delay time in the Linux Ubuntu than in Windows. The fastest browser with this software is Opera. The CPU use varies between 15% & 100%.

Tables indicate that OpenEMR has less delay time in Linux Ubuntu than in Windows. The Opera browser is faster than the others Web browsers for

Table 6. Measurement parameters

Parameters	Time (seconds)	Percentage CPU use
Initial CPU use	*	18%
The reboot time of the server	85,6	**
The startup time of tomcat	4,9	100%
The shutdown time of tomcat	102	100%
The reboot time of the apache	18,6	100%
The reboot time of MySQL	7,5	20%
The startup time of XAMP	0,6	20%

*In the initial CPU use the time is irrelevant.

** In the reboot time of the server, the percentage CPU use varies between 0% & 100%.

Table 7. OpenMRS on Windows operating systems

Parameters	OpenMRS				
	Firefox	Chrome	Internet Explorer	Opera	Safari
Request Web time	5,9	2,07	5,2	1,5	1,4
CPU use	95%	100%	80%	85%	95%
Log in time	10,1	1,38	2,1	1,2	1,3
CPU use	98%	100%	80%	50%	55%
Patient search time	1,06	0,730	2,8	0,704	1,2
CPU use	65%	95%	85%	60%	78%
Time for create new patient	15,35	3,43	3,4	1,5	2,2
CPU use	100%	100%	85%	60%	90%
Time for change of patient	7,55	6,66	12,2	4,1	5,4
CPU use	90%	100%	95%	95%	100%
The average time navigating for the main menu	0,200	0,140	0,307	0,125	0,225
CPU use	40%	40%	60%	15%	38%
Log out time	1,77	0,998	1,4	0,581	0,825
CPU use	100%	100%	60%	40%	62%

Note: time is in seconds.

Table 8. OpenEMR on Windows operating systems

Parameters	OpenEMR				
	Firefox	Chrome	Internet Explorer	Opera	Safari
Request Web time	2,4	2,66	4,121	1,5	1,9
CPU use	80%	80%	95%	80%	80%
Log in time	27,19	7,63	8,6	5,5	6,3
CPU use	100%	100%	95%	100%	100%
Patient search time	10,06	8,56	5,1	7,3	8,831
CPU use	70%	70%	95%	90%	90%
Time for create new patient	17,58	15,03	16,27	12,04	13,91
CPU use	80%	80%	95%	98%	95%
Time for change of patient	7,96	5,82	6,23	3,95	5,32
CPU use	90%	90%	90%	80%	70%
The average time navigating for the main menu	4,93	2,14	3,18	1,75	2,34
CPU use	40%	40%	50%	60%	50%
Log out time	2,74	2,18	1,8	0,98	2,15
CPU use	80%	80%	95%	90%	95%

Note: time is in seconds.

Table 9. OpenVistA on Windows operating systems

Parameters	OpenVistA
	OpenVistA CIS
Request Web time	Not based on Web
CPU use	Not based on Web
Log in time	11,1
CPU use	100%
Patient search time	2,1
CPU use	80%
Time for create new patient	5,3
CPU use	85%
Time for change of patient	9,2
CPU use	70%
The average time navigating for the main menu	1,7
CPU use	90%
Log out time	3,9
CPU use	100%

Note: time is in seconds.

use of this program. The CPU use varies between 40% & 100%.

On the other hand OpenVista has less delay time in Windows than in Linux Ubuntu. The CPU use in this case varies between 70% & 100%.

CONCLUSION

To support the EHR integrated systems may be introduced. The systems must be stable, modular, configurable, versatile, safe and comprehensive. In this chapter we review a set of software that enables the proper management of EHR, which common feature is to be open source and to offer the best opportunities in health care to developing countries.

We have carried out a major analysis of the main applications of free software which exist worldwide. The choice of analyzing those health management applications is due to its importance in terms of number of patients managed, number of sites that use the application, heterogeneity of the clinics where they are used, higher level of software development, number of the functions available to professionals of the medicine, core technology, programming language which implements the application interface, language of the interaction with database, etc. Unfortunately the information available for do the review of such applications is not always accessible and has only been possible to analyze certain aspects.

Finally we focus on the description of the three open source applications most used in hospitals and clinics around the world (OpenMRS, OpenEMR, and VistA) by its technological development, rapid development and efficient implementation.

Taken into account that the main advantage of using free software has no economic cost in terms of copyright, which is a common feature in the assessed applications, we compared several characteristics of the three aforementioned programs related to core technology, interaction with the database, interface type, operating systems, level of development, etc.

The chapter showed how OpenMRS is covering all the needs in medical institutions at the moment and is successfully answering to first expectations in the places where it was installed. Even if it has been running for a shorter time than VistA and OpenEMR, it has proved to be very complete and effective, and able to answer positively in the management of EHR.

From our point of view, the evolution of OpenMRS is meteoric due to the great development during the short lifetime of the project, what came from the need of a fast evolution in the places where the software is being implemented. In the coming years, it will be noticed how OpenMRS is likely to become the best, most used program to manage medical records in disaster areas or pandemics.

REFERENCES

Allen, C., Jazayeri, D., Miranda, J., Biondich, P. G., Mamlin, B. W., & Wolfe, B. A. (2007). Experience in implementing the OpenMRS medical record system to support HIV treatment in Rwanda. *Studies in Health Technology and Informatics, 129*(1), 382–386.

Allen, C., Manyika, P., Jazayeri, D., Rich, M., Lesh, N., & Fraser, H. (2006). Rapid deployment of electronic medical records for ARV rollout in rural Rwanda. In *Proceedings of the AMIA Annual Symposium*, (p. 840). AMIA.

Biondich, P. G., Anand, V., Downs, S. M., & McDonald, C. J. (2003). Using adaptive turnaround documents to electronically acquire structured data in clinical settings. In *Proceedings of the AMIA Annual Symposium*, (pp. 86-90). AMIA.

BIRT. (2010). *Web page*. Retrieved December 14, 2010, from http://www.eclipse.org/birt/phoenix.

ClearHealth. (2011). *Web page*. Retrieved May 12, 2011, http://en.wikipedia.org/wiki/ClearHealth.

Community Health Information Tracking System. (2011). *Web page*. Retrieved May 12, 2011, from http://www.chits.ph/web.

Department of Veterans Affairs. (2011). *Web page*. Retrieved January 15, 2011, from http://www.va.gov/vista_monograph.

Diero, L., Rotich, J. K., Bii, J., Mamlin, B. W., Einterz, R. M., Kalamai, I. Z., & Tierney, W. M. (2006). A computer-based medical record system and personal digital assistants to assess and follow patients with respiratory tract infections visiting a rural Kenyan health centre. *BMC Medical Informatics and Decision Making, 6*, 21. doi:10.1186/1472-6947-6-21

Elemental Clinic. (2011). *Web page*. Retrieved May 12, 2011, from http://directory.fsf.org/project/elemental_clinc.

FFEHR. (2011). *Web page*. Retrieved May 12, 2011, from http://trac.afterfivetech.com/ffehr.

Fraser, H. S., Biondich, P., Moodley, D., Choi, S., Mamlin, B. W., & Szolovits, P. (2005). Implementing electronic medical record systems in developing countries. *Informatics in Primary Care, 13*(2), 83–95.

Fraser, H. S., Blaya, J., Choi, S. S., Bonilla, C., & Jazayeri, D. (2006). Evaluating the impact and costs of deploying an electronic medical record system to support TB treatment in Peru. In *Proceedings of the AMIA Annual Symposium*, (pp. 264–268). AMIA.

Fraser, H. S., Jazayeri, D., Nevil, P., Karacaoglu, Y., Farmer, P. E., & Lyon, E. (2004). An information system and medical record to support HIV treatment in rural Haiti. *British Medical Journal, 329*(7475), 1142–1146. doi:10.1136/bmj.329.7475.1142

FreeMED. (2011). *Web page*. Retrieved May 12, 2011, from http://freemedsoftware.org.

FreeMedForms. (2011). *Web page*. Retrieved May 12, 2011, from http://www.freemedforms.com/en/start.

GNUmed. (2011). *Web page*. Retrieved May 12, 2011, from http://wiki.gnumed.de/bin/view/Gnumed.

HL7. (2010). *Web page*. Retrieved December 14, 2010, from http://www.hl7.org.

Häyrinen, K., Saranto, K., & Nykänen, P. (2008). Definition, structure, content, use and impacts of electronic health records: A review of the research literature. *International Journal of Medical Informatics, 77*(5), 291–304. doi:10.1016/j.ijmedinf.2007.09.001

HealthForge. (2011). *Web page*. Retrieved May 12, 2011, from http://healthforge.codeplex.com.

Hibernate. (2010). *Web page*. Retrieved December 14, 2010, from http://www.hibernate.org.

Hospital, O. S. (2011). *Web page*. Retrieved May 12, 2011, from http://www.hospital-os.com/en.

HOSxP. (2011). *Web page*. Retrieved May 12, 2011, from http://hosxp.net.

HTML. (2010). *Web page*. Retrieved December 14, 2010, from http://www.w3.org/html.

Indivo. (2011). *Web page*. Retrieved May 12, 2011, from http://indivohealth.org.

Java. (2010). *Web page*. Retrieved December 14, 2010, from http://www.java.com/es.

Littlejohns, P., Wyatt, J. C., & Garvican, L. (2003). Evaluating computerised health information systems: Hard lessons still to be learnt. *British Medical Journal, 326*(7394), 860–863. doi:10.1136/bmj.326.7394.860

Mamlin, B. W., & Biondich, P. G. (2005). AMPATH medical record system (AMRS): Collaborating toward an EMR for developing countries. In *Proceedings of the AMIA Annual Symposium,* (pp. 490–494). AMIA.

Mamlin, B. W., Biondich, P. G., Wolfe, B. A., Fraser, H., Jazayeri, D., & Allen, C. … Tierney, W. M. (2006). Cooking up an open source EMR for developing countries: OpenMRS - A recipe for successful collaboration. In *Proceedings of the AMIA Annual Symposium,* (pp. 529–533). AMIA.

McMaster, O. S. C. A. R. (2011). *Web page*. Retrieved May 12, 2011, from http://en.wikipedia.org/wiki/OSCAR_McMaster.

Medical. (2011). *Web page*. Retrieved May 12, 2011 from http://medical.sourceforge.net.

Microsoft Infopath. (2010). *Web page*. Retrieved December 14, 2010, from http://office.microsoft.com/en-us/infopath.

Murray, C. J. L., Lopez, A. D., & Wibulpolprasert, S. (2004). Monitoring global health: Time for new solutions. *British Medical Journal, 329*, 1096–1100. doi:10.1136/bmj.329.7474.1096

MySQL. (2010). *Web page*. Retrieved December 14, 2010, from http://www.mysql.com.

Noor, A. M., Gikandi, P. W., Hay, S. I., Muga, R. O., & Snow, R. W. (2004). Creating spatially defined databases for equitable health service planning in low-income countries: The example of Kenya. *Acta Tropica, 91*, 239–251. doi:10.1016/j.actatropica.2004.05.003

Open Healthcare. (2011). *Web page*. Retrieved May 12, 2011, from http://www.openhealth.org.

OpenEMR. (2011). *Web page*. Retrieved January 15, 2011, from http://www.oemr.org.

OpenMRS. (2010). *Web page*. Retrieved December 14, 2010, from http://www.openmrs.org.

OpenVista. (2011). *Web page*. Retrieved January 15, 2011, from http://worldvista.sourceforge.net/openvista/index.html.

Partners in Health. (2010). *Electronic medical records*. Retrieved December 14, 2010, from http://www.pih.org/pages/electronic-medical-records.

Partners in Health. (2010). *Electronic medical records publications*. Retrieved December 14, 2010, from http://www.pih.org/pages/electronic-medical-records-publications.

Sainz, B., de la Torre, I., Bermejo, P., García, E., Díaz, F. J., Díez, J. F., … de Castro, C. (2010). Evolución, beneficios y obstáculos en la implantación del historial clínico electrónico en el sistema sanitario. *Revista esalud.com, 6*(22).

Seebregts, C. J., Mamlin, B. W., Biondich, P. G., Fraser, H. S., Wolfe, B. A., & Jazayeri, D. (2009). The OpenMRS implementers network. *International Journal of Medical Informatics, 78*(11), 711–720. doi:10.1016/j.ijmedinf.2008.09.005

Siika, A. M., Rotich, J. K., Simiyu, C. J., Kigotho, E. M., Smith, F. E., & Sidle, J. E. (2005). An electronic medical record system for ambulatory care of HIV-infected patients in Kenya. *International Journal of Medical Informatics*, *74*(5), 345–355. doi:10.1016/j.ijmedinf.2005.03.002

SmartCare. (2011). *Web page*. Retrieved May 12, 2011, from http://www.smartcare.org.zm.

SQL. (2010). *Web page*. Retrieved December 14, 2010, from http://www.sql.org.

Stansfield, S. (2005). Structuring information and incentives to improve health. *Bulletin of the World Health Organization*, *83*, 562.

Tolven Healthcare. (2011). *Web page*. Retrieved May 12, 2011, http://www.tolven.org.

Tomasi, E., Facchini, L. A., & Maia, M. F. (2004). Health information technology in primary health care in developing countries: A literature review. *Bulletin of the World Health Organization*, *82*(11), 867–874.

Trusted Opensource Records for Care and Health. (2011). *Web page*. Retrieved May 12, 2011, from https://launchpad.net/trusted. XML. (2010). *Web page*. Retrieved December 14, 2010, from http://www.w3.org/XML.

ZEPRS. (2011). *Web page*. Retrieved May 12, 2011, from http://www.ictedge.org/zeprs.

KEY TERMS AND DEFINITIONS

Electronic Health Records (EHR): Is an evolving concept defined as a systematic collection of electronic health information about individual patients or populations.

Free Software: Is software that can be used, studied, and modified without restriction, and which can be copied and redistributed in modified or unmodified form either without restriction, or with restrictions that only ensure that further recipients can also do these things and that manufacturers of consumer-facing hardware allow user modifications to their hardware.

OpenEMR: Generic system for the management of medical records that may assist on patients healthcare, collection of observations, visits to specialists, explanatory notes on individual patients, and other necessary data for diagnosis.

OpenMRS: Is an open source medical record system platform for developing countries with a focus on improving the lives of underprivileged people worldwide through health care service.

Open Source: Access to the source code with the following criteria; free redistribution, include source code, allow modifications and derived works, integrity of the author's source code, no discrimination against persons or groups, no discrimination against fields of endeavor, distribution of license, license must not be specific to a product, license must not restrict other software and license must be technology-neutral.

Pandemic: Is an epidemic of infectious disease that is spreading through human populations across a large region; for instance multiple continents, or even worldwide.

Patients: People who are receiving medical treatment.

Software Licenses: Is a legal instrument governing the usage or redistribution of software.

Undeveloped Countries: Is a country with a low standard of industrialization and low level of well being. Many undeveloped countries also have low standards of democratic governments, industrialization, social programs, and a poor human rights record.

VistA: Software for the management of medical records. It is built on a client-server architecture, which ties together workstations and personal computers with graphical user interfaces at Veterans Health Administration (VHA) facilities, as well as software developed by local medical facility staff.

Chapter 13
RFID in E–Health:
Technology, Implementation, and Security Issues

Peter J. Hawrylak
The University of Tulsa, USA

Nakeisha Schimke
The University of Tulsa, USA

John Hale
The University of Tulsa, USA

Mauricio Papa
The University of Tulsa, USA

ABSTRACT

Electronic healthcare or E-Health promises to offer better care at lower cost. This is critical as the cost of healthcare continues to increase and as the population ages. Radio Frequency Identification (RFID) technology is one form of wireless technology that will be part of the E-Health environment. RFID provides the ability to identify, track, and monitor patients and staff members. This enables better resource allocation, reduction of medical errors, and increased independence for patients. One part of E-Health is the Electronic Medical Record (EMR). New developments in RFID technology now enable the storage of all or part of the EMR on an RFID tag that remains with the patient. This chapter investigates the use of RFID in E-Health, how RFID can be used to store the EMR, and the security and privacy risks associated with using RFID to store the EMR.

INTRODUCTION

This chapter focuses on the use of Radio Frequency Identification (RFID) technology in E-Health applications and on the privacy issues related to

this. RFID is a wireless technology that can be used not only to identify a patient, but also to store information about that patient. This information can be incorporated into many hospital activities to improve performance and quality of care. Most RFID systems provide both write and re-write

DOI: 10.4018/978-1-4666-0888-7.ch013

capability. This is ideal for storing and updating a key parts of a patient's medical information. RFID tags are often included in patient wristbands and this enables their medical information to travel with them.

The first part of this chapter provides a brief overview of RFID describing the differences between general classes of RFID systems and a brief explanation of the physics behind passive RFID technology. Next, example cases of applications using RFID in the medical environment to monitor patents and medical staff are presented. These example cases focus on using RFID in applications beyond simply identifying the patient. The third part describes on how RFID can be used to store patient information such as the Electronic Medical Record (EMR). The EMR allows the development of systems to monitor patient activities remotely enabling the patient to be more independent while maintaining constant monitoring by medical personnel. Methods for storing this information are presented along with which classes of RFID technology are best suited to each method. However, significant security and privacy risks associated with this type of a system exist. The fourth part of the chapter presents security requirements for these systems to ensure that the patient's privacy is protected.

BACKGROUND

RFID has been around for a long time, with initial applications being in the areas of automatic toll collection and airline baggage handling systems (Landt, 2001; Landt, 2005). Hawrylak, Mickle, and Cain present the background and history of the technological development of RFID (Hawrylak, Cain, & Mickle, 2008). RFID is composed of three components: RFID tags, RFID readers, and middleware/backend software. RFID tags are attached to an asset or person. The RFID tag identifies the asset or person and provides a medium to store additional data about the asset

or person. This memory is commonly referred to as *user memory*. The RFID reader serves as the link between the middleware/backend software and the RFID tag. The RFID reader is responsible for communicating with the RFID tag and transferring information between the middleware/backend software and the RFID tag. The middleware/backend software represents two software components that are sometimes merged together. The middleware provides the glue logic, similar to a device driver, to connect the RFID reader to the backend system responsible for process control. Some advanced middleware platforms incorporate filtering and data processing capabilities to reduce the amount of data and requests sent to the backend software. The middleware connects to the backend software. In some RFID systems the middleware component is built into the RFID reader. The backend software provides the process control for the larger system. An Enterprise Resource Planning (ERP) system is one example of a backend system. Figure 1 illustrates the four major components in an RFID system.

RFID enhances a traditional ERP system by providing better visibility and insight in the real-time operation of the system or process being managed. In the medical environment RFID can provide better inventory management, inventory locating capability, improve patient throughput, and improve patient safety.

RFID Readers and Tags

RFID readers and tags provide the *last mile* connectivity between the backend system and the asset or person. RFID provides a wireless means to identify, track, and monitor the asset or person.

A barcode based identification system requires a line of sight between the barcode and the barcode scanner. While this is acceptable for supermarket and retail applications, the need for a line of sight causes problems in a number of environments including hospitals. Another drawback of barcodes is related to the fact that they are read using an

Figure 1. Overview of a typical RFID system

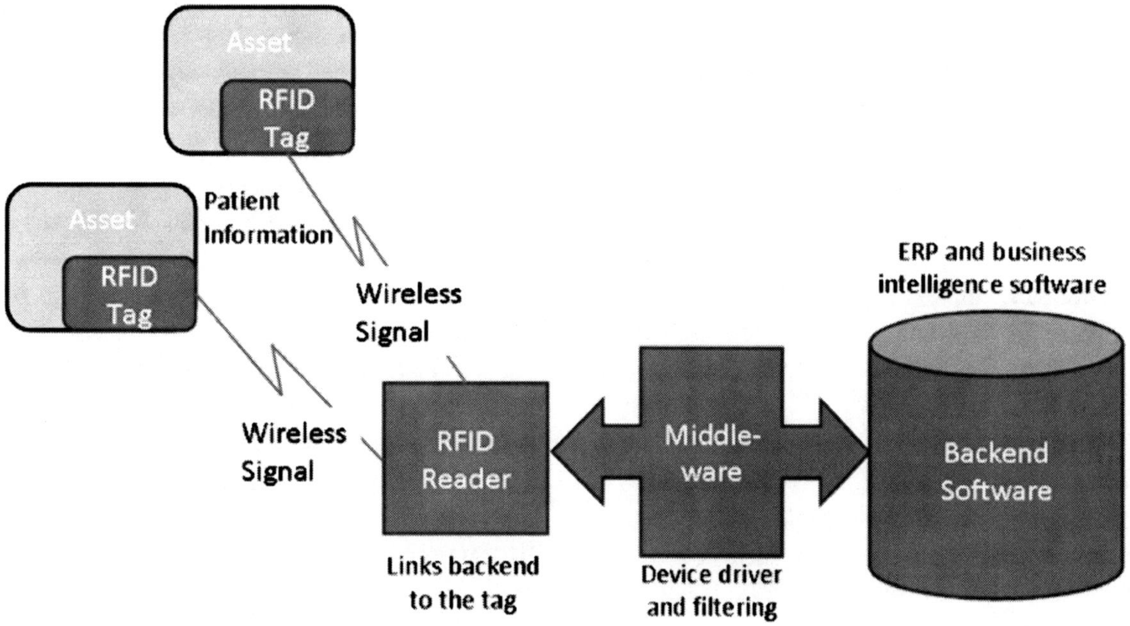

optical scanner. If the barcode becomes dirty or is damaged the optical scanner may interpret the barcode incorrectly or not be able to read it at all. The inability to read barcodes is cited as a significant issue identified in a survey of research studies into electronic versions of patient's medical records (Harrington, Kennerly, & Johnson, 2011).

On the other hand, RFID's wireless communication overcomes these problems and includes error detection capabilities, e.g. Cyclic Redundancy Check (CRC). More importantly, RFID does not require a line of sight between the RFID reader and RFID tag to establish communication. This is beneficial because the patient does not have to be disturbed (e.g. they are asleep) if their RFID tag is not visible to the medical staff. Most importantly, the user memory that is included with nearly all modern RFID tags enables data to be written and updated without adding additional area (volume) to the RFID tag. Barcodes cannot support updating already stored information as there is no method to erase or rewrite data already printed (e.g. correct mistakes) on the barcode (save

by physical erasure). Barcodes do support the addition of information but this requires more area because new barcode symbols must be printed on the barcode. The user memory in the RFID tag can be built using standard memory cells similar to those used in Flash sticks and RAM (random access memory) chips that are very compact and space efficient.

The RFID reader provides the communication link between the middleware/backend system and the RFID tag. In the case of passive RFID systems, the RFID reader also provides power to the RFID tag. RFID readers typically communicate with several RFID tags and cover large areas, such as a room, corridor, or medical supply cabinet.

Traditional RFID systems are reader-talk-first meaning that the RFID reader initiates all exchanges with the RFID tags. However, some systems such as the tag-talks-only-after-listening (TOTAL) variation of the ISO 18000-6 Type C UHF (860 MHz–960 MHz) passive RFID protocol (ISO 18000-6:2010, 2010) and some active RFID systems allow tags to initiate communication. In an active RFID system, tags initiate communication to issue alerts, alarms, or to relay messages as part of a mesh network infrastructure (e.g. ZigBee).

In a typical application, the RFID reader begins the exchange by identifying which RFID tags are within range. This process is termed *inventorying* and enables the RFID reader to retrieve the Unique Identifier (UID) from each RFID tag. The RFID reader carries out further communication with specific RFID tags as they are identified.

There are three categories of RFID tags: passive, Battery Assisted Passive (BAP), and active. Passive RFID tags have no on-board power supply (battery) and harvest their operating energy from the RFID reader's RF (radio frequency) transmission. These tags are widely used in the retail environment because of their low cost. Most patient identification applications will use passive tags because their low cost makes them a disposable item and minimizes any additional cost resulting from system deployment to the patient. For example, WalMart is currently using passive RFID tags to track the inventory of blue jeans currently on store shelves (Bustillo, 2010) and this model can easily be applied to patient or asset tracking in the hospital. Passive RFID tags use backscatter communication to send information back to the RFID reader.

Backscatter communication is based on the same principles as RADAR. In a RADAR system radio waves are transmitted that will be reflected back to the transmitter (source) by objects (e.g. airplanes). The amount of RF energy reflected back to the transmitter is determined by how well the object (e.g. an airplane) absorbs the RF energy. For example, a Boeing 737 jet will absorb very little energy and reflect most of the RF energy back to the transmitter, while a stealth fighter will absorb most of the energy and reflect very little energy back to the transmitter. Like airplanes, RFID tags reflect RF waves (energy) back to the RFID reader and backscatter communication uses the reflection to encode information. The amount of energy reflected back to the RFID reader is

determined by how well the antenna on the RFID tag is matched to the RFID tag electronics. A matched antenna will reflect very little energy, while an unmatched antenna will reflect most of the energy. The RFID tag can easily control the matching/unmatching of the antenna. Typically, this is accomplished by using a transistor (switch) to short the tag antenna to cause the unmatched condition. An overview of the design of a passive UHF RFID tag is provided by Ricci *et al.* (2010). By matching or unmatching the antenna, the RFID tag can encode information that is sent to the RFID reader by controlling the amount of energy reflected back to the RFID reader. Backscatter communication is useful because the RFID tag does not have to power a transmitter. Thus, the RFID tag can be energized (powered) by the RFID reader at a greater distance or in more unfavorable conditions. The typical communication range for passive RFID tags is between one and 15 meters depending on the type of tag.

BAP RFID tags (sometimes termed semi-passive tags) are a passive RFID tag with an on-board battery. The battery powers the intelligence (microprocessor) and/or sensors incorporated with the RFID tag. Typical uses of BAP RFID tags are in applications where sensor readings are required between reads. One example is a BAP RFID tag with an attached temperature sensor that is used to monitor the temperature of frozen food items or for pharmaceutical drugs. In comparison, a passive RFID would only be able to record the temperature when it was energized (read) by the reader, but a reader may not be available in a tractor-trailer during transit. BAP RFID tags use backscatter to respond to the RFID reader. In comparison to a passive RFID tag, a BAP RFID tag offers increased functionality while the battery lasts and then reverts to the functionality of a passive RFID tag after the battery is depleted. By reverting to a passive RFID tag after the battery is depleted, the BAP RFID tag can still interact with backend system although at a reduced level of functionality. One benefit of this is that the sensor

Table 1. RFID ISO protocols for each type of tag

Tag Type	ISO Protocols
Active	ISO 18000-7 (433 MHz)
BAP	ISO 18000-6 Type C (860 MHz – 960 MHz) using BAP extensions defined in ISO 18000-6
Passive	ISO 18000-2 (125-135 kHz) ISO 18000-3 (13.56 MHz) ISO 18000-6 (860 MHz – 960 MHz)

readings can be retrieved from the BAP RFID tag even after the battery is depleted. This information is still of value because it may contain an alarm condition that would indicate that the item may have been compromised. BAP RFID tags have a communication range slightly greater than passive RFID tags because all of the energy transmitted by the RFID reader can be used for communication. This results in a stronger backscatter signal that can travel farther, or be detected through higher levels of interference.

Active RFID tags have an on-board battery and communicate using an active or battery powered transmitter and receiver. Active RFID tags can communicate over ranges of several hundred meters. Active RFID tags are often used in environments that are unfriendly to passive or BAP RFID tags such as on board a container ship. Tracking and monitoring Twenty-Foot Equivalent Unit (TEU) cargo containers is one typical application for active RFID tags.

The International Organization for Standardization (ISO) has defined a set of standards for RFID, ISO 18000-*X*, where *X* denotes a particular operating frequency. Table 1 lists the ISO standards for the various types of RFID systems and frequencies in use today. Other RFID systems exist, but those use propriety protocols. The Table 1 lists the major RFID protocols for each tag type defined by ISO.

RFID tags contain memory that can be used to store information. All tags contain memory to hold at least the UID. The UID is often stored in a Read-Only Memory (ROM) at the time of tag manufacture. Re-writable memory is also in-

cluded in differing quantities in tags. This memory is divided into memory segments whose contents are defined by the protocol and the standard the tag complies with, and user memory. User memory is a blank piece of memory whose data and contents are determined by the user or application and is ideal for containing all or part of the EMR.

Passive tags typically have small user memories because of their powering restrictions. Larger memories require more power to operate and this means that the passive tag will have to harvest more energy from the reader and that there is less energy left over for the tag to backscatter its response back to the reader. This will reduce the maximum distance that communication can occur between the reader and tag. BAP tags can support larger memories than passive tags can because the memory can be powered from the battery. Active tags support the largest memories because of they are powered by high performance batteries.

The user memory in passive tags are typically designed to hold values such as an expiration date, for food or medical items, or a lot number, for retail goods. Passive tag supporting larger memories in the kilobyte range (KB) are available and being used in the airline industry (Swedberg, 2010b; Wessel, 2010). These high memory tags could also be used to store critical parts of the EMR. BAP tags typically use their memory to store sensor readings. Often BAP tags incorporate temperature sensors to monitor pharmaceuticals or frozen food temperatures (RFID Journal, 2010). Active tags may contain databases (e.g. ISO 18000-7 tags) and have large memories to store cargo manifests and sensor readings. Coupling sensors with RFID tags provides a useful platform for monitoring patients (Hoque, Dickerson, & Stankovic, 2010).

Physics of RFID

Passive RFID tags derive their operating power from the RFID reader's transmission by converting the Electro-Magnetic (EM) waves (wireless communication signal) into electrical energy. An antenna provides the conversion between EM waves and electrical energy and vice versa. Therefore, the amount of RF energy that a passive RFID tag can harvest is determined by the amount of energy that the RFID reader transmits and the amount of energy that the RFID tag's antenna can capture. The amount of energy that the RFID tag can harvest depends on a number of factors but the primary factors are (1) the amount of energy transmitted by the RFID reader; (2) the characteristics of the RFID tag antenna; and (3) the propagation effects, e.g. absorption, diffraction, and reflection, caused by the operating environment.

First, the amount of energy transmitted by the RFID reader defines how much total energy is available for the tag to harvest. The amount of energy that can be obtained typically decreases very quickly as the distance between the transmitting antenna and the receiving antenna increases. The simplified version of the Friis equation defines the amount of energy that can be received, P_R, based on wavelength, λ, (derived from the frequency of operation), distance between receiver and transmitter, r, gain of the receiving, G_R, and transmitting, G_T, antennae, and the transmitter power level, P_T. The Friis equation, Eq. (1), is valid only in the far field region of operation and in free space (outdoors).

$$P_R = \frac{P_T G_T G_R \lambda^2}{(4\pi r)^2} \qquad (1)$$

Second, the RFID tag antenna characteristics determine the volume from which the tag's antenna can collect the energy transmitted by the RFID reader. The larger this volume is, the greater the amount of energy that can be collected. This volume is referred to as the *electrical area* of the antenna. A common model for a transmitter is the isotropic model, which defines a single point in space as the emitter (transmitter). In the isotropic model the emitter transmits a signal, or energy, that radiates away from the emitter in all directions. This forms a sphere that grows over time as the EM waves travel away from the emitter and is reflected in the 4π quantity of the Friis equation above. The electrical area of the antenna also determines the frequency range (band) in which the antenna will operate in optimal condition. If one moves outside of this frequency band, a large percentage of the transmitted energy is not harvested. The shape of the antenna determines the impedance of the antenna. The antenna impedance determines how well the antenna transfers energy from the antenna to the attached Integrated Circuit (IC) or digital electronics, and what frequency band the antenna is optimize or tuned to. Matching the antenna impedance to the input impedance of the IC yields maximum power transfer between the IC and antenna, but may result in a smaller electrical area of the antenna.

Magnetic coupling between the reader and tag occurs in the *near field* and is different from the far field. In the near field, the tag and reader behave as an air core transformer. The reader acts as the primary coil and the tag as the secondary coil. The power received by the tag is proportional to the number of lines of magnetic flux that the tag antenna intersects or cuts. Near field systems are less susceptible to orientation issues than a far field system. In the far field for optimal power transfer, the orientation of the reader and tag antennae must be identical, e.g. either both horizontal or both vertical. This is determined by the polarization (vertical or horizontal) of the antennae. If the orientation of the two antennae is

Table 2. Frequency range for ISO standardized RFID protocols

Protocol	Frequency	Typical Range
ISO 18000-2	125-135 kHz	35 cm
ISO 18000-3	13.56 MHz	1 m
ISO 18000-6	860 MHz – 960 MHz	3-10 m
ISO 18000-7	433 MHz	100+ m

not optimal then some of the transmitted power will not be received by the tag and is lost. Near field systems are not as sensitive to orientation because the lines of flux wrap around the reader antenna forming a cylindrical volume inside which the tag can harvest energy by cutting the lines of flux at nearly any orientation. For this reason, HF systems are often used in applications where the orientation of the RFID tags is unknown or uncontrollable. HF systems are heavily used in pharmaceutical industry because orders consist of many different types of items and are filled in plastic totes and the tag orientation is not constant throughout the tote.

Third, the RF propagation effects alter the characteristics of the antenna and thus alter the behavior of the RFID tag. The composition of the item that the RFID tag is attached to can alter the impedance of the antenna and adjust the optimal frequency band for that antenna. As a result, RFID tags exist for specific products by optimizing the antenna for a frequency band above or below the desired operating band. When this RFID tag is applied to the product in question, the interaction between the product and antenna will adjust the optimal frequency band to the desired frequency band. In other cases, the item composition will absorb RF energy (RFID signals) reducing the amount of energy available to the RFID tag. Liquids, especially water, are particularly problematic. Water is problematic for UHF RFID systems because the water molecules are polar and the EM waves of the RFID signal cause these molecules to rotate. As a result, the water molecules absorb the EM waves and this rotation causes friction,

which generates heat. This is the same process used by microwave ovens to heat food. Low Frequency (LF) and High Frequency (HF) systems operate using magnetic, or near-field, coupling verses electrical coupling (used by UHF RFID) and have better performance around liquids. Magnetic coupling offers a shorter operating range (1 meter) than electrical coupling (3-10 meters). A comparison between HF RFID and near-field UHF systems is provided by Turner and Mickle (2007). An analysis was conducted by Fuschini *et al.* of near field UHF tags showing that there was little improvement in performance with respect to environmental conditions verses far field UHF tags (Fuschini, Piersanti, Sydanheimo, Ukkonen, & Falciasecca, 2010).

Wireless Interference

RFID is one of many wireless applications present in today's world. The majority of common RFID systems operate in one of the Industrial, Scientific, and Medical (ISM) frequency bands. ISM bands are provided for use by industry, scientific, and medical applications for free and without a license. The ISM bands used by RFID are 135 kHz, 13.56 MHz, 433 MHz, and 860 MHz to 960 MHz and the associated protocols are listed in the Table 2.

The operating frequency directly affects the range at which a reader and tag can communicate because the wavelength, λ, in Eq. (1) depends on the frequency. The operating range is directly proportional to the frequency. The range of the system is important when the RFID system is used to locate assets or patients.

Interference with other wireless systems is another important issue. Hospitals typically employ a Wi-Fi network to connect Personal Data Assistant (PDA) type devices and medical equipment to the hospital network. RFID systems are typically added afterward and must be selected so that their frequency of operation does not interfere with other wireless systems already in place. This issue must be studied carefully before deployment by a hospital's Information Technology (IT) group. Interference of a wireless device (e.g. cell phones) with medical devices and instruments must be carefully studied.

RFID Applications in the Medical Space

RFID provides increased visibility into processes that can be used to reduce operating costs and improve quality of care and patient safety. The use of RFID in medical environments falls into three categories, (1) identification of assets and people, (2) locating assets and people, and (3) providing data input into systems to improve patient quality of care.

The initial uses of RFID in hospitals paralleled the retail model for RFID to simply identify assets and extended the retail model to identify patients and staff members rather than just assets (Swedberg, 2011b; Lahtela, 2009; Nursing, 2006; Roark & Miguel, 2006). However, tailoring RFID systems to track medical supplies is still very useful, providing significant savings through better inventory management, lower labor costs to manage that inventory, and more accurate billing of patients (O'Connor, 2011a; O'Connor, 2011b). Distribution of medication in hospitals was an early application of RFID to improve quality of care. Hospitals typically dispense medication from a central pharmacy into small containers that are then given to nurses for delivery to the patients. Such a process can be very error prone, especially when hospitals have many patients. RFID has been used to prevent a patient from getting the wrong medication by tracking the medication and identifying the patient, with the backend system matching the patient to the medication and alerting the nurse to any discrepancy (Lai, Chien, Chang, Chen, & Fang, 2007). This type of system can be extended by storing a patient's drug information in the RFID tag and then checking that information against the new medication for harmful interactions (Ting, Tsang, Ip, & Ho, 2011). RFID can also be incorporated into automated medication dispensing equipment to identify the medication being retrieved. RFID can be combined with other technologies to link into the larger hospital information system. One such application uses RFID to identify a patient using a hand-held RFID reader and then provides a ZigBee connection to the central hospital information system (Jacob & Reddy, 2011).

Another example of RFID involves both inventory management and improving quality of care. Contrast agents, used in medical imaging procedures, are provided in specific volumes to specific patients. One system uses RFID tags to record the volume of available contrast agent in each syringe (Lavine, 2008). This system provides additional safeguards against using the wrong contrast agent for a patient or for using a syringe that cannot provide the necessary volume, potentially resulting in air being injected into the patient possibly leading to a fatality. Such a system can easily be incorporated into an inventory management system.

RFID can be used to identify medical staff members to patients. This helps patients identify whom they are talking with and is especially useful for those patients suffering from memory loss. Alternatively, a medical staff member can use RFID to retrieve a patient's medical history and then display that information on a PDA, smart phone, or computer screen (Kim & Jo, 2009). Other systems use RFID tags to track medical staff members' adherence to hand washing guidelines (Swedberg, 2010a). Infections can be quickly and easily spread among patients when proper hand washing is not observed.

In one application, RFID tags were used to store information for treatment of diabetes (Jara, Zamora, & Skarmeta, 2011). This application used the RFID tag to store dosage information that could be used by the patient and/or medical staff to adjust their medication and dosage. The RFID system provided the patient to system connection with other wireless technology connecting the system to medical devices and the hospital or doctor's office.

RFID tags can incorporate sensor devices that provide information about the surrounding environment. Such sensor equipped RFID tags can provide additional information about patients and enable some patients to remain independent. In one proposed system RFID tags would encode behavior rules for a given patient (Chen, Gonzalez, Leung, Zhang, & Li, 2010). In this system, the patient's activities are monitored through a variety of sensors and any violation of the behavior rules would generate an alert sent to the caregiver. Another important aspect of patient care is ensuring that the patient properly follows the medical guidance with respect to medications. RFID can be employed to monitor a patient's compliance with the prescribed treatment. One example of such a system is to monitor a patient's medicine intake to ensure that they are following the prescribed regime. If the patient has to take a large number of medications, it is easy for them to forget one or two. One system uses a special drawer equipped with RFID readers and pill bottles with RFID tags attached to log when a patient removes a bottle from the drawer (Becker, et al., 2009). This system assumes that the removal of the pill bottle indicates that the patient has taken the proper dose, and a later version incorporates a scale to weigh the pill bottles to verify if the proper dose was taken (Vinjumur, Becker, Ferdous, Galatas, & Makedon, 2010).

RFID also provides a platform for implantable devices as part of a body area network. Orthopedic implants are one example of implantable devices that are difficult to identify and monitor once installed. Physicians could provide better care by having access to physiological information relating to the implant, such as temperature and PH levels. This information would enable the physician to identify complications with the implant earlier and start treatment before the situation becomes severe. A team at the University of Pittsburgh, headed by Prof. Mickle, has developed technology to communicate with an RFID tag equipped with sensors on in orthopedic joint (Swedberg, 2011a).

Locating patients, staff members, and assets is another advantage offered by RFID. RFID location systems can be used to monitor and improve workflow, to find needed equipment, and to improve quality of care (Cangialosi, Monaly, & Yang, 2007; Hanser, Gruenerbl, Rodegast, & Lukowicz, 2008; Lee & Cho, 2007; Sanders, et al., 2008; Xiong, Seet, & Symonds, 2009). There are four general methods to determining location based on RFID or RF (radio frequency) communication. First, the knowledge that a tag was read by a particular reader can provide location. Because RFID systems have a limited range of a few meters in most indoor conditions a tag can be assumed to be within a few meters of the reader when it is read. A number of factors including the transmitter power level of the reader and environmental factors define the volume of this vicinity. Most readers have an adjustable transmitter power level that can be used to restrict the read range to only the desired volume such as an entrance or exit point. Linking the date and time of the read enables the system to locate the person or asset at a specific time.

The second method uses the time it takes for the wireless message to travel from the reader to the tag and then back to the reader. This method is known as Time-Of-Arrival (TOA) and provides a maximum distance away from the reader. The speed of the RF wave (signal) is approximately the speed of light in free space. Thus, based on the time and velocity of the RF wave the distance between transmitter and receiver can be determined.

However, this distance is the straight-line distance between the two and this assumption may not be correct indoors because the RF signal can bend around corners as a result of reflections. Thus, the accuracy of the TOA method is limited, but is usually sufficient to provide an accurate location to the room level.

The third method estimates the distance the tag is from the reader based on the amount of power in the message the tag transmits to the reader. This method is known as received signal strength (RSS). RSS is based on the fact that in free space the signal strength will increase as the tag moves closer to the reader. However, indoors this may not be the case due to the multipath effect caused by the RF signal reflecting off objects (e.g. walls and equipment). Multipath can introduce significant error into the location based on RSS methods. The RSS of a tag's reply is a commonly provided as an output by RFID readers and can easily be incorporated into location determination software.

A fourth option combines two or more of the previous three methods in a hybrid method. By combining multiple methods, the inaccuracies of each method can be addressed to some level by the other method(s). The later three methods involve signal processing and require complex software. The first method provides a coarse location, approximately to the room level, but requires only a database to hold the read area of each reader and the ability to overlay that area on a floor plan of the medical facility.

Angle Of Arrival (AOA) is one method to determine direction of the tag relative to the reader based on the angle the signal arrived at the reader antenna. Reflectors can be placed on the antenna to limit the angle from which it can receive signals or an antenna array (e.g. a phased array antenna) can be used to construct a steerable antenna. The antenna array option is complex and too expensive, and while the reflector option can be constructed more economically, it requires multiple antennae. Reflectors are often used when the reader is placed next to a wall to prevent the reader from

identifying tags through the wall that are outside of the room. Such reflectors are economical because multiple antennas are not needed as there is no need to read tags on the other side of the wall (outside the room) and improve the accuracy of the reported location.

Linking an RFID Tag to Patient Information

RFID tags contain a Unique Identifier (UID) or serial number. This UID can be used as a key to index a central database to retrieve information associated with that UID (RFID tag). The UID can be used by a hospital to retrieve the patient's information from the hospital's central database, as illustrated in Figure 2. The staff member (e.g. doctor or nurse) would have access to the RFID reader or computer terminal connected to the reader in order to access the EMR retrieved from the patient database. This works well within the same facility or at a facility within the same network, e.g. same health-insurance network. However, this system breaks down when the patient goes to two or more medical facilities that maintain separate central databases and do not share their databases with each other. Another issue is the frequency of updates to the central database. The patient may be seen by one doctor and then a second doctor before the first doctor's diagnosis and recommendations have been entered into the system and have had time to propagate through to the central database. This could lead to the second doctor having incomplete or inaccurate information resulting in the second doctor potentially prescribing conflicting and/or harmful treatments.

Synchronization of patient information is identified as an issue with EMRs that can be solved by storing the EMR with the patient (Harrington, Kennerly, & Johnson, 2011). This could be the complete EMR or critical parts of the EMR such as name, date of birth, and drug allergies. Storing the EMR in the patient's RFID is a better solution

Figure 2. Tag UID used to index patient database

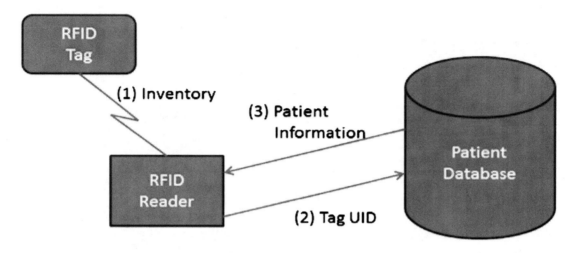

and provides a backup in the event of a failure of the central database. This option addresses the above problem and allows the patient's medical record to travel with the patient. The tag may contain all or part of the patient's EMR. The system where the entire EMR is stored on the tag is illustrated in Figure 3(a) and the case where only part of the EMR is stored on the tag is illustrated in Figure 3(b). Ting *et al.* (Ting, Tsang, Ip, & Ho, 2011) developed the RF-MediSys system which stored core patient and medical information in a RFID enabled smart-card carried by the patient.

This system enabled the patient to have their medical information available to any doctor. Results of the one month test deployment of the RF-MediSys system were very positive. Storing only the critical parts of the EMR on the tag, e.g. patient name and drug allergies, enables the use of tags with less memory that have a lower cost.

Storing the EMR in the RFID tag requires standardization of the data format to enable any medical facility to read the EMR. RFID tags provide a blank memory system but do not provide a file system as is provided by a typical Operating

Figure 3. (a) Entire EMR stored on the tag; (b) partial EMR stored on the tag

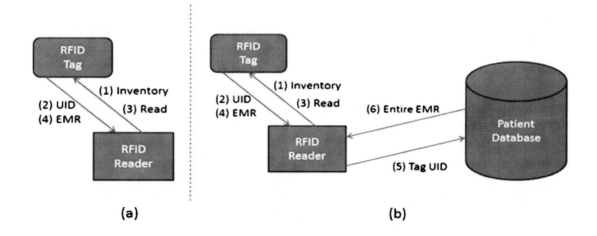

Figure 4. Data storage methods: (a) delimiter method, (b) directory method, and (c) hybrid method

Name	8$	Date of Birth	8$	Medications	8$	...

(a)

Address:	0	4	8	12	50	60	...
	Name: 12	Date of Birth: 50	Medications: 60	Name	Date of Birth	Medications	

(b)

Address:	0	1	38	39	40	...
	Name	37	Date of Birth	49	Medications	

(c)

System (OS). As a result, a means to denote where one piece of information begins and ends in the RFID tag's memory is important. Encoding the location of the beginning and end of each field or file results in overhead and reduces the amount of memory available for the EMR in the RFID tag. The ideal solution will be able to handle a variety of data types including medical images with very low overhead.

One method to separate data fields is to use a set delimiter. For example, for text data the sequence of characters "8$" may never appear and could be used as the delimiter. This method is illustrated in Figure 4(a). This is a simple and low overhead solution but will not work for the EMR. The EMR may need to contain medical images (e.g. x-rays) or other data that are stored in binary format and cannot guarantee that the pattern "8$" will never appear within the medical image. If that pattern were present in a medical image, it would appear to be two separate data fields rather than one data field. Longer length delimiters can be employed to reduce the frequency of matching a piece of data but this can never be guaranteed.

Another solution is to provide a directory for the data fields and is illustrated in Figure 4(b). A directory can be viewed as a simple file system for the tag memory. The directory is stored in a specific memory location in the RFID tag memory. One option is for the directory to maintain the beginning and ending addresses of each data field. The directory must be allocated enough memory to grow. The memory space allocated for the directory will determine the maximum number of data fields that can be stored in the tag.

A hybrid between the directory and the delimiter method is to store the directory information (end address of the data item) with each data field. The ending address of the data item could be stored as the first *n* bits of the data item. An alternative implementation would store the length of the data item in terms of bits or bytes depending on the data standard instead of the end address. This is preferable if the length of most data items can be stored, using fewer bits than the ending address would require and is illustrated in Figure 4(c). This overcomes the problem of needing to set aside memory for the directory and allows the tag memory to be used efficiently for both large numbers of small data items or small numbers of large data items. Searching for a particular data field in memory must be done serially (one at a time) with this method because there is no central map of the data fields in memory. Rather, each data item must be read to identify if it is desired item and if not to determine the starting address of the next data item. Encoding a type field with the address of the next data item simplifies searching because if the type does not match the desired type there is no need to read more data other than the address of the next data item. However, adding a type field increases the overhead of the data management system.

The hybrid method is probably the best method for data mapping because of the low overhead and flexibility with the type and size of data items. The hybrid method will maximize memory storage space because memory is stored serially in the tag from beginning to end.

Active tags complying with the ISO 18000-7 standard (ISO/IEC 18000-7:2009, 2009) support database functionality, including support for database queries. The database structure can be used to store the EMR. However, active tags typically, cost significantly more than passive tags and may not be economical for patient identification. The issue of replacing batteries in active tags is another downside to their use for patient identification. Active tags will not function after the battery is depleted and this can be problematic for a patient identification system. However, the database query capability simplifies information retrieval.

The time required to search the tag memory to retrieve the desired data items must be taken into account (Ogirala, Murari, Hawrylak, & Mickle, 2011). There are three different general methods to retrieve data items from the tag. The first is to read the contents of the entire tag memory and parse the information on the reader, middleware, or backend. This is very time consuming for tags with large memories and is inefficient if only a few data items are required (e.g. patient name and

date of birth). However, this method simplifies the structure and format of the data being stored in the tag because no directory or other information is required to be maintained in the tag. The delimiter storage method requires that the interrogator to read each data item serially until the desired item is located. Searching in this manner requires time proportional to the location of the requested data item. There is no need to start at the lowest memory address and work toward the higher memory addresses. The interrogator can start at the middle and read in either direction, or start at the highest address and read toward the lowest address.

The majority of tags support the ability to read memory starting at an arbitrary address or offset that is included with the read command issued by the reader. The second method leverages this capability to access the request data item directly. If the memory layout is known a priori then the interrogator can request the data item directly without having to retrieve the earlier items. The directory collects this information in a known location, usually in the lower address range. This provides an efficient means to locate and retrieve required information. The interrogator can retrieve the directory to obtain the starting and ending address of the requested data. Using this information the interrogator can use the read operation to retrieve the data directly.

The third method is similar to the serial search (first method) but with the data stored in the hybrid format. The interrogator can read the first few bytes of a particular data item to determine if it is of interest. If the data is not of interest the interrogator has the starting address of the next data item (see Figure 4[c]) and can move quickly to the next data item. This method requires multiple memory read exchanges between the interrogator and tag and may be more efficient than the serial searching using the delimiter if the data items are large. If the data are small then a single read command would be able to read multiple data items in one exchange. The overhead required for each read exchange must be considered to determine which method is better. In the case of small data items, the overhead for the multiple exchanges may be more than the savings provided by the hybrid method.

Data Items Making up the EMR

The EMR is composed of a number of standard data items. Common to all EMRs is the patient name and ID assigned by the hospital. Each RFID tag has a *unique* serial number associated with it. Typically, the UID is the unique serial number that is stored in the RFID tag, which is a good choice because this number is meaningless and is not linked to any personal identification such as a Social Security Number (SSN) or driver's license number. The link between the tag UID and the patient's personal information is made in the backend software (see Figure 1). Thus, the patient's personal information can be secured using accepted and well-understood network security procedures. When storing EMR data with the patient sensitive information such as the SSN could be either encrypted or stored only in the backend software. The majority of queries about the patient will start by checking the patient's name and UID so these items should be stored at the beginning of the EMR so they can be retrieved quickly without having to search through a number of fields. Other important and frequently used information, such as current medications, drug allergies, date of birth, physical condition, and emergency contact person should be stored after the name and UID. Specific items such as x-ray images and diagnoses can be stored item by item. These items are likely to be used relatively infrequently by specialists and can be stored in locations requiring longer search times and if there is space in the tag memory.

Security Features of Tag Data Memory

Passive RFID tags following the ISO 18000-6 Type C standard have memory banks that can be individually locked. This locking feature enables each memory bank to require a password before it can be written to, or writing can be disabled completely (ISO/IEC 18000-6:2010, 2010). This functionality needs to be extended to support limiting read access as well as write access. By extending this functionality to include both read and write access, both privacy and data integrity can be achieved. Privacy is achieved because the data cannot be read unless the correct password is provided, and integrity because the data cannot be modified without the proper password. Existing and accepted password management, distribution, and storage methods can be implemented to secure passwords.

Currently, ISO 18000-6 Type C allows locking only the entire user memory, but in the case where the EMR is stored in the tag, this is not sufficient. For the EMR individual items must be secured and different users given specific access rights similar to the access rights (e.g. read, write, and execute) to files on a shared computer. Therefore, future RFID tags must support the ability to lock individual sections, even down to the byte level, to support multiple users.

One important consideration using a password to protect the memory data is to prevent a replay attack. In a replay attack, the attacker records a previous exchange where a legitimate user accesses a tag with a valid password. The attacker later uses this password to access that memory area on the tag. By locking individual sections of the tag with different passwords, the attacker will be limited to what data they can access. Ideally, changing the passwords or using a public-private key system to exchange passwords will thwart the replay attack. However, changing passwords is difficult to manage in practice because the new password must be propagated to the tag and all readers in the facility. The public-private key infrastructure is problematic for passive tags because of the added energy requirement for the encryption routines. In addition, the key management system must be implemented correctly to prevent that from being a source of compromise for the overall system.

Encryption of the information before it is written to the tag is another option. The encryption and decryption routines would be performed on the reader, middleware, or backend systems. Thus, the tag does not have to support the advanced processing capabilities required for encryption algorithms such as public-key encryption. Different encryption keys could be used to enable different levels of access to the data. For example, doctors may have access to the nurse and staff keys to read the information they write to the tag. If public key cryptology is used read access and write access can be separated because the public key could be shared with authorized users, e.g. doctors, nurses, or medical staff, while the private key would only be available to member of a particular group, e.g. nurses.

Passive and BAP tags typically cannot support the required advanced processing capabilities required for public-key encryption due to power and cost constraints. While these capabilities could be added, the resulting tags would not meet the customer's requirements and would thus not be economical. While active tags can support advanced encryption techniques, e.g. public-key encryption, if this functionality can be moved to the reader side the tag's battery will last longer. Thus, the lifetime of the active tag will increase.

Encrypting the data before the data are written to the tag also simplifies key distribution issues. Key distribution is required to pass the private or secret keys to authorized devices so that they can decrypt information from the tags. However, the key distribution systems are often the Achilles heel of security systems. If an attacker compromises the key distribution system, they can obtain all of the private or secret keys that are sent through the key distribution network. Therefore, it is imperative that proper and accepted security practices be applied to the key distribution system. Limiting the number of machines that perform the encryption simplify the key distribution network and the task of securing the key distribution network.

In the data encryption method, each group could share a common secret key that is used to encrypt the information. A group could be all medical staff members within one health insurance plan or all staff members within a specific doctor's office. Multiple groups can place information on the tag and only those with access to their secret key can decode and read that information. Thus, the encryption method can be applied to any tag with sufficient memory and all of the multi-user capability is off-loaded to the reader/middleware/backend side.

PRIVACY AND SECURITY RISKS OF RFID

Privacy is an important concern in medical environments. In the US, healthcare providers must comply with privacy guidelines in the Health Insurance Portability and Accountability Act of 1996 (HIPAA). The HIPAA Privacy Rule establishes Protected Health Information (PHI) fields and how they must be handled (U.S. Department of Health and Human Services, 2011). The HIPAA Security Rule creates security standards for transmitting and storing patient data through administrative, physical, and technological measures. Any automated EMR system must follow these guidelines to ensure privacy and put in place security features to prevent the disclosure of confidential information to unauthorized individuals. These features must be implemented at every level of the RFID architecture, including the middleware and backend solutions.

Special privacy considerations may be required when storing the EMR locally on the RFID tag (Ting, Kwok, Tsang, & Lee, 2011). These tags may contain a wealth of personal and medical information about the patient. Local storage can improve data integrity as well as the battery life of the tag by reducing the need for frequent data federation, but an attack need only access the tag to discover EMR data. Healthcare providers must also be able to detect and report data breaches.

The preservation of patient privacy is principally a function of healthcare information system security. Security practices can be categorized as focusing on three general properties: integrity, confidentiality, and availability. Any security function or control incorporated within a system serves to promote one or more of these three core properties. Integrity is concerned with maintaining correct data in the system, so that the information recorded in the system is accurate. Confidentiality focuses on preventing data from being disclosed to unauthorized users. Availability requires that system resources—services and data—be accessible by authorized users when needed and in a timely manner.

The three security properties of integrity, confidentiality, and availability may come into conflict with each other and accordingly must be balanced by the control set to harmonize with the operational and mission objectives of the system. These properties are often depicted as a triangle where each point within the triangle represents a combination of the three (Krutz & Vines, 2003).

In the medical setting integrity and confidentiality are the prevailing concerns; availability, while beneficial, is not regarded as critical because backup systems, e.g. a computer terminal or paper chart, are commonly in place and can be used if the RFID EMR functionality is not available. Availability can be disrupted within the hospital or medical facility site with very limited impact on patient care because patients are treated by the staff at that particular location. It is important to note, however, that as a service such as RFID-based patient monitoring becomes deeply integrated within an information system to the extent that the system relies on it to function, availability emerges as an overriding concern. The general strategy for mitigating risks associated with threats to availability is system redundancy and resiliency as implemented by backup and failover solutions that exhibit qualities of graceful service degradation.

During treatment, ensuring data integrity is critical to prevent medical mistakes being made due to incorrect information stored in the tag. Inaccurate medical records can also negatively impact a patient's treatment schedule and their ability to obtain private health insurance, and can even introduce billing errors. To mitigate the risk of threats to data integrity in RFID (by both intentional and unintentional acts), data on the tag should be protected by an error detection scheme such as a checksum or a CRC. The error detection mechanism will alert the system to errors present in the data due to transmission errors or physical errors with the tag's memory. Where computing power and bandwidth will permit, more robust and cryptographically based Message Authentication Codes (MACs) may be employed to offer a higher degree of assurance and to support data origin authenticity. (It should be stated that such schemes require a key management solution and infrastructure that could unduly burden an otherwise lightweight RFID deployment.)

While integrity promotes the accuracy of information, confidentiality is focused on protecting information from disclosure to unauthorized individuals. Confidentiality can be breached many ways: both intentional and unintentional (e.g. where a patient's files are accidentally discarded). It is natural to consider personal health information as the primary target in an attack on confidentiality, but other kinds of data may be targets as well. System passwords and configuration data may be equally valuable to an adversary conducting network reconnaissance in building a subsequent attack plan over a healthcare information system. Depending on the specific implementation, harvesting this kind of information from RFID systems may yield knowledge particularly damaging to an information system's security posture. Access control, backed by a practical authentication service that binds identities to subjects and processes, is a core service that promotes data confidentiality. Access control services are composed of policy and enforcement elements. An access control policy language expresses which subjects can access what data and how (e.g., read, write or execute). An access control enforcement engine uses reference monitors, along with physical and cryptographic isolation strategies to prevent unauthorized disclosure of data.

RFID Attack Vectors

Attack vectors for RFID systems fall into one of four categories, (1) interception, (2) interruption, (3) modification, and (4) fabrication. All four categories have corresponding implications for privacy and security. In RFID systems, interception occurs when the adversary listens to the exchanges between the reader and tag. The general term for such an attack is *eavesdropping*. Because the reader-to-tag link is wireless the exchange can easily be observed by a third party within range of the reader and is often termed *sniffing*. Interruption deals with the methods available to the adversary to reduce the quality of service for the RFID network by blocking messages in the network. This may adversely affect service or, in extreme cases, cause a complete Denial of Service (DoS). While in certain cases a DoS attack may have little impact on privacy, it could be used as part of a larger attack to obtain confidential information. Forcing the healthcare provider into relying on the failover mechanism (in response to a DoS attack) could potentially expose patient data and interrupt the delivery of service. Modification is when the adversary attempts to alter data on the tag or in the main system using the tag as an entry point to carry out the modification. With respect to security, this type of attack could be used to elevate the privileges of the attacker to enable them to access confidential information or to impersonate a reader with a tag. Fabrication deals with the insertion of messages in the network. They can be used in conjunction with fake credentials or identity to obtain elevated access

privileges. As with modification, fabrication attacks are typically used to elevate the attacker's access level to provide them access to confidential information. A *Man-In-The-Middle* (MITM) attack is one common form of fabrication attack.

Sniffing or eavesdropping is a common security threat to all wireless systems. The adversary can obtain additional information by monitoring the reader/tag exchange. For example, the ISO 18000-6 Type C protocol, based on the EPC Gen-2 protocol (EPCglobal Inc., 2008), defines a series of three steps to access an RFID tag; (1) selection, (2) inventory; and (3) access (ISO 18000-6:2010, 2010). During the selection phase, the set of tags that will participate in the inventory phase is determined. The Select command provides the reader the ability to include or exclude tags based on their UID or data stored in their user memory areas. During the inventory phase, the UID from each participating tag is obtained. An eavesdropper observing a series of Select commands and the subsequent inventory phase can potentially link patient information, such as medical condition, to particular tags. Hawrylak and Mickle present an overview of Gen-2 protocol and the use of the Select command (Hawrylak & Mickle, 2010). Ultimately, the eavesdropper can link those tags to a particular individual. This scenario requires the adversary to know the format and layout of the EMR stored in the RFID tag and this is feasible because the EMR format and layout will most likely be standardized in the near future.

Alternatively, the adversary can observe data read/write messages between the reader and tag to obtain the EMR. If the data is unencrypted the adversary can learn part or all of the patient's EMR.

Typical ISO 18000-6 Type C tags cannot economically support public key style encryption capability. Using a centralized approach can help alleviate this problem by reducing the computational burden on the tags. On the other hand, this would limit Select commands to working with a single tag unless multiple tags share the same key, which would considerably weaken the public key security. This tradeoff of encryption strength versus usability must be investigated and the appropriate level determined on a case-by-case basis. A centralized solution may help to solve the key distribution problem (often the Achilles heel of public key encryption systems) and encryption/decryption processing requirements.

Tracking is another major privacy concern. The UID associated with each RFID tag can be used by the adversary to track the location of the tag and person associated with that tag. However, tracking using RFID requires the adversary to either gain access to the RFID infrastructure in the facility or to install their own RFID readers throughout the facility. Adequate network and system security can prevent the former while adequate physical security can prevent the latter. The adversary would have to place their own reading devices within a few meters of the areas they wished to monitor because most RFID patient identification systems will be based on passive technology. The requisite level of network security and access control is typically found in most doctor's offices and hospitals.

Clandestine reading of a RFID tags is a significant threat to privacy. Such an attack requires the adversary to have their own reader or to have access to an existing reader. Clandestine reading can be used to link a tag UID to a particular individual in order to track that individual. More intrusive attacks would allow the adversary to obtain information about the individual from the tag. For example, the Select command (ISO 18000-6:2010, 2010) can be used by the adversary to search for patients with a particular medical condition, e.g. cancer. The adversary would then conduct the inventory round to determine if any of the patients within range match the criteria in the Select command. Only those tags that match the Select command criteria will participate in the subsequent inventory round. Conversely, the adversary can obtain information and draw inferences from knowing what information is not present on the tag.

Clandestine reading and tracking can be addressed in a number of ways. First, sensitive information can be encrypted to prevent unauthorized third parties from reading sensitive data. However, this does not address tracking because each tag will still have a UID, whether encrypted or not, that can be used to track the individual. Jamming is one method that can be employed to prevent tracking. Solutions such as the Blocker Tag (Juels & Brainard, 2004; Juels, Rivest, & Szydlo, 2003) can prevent the reader from reading any tag. This type of solution would not be acceptable in most cases. While it may help protect privacy, jamming countermeasures render legitimate uses of RFID unusable. Other methods include having a tag that responds only to authorized readers. Authorization could be performed through a challenge-response exchange or by the tag maintaining a list of authorized readers. The latter method is less flexible because legitimate new readers will not be viewed as authorized by the tag, and a fake reader could impersonate a legitimate reader by using the same reader ID.

Adequate physical security is key to preventing the vast majority of clandestine reading and tracking attacks. Physical security may include detective controls such as video cameras and sensors, as well as locks, doors and shielded walls to limit access to a location. Detective controls are useful for minimizing the impact of a threat—once detected, an attack can quickly be handled. Controls that limit access to physical space minimizes the likelihood of a reading or tracking attack because an adversary must be able to place the necessary readers to track or read the tags proximal to their location.

The National Industrial Security Program Operators Manual provides guidance on implementing a physical security program from the perspective of protecting classified information (Department of Defense, 2006). While the operational context and security model is different, the solutions, procedures, and processes described therein are also largely applicable to protecting medical information flowing across a RFID system. NIST

SP 800-98 also offers some guidance on physical access controls for RFID systems (Karigiannis, Eydt, Barber, Bunn, & Phillips, 2007).

Man-in-the-middle attacks are not considered a major threat to patient privacy due to the specific features of the physical and data-link layers in the RFID environment. This type of attack attempts to trick the legitimate RFID tag and reader into thinking that they are in close physical proximity while they are really very far apart. This main use for this type of attack would be to circumvent access control and to gain entry to restricted areas. For instance, an adversary may try to gain access to the medical records room to steal personal information by impersonating an IT staff member. The attacker would have to obtain privileged data from a valid IT badge and then use that information to impersonate the staff with that ID to an RFID-enabled door.

Relay attacks are conducted using a fake interrogator and a fake tag to relay messages between a legitimate interrogator and a legitimate tag. The only requirement is that the fake interrogator and fake tag be able to communicate information fast enough to fit within the time window required by the protocol. Passive RFID systems are very slow compared to other wireless technology such as Wi-Fi or a cellular modem. This is a result of the tag needing to be energized by the reader before it can compute the response. Thus, there is sufficient time in the RFID protocols for the fake tag and fake interrogator to communicate and still respond to the legitimate device before it times out.

CONCLUSION

RFID provides a number of benefits to the medical environment. The advent of passive tags with a large memory enable the storage of part or all of the EMR in the RFID tag. Thus, the EMR can follow the patient throughout their hospital stay. Having this information reside with the patient provides the medical staff with immediate access to the patient's medical record and will reduce medical errors and improve the quality of care.

The formatting and storage of the EMR in the RFID tag's memory is an important consideration and should be standardized to provide interoperability among healthcare providers and lower cost. This will simplify searching and retrieval of information from the EMR. Methods to enforce access rights to the individual sections of the EMR are required as multiple users will need to access the EMR. HIPAA requirements must also be investigated and enforced in any system.

In summary, eavesdropping, tracking, and malicious reading of tags are the chief privacy concerns relating to RFID for storing a patient's medical information. Employing standard physical and network security practices can eliminate most of these threats. Physical security is the most effective means to combat these threats and is inherently provided in doctor's offices and hospitals. Thus, RFID provided significant opportunities to improve the quality of patient care by storing the EMR on the patient.

REFERENCES

Becker, E., Metsis, V., Arora, R., Vinjumur, J., Xu, Y., & Makedon, F. (2009). SmartDrawer: RFID-based smart medicine drawer for assistive environments. In *Proceedings of the 2nd international Conference on Pervsive Technologies Related To Assistive Environments (PETRA 2009)*, (pp. 1-8). New York, NY: ACM Press.

Bustillo, M. (2010, July 23). Wal-Mart radio tags to track clothing. *Wall Street Journal*. Retrieved Feb. 18, 2011, from http://online.wsj.com/article/SB10001424052748704421304575383213061198090.html.

Cangialosi, A., Monaly, J. E., & Yang, S. C. (2007). Leveraging RFID in hospitals: Patient life cycle and mobility perspectives. *IEEE Communications Magazine, 45*(9), 18–23. doi:10.1109/MCOM.2007.4342874

Chen, M., Gonzalez, S., Leung, V., Zhang, Q., & Li, M. A. (2010). 2G-RFID-based e-healthcare system. *IEEE Wireless Communications, 17*(1), 37–43. doi:10.1109/MWC.2010.5416348

Department of Defense. (2006). *National industrial security program operating manual.* Washington, DC: Department of Defense.

EPCGlobal Inc. (2008). *EPC™ radio-frequency identity protocols class-1 generation-2 UHF RFID protocol for communications at 860 MHz – 960 MHz version 1.2.0.* New York, NY: EPCGlobal, Inc.

Fuschini, F., Piersanti, C., Sydanheimo, L., Ukkonen, L., & Falciasecca, G. (2010). Electromagnetic analyses of near field UHF RFID systems. *IEEE Transactions on Antennas and Propagation, 58*(5), 1759–1770. doi:10.1109/TAP.2010.2044328

Hanser, F., Gruenerbl, A., Rodegast, C., & Lukowicz, P. (2008). Design and real life deployment of a pervasive monitoring system for dementia patients. In *Proceedings of the Second International Conference on Pervasive Computing Technologies for Healthcare*, (pp. 279-280). IEEE.

Harrington, L., Kennerly, D., & Johnson, C. (2011). Safety issues related to the electronic medical record (EMR): Synthesis of the literature from the last decade, 2000-2009. *Journal of Healthcare Management, 56*(1), 31–43.

Hawrylak, P. J., Cain, J. T., & Mickle, M. H. (2008). RFID tags. In Yan, L., Zhang, Y., Yang, L. T., & Ning, H. (Eds.), *The Internet of Things: From RFID to Pervasive Networked Systems* (pp. 1–32). Boca Raton, FL: Auerbach Publications, Taylor & Francis Group. doi:10.1201/9781420052824.ch1

Hawrylak, P. J., & Mickle, M. H. (2010). EPC gen-2 standard for RFID. In Yan, L., Zhang, Y., Yang, L. T., & Chen, J. (Eds.), *RFID and Sensor Networks: Architectures, Protocols, Security, and Integrations* (pp. 97–123). Boca Raton, FL: Auerbach Publications, Taylor & Francis Group.

Hoque, E., Dickerson, R. F., & Stankovic, J. A. (2010). Monitoring body positions and movements during sleep using WISPs. In *Proceedings of Wireless Health, 2010*, 44–53.

ISO/IEC 18000-6. (2010). *Information technology -- Radio frequency identification for item management -- Part 6: Parameters for air interface communications at 860 MHz to 960 MHz.* Geneva, Switzerland: International Organization for Standardization.

ISO/IEC 18000-7. (2009). *Information technology — Radio frequency identification (RFID) for item management — Part 7: Parameters for active RFID air interface communications at 433 MHz.* Geneva, Switzerland: International Organization for Standardization.

Jacob, N., & Reddy, K. T. V. (2011). Smart hospital using RFID and ZigBee technology. In *Proceedings of the International Conference & Workshop on Emerging Trends in Technology (ICWET 2011)*, (pp. 987-989). New York, NY: ACM Press.

Jara, A. J., Zamora, M. A., & Skarmeta, A. F. (2011). An internet of things--Based personal device for diabetes therapy management in ambient assisted living (AAL). *Personal and Ubiquitous Computing, 15*(4), 431–440. doi:10.1007/s00779-010-0353-1

Journal, R. F. I. D. (2010). RFID news roundup – March 15, 2010. *RFID Journal.* Retrieved February 19, 2011, from http://www.rfidjournal.com/article/view/7492.

Juels, A., & Brainard, J. (2004). Soft blocking: Flexible blocker tags on the cheap. In *Proceedings of the 2004 ACM Workshop on Privacy in the Electronic Society*, (pp. 1-7). ACM Press.

Juels, A., Rivest, R. L., & Szydlo, M. (2003). The blocker tag: Selective blocking of RFID tags for consumer privacy. In *Proceedings of the 10th ACM Conference on Computer and Communications Security*, (pp. 103-111). ACM Press.

Karigiannis, T., Eydt, B., Barber, B., Bunn, L., & Phillips, T. (2007). *Special publication 800-98 guidelines for securing radio frequency identification (RFID) systems*. Washington, DC: National Institute of Standards and Technology.

Kim, Y., & Jo, H. (2009). Patient information display system in hospital using RFID. In *Proceedings of the 2009 International Conference on Hybrid Information Technology*, (pp. 397-400). New York NY: ACM Press.

Krutz, R. L., & Vines, R. D. (2003). *The CISSP® prep guide: Gold edition*. Indianapolis, IN: Wiley Publishing, Inc.

Lahtela, A. (2009). A short overview of the RFID technology in healthcare. In *Proceedings of the Fourth International Conference on Systems and Networks Communications*, (pp.165-169). IEEE.

Lai, C.-H., Chien, S.-W., Chang, L.-H., Chen, S.-C., & Fang, K. (2007). Enhancing medication safety and healthcare for inpatients using RFID. In *Proceedings of the Portland International Center for Management of Engineering and Technology*, (pp. 2783-2790). Portland, OR: Portland International Center for Management of Engineering and Technology.

Landt, J. (2001). *Shrouds of time*. New York, NY: AIM Inc.

Landt, J. (2005). The history of RFID. *IEEE Potentials, 24*(4), 8–11. doi:10.1109/MP.2005.1549751

Lavine, G. (2008). RFID technology may improve contrast agent safety. *American Journal of Health-System Pharmacy, 65*(15), 1400–1403. doi:10.2146/news080064

Lee, S.-Y., & Cho, G.-S. (2007). A simulation study for the operations analysis of dynamic planning in container terminals considering RTLS. In *Proceedings of the Second International Conference on Innovative Computing, Information and Control (ICICIC 2007)*, (p. 116). IEEE.

Nursing. (2006). Replacing bar coding: Radio frequency identification. *Nursing, 36*(12), 30.

O'Connor, M. C. (2011a). Study determines optimized, RFID-enabled resupply system for nurse stations. *RFID Journal*. Retrieved July 1, 2011 from http://www.rfidjournal.com/article/view/8552.

O'Connor, M. C. (2011b). Saint Luke's hospital of Kansas City saves thousands with RFID. *RFID Journal*. Retrieved July 1, 2011 from http://www.rfidjournal.com/article/view/8560.

Ogirala, A., Murari, A., Hawrylak, P. J., & Mickle, M. H. (2011). Gen 2 timing analysis in state plane: Optimum parameter and command configuration for memory operations. *Journal of Computer Technology and Application, 3*(3).

Revere, L., Black, K., & Zalila, F. (2010). RFIDs can improve the patient care supply chain. *Hospital Topics, 88*(1), 26–31. doi:10.1080/00185860903534315

Ricci, A., Facen, A., Grisanti, M., Boni, A., Munari, I. D., Ciampolini, P., & Morandi, C. (2010). Low-power transponders for RFID. In Yan, L., Zhang, Y., Yang, L. T., & Chen, J. (Eds.), *RFID and Sensor Networks: Architectures, Protocols, Security, and Integrations* (pp. 59–95). Boca Raton, FL: Auerbach Publications, Taylor & Francis Group.

Roark, D. C., & Miguel, K. (2006). RFID: Bar coding's replacement? *Nursing Management, 37*(2), 28–31. doi:10.1097/00006247-200602000-00009

Sanders, D., Mukhi, S., Laskowski, M., Khan, M., Podaima, B. W., & McLeod, R. D. (2008). A network-enabled platform for reducing hospital emergency department waiting times using an RFID proximity location system. In *Proceedings of the International Conference on Systems Engineering (ICSENG 2008)*, (pp. 538-543). ICSENG.

Swedberg, C. (2010a). RFID-based hand-hygiene system prevents health-care acquired infections. *RFID Journal*. Retrieved June 11, 2010, from http://www.rfidjournal.com/article/view/7660.

Swedberg, C. (2010b). Boeing, Fujitsu to offer airlines a holistic RFID solution. *RFID Journal*. Retrieved February 19, 2011, from http://www.rfidjournal.com/article/view/8099.

Swedberg, C. (2011a). Pittsburgh researchers develop implantable RFID for orthopedic device. *RFID Journal*. Retrieved June 20, 2011, from http://www.rfidjournal.com/article/view/8538.

Swedberg, C. (2011b). Wi-Fi system monitors health of cardiac patients. *RFID Journal*. Retrieved July 1, 2011, from http://www.rfidjournal.com/article/view/8535.

Ting, J. S. L., Tsang, A. H. C., Ip, A. W. H., & Ho, G. T. S. (2011). Professional practice and innovation: RF-MediSys: A radio frequency identification-based electronic medical record system for improving medical information accessibility and services at point of care. *Health Information Management Journal, 40*(1), 25–32.

Ting, S. L., Kwok, S. K., Tsang, A. H. C., & Lee, W. B. (2011). Critical elements and lessons learnt from the implementation of an RFID-enabled healthcare management system in a medical organization. *Journal of Medical Systems, 35*(4), 657–669. doi:10.1007/s10916-009-9403-5

Turner, L., & Mickle, M. H. (2007). Overview primer on near-field UHF versus near-field HF RFID tags. *International Journal of Radio Frequency Identification Technology and Applications, 1*(3), 291–302. doi:10.1504/IJRFITA.2007.015852

U.S. Department of Health and Human Services. (2011). *Health information privacy*. Retrieved March 13, 2011, from http://www.hhs.gov/ocr/privacy.

Vinjumur, J. K., Becker, E., Ferdous, S., Galatas, G., & Makedon, F. (2010). Web based medicine intake tracking application. In *Proceedings of the 3rd International Conference on Pervasive Technologies Related To Assistive Environments*. IEEE.

Wessel, R. (2010). Airbus signs contract for high-memory RFID tags. *RFID Journal*. Retrieved February 19, 2011, from http://www.rfidjournal.com/article/view/7323.

Wicks, A. M., Visich, J. K., & Li, S. (2006). Radio frequency identification applications in hospital environments. *Hospital Topics, 84*(3), 3–8. doi:10.3200/HTPS.84.3.3-9

Xiong, J., Seet, B.-C., & Symonds, J. (2009). Human activity inference for ubiquitous RFID-based applications. In *Proceedings of the 2009 Symposia and Workshops on Ubiquitous, Autonomic and Trusted Computing*, (pp. 304-309). IEEE.

Chapter 14
Public Health ICT Based Surveillance System

Josipa Kern
University of Zagreb, Croatia & Andrija Štampar School of Public Health, Croatia

Slavica Sović
University of Zagreb, Croatia & Andrija Štampar School of Public Health, Croatia

Marijan Erceg
Croatian National Institute of Public Health, Croatia

Kristina Fišter
University of Zagreb, Croatia & Andrija Štampar School of Public Health, Croatia

Tamara Poljičanin
Merkur Clinical Hospital, Croatia

Davor Ivanković
University of Zagreb, Croatia & Andrija Štampar School of Public Health, Croatia

Silvije Vuletić
University of Zagreb, Croatia & Andrija Štampar School of Public Health, Croatia

ABSTRACT

The Public Health Surveillance System (PHSS) is defined as the ongoing, systematic collection, analysis, interpretation and dissemination of health-related data essential to the planning, implementation, and evaluation of public health practice. It serves as an early warning system, guides public health policy and strategies, documents the impact of an intervention or progress towards specified public health targets/ goals, and understands and monitors the epidemiology of a condition to set priorities and guide public health policy and strategies. For this purpose, the PHSS should: be ICT-based and comprehensive with clearly defined sources, volumes, and standards of data; include all the stakeholders with information they produce, with enough flexibility in the dynamic of constructing indicators; be safe and able to produce information on demand and on time; and be able to act as a risk management system by providing warnings/reminders/alerts to prevent unwanted events.

DOI: 10.4018/978-1-4666-0888-7.ch014

INTRODUCTION

The chapter is dealing with problems of acquiring information needed to make better public health decisions. Although some intuitive decisions can be made in public health and elsewhere, we believe that public health decision making should mostly be guided by the information gathered about the health system, health policy, and strategies, setting public health priorities, and taking actions to improve the health of the population. Being spread around a number of health institutions such as primary health care, hospitals, laboratories, etc., health data are not easy to link, to analyze, and interpret, and most importantly, there is often a delay in health data reaching the public health system, which hampers making quality, on-time decisions. Contemporary health information systems, although based on modern Information and Communication Technology (ICT), are often fragmented and unable to merge the information coming from various sources.

On the other hand, as a general rule, good decisions should be based on evidence, on information reflecting the reality. Which important decisions are made in health care systems? Whereas in developed or less developed countries, however a system is organized—based on primary health care (e.g. family practice is the "gate" of the health care system in some countries) or not, health care systems are exceedingly complex. Human resources or the health workforce are the core blocks of every health care system. Other health resources, material resources such as health technology, hospital beds, etc. are also very important, enabling the system to be effective and efficient. Diseases or health of individuals and populations are the major challenges for health care systems and the reasons for its existence. Answering the question of "how to handle the health care system to be good enough" requires knowing the system, having information about the system, using data processing or data mining techniques, and interpreting the results in the framework of harmony

or excess in the health care system. Knowledge about the health care system (human and material resources, health status of the population, and relations between them) enables making better decisions in terms of management and planning.

The chapter's objectives can be described as: (1) what is public health, what is a surveillance system, (2) what should be kept under public health surveillance, and why, (3) what are the problems with existing public health surveillance systems worldwide, (4) proposals for the development of effective and efficient public health surveillance systems.

BACKGROUND

Definitions or "What is What"

Public health is defined as "the science and art of preventing disease, prolonging life and promoting health through the organized efforts and informed choices of society, organizations, public and private, communities and individuals" (Winslow, 1920). To be up-to-date and able to act in such direction, the public health is "crying" for information: its action should be based on evidence, and evidence is implied by data and information. Therefore, the continuous monitoring of population health, health care services, and effect of their actions and interventions has been needed. This means that a public health surveillance system is the inevitable tool for effective public health practice.

The concept of public health surveillance can sometimes be confused with other uses of the word surveillance. The Oxford English Dictionary defines surveillance as "close observation, especially of a suspected spy or criminal." The origin of the word is French, from *sur-* 'over' + *veiller* 'watch' (from Latin *vigilare* 'keep watch'). With regard to medicine, surveillance for long was considered as a branch of epidemiology, and was defined as close observation of persons exposed to a communicable disease. However, in the past few decades, surveillance has developed into a discipline within public health, with its own objectives and methodologies.

In this context a *public health surveillance system* can be defined as the ongoing, systematic collection, analysis, interpretation (and dissemination) of health-related data essential to the planning, implementation, and evaluation of public health practice (Teutsch & Churchill, 2000; http://www.who.int/immunization_monitoring/burden/routine_surveillance/en/index.html). It should:

- serve as an early warning system
- guide public health policy and strategies
- document impact of an intervention or progress towards specified public health targets/goals

- understand and monitor the epidemiology of a condition to set priorities and guide public health policy and strategies.

The term *surveillance system* is not yet part of the MeSH database, and neither is *public health surveillance*. We have identified only *Behavioral Risk Factor Surveillance System* defined as *"Telephone surveys are conducted to monitor prevalence of the major behavioral risks among adults associated with premature MORBIDITY and MORTALITY. The data collected is in regard to actual behaviors, rather than on attitudes or knowledge. The Centers for Disease Control and Prevention (CDC) established the Behavioral Risk Factor Surveillance System (BRFSS) in 1984."* The term was included in the MeSH database in 2003.

Figure 1 shows three MeSH trees that contain the term *behavioral risk factor surveillance system.*

Figure 1. MeSH trees containing the term behavioral risk factor surveillance system

All MeSH Categories
    Analytical, Diagnostic and Therapeutic Techniques and Equipment Category
        Investigative Techniques
            Epidemiologic Methods
                Data Collection
                    Health Surveys
Behavioral Risk Factor Surveillance System

All MeSH Categories
    Health Care Category
        Health Care Quality, Access, and Evaluation
            Quality of Health Care
                Health Care Evaluation Mechanisms
                    Data Collection
                      Health Surveys
Behavioral Risk Factor Surveillance System

All MeSH Categories
    Health Care Category
        Environment and Public Health
            Public Health
                Epidemiologic Methods
                  Data Collection
                    Health Surveys
Behavioral Risk Factor Surveillance System

Figure 2. MeSH trees containing the term public health

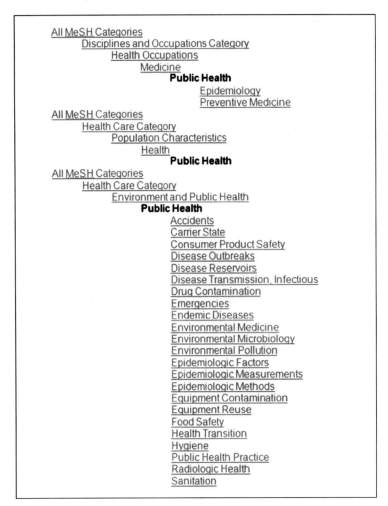

Considering this definition, we found that surveillance is related to risks for diseases only. Other aspects of public health activities (like surveillance of human resources for health) are not covered by this definition. In fact, the term *surveillance system* as such is not yet included in the MeSH database.

Looking at *Public health* as a MeSH term and at the corresponding MeSH trees, we found *Public Health* as a subcategory of *Medicine* (the 1st tree), of *Health* (the 2nd tree) and of *Environment and Public Health* (the 3rd tree). It is apparent that the first two trees are related to disease or health of populations, with a person / patient / examinee) as the entity under consideration (see Figure 2).

It is also apparent that most of the subcategories of *Public Health* in the third tree also put the patient / person / examinee as the leading entity; however, several of them rely on other entities such as sample of water, bacteria, equipment, method, etc. Of course, the role of all of them is in how to preserve health or prevent disease, but most of them could (or should) also be under surveillance of public health.

It seems that *Public Health* as a field is insufficiently developed in the MeSH database—namely some subcategories of public health are missing. It is apparent, for example, that the health workforce is one key object of public health consideration yet it is not mentioned.

Public Health Surveillance Systems: What Do They Do?

As a term, the public health surveillance was described previously (for example, Teutsch & Churchill, 2000). However, the methodology most often utilized in papers reporting on public health surveillance are surveys, usually cross-sectional and performed on samples (random or not) of target populations. Some of the most recent papers, published in last two years, and having "surveillance" in their titles were Nangkynrih and coauthors (Nongkynrih, Anand, Pandav, & Kapoor, 2010), Aboobakur and coauthors (Aboobakur, Latheef, Mohamed, Moosa, Pandey, Prabhakaran, et al., 2010), Ng and coauthors (Ng, Hakimi, Van Minh, Juvekar, Razzaque, Ashraf, et al., 2009). The authors have chosen a well-defined health problem, selected a sample, collected data, conducted analysis and provided the interpretation with conclusion based on the results, being more or less generalizable. Quite a different paper is the paper written by Woods and coauthors (Woods, Coleman, Lawrence, Rashbass, Berrino, & Rachet, 2011). Studying cancer survival statistics, the authors pointed to the problem of registrations in the National Cancer Registry (NCR). Remarkable differences in survival between the UK and other countries have led Woods and collaborators to hypothesize that "UK cancer survival statistics are misleading." They applied simulation methodology by including potential bias regarding the registration in NCR (registration by date of recurrence—not the date of diagnosis, and failure in registration of long-term survivals), simulate registration and analyzed results. However, they could not explain the differences in survival between the UK and other European countries. The problem was therefore not solved. Data quality remains questionable, at least in the methodology of data collection (being non-adequate or not the same in all the countries compared). A large number

of studies, in fact more than 60, were cited in PubMed in year 2011 as registry-based studies (Dadvand, Rankin, Rushton, & Pless-Mulloli, 2011). Some of these registry based studies on public health surveillance issues pointed to problems of data quality in registries—for example Gholiha and coauthors (Gholiha, et al, 2011), and Rakowitz (2011).

The Canadian Integrated Public Health Surveillance system (CIPHS) is an extraordinary example of surveillance systems in the world today. The Canadian system is based on the principle that the "custom tools are being designed to support the systematic collection and collation of health surveillance data as a by-product of the normal work of public health professionals" (http://www.phac-aspc.gc.ca/php-psp/ciphs-eng.php). For example, vaccination is business as usual for public health professionals. Vaccination data should therefore be part of patient records and, in the case of an integrated information system, this data could then be used for estimating rates of vaccination in the population under consideration. Similarly, this data can also be used to support evidence-based public health decisions (http://www.phac-aspc.gc.ca/php-psp/ciphs-eng.php). CIPHS is described as the "integrated business system," allowing "capture, integration, and forwarding of data as a by-product of front-line workers doing their normal work." Such system enables public health professionals to use the same data without re-entering them into another information system.

The priorities of CIPHS were "health surveillance in communicable diseases, immunization, and vaccine associated adverse events." However, the next important step of CIPHS development is directed towards establishing the public health components of the Electronic Health Record (EHR), enabling communication with other parts of the health system, such as various kinds of health registries (e.g. cancer registry).

Health-EU—the Public Health Portal of the European Union—serves in a way as a public health surveillance system that disseminates information on health and health related issues for all European countries, and internationally: "the main objective of this thematic Portal is to provide European citizens with easy access to comprehensive information on Public Health initiatives and programmes at EU level. The portal is intended to help meet EU objectives in the Public Health field, it is an important instrument to positively influence behavior and promote the steady improvement of public health in the 27 EU Member States" (http://ec.europa.eu/health-eu/about_en.htm).

Europe has a high prevalence of non-communicable diseases, which are all attributable to the interaction of various genetic, environmental, and lifestyle factors such as unhealthy diets, physical inactivity, obesity, smoking, and alcohol abuse. For that reason, European Union recommends addressing avoidable diseases by developing strategies and mechanisms for prevention as well as exchanging information on and responding to non-communicable disease threats and besides raising public awareness, reinforcing preventive measures and improving knowledge plan to support actions by setting up networks and information systems across the Member States to generate a flow of information, analysis and exchange of best practice in the public health field (http://ec.europa.eu/health-eu/health_problems/other_non-communicable_diseases/index_en.htm).

Sources of information gathered by the Health-EU are the European countries and their public health surveillance systems: "National-level information is provided by the Member States concerned and Member States are solely responsible for the accuracy of the information."

Data collection is the most costly and most difficult component of a public health surveillance system. The quality of a system is dependent on the quality of its input; or, the system is only as good as the data collected. Diversity in needs and sources may require different procedures for data collection. Depending on this, passive and active

surveillance has been defined and described (Vogt, Larue, Klaucke, & Jillson, 1983).

In the so-called *passive* surveillance, the system data recipient has to wait for the data in order to deal with providers. The reports are coming from hospitals, clinics and other sources. Sometimes, as in registries or laboratory reporting, the providers are obliged by law to produce and report information relevant for public health surveillance. In spite of obligation in reporting, the passive surveillance system has limitations like delay and/or incompleteness of data and information important for surveillance, especially for interventions based on them. Being relatively inexpensive but limited in their functioning, the passive surveillance system should be replaced in practice (Nsubuga, et al., 2006). Trying to overcome the limitations of passive surveillance, *active* surveillance systems should enter into the practice of public health surveillance.

Active public health surveillance systems employ staff who are contacting health care providers and reach into the population, or selected targeted groups or networks put together for specific purposes, and regularly collect data and information (Bern, Maguire, & Alvar, 2008). Active systems are much more costly. In practice, they usually cover a subset of the population like cases with rare diseases (Nsubuga, White, Thacker, et al., 2006). The Canadian CIPHS is one example of an active public health surveillance system.

Sentinel surveillance, which can also be considered a form of active surveillance, relies on an arranged sample of reporting sources (sites such as e.g. hospitals, individuals like e.g. GPs, or events like e.g. disease) who report all the cases of one or more conditions. This type of surveillance is considered as only worthwhile for common diseases (Gauci, Melillo Fenech, Gilles, O'Brien, Mamo, Stabile, et al., 2007).

Syndromic surveillance is based on large amounts of routinely acquired health data, which are individually identifiable and able to predict outbreak of disease (Stoto, 2008). Infodemiology (Eysenbach, 2006) points to a new approach to syndromic surveillance by using web technology and Internet searching. He found a correlation between influenza-related searches on Google and influenza cases occurring in the following week in Canada.

Epidemic field investigation, or surveys, and use of available data sets could also be considered as collection methods in public health surveillance. Most of papers reporting on public health surveillance relating to a variety of health problems were exactly of the same kind.

Generally, data collection for public health surveillance can be presented by a scheme as in Figure 3. According to the available literature, the Canadian CIPHS is the only exception.

Usual practice in the health care systems worldwide used to be to ask health care services to make reports on their work (for example, if they found a person with malaria, HIV-infection, heart attack, or other infectious or chronic, non-infectious diseases). Based on the frequency of such cases, the public health has to identify epidemic or other public health problem, and the need for intervention. Interventions based on individual (e.g. person with HIV infection) or

statistically identified cases (e.g. high prevalence or incidence) should be monitored and evaluated.

Usually, the public health practice has not been satisfied with these procedures, regardless of their global presence; they have been criticized as not being up-to-date, sometimes inaccurate, and not available fast enough. The fact is that old paper based technology as well as not appropriately organized the ICT based solutions has not have the proper solution for such problems.

The fact is that contemporary ICT, technology of today, could be more effective—the Canadian approach is a good example. Unfortunately, despite their potential, the existing health information systems are mostly not designed in a way that would enable efficient surveillance. Most of them act as passive surveillance systems, and collect data isolated of daily work of health professionals. Health professionals are obliged to make reports on their daily work and to send them to public health units or public health institutes. Such data should be entered into computer systems to be processed and analyzed. Sometimes, such data were used to "feed" the registries of various diseases as the collections of data related to patients with a specific diagnosis, condition, or procedure (Wikipedia). They played an important role in

Figure 3. Sources of data for public health surveillance

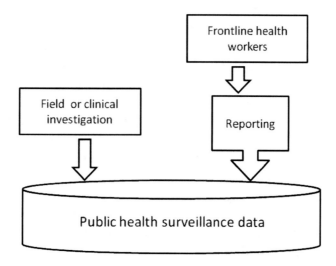

surveillance, whatever the aims of the specific registry were. This approach with re-entering the data into computer (at least) doubles (or even multiplies) the human work, implies errors or missing data, and, finally, information needed for empowering public health decision making become overdue.

Croatian Diabetes Registry as a Good Case Example of Surveillance System

The aim of establishing the Croatian Diabetes Registry was to enable promotion of diabetes care, assessment of the prevalence and incidence of diabetes, its acute and chronic complications, and to follow-up morbidity, mortality, and basic clinical indicators on a national level. All the physicians providing diabetes care were obliged to supply data on their patients to referral diabetes centre. It uses to analyze data and send report to the Croatian National Public Health Institute on the annual basis.

Data collecting is based on BIS (*Basic Information Sheet*) internationally recognized as the optimal data form for follow-up and improvement of diabetes care (WHO, 1990). Different methods of data collection were applied, depending on the level of informatization of the specific level of care. Some of them use to complete BIS by CroDiab NET system (Poljicanin, Pavlić-Renar, Metelko, 2005). Other, most secondary and all primary health centers use to complete BIS by CroDiab Web system (Poljicanin, Šekerija, & Metelko, 2010). Users without access to Internet complete and mail the paper BIS forms.

CroDiab NET system integrates electronic patient records. It is able to generate discharge summaries of the patient and send his/her data to the registry in the same time. Central CroDiab NET module is BIS. It is composed of anamnestic data including risk factors, self-monitoring results, data on chronic complications and treatment as well as individual treatment goals. Possibility of using drug registry, ICD-10 classification, trends

of laboratory parameters for individual patients and basic statistical analyses with graphical display are only some of CroDiab NET's features that made it well-suited and accepted in routine clinical practice.

On the other hand, the CroDiab Web is the system developed for data collecting via Internet, created and adjusted to family physicians need. The CroDiab Web's additional facilities: faster and more efficient co-operation with diabetes specialists and registry personnel, as well as analysis of basic clinical and public health indicators for their patients.

All the data in the central registry database are merged on the patient level. To ensure the accuracy of data, the national mortality database, as well as national physician registry is regularly imported to the registry database. Organization and data flow in CroDiab registry is presented in Figure 4.

The regular implementation of CEZIH data is the current improvement that the CroDiab is working on. The CEZIH is a central Croatian IT based primary health care information system. It collects the patients data from all the general practice offices, other primary health care units (like pediatrics, gynecology, dentistry, etc.), pharmacy, and laboratories enabling e-transfer of medical data to national insurance company and some public heath institutions including registries (Končar, Gvozdanović, 2006; Gvozdanović, et al., 2007). Regular link of CEZIH and CroDiab data enables to cover the persons with diabetes mellitus completely. Extraction of data regarding hospitalization, sick leaves, and treatment and laboratory measurements becomes possible.

The IT structure of CroDiab ensures data protection on several levels. Data transfer via Internet is protected by means of SSL and 128-bit encryption and user authentication. Access to patient data is regulated and limited only to personal data available from official records. Accessibility of data is enabled only to authorized users. Daily back up of database includes encryption by a 128-bit key.

Diabetes quality indicators have been created annually. The major indicators are:

Figure 4. CroDiab registry – organization and data flow

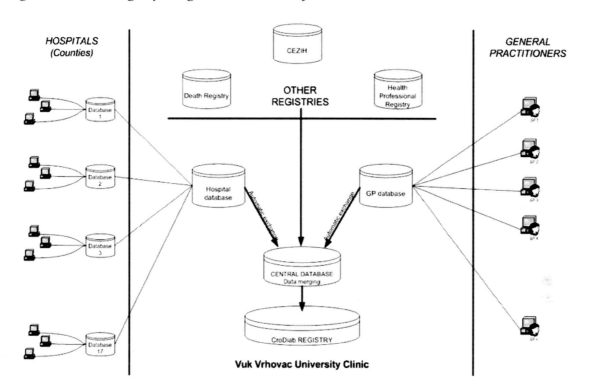

- Clinical characteristics - diabetes status, type of diabetes, duration of disease
- Risk factors – BMI, smoking, systolic and diastolic blood pressure, total cholesterol, LDL-cholesterol, HDL-cholesterol, triglycerides, micro albumin, creatinine, HbA1c
- Diabetes complications – myocardial infarction, stroke, hypertension, retinopathy, polineurophathy, and end-stage of renal failure, foot ulcer, and amputation
- Processes (at least one measurement in 12 months) – measurements – blood pressure, lipids, micro albumin, HbA1c, foot examination, eye examination,
- Treatment (at least one medication in 12 months) – antihypertensive, lipid lowering, glucose lowering treatment and type of treatment (diet, tablets, insulin)
- Process Quality – percentage of patients with at least one test during the last 12 months – HbA1c, microalbuminuria, fun-

doscopy, foot examination, smoking status, BMI, blood pressure
- Outcome quality – intermediate outcomes – percentage of patients with most recent values of HbA1c > 7.5 and 6.5%, blood pressure > 130/80 mmHg, total cholesterol>5 mmol/l, LDL-cholesterol >2.5 mmol/l, triglycerides > 1.7 mmol/l, smokers, foot ulceration
- Outcome quality – terminal outcomes – myocardial infarction, stroke, Blindness, end-stage of renal failure

Example of annual report is presented in Figure 5. The total number of patients registered in the CroDiab registry is 103,730. In 2009 data for 41,362 patients were collected. There were 6.11% of patients with type 1 diabetes, 92.91% with type 2 and 0.98% of those with other specific types of diabetes mellitus. 53% of patients were treated with oral antidiabetic agents, 15% with oral antidiabetics and insulin, 29% with insulin alone,

Figure 5. Excerpt from the annual CroDiab registry report

RIZIČNI FAKTORI ZA RAZVOJ KOMPLIKACIJA (U OSOBA SA ŠEĆERNOM BOLEŠĆU) – RISK FACTORS FOR COMPLICATIONS (IN PEOPLE WITH DIABETES)		
HbA1c: Udio bolesnika sa vrijednostima u posljednjih 12 mjeseci – HbA1c: Percent tested in last 12 months	CroDiab (DiabCare System)_2009	42,47%
HbA1c: Udio bolesnika sa HbA1c >7.5% u posljednjih 12 mjeseci - HbA1c: Percent >7,5% in last 12 months	CroDiab (DiabCare System)_2009	31,96%
Lipidi: Udio bolesnika sa profilom lipida u posljednjih 12 mjeseci - Lipids: Percent with lipid profile in last 12 months	CroDiab (DiabCare System)_2009	35,60%
Lipidi: Udio bolesnika sa vrijednostima ukupnog kolesterola >5 mmol/l – Lipids: Percent of those tested with total cholesterol >5 mmol/l	CroDiab (DiabCare System)_2009	65,22%
Lipidi: Udio bolesnika sa vrijednostima LDL >2.6 mmol/l – Lipids: Percent with LDL >2.6 mmol/l	CroDiab (DiabCare System)_2009	71,39%
Lipidi: Udio bolesnika sa vrijednostima HDL <1.15 mmol/l – Lipids: Percent with HDL <1,15 mmol/L	CroDiab (DiabCare System)_2009	31,70%
Lipidi: Udio bolesnika sa vrijednostima triglicerida >2.3 mmol/l – Lipids: Percent with triglycerides >2,3 mmol/l	CroDiab (DiabCare System)_2009	34,24%
Mikroalbuminurija: Udio bolesnika testiranih u posljednjih 12 mjeseci – Microalbuminuria: Percent tested in last 12 months	CroDiab (DiabCare System)_2009	6,38%
Mikroalbuminurija: Udio bolesnika sa mikroalbuminurijom u posljednjih 12 mjeseci – Microalbuminuria_ Percent with microalbuminuria in last 12 months	CroDiab (DiabCare System)_2009	28,08%
Krvni tlak: Udio bolesnika sa vrijednostima u posljednjih 12 mjeseci – Blood pressure: Percent tested in last 12 months	CroDiab (DiabCare System)_2009	75,79%
Krvni tlak: Udio bolesnika sa RR>140/90 u posljednjih 12 mjeseci – Blood pressure: Percent with BP >140/90 in last 12 months	CroDiab (DiabCare System)_2009	32,06%
Udio bolesnika koji puše – Percent of persons with diabetes who are smoking	CroDiab (DiabCare System)_2009	11,70%
Udio bolesnika sa ITM≥25 kg/m² (≥30 kg/m²) – Percent with BMI ≥25 kg/m² (≥30 kg/m²)	CroDiab (DiabCare System)_2009	83,08% (40,72%)

while 3% of patients were treated only with diet and physical activity. Glycemic regulation (HbA1c<6.5%) was good in 37.06% of cases, intermediate (6.5%< HbA1c<7.5%) in 30.98% and poor (HbA1c>7.5%) in 31.96% of patients with average value (mean±standard deviation) of HbA1c being 7.10±1.47, fasting glucose 9.13±3.11, and postprandial glucose 11.48±4.07.

The CroDiab data analyses have been made periodically, according to health care level and counties, and discussed on semi-annual national meetings of diabetologists. Audit of data has been performed on each the individual report basis. Written feedback has to be sent to every general practitioner who reported data for his patients. After analysis the standard reports are submitted to the Croatian Institute of Public Health on an annual basis.

CroDiab data analysis showed that maintaining the diabetes registry facilitates and monitoring the epidemiological situation, can contribute to better regulation of patients' risk factors.

Since the last year, the CroDiab registry has been the partner in European quality of care initiatives, projects that have promoted meaningful international comparisons of the quality of diabetes care. After voluntary participation in European Core Indicators in Diabetes (EUCID) project, CroDiab was included in currently ongoing project on quality of diabetes care, i.e. European registry - EUBIROD. Developed set of indicators and data system is now being rolled out to sites in 22 European countries. These initiatives have managed to report on quality of care to a great extent in majority of European countries, there is still need to enlarge this project to the continuous European diabetes surveillance system.

Other Case Examples of Public Health Surveillance Systems in Croatia

Communicable Disease Surveillance in Croatia

The Croatian National Institute of Public Health (CNIPH) is in charge of communicable disease surveillance in Croatia. The Croatian Health Care Act, the Act on the Protection of the Population form Communicable Diseases and eleven related ordinances represent the current legal framework in the area of communicable disease surveillance in Croatia. Croatian *networks on communicable diseases surveillance and control,* including *the early warning and response system,* are mostly compatible with those of the EU and operational for reporting to the World Health Organization's (WHO) Centralized Information System for Infectious Diseases (CISID). Data collection is based on daily, monthly, and annual reports and/or telephone communications in case of emergency. The implementation of CEZIH has enabled collection of such information directly from primary health care units.

Registries under the CNIPH

Most of Croatian public health registries under auspices of the Croatian National Institute of Public Health are organized in the same way—on reports based data collection.

The CNIPH has organized registries as follows:

- Registry of health workforce
- Registry of drug addicts under treatment
- Registry of psychosis
- Registry of committed suicides
- National cancer registry
- Registry of disabled persons
- Registry of Legionellosis
- Registry of tuberculosis
- HIV registry

Registry of health workforce: besides the age and gender, the professional and scientific achieved status, as well as the place of work, was recorded chronologically. Based on approval from the Ministry of Health and Welfare, the information on health professional license was also noticed for every health professional. All the workforce statistical data use to be published annually in the official publication of CNIPH.

Registry of drug addicts under treatment: includes all people with drug addiction, regardless if they were under treatment in hospital or as outpatients. Pompidou form created by the Pompidou group of the Council of Europe enables to compare the Croatian data with data coming from other countries in Europe. All the drug addicts have been followed in health care institutions, and every year their individual set of data has to be sent to the registry.

Registry of psychosis: as attributes, the treatment of schizophrenia patients, their somatic diseases, number of days in the hospital, and, in case of death, cause of death was recorded. Also, age and gender, county where the patient was born, and where he/she lives, as well as the hospital where the patient was under treatment, were included.

Registry of committed suicides: contains the following variables - month, day, method and place of committed suicide, socioeconomic variables such as gender, age, marital status, employment, education, and psychiatric or medical characteristic. Number of suicides is varying in time; there are some differences according to age, gender and method of suicide. Having the Registry, analysis of such differences and trends become possible. Consequently, intervention and prevention could be undertaken.

National cancer registry: starting with 1968 this Registry is computerized. In 1994 the National cancer registry became a full member of the International Association of Cancer Registries - IACR (Lyon, France).

379

Through the membership in the European Network of Cancer Registries – ENCR, the Croatian cancer registry data entered into EUROCIM database talking on incidence and mortality of cancer in different European countries. National cancer registry data have been used a lot. Till now, the 31 paper based on data from National cancer registry in Croatia was cited in Medline database. The newest one, talking on skin cancer, was published in 2010 (Lipozencić, et al., 2010).

Registry of disabled persons: in 2001, the Croatian parliament promoted the Act of the Croatian registry of disabled persons. This Registry was consequently implemented in 2002 as the service of the Department of epidemiology of chronic diseases. The newest report based on the Registry of disabled persons was published in 2011 (Benjak, 2011).

Registry of Legionellosis, Registry of tuberculosis and HIV registry are relatively new registries in the Croatian National Institute of Public Health. All of them were computerized and based on data reported by health institutions where cases were identified.

MAIN FOCUS OF THE CHAPTER

Issues, Controversies, Problems

What Should be under Public Health Surveillance?

Historically, surveillance started with surveillance of *diseases* from the epidemiological point of view. Currently, the European Centre for Disease Prevention and Control (ECDC) established in 2005, seated in Stockholm (Sweden), is aimed at strengthening Europe's defenses against infectious diseases (http://www.ecdc.europa.eu/en/aboutus/Mission/Pages/Mission.aspx). In 1968, WHO listed ten key sources of surveillance data: mortality data, morbidity data, epidemic reporting, laboratory reporting, individual case reports, epidemic field investigation, surveys, animal reservoir and vector distribution studies, demographic data, and environmental data. Since 1968, additional data have become available. Some of them are collected for other purposes: hospital and medical care statistics, networks of GP offices, public health laboratory reports, diseases registries, drug and biologics utilization and sales data, absenteeism from work and school, even newspaper and news broadcasting reports (Declich, Carter, 1994; WHO, 2011). However, it is generally known that the most reliable data come from the primary source, that is, from the site where there emerge. Consequently, the most reliable sources of data on diseases are not reports, but patient health or medical records. The same is with drugs utilization, adverse effects, etc.

Not only diseases, but also *health behaviors* such as smoking, alcohol consumption, dietary habits, physical activity, and addiction should be (and are) under public health surveillance worldwide. One such surveillance system was the Behavioral Risk Factor Surveillance System (BRFSS), a US state-based system established in 1984 by CDC and state health departments (Mokdad, Stroup, & Giles, 2003). Surveillance was based on a representative sample of adults, data were collected monthly in all 50 states, the District of Columbia, Puerto Rico, the Virgin Islands, and Guam, and the survey was conducted by telephone. Also, other health related behaviors can be of interest for surveillance. Ortiz and co-authors reported on sexual behavior among adults in Puerto Rico (Ortiz, Soto-Salgado, Suárez, Del Carmen Santos-Ortiz, Tortolero-Luna, Pérez, 2011). It was a cross-sectional population based survey.

Health workforce or human resources for health, health technology such as equipments and procedures, and health organizational units such as hospitals, clinics etc. as the healthcare resources in general are also of interest of public health and should be under surveillance. WHO (2011) described the Kenya Health Workforce Information System which represents one of the longest running and comprehensive human resources information systems in sub-Saharan Africa. Using health workforce information collated in electronically linked databases, it has successfully informed workforce planning and management in various contexts. Settle (2010) pointed to the need to approaches to develop the science and methodologies of workforce surveillance based on appropriate and effective information systems. Surveillance of human resources holds the potential to strengthen a health system on the whole.

Environmental factors potentially related to health, such as water, food, air, noise, etc. should also be subjects of public health surveillance.

Public health is also interested in *health interventions* and their outcomes. The most interesting is the effect of such interventions to health of population or population subgroups.

Health workforce and health equipment data have their primary source in health institutions; environmental data (water, food, etc.) have their source in laboratories, and health interventions in public health institutions undertaking these interventions. Other sources, like the education system, politics and legislation, industry and economy, or agriculture should not be neglected as important sources of data for health surveillance, at least as sources of accounting for various confounding variables that represent a noise in analyzing, e.g. the effects of a public health intervention or just to recognize the current status in issue under interest.

What is the Purpose of a Public Health Surveillance System?

The purpose of a public health surveillance system is to form the basis for quality planning, implementation and evaluation of public health practice, taking into account as many possible influences as possible.

According to WHO (http://www.who.int/topics/public_health_surveillance/en/) a surveillance system can serve as an early warning system for

impending public health emergencies; document the impact of an intervention, or track progress towards specified goals; and monitor and clarify the epidemiology of health problems, to allow priorities to be set and to inform public health policy and strategies.

It can be added:

- Risky health behavior is an important part in the chain of the development of cardio and cerebrovascular diseases; surveillance of health behaviors can therefore serve as a warning system for these unhealthy behaviors;
- Surveillance of health workforce enables to take a look at existing human resources and plan their education and employment; also, knowing the status (number and specialties) enables organize them to intervene in specific circumstances (in case of outbreak, bioterrorism, or similar);
- Surveillance of material resources enables to establish more appropriate health networks, better geographical distribution of health organizational units (hospitals, polyclinics, network of specific laboratories, etc.);
- Monitoring the quality of water, food, air, noise, etc. can ensure the healthier environment, prevent health problems, and reduce the cost of health system.

It is clear that only good quality of the data and their timeliness are the major and necessary postulates. Including all the relevant data, the public health surveillance system can serve as a basis for Evidence Based Public Health Practice (EBPHP).

How to Make an Effective Public Health Surveillance System

To avoid problems such as not being up-to-date, not being accurate and missing some important data, as well as not being timely enough, the following axiom could be proposed: *Health care system must integrate information originating in it, but also be able to communicate with other sectors.*

Integration (from the Latin *integer*, meaning whole or entire) generally means combining parts so that they work together or form a whole (http://searchcrm.techtarget.com/definition/integration). Integration of health care means "to ensure that services provided by various professionals in various locations or organizations, meet the specific needs, over time, of each patient given the knowledge and technology available" (Contandriopoulos, Denis, Touati, Rodriguez, 2003). A number of definitions and explanations for this term can be found in the literature (Kodner, 2002).

Integration of health information (or integrated health information system) means integration of health care system in a way that every stakeholder working at his first line (primary health care, hospital, laboratory, etc.) generate information that:

- Can be communicated to others stakeholders automatically (without specific reporting),
- Should be standardized (based on international standards),
- Should be protected from unauthorized use,
- Should be based upon clear strategy for privacy protection (to avoid breaching current regulations and future concerns).

Regarding the data collecting such an integrated information system can ensure that the public health surveillance can act as an active surveillance system. Of course, the prerequisite for that is that the integrated health information system be based on information and communication technology. Availability of data based on ICT has broadened the potential for data analysis, and enabled quick return of information, on-line access to information, and development of mathematical models to study dynamic and forecast surveillance objectives.

Standards and Standardization in Public Health Surveillance

Generally speaking, a standard is a set of rules and definitions that specifies how to carry out a process or produce a product, whereas the standardization is a process of creating standards (Kern, 2006). A standard is achievable as a document, made by standardization bodies or organizations (e.g. ISO—International Organization for Standardization, CEN—European Committee for Standardization, etc.), their Technical Committees (TC), e.g. ISO/TC215—standardization in medical/health informatics in ISO, CEN/251—standardization in medical/health informatics in CEN, etc., sometimes Sub-Committees (SC) and corresponding Working Groups (WG). A standard is a voluntary and dynamic category. As a rule, it should be changed time after time, by considering the needs of the branch in which it should be applied, and advancement in science and practice.

The intention of standardization is in compatibility of products (wherever, and by whom they have been produced), equalization of procedures (wherever, and by whom they have been conducted), and better understanding between people or systems (whatever they are). Considering the term "better understanding" terminology in particular discipline is the first issue that should be standardized.

In addition to international standardization bodies, the national bodies exist, and having similar functions at the national levels. They take part in creating the international standards, use to accept international standards, or make standards for local (national) level needs.

Medical guidelines made by international or national medical and health associations can also be considered as standards (standards of diagnosing and treatment, e.g. hypertension, diabetes, etc.). Classifications such as ICD (International Code of

Diseases) are also standards enabling to compare, for example, morbidity (in different countries) according to diagnoses coded and defined in the same way (no matter which language were used).

An example of a public health standard is the air quality standard for nitrogen dioxide (NO2). Namely, the American Lung Association in New York calls on the U.S. Environmental Protection Agency (EPA) to strengthen the national ambient air quality standards for NO_2 that has remained unchanged since 1971 (http://www.lungusa. org/associations/states/new-york/pressroom/ news-releases/2010-2011/tighter-no2-standard. html). This notice illustrated the dynamics in the development of standards, in this case because "this harmful pollutant which can irritate the lungs and aggravate asthma"; the environment has been changed because the traffic and power plants were changed and they are "the two major sources of NO_2." What has been demanded? The "new official limit on this air pollutant that each county in the nation must meet," i.e. new standard, because the "scientific research shows that the current NO_2 standard fails to protect the public health."

Standardization is needed also in public health action or intervention, e.g. in case of disasters. McCann and Cordi (2011) recommended the development of *international standards for disaster preparedness and response*. While developing such standards, they suggested implementation of recommendations of Bar-Dayan (2008). These recommendations are as follows:

- To develop an international common terminology for disaster work,
- To create an international disaster preparedness and response organization, which would coordinate response from multiple member states and NGOs—the organization would develop plans for use of existing resources, equipment, and infrastructure,

- To develop an international command-and-control system for response personnel from multiple countries (such as the Incident Command System used in the United States),
- To develop and implement international disaster education programs,
- To develop and implement international disaster drills to improve response force coordination.

Standardization is linked not only to development of public health surveillance systems but also to its functioning. For example, standard ISO 31000:2009 is dealing with risk management. The standard ISO 31000:2009 provides principles and generic guidelines on risk management (http:// www.iso.org/iso/iso_catalogue/catalogue_tc/ catalogue_detail.htm?csnumber=43170). It can be applied to a wide range of activities, including strategies and decisions, operations, processes, functions, projects, products, services and assets, and to any type of risk, whatever its nature, whether having positive or negative consequences. It should be mentioned that ISO 31000:2009 is not intended for the purpose of certification.

Electronic health record, consisting of patient information and being a base for public health disease surveillance, could and should be standardized. Dealing with electronic health records the following standards should be taken into account:

- ISO 13606-1:2008 Electronic health record communication—Part 1: Reference model

ISO 13606-1:2008 will predominantly be used to support the direct care given to identifiable individuals, or to support population monitoring systems such as disease registries and public health surveillance. Use of health records for other purposes such as teaching, clinical audit, administration and reporting, service management, research and epidemiology, which often require anonymization or aggregation of individual records, are not the focus of ISO 13606-1:2008 but such secondary uses might also find this document useful (http://www.iso.org/iso/iso_catalogue/catalogue_tc/catalogue_detail.htm?csnumber=40784).

- ISO 13606-2:2008 Electronic health record communication -- Part 2: Archetype interchange specification

ISO 13606-2:2008 specifies the information architecture required for interoperable communications between systems and services that need or provide EHR data. The subject of the record or record extract to be communicated is an individual person, and the scope of the communication is predominantly with respect to that person's care. Uses of healthcare records for other purposes such as administration, management, research and epidemiology, which require aggregations of individual people's records, are not the focus of ISO 13606-2:2008 but such secondary uses could also find this document useful (http://www.iso.org/iso/iso_catalogue/catalogue_tc/catalogue_detail.htm?csnumber=50119).

- ISO 13606-3:2008 Electronic health record communication—Part 3: Reference archetypes and term lists

ISO 13606-3:2009 is for the communication of part or all of the Electronic Health Record (EHR) of a single identified subject of care between EHR systems, or between EHR systems and a centralized EHR data repository. It may also be used for EHR communication between an EHR system or repository and clinical applications or middleware components (such as decision support components) that need to access or provide EHR data, or as the representation of EHR data within a distributed (federated) record system (http://www.iso.org/iso/iso_catalogue/catalogue_tc/catalogue_detail.htm?csnumber=50120).

- ISO 13606-4:2008 Electronic health record communication—Part 4: Security

ISO/TS 13606-4:2009 describes a methodology for specifying the privileges necessary to access EHR data. This methodology forms part of the overall EHR communications architecture defined in ISO 13606-1. ISO/TS 13606-4:2009 seeks to address those requirements uniquely pertaining to EHR communications and to represent and communicate EHR-specific information that will inform an access decision. It also refers to general security requirements that apply to EHR communications and points at technical solutions and standards that specify details on services meeting these security need (http://www.iso.org/iso/iso_catalogue/catalogue_tc/catalogue_detail.htm?csnumber=50121).

- ISO 13606-5:2008 Electronic health record communication—Part 5: Interface specification

ISO 13606-5:2010 specifies the information architecture required for interoperable communications between systems and services that need or provide EHR data. The subject of the record or record extract to be communicated is an individual person, and the scope of the communication is predominantly with respect to that person's care (http://www.iso.org/iso/iso_catalogue/catalogue_tc/catalogue_detail.htm?csnumber=50122).

Collecting data for surveillance demands telecommunications. Some of relevant standards are:

- ISO/TR 16056-1:2004 Interoperability of telehealth systems and networks – Part 1: Introduction and definitions

ISO/TR 16056-1:2004 gives a brief introduction to interoperability of telehealth systems and networks, along with definitions of telehealth and related terms (http://www.iso.org/iso/

iso_catalogue/catalogue_tc/catalogue_detail.
htm?csnumber=37351).

- ISO/TR 16056-2:2004 Interoperability of telehealth systems and networks—Part 1: Real-time systems

ISO/TR 16056-2:2004 builds on the introduction to telehealth described in Part 1: *Introduction and definitions*, and focuses on the technical standards related to real-time applications (including video, audio, and data conferencing) and interoperability aspects of telehealth systems and networks (http://www.iso.org/iso/iso_catalogue/catalogue_tc/catalogue_detail.htm?csnumber=37352).

The fact is that some kind of Electronic Health Record has existed in many health information systems, but the final EHR internationally (even neither nationally) compatible has been under development yet.

Effectiveness and Efficiency of a Public Health Surveillance System

The *efficiency* refers to how well you do something, whereas *effectiveness* refers to how useful it is (http://www.diffen.com/difference/Effectiveness_vs_Efficiency), or "effectiveness: being effective is about doing the right things; efficiency: being efficient is about doing the things in the right manner." Effectiveness is goal oriented – if someone achieved the goal, he/she is effective, no matter of how he/she did it.

Is our existing public health surveillance system *efficient* or *effective*? Do we want to have an *efficient* or *effective* public health surveillance system?

Example 1.

On 8 December 2010, the WHO endorsed a new rapid test for tuberculosis that can provide an accurate diagnosis for many patients in as little as 100 minutes, compared with the current gold standard test which takes up to three months (WHO, 2010). The test is a fully automated NAAT (nucleic acid amplification test), and after a rigorous assessment, it showed to be *effective* in the early diagnosis of tuberculosis (especially for multidrug-resistant tuberculosis and tuberculosis complicated by HIV infection). The technology also allows testing of other diseases, which should further increase *efficiency*.

This example is a good illustration of both terms: effectiveness and efficiency. Achieving better test accurtacy in the diagnosis of tuberculosis means that this test is more *effective* than the previous test, which was based on sputum smear microscopy (more accurate in achieving the goal: diagnosis of tuberculosis). On the other side, being quicker and allowing for the testing of other diseases, this test offers to increase its *efficiency*.

Example 2.

Haynes and co-authors (Haynes, Linkin, Fishman, Bilker, Strom, Pifer, & Hennessy, 2011) described hospital surveillance. They analyzed the *effectiveness* of an information technology intervention to improve prophylactic antibacterial use in the postoperative period (Haynes, Linkin, Fishman, Bilker, Strom, Pifer, & Hennessy, 2011). In this paper, their "report from the Centers for Medicare and Medicaid Services and the Centers for Disease Control Surgical Infection Prevention program indicated that only 41% of prophylactic antibacterials were correctly stopped within 24 h following the end of surgery. Electronic order sets have shown promise as a means of integrating guideline information with electronic order entry systems and facilitating safer, more effective care." The objective of research was "to study the effectiveness of a computer-based antibacterial order set on increasing the proportion of patients who have antibacterial wound prophylaxis discontinued in the appropriate time frame." After the analysis and results "the computer-based order intervention significantly improved the proportion of surgeries with timely discontinuation of antibacterials from 38.8% to 55.7% (p<0.001) in the intervention hospital, whereas the control hospitals remained at 56–57% (p=0.006 for the difference between treated and control hospitals) the conclusion was "a computer-based electronic order set intervention increased timely discontinuation of postoperative antibacterials," or the system showed to be more effective after introducing the computer-based electronic order set. In this case, the *effectiveness* was the issue of relevance.

Example 3.

Choubert and co-authors (Choubert, et al., 2011) assessed "the *efficiency* of different types of primary, secondary and tertiary processes for the removal of more than 100 priority substances and other relevant emerging pollutants through on-site mass balances over 19 municipal wastewater treatment lines" and concluded secondary biological processes proved to be in average 30% more efficient than primary settling processes."

Here the authors compared secondary and primary processes, willing to find out which process is better in removal pollutants, or to find out the more *efficient* process/procedure.

More deeply analysis of what process of removal pollutant is more efficient, the authors concluded that "the activated sludge process (AS) led to a significant reduction of pollution loads (more than 50% removal for 70% of the substances detected). Biofilm processes led to equivalent removal efficiencies compared to AS, except for some pharmaceuticals. The Membrane Bioreactor (MBR) process allowed upgrading removal efficiencies of some substances only partially degraded during conventional AS processes. Preliminary tertiary processes like tertiary settling and sand filtration could achieve significant removal for absorbable substances. Advanced tertiary processes, like ozonation, activated carbon and reverse osmosis were all very efficient (close to

100%) to complete the removal of polar pesticides and pharmaceuticals; less polar substances being better retained by reverse osmosis."

There are also other examples describing the problem of efficiency or effectiveness (e.g. Morgan, Day, Furuno, Young, Johnson, Bradham, Perencevich, 2010).

Trying to answer questions being put at the beginning of the paragraph about efficiency and effectiveness of public health surveillance systems—do we want an *efficient* or *effective* public health surveillance system—we can say: we want both—achieve the goal (effectiveness) and do it in a good way (efficiency).

Recently, CDC gave guidelines (German, 2011) on how to evaluate a public health surveillance system to achieve its efficiency and effectiveness.

Evidence Based Public Health Practice

"Evidence-based" is very popular term today, and not only in public health. Known terms are Evidence Based Medicine (EBM), Evidence Based Dentistry (EBD), etc. The reason of "evidence-based" popularity in public health is in our will to make decisions providing good outcome to population and individual himself/herself. Generally, the paradigm "evidence-based" meaning "based on information we got by applying scientific methodology" relies to real practice, to decision making in solving a particular problem, promote healthy behavior, or make a reform of health system existing in a country (like intervention in population in order to reduce alcohol consumption, or action to promote healthy diet in adult population, etc.). Evidence based public health practice, relating to particular public health problem (or decision about intervention), includes:

- Experience of public health workers
- Systematic search of scientific evidence relating to the problem under consideration

Table 1. Papers on EBPH published in journals cited in Pubmed

Year of publishing	Number of papers	Topic
1997	3	General
1999	3	General; tobacco control
2000	1	Knowledge discovery
2002	2	General; Quality & quantity of evidence
2003	7	General; Cochran; Randomized controlled trial; Evaluation of programs
2004	5	EBPH glossary; EBPH education; Health promotion; Intervention; Randomized trials
2005	6	General; EBPH education; PH policy; Nutrition
2006	7	General; PH policy; Health assessment in disasters; Breastfeeding promotion; Qualitative research in EBPH practice
2007	3	General; Making decisions; Colorectal cancer screening program
2008	7	General; EBPH education; Interventions; Prevention & health promotion; Benefits to community
2009	4	General; EBPH education; PH policy; Air pollution
2010	4	Malaria; Pandemic flu; PH guidance; Injury priorities & prevention
2011	1	General

- Priorities of population (or attitudes to relating problem).

Generally speaking, the Evidence-Based Public Health Practice is the careful, intentional and sensible use of current best scientific evidence in making decisions about the choice and application of public health interventions (http://ibis.health.state.nm.us/resources/EvidenceBased.html).

The "Evidence based public health" has not been recognized as the MeSH term yet. Therefore, searching the Pubmed by using "Evidence based public health" as a key in a field *Title* was done. 53 papers were published in period 1997-2011 were found. The topics the papers discuss are shown in Table 1.

Clearly, most papers (18 papers in the whole period) discussed the EBPH as a topic *per se.* However, there are several papers discussing the methodology (randomized trials, knowledge discovery, quality and quantity of evidence, qualitative research, making decision, Cochrane), and a great number of them addressing real public health problems and processes that demand surveillance (like tobacco control, nutrition, ma-

laria, pandemic flu, injury, colorectal cancer etc., or prevention, health promotion, public health policy, etc.). It can be concluded that evidence based public health practice needs a surveillance system as the primary source of information.

Solutions and Recommendations

Considering the previously mentioned demands on development of public health surveillance system, like its purpose, goal and functionality (i.e. contents or issues under surveillance, applying standards for integrity and interoperability of all the system components, achieving effectiveness and efficiency as well as applicability of EBPH practice) the following subsystems should be considered:

Disease Surveillance Subsystem

Figure 6 shows disease surveillance subsystem with electronic health records as data sources relevant for surveillance. The electronic health records were coming from all the subsystems. It is supposed that electronic health records follow appropriate standards to be compatible wherever

Figure 6. Scheme of data sources for disease surveillance

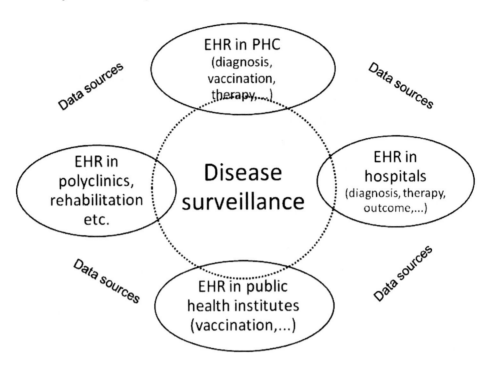

they come from (possibly ISO 13606). Coming from different sources through different network (telehealth communication) the appropriate standards are needed (possibly ISO/TR 16056). Data flow from electronic health records to surveillance system should be automatic and continuous process.

Health Workforce Surveillance Subsystem

Figure 7 shows the health workforce surveillance subsystem with several sources of data relevant for surveillance: Schools of medicine, where health professionals were educated (MD diploma as the collection of data), Ministry of health and professional chambers as the authority dealing with licensing and relicensing (license examination, health professional licenses, long life education programs), health, and other institutions where health professionals are employed.

Materials and Technology Surveillance Subsystem

Figure 8 shows material and technology surveillance subsystem with several sources of data relevant for surveillance: health institutions where the equipment have been installed, authorities as owners of health institutions, industry as vendors of equipments, ministry of health, agencies for drugs, and health insurance as relevant institutions for health care delivery.

Public Health Intervention Surveillance Subsystem

Figure 9 shows public health intervention surveillance subsystem with sources of data relevant for surveillance (institutions defining programs of interventions and those delivering these programs and interventions). Disease surveillance system should be necessarily linked to this subsystem because the outcomes of intervention and impact

Figure 7. Scheme of data sources for health workforce surveillance

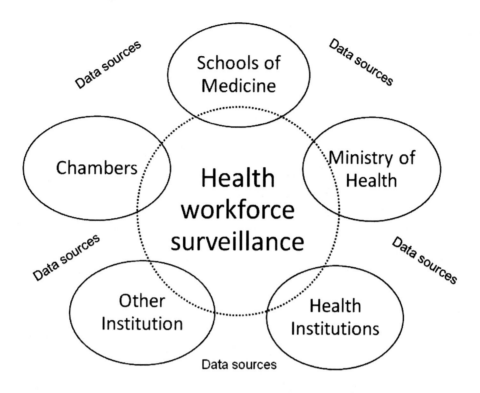

Figure 8. Scheme of data sources for material and technology surveillance

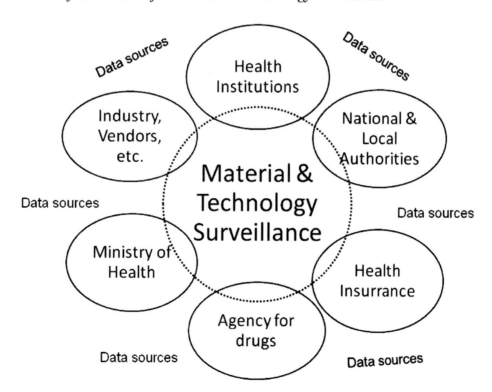

Figure 9. Scheme of data sources for public health intervention surveillance

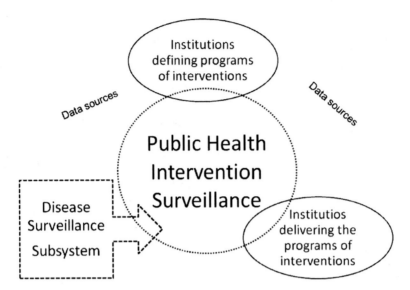

of the program must be evaluated only based on data get from patient data (no matter if it is dealing with diseases or behavior). Such a surveillance system does not exist as yet, or perhaps exists but in fragments only.

FUTURE RESEARCH DIRECTIONS

It is obvious that the era of paper archives is disappearing. Information and communication technology and their use in health care are coming. The leading problem is how to implement the ICT aiming to ensure not only fragmented goals but also the holistic one. Achieving the holistic goal, integration of health and health related information in a health information system, could empowering decisions in public health and in the whole health system. Having available information on patients, population, human, and other health resources, as well as information on initiatives, reforms, and interventions in health system and their outcomes, it will be possible: (1) the scientists to keep on searching and investigate new knowledge; (2) health professionals, managers and authorities to act based on evidences; (3) population to be

informed and more educated about their health and how to preserve it.

The implementation of ICT in future health care systems should be based on the following principles:

- Use of integrated electronic health records in all segments of health care system,
- Electronic health records should be in full functionality, protected of abuse by unauthorized persons, and interoperable between primary health care, policlinics and hospitals (EHR should be in meaningful use),
- Data on disease and behavior as well as use of drugs and drug adverse effects should be extracted from electronic health record automatically (data for surveillance should be simply a by-product of health professionals' daily practice),
- Standardization wher ever possible,
- Data about health workforce and equipment in health institutions and data from electronic health records (with anonymized patient data) should be achievable from a public health unit,

- Defining appropriate indicators (e.g. indicators of quality) and reminders,
- All the data should be up-to-date enabling up-to-date information and making decisions in the direction of better health, better organization of health care, and decrease of health risks.

Future trends in public health surveillance systems can be (Nsubuga, et al., 2006):

- Transformation of the surveillance of present health statistics to modern risk management by achieving full collaboration with all public health agencies and Ministries of health,
- The present surveillance system has to change from "after-the-fact-statistics" to: making meaningful measures that provide accountability for local health status community and deliver "real-time early warning" for critical events in health care
- Consensus on critical surveillance content from all stakeholders
- Commitment on the part of countries funding partners
- Matching surveillance with high data source paying attention to country/region/community specific circumstances while maintaining global attention to data content needs
- Automatic e-transmission should be sent to public health authorities with relevant information to public health jurisdiction.

All this could be done only with the use of information technology. Informatics comparable standards should be used or, in case of non existence, they should be established.

This vision of the future assumes a coherent, integrated approach to surveillance systems that is based on matching the surveillance objective with the right data source and modality and on paying attention to country-specific circumstances while maintaining global attention to data content needs.

The European parliament and the Council cited: An overall strategy for health information should therefore focus on generating, disseminating and applying the best information and evidence available to support the health strategy in improving health overall, and in achieving these three specific objectives.

CONCLUSION

A holistic public health surveillance system forms the basis for evidence based public health practice. Evidence Based Public Health (EBPH) is defined as the process of integrating science-based interventions with community preferences to improve the health of populations (Kohatsu, Robinson, & Torner, 2004), or "Evidence-based public health practice is the careful, intentional and sensible use of current best scientific evidence in making decisions about the choice and application of public health interventions" (NM-IBIS, 2011).

Most of current public health surveillance systems are not effective enough. Paper based data (e.g. in the form of reports, even if in the e-format) that is collected by public health units and requires to be entered into a computer system have a number of limitations (inconsistency, inaccuracy, incompleteness, untimeliness). As such, the existing public health surveillance systems are not able to provide up-to-date information, nor to alert in time to possible risks, nor to provide the real information of value of intervention and its impact in reality.

Being able to serve as the basis for EBPH, a surveillance system must be ICT based, comprehensive (holistic) with clearly defined sources, volumes and standards (format) of data; it should include all the stakeholders with information they produce, with enough flexibility in the dynamic of constructing indicators (e.g. measures of quality); it should be safe and able to produce information on demand (ad hoc) and on time; able to act as a modern risk management system by using warnings, reminders and alerts to prevent the unwanted events (disasters, epidemics, etc.). Evaluating interventions, the public health underwent, and entering information about it into its repository (database), the appropriate surveillance system enables to public health authorities to practice evidence based public health practice.

Doing surveillance is also a political goal. Willing to develop a new surveillance system the arts-based methodology should be applied (Finley, 2008). Rather than following the scientific model of objectivity, certain qualitative social inquiry is needed. It takes its form through interpersonal, political, emotional, and ethical relational skills that are developed and shared between those who are professionally engaged (researcher and enterprises) in surveillance project and other authorities, and particularly community partners.

Namely all those who are engaged in the process of surveillance need to learn a variety of social skills. These social skills were characterized by Felshin (1995).

To address issues of sociopolitical and cultural significance, the following are needed:

- Encourage a community and participants in arts-making as a means of effecting data surveillance research
- Promoting voices and visibility among participants and of making the personal political
- Use of mainstream media techniques (e.g. posters, advertising, newspaper inserts and other) to connect to a wider audience and to subvert the usual uses of commercial forms
- Immersion in community for collaboration among communities/constituencies that share the surveillance system
- Conscious use of public space to contextualize artworks and to encourage audience to define themselves not as passive spectators of the surveillance system,

but rather as active participants in the artworks.

The surveillance system is the Enlightening Eye, not the Big Brother. A major dilemma for surveillance researchers has emerged around the definition of quality criteria.

What makes for good public health surveillance? Good public health surveillance is an effective and efficient system, a system able to provide up-to-date information, information of meaningful use and relevant for making decisions in public health. Also, it should be automated, with no (or minimum) delay in giving information, alerts or reminders. It should extract data from the place where the data emerged. Surveillance systems should be based on international standards and continuously evaluated and upgraded.

REFERENCES

Aboobakur, M., Latheef, A., Mohamed, A. J., Moosa, S., Pandey, R. M., & Prabhakaran, D. (2010). Surveillance for non-communicable disease risk factors in Maldives: Results from the first STEPS survey in male. *International Journal of Public Health*, *55*(5), 489–496. doi:10.1007/s00038-009-0114-y

American Lung Association. (2011). *More protective air quality standard would reduce pollution in NY*. Retrieved March 28, 2011, from http://www.lungusa.org/associations/states/new-york/pressroom/news-releases/2010-2011/tighter-no2-standard.html.

Bar-Dayan, Y. (2008). International collaboration in disaster medicine—It is time for the "big step" in disaster preparedness. *Prehospital and Disaster Medicine*, *23*, 280–281.

Benjak, T. (2011). *Report on disabled persons in Croatia.* Retrieved March 26, 2011, from http://www.hzjz.hr/epidemiologija/kron_mas/invalidi10.pdf.

Bern, C., Maguire, J. H., & Alvar, J. (2008). Complexities of assessing the disease burden attributable to Leishmaniasis. *PLoS Neglected Tropical Diseases, 2*(10), 313. doi:10.1371/journal.pntd.0000313

Choubert, J. M., Martin Ruel, S., Esperanza, M., Budzinski, H., Miège, C., Lagarrigue, C., & Coquery, M. (2011). Limiting the emissions of micropollutants: What efficiency can we expect from wastewater treatment plants? *Water Science and Technology, 63,* 57–65. doi:10.2166/wst.2011.009

Contandriopoulos, A. P., Denis, J. L., Touati, N., & Rodriguez, C. (2003). *The integration of health care: Dimensions and implementation.* Working Paper (N04-01). Montreal, Canada: Universite de Montreal.

Dadvand, P., Rankin, J., Rushton, S., & Pless-Mulloli, T. (2011). Ambient air pollution and congenital heart disease: A register-based study. *Environmental Research, 111*(3), 435–441. doi:10.1016/j.envres.2011.01.022

Declich, S., & Carter, A. O. (1994). Public health surveillance: Historical origins, methods and evaluation. *Bulletin of the World Health Organization, 72,* 285–304.

Eysenbach, G. (2006). Infodemiology: Tracking flu-related searches on the web for syndromic surveillance. In *Proceedings of the AMIA Annual Symposium,* (pp. 244-248). AMIA. Retrieved from http://www.pubmedcentral.nih.gov/articlerender.fcgi?tool=pubmed&pubmedid=17238340.

Felshin, N. (Ed.). (1995). *But is it art? The spirit of art as activism.* Seattle, WA: Bay Press.

Finley, S. (2008). Arts-based inquiry: Performing revolutionary pedagogy. In Denzin, N. K., & Lincoln, Y. S. (Eds.), *Collecting and Interpreting Qualitative Materials* (pp. 75–113). Los Angeles, CA: Sage Publications, Inc.

Gauci, C., Melillo Fenech, T., Gilles, H., O'Brien, S., Mamo, J., & Stabile, I. (2007). Sentinel surveillance: An option for surveillance of infection intestinal diseases. *Eurosurveillance, 12,* 129–132.

German, R. R., & the CDC Guidelines Working Group. (2011). *Updated guidelines for evaluating public health surveillance system.* Retrieved March 18, 2011, from http://www.cdc.gov/mmwr/preview/mmwrhtml/rr5013a1.htm.

Gholiha, A., Fransson, G., Fürst, C. J., Heedman, P. A., Lundström, S., & Axelsson, B. (2011). Big gaps in documentation of end-of-life care: Incomplete medical records reported to the Swedish registry of palliative care. *Lakartidningen, 108*(16-17), 918–921.

Gvozdanović, D., Koncar, M., Kojundzić, V., & Jezidzić, H. (2007). National healthcare information system in Croatian primary care: The foundation for improvement of quality and efficiency in patient care. *Journal of Informatics in Primary Care, 15,* 181–185.

Haynes, K., Linkin, D. R., Fishman, N., Bilker, W. B., Strom, B. L., Pifer, E. A., & Hennessy, S. (2011). Effectiveness of an information technology intervention to improve prophylactic antibacterial use in the postoperative period. *Journal of the American Medical Informatics Association, 18,* 164–168. doi:10.1136/jamia.2009.002998

Ibis. (2011). *Evidence based public health practice.* Retrieved March 19, 2011, from http://ibis.health.state.nm.us/resources/EvidenceBased.html.

Kern, J. (2006). Standardization in health and medical informatics. In Lazakidou, A. A. (Ed.), *Handbook of Research on Informatics in Healthcare and Biomedicine* (pp. 44–50). Hershey, PA: IGI Global. doi:10.4018/978-1-59140-982-3. ch006

Kodner, D. L. (2002). Integrated care: Meaning, logic, applications, and implications – A discussion paper. *International Journal of Integrated Care, 2*, 12.

Kohatsu, N. D., Robinson, J. G., & Torner, J. C. (2004). Evidence-based public health: An evolving concept. *American Journal of Preventive Medicine, 27*, 417–421. doi:10.1016/S0749-3797(04)00196-5

Končar, M., & Gvozdanović, D. (2006). Primary healthcare information system—The cornerstone for the next generation healthcare sector in Republic of Croatia. *International Journal of Medical Informatics, 75*, 306–314. doi:10.1016/j.ijmedinf.2005.08.007

Lipozencić, J., Celić, D., Strnad, M., Toncić, R. J., Pasić, A., Rados, J., & Znaor, A. (2010). Skin cancers in Croatia, 2003-2005: Epidemiological study. *Collegium Antropologicum, 34*, 865–869.

McCann, D. G. C., & Cordi, H. P. (2011). Developing international standards for disaster preparedness and response: How do we get there? *World Medical & Health Policy, 3*, 5. Retrieved March 29, 2011, from http://www.psocommons.org/wmhp/vol3/iss1/art5.

Mokdad, A. H., Stroup, D. F., & Giles, W. H. (2003). Public health surveillance for behavioral risk factors in a changing environment recommendations from the behavioral risk factor surveillance team. *Recommendation and Reports, 52*, 1-12. Retrieved from http://www.cdc.gov/mmwr/Preview/Mmwrhtml/rr5209a1.htm.

Morgan, D. J., Day, H. R., Furuno, J. P., Young, A., Johnson, J. K., Bradham, D. D., & Perencevich, E. N. (2010). Improving efficiency in active surveillance for methicillin-resistant Staphylococcus aureus or vancomycin-resistant Enterococcus at hospital admission. *Infection Control and Hospital Epidemiology, 31*, 1230–1235. doi:10.1086/657335

Ng, N., Hakimi, M., Van Minh, H., Juvekar, S., Razzaque, A., & Ashraf, A. (2009). Prevalence of physical inactivity in nine rural indepth health and demographic surveillance systems in five Asian countries. *Global Health Action, 28*, 2.

NM-IBIS. (2011). *Evidence based public health practice.* Retrieved March 19, 2011, from: http://ibis.health.state.nm.us/resources/EvidenceBased.html.

Nongkynrih, B., Anand, K., Pandav, C. S., & Kapoor, S. K. (2010). Introducing regular behavioural surveillance into the health system in India: its feasibility and validity. *The National Medical Journal of India, 23*(1), 13–17.

Nsubuga, P., Nwanyanwu, O., Nkengasong, J. N., Mukanga, D., & Trostle, M. (2010). Strengthening public health surveillance and response using the health systems strengthening agenda in developing countries. *BMC Public Health, 3*, 10.

Nsubuga, P., White, M. E., Thacker, S. B., Anderson, M. A., Blount, S. B., & Broome, C. V. ... Trostle, M. (2006). Public health surveillance: A tool for targeting and monitoring intervention. In *Disease Control Priorities in Developing Countries* (2nd Ed), (pp. 997-1018). New York, NY: Oxford University Press.

Ortiz, A. P., Soto-Salgado, M., Suárez, E., Del Carmen Santos-Ortiz, M., Tortolero-Luna, G., & Pérez, C. M. (2011). Sexual behaviors among adults in Puerto Rico: A population-based study. *Journal of Sexual Medicine, 8*(9), 2439–2449. doi:10.1111/j.1743-6109.2011.02329.x

Poljicanin, T., Pavlić-Renar, I., & Metelko, Z. (2005). CroDiab net--Electronic diabetes registry. *Acta Medica Croatica, 59*, 185–189.

Poljicanin, T., Šekerija, M., & Metelko, Z. (2010). CroDiab web and improvement of diabetes care at the primary health care level. *Acta Medica Croatica, 64*, 349–354.

Rakowitz, B. (2011). How (in-)complete are study reports? *Deutsche Medizinische Wochenschrift, 136*(15), 752.

Settle, D. (2010). Greater than the sum. *Global Health.* Retrieved from http://www.global-healthmagazine.com/top_stories/greater_than_the_sum/.

Stoto, M. A. (2008). Public health surveillance in the twenty-first century: Achieving population health goals while protecting individuals' privacy and confidentiality. *The Georgetown Law Journal, 96*, 703–719.

Teutsch, S. M., & Churchill, R. E. (Eds.). (2000). *Principles and practice of public health surveillance.* New York, NY: Oxford University Press.

Vogt, R. L., Larue, D., Klaucke, D. N., & Jillson, D. A. (1983). Comparison of an active and passive surveillance system of primary care providers for Hepatitis, Measles, Rubella, and Salmonellosis in Vermont. *American Journal of Public Health, 73*, 795–797. doi:10.2105/AJPH.73.7.795

WHO. (1990). Diabetes care and reasearch in Europe: The Saint Vincent declaration. *Diabetes Mellitus, 7*, 360.

WHO. (2010a). *WHO endorses new rapid tuberculosis test: A major milestone for global TB diagnosis and care.* Retrieved March 29, 2011, from http://www.who.int/mediacentre/news/releases/2010/tb_test_20101208/en/.

WHO. (2010b). *Surveillance recommendations for member states in the post-pandemic period.* Retrieved March 20, 2011, from http://www.who.int/csr/resources/publications/swineflu/surveillance_post_pandemic_20100812/en/.

WHO. (2011a). *Health topics.* Retrieved March 20, 2011, from http://www.euro.who.int/en/what-we-do/health-topics.

WHO. (2011b). *Establishing a robust and sustainable human resources information systems in Kenya.* Retrieved from http://www.who.int/workforcealliance/forum/2011/hrhawardscs5/en/index.html.

Winslow, C. E. A. (1920). The untilled fields of public health. *Science, 51*, 23. doi:10.1126/science.51.1306.23

Woods, L. M., Coleman, M. P., Lawrence, G., Rashbass, J., Berrino, F., & Rachet, B. (2011). Evidence against the proposition that "UK cancer survival statistics are misleading": Simulation study with national cancer registry data. *British Medical Journal, 342*, 399. doi:10.1136/bmj.d3399

ADDITIONAL READING

Arzt, N. H. (2007). *Evolution of public health information systems: Enterprise-wide approaches: A consultation paper for the state of Utah department of health.* Retrieved July 21, 2011. http://health.utah.gov/phi/publications/UT_White_Paper.pdf.

Di Iorio, C. T., Carinci, F., Azzopardi, J., Baglioni, V., Beck, P., & Cunningham, S. (2009). Law, ethics and medicine: Privacy impact assessment in the design of transnational public health information systems: The BIRO project. *Journal of Medical Ethics, 35*, 753–761. doi:10.1136/jme.2009.029918

Government Health IT. (2011). *CDC to build public health surveillance via EHR data*. Retrieved July 22, 2011 from http://govhealthit.com/news/cdc-will-build-public-health-surveillance-through-ehr-data.

Healthcare, I. T. News. (2011). *ONC: Adoption of public health surveillance specifications 'made in error'*. Retrieved July 22, 2011 from http://www.healthcareitnews.com/news/onc-adoption-public-health-surveillance-specifications-made-error.

Hinman, A. R., & Davidson, A. J. (2009). Linking children's health information systems: Clinical care, public health, emergency medical systems, and schools. *Pediatrics, 123*, 67. Retrieved July 21, 2011 from http://pediatrics.aappublications.org/content/123/Supplement_2/S67.full.pdf+html.

Kass-Hout, T. A. (2011). *Novel approaches in public health surveillance*. Paper presented at the meeting International Meeting on Emerging Diseases and Surveillance. Vienna, Austria.

Lombardo, J. S., & Buckeridge, D. L. (Eds.). (2007). *Disease surveillance: A public health informatics approach*. Hoboken, NJ: John Wiley & Sons.

Public Health Agency of Canada. (2011). *Surveillance*. Retrieved July 22, 2011 from http://www.phac-aspc.gc.ca/surveillance-eng.php.

Quin, J. (2011). *Meaningful use - HL7 version 2*. Paper presented at the Meeting on HL7 Version 2 & Surveillance Reporting, HIMSS. Orlando, FL.

Wisconsin Department of Health Services. (2011). *Public health meaningful use*. Retrieved July 22, 2011 from http://www.dhs.wisconsin.gov/ehealth/PHMU/index.htm.

Youde, J. (2010). *Biopolitical surveillance and public health in international politics*. New York, NY: Palgrave Macmillan. doi:10.1057/9780230104785

Zaletel-Kragelj, L., & Božikov, J. (Eds.). (2010). *Methods and tools in public health*. Lage, Germany: Hans Jacobs Verlag.

KEY TERMS AND DEFINITIONS

Effective Health Surveillance System: the health surveillance system doing the right things

Efficient Health Surveillance System: the health surveillance system doing the things in the right manner

Monitoring of Health: having oversight on health continuously

Population Health: health of population being described by prevalence and/or incidence of certain diseases

Public Health: science and art of preventing disease, prolonging life and promoting health through the organized efforts and informed choices of society, organizations, public and private, communities and individuals (Winslow, 1920)

Public Health Informatics: development, application and evaluation of information and communication technology in public health

Public Health Surveillance System: surveillance system related to public health practice

Surveillance System: systematic collection, analysis, and interpretation of data essential for planning, implementation, and evaluation of practice the data are related to

Chapter 15
Digital Economy and Innovative Practices in Healthcare Services

Riccardo Spinelli
Università degli Studi di Genova, Italy

Clara Benevolo
Università degli Studi di Genova, Italy

ABSTRACT

In this chapter, the authors analyze the impact of the new ICT-driven economic paradigm—the digital economy—on healthcare services. The increasing adoption of ICT in healthcare has been very fruitful and has led to the innovative approach to healthcare practice commonly known as e-health. Here the authors first propose a framework, consisting of six elements, whose mutual interaction outlines the structure and the dynamics of the digital economy. Then, a classification scheme of services is presented, which considers their characteristics and their delivery modes; this scheme supports understanding the way in which the adoption of ICT impacts healthcare services. Finally, an overall explanatory outline is constructed that allows one to analyze and understand the origins, implications, and future perspectives of the changes that ICT has brought to healthcare services. Examples of e-health applications are traced back to the building blocks of the framework, isolating the impact of each driver on their structure, configuration, and delivery modes.

INTRODUCTION

The advent of the so-called "ICT revolution" can be undoubtedly considered a turning point in economic history, due to the strong impact it has had on the structure of the economic system and on the way business is done. Many authors—see, among others, Castells (2000), Porter (2001), Rullani (2001), and Burman (2003)—have theorized the progression from the traditional industrial economic paradigm to the so-called "digital economy," stressing the central role that ICT and digital technologies play in this progression. Underlying this shift in paradigms has been the

DOI: 10.4018/978-1-4666-0888-7.ch015

increasing digitalization of information—that is the process of representing any kind of information as a sequence of *bit,* that is *binary digits*—which has come into conflict with real world processes that remained substantially analog based (Tocci, 1988) and not always reducible to binary storage. However, modern digital technologies allow for an accurate digitalization of information from many different sources (words, sounds, images, etc.), without losing any relevant aspect of the processed information. In other words, more and more typologies of data and information can be properly turn to the digital format or, in short, "digitalized" (Aldrich & Masera, 1999).

Coming back to the concept of the digital economy, Atkinson and McKay (2007) state that it "represents the pervasive use of IT (hardware, software, applications, and telecommunications) in all aspects of the economy, including internal operations of organizations (business, government, and non-profit); transactions between organizations; and transactions between individuals, acting both as consumers and citizens, and organizations" (p. 7). While we recognize the value of this technology-focused definition; nevertheless, the advent of the digital economy has not only a technological origin, but is also the result of several more complex dynamics, which—together with the innovation in ICT—contribute to shape the new economic paradigm. Consequently, there is the need for a more articulated analysis on the constituents of the digital economy, which we propose later in this chapter.

The consequences of the evolution from the traditional to the digital economy are deep and involve almost every aspect of economic activities. In this chapter, the attention is focused on how the development of the digital economy influences one of the most important service sectors that is the healthcare industry.

Over the last decades, the economic scenario and the structural and operative conditions of service firms have deeply changed. First, deregulation, liberalization, and globalization processes

have had an impact on the general environment; the healthcare industry has been certainly involved in this processes, even if the industry has been "partially protected" by some structural peculiarities (in particular the significant presence of national public operators along with national public policies and regulations) which have keep it somewhat protected from the new and more intense forms of competition. Then, industrialization, digitalization, IT networks, evolution in communication and transport, virtualization demand-side changes have strongly modified the way of conceiving, producing and delivering services (Javalgi, Martin, & Todd, 2004; Rahman, 2004). In particular, "the industrialization of at least some processes and the digitalization of information [have changed] the options about 'how' to produce and deliver services (e.g. reducing the contact with the consumer) and 'where' (from a distance or across the borders)" (Benevolo & Spinelli, 2011, p. 252).

This process has certainly involved healthcare services too; in fact, the increasing adoption of ICT in that industry has been very fruitful and has led to the innovative approach to healthcare services commonly known as e-health.

Our opinion—which motivates the present study—is that to fully appreciate the origins, the structure and the great potential of e-health applications it is important to understand their deep drivers; we refer to those economic, technological, and social phenomena which lead to the creation of those applications and which condition the way in which they are performed. If those underlying forces are not made clear, the development of innovative practices in healthcare may suffer strategically.

The main objective of the chapter is accordingly to support the understanding of the digitalization process of healthcare services, by tracing them back to the drivers of the evolution towards a digital configuration of the economic system as a whole.

To this purpose, after discussing the key features of e-health we identify these drivers and include them in an overall framework of the digital economy. Then, we present a scheme, which classifies services in accordance with their characteristics and their delivery modes. This scheme helps to analyze and understand origins, implications, and future perspectives of the changes that ICT have originated in healthcare services. Finally, we apply the framework to healthcare services by connecting examples of e-health applications to the building blocks of the framework, and isolating the impact of each driver on the structure, configuration, and delivery modes of the services.

BACKGROUND

In this section, we first look for a suitable definition for e-health, which embraces the most relevant elements of this phenomenon. Then, the main objectives associated with the development of e-health are illustrated, to show its great potential in terms of efficiency, effectiveness, innovation, relationships, etc. Finally, e-health is contextualized within an overall outline of the digital economy, to evaluate the extent to which the adoption of ICT has taken place in the healthcare industry.

Definition and Objectives of e-Health

The most commonly accepted definition of e-health is Eysenbach's (2001) one, who defines e-health as:

an emerging field in the intersection of medical informatics, public health and business, referring to health services and information delivered or enhanced through the Internet and related technologies. In a broader sense, the term characterizes not only a technical development, but also a state-of-mind, a way of thinking, an attitude, and a commitment for networked, global thinking, to improve health care locally, regionally, and worldwide by using information and communication technology. (p. e20)

Nevertheless, several more definitions of e-health have been proposed, as Oh et al. (2005) report. Their analysis of 51 definitions confirms that the term e-health encompasses a wide set of concepts, including health, technology, and commerce. A very important conclusion they come to is that "most commonly, the word health [is] used in relation to health services delivery which suggests that eHealth may refer more to services and systems rather than to the health of people"; furthermore, "health, as used in these definitions, usually [refers] explicitly to health care as a process, rather than to health as an outcome."

Furthermore, a major importance is given to the communication between the subjects involved in healthcare processes: patients and relatives/friends, hospitals, practitioners, local and central public authorities, private corporations, etc. With respect to this topic, we make reference to Pagliari et al. (2005), who—in another review of e-health definitions—found that:

the majority of definitions [...] specify the use of networked information and communications technologies, primarily the Internet, and digital data, thus differentiating eHealth from the broader field of medical informatics, which incorporates 'harder' technologies, such as scanning equipment, and bioinformatics research which tends to take place in isolation and is less directly applicable to health care service delivery (p. e9).

The view of e-health as process-centered and the importance of the communication features are very consistent with the approach we are adopting; indeed, our attention is concentrated on the role of ICT in performing healthcare services and in supporting effective communication between the subjects involved in healthcare processes.

In particular, three major healthcare macro-processes can be identified, which are increasingly supported by ICT applications (Osservatorio ICT in Sanità, 2008):

- primary processes, directly related to the main steps in the process of caretaking of the patient: admission, diagnosis, treatment and discharge;
- support processes to caretaking activities, such as quality and risk management, public relations, facility management, programming and controlling, human resource management, etc;
- network processes, associated with the whole assistance process in a broad sense; the perspective is the "continuing assistance" view, which goes beyond the moment of hospitalization or of the treatment for acute disease and include a continuing relation between the individual and the healthcare system, to exchange information, monitor the patient's health, prevent future disease, support healthier behavior, etc.

Even if conceptually distinct, in practice the three processes are deeply connected and mutually crossing, to such an extent that it would be reductive to identify e-health applications specific for each process, as a great part of the value added by these applications lie exactly in their cross-process nature.

A more general but useful list of the main groups of e-health applications is the one created in 2005 by the World Health Organisation for the surveys of the *WHO Global Observatory for eHealth*. The list includes the following tools (WHO, 2006a, p. 15):

- electronic health records, including patient's clinical history, test results, medication, etc.;
- patient information systems, which contain information about a hospitalized patient and are used to support both the administrative and clinical activities in a hospital;
- hospital information systems, that support information processing within a hospital

in areas such as administration, appointments, billing, planning, budgeting and personnel;
- general practitioner information systems, that support the work of a general practitioner often link to other health care systems such as billing, GP reimbursement, or laboratory results reporting systems;
- national electronic registries, which contain data on specific medical subjects such as births, mortality, cancer, diabetes, or other subjects of medical or epidemiological interest;
- national drug registries, containing national pharmaceutical information;
- directories of healthcare professional and institutions;
- decision support systems, that is automated or semi-automated systems that support decision-making in a clinical environment;
- telehealth, which relate with the use of ICT to either support the provision of health care or as an alternative to direct professional care and encompasses telemedicine and the use of remote medical expertise;
- geographical information systems, which capture, integrate, analyze and display data related to geographic coordinates.

The list does not pretend to be exhaustive and could be subject to obsolescence, due to the rapid development of new technologies, but its value is undoubted, as it provides a general overview of the various areas in which the application of ICT to healthcare can contribute.

Our interest in this topic—and the relevance of the study too—is justified by the great potential associated with the huge adoption of ICT in healthcare services (Commission of the European Communities, 2004; Stroetmann, Jones, Dobrev, & Stroetmann, 2006; WHO, 2006a & 2006b). Healthcare costs are growing at an unsustainable rate throughout much of the world, due to factors such as the aging process of population, the request for better and more effective healthcare services, the introduction of more sophisticated technologies in caretaking processes (Haux, Ammenwerth, Herzog, & Knaup, 2002). In response, "many governments are taking steps to prod the health care industry to aggressively expand its use of IT" (Kennedy & Berk, 2011, p. 1).

In fact, an increasing number of studies show the potential benefits and limitations of multifunctional clinical ICT systems (Shekelle & Goldzweig, 2009); even if data on cost and cost-effectiveness remains limited, there is a general consensus that health ICT has the potential to dramatically transform healthcare.

According to the OECD (2010), the use of health information technology can improve the efficiency, cost-effectiveness, quality and safety of medical care delivery; indeed, the potential benefits that can result from ICT implementation in this industry can be traced back to four broad, inter-related categories of objectives (p. 32) (see Figure 1):

1. increasing quality of care and efficiency;
2. reducing operating costs of clinical services;
3. reducing administrative costs;
4. enabling entirely new modes of care.

Objective 2 and 3 focus mainly on the efficiency gain obtainable through ICT application to core and ancillary healthcare activities. Nevertheless, this view alone would be quite reductive; "if greater investment in health IT simply automates a broken health care system, vital opportunities for transformation will be missed" (Frisse, 2009, p. w380). Objective 1, on the contrary, is centered on cost-effectiveness, quality and safety and is consequently more demanding than simply cutting expenses. It is worth underlining that this objective jointly focuses on two complementing elements: on the one side, the direct savings and quality improvements obtainable through a new ICT-intensive way of performing health-related activities; on the other side, the equally important

Figure 1. The main objectives of e-health

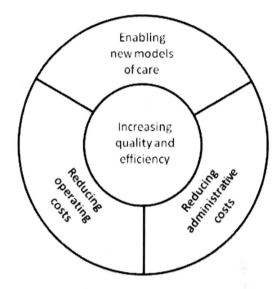

Source: Constructed by the authors.

indirect savings which derive from the more intensive and effective prevention initiatives which ICT make possible, for example the reduction of the incidence of chronic disease attributable to prevention. Indeed, the payoff of some types of preventive care, such as for diabetes and heart failure, can be very high, as they reduce the need for very expensive and long-term treatments.

Finally, objective 4 casts light on the most innovative scenario, which is the development of new ways of taking care of people's health—again, with respect to both patient treatment and prevention—thanks to the comprehensive application of ICT to the whole care process, from the administrative side to the clinical one.

Another interesting approach to e-health benefits for healthcare organizations is the taxonomy proposed by Osservatorio ICT in Sanità (2008), where four main drivers (divided into sub-drivers) of benefit from ICT application to healthcare processes are proposed (p. 19):

• efficiency, declined into staff productivity, equipment usage, cost control;

- quality, with respect to diagnosis, cure, clinical risk and processing time;
- relationship, with both the patient (in terms of service personalization and access) and other organizations;
- monitoring and control of the healthcare organization, which includes regulations accomplishment and the monitoring of performance and processes.

This articulated approach is particularly useful because it allows for a more precise identification—for each area of activity—of the potential and actual benefits from e-health. The contribution of ICT to healthcare services seems to be already relevant to all the considered dimensions; nevertheless, a large gap is still present between actual and potential contribution, especially in areas such as clinical risk control, service accessibility, and process monitoring.

The E-Health in the Digital Economy

To contextualize the development of e-health within the ICT-driven evolution of the whole economy, it is useful to recall that the extent of development of the digital economy is rather uneven on an industry basis. Similar observations could be made about differences in the development of the digital economy on a geographical basis, as not all countries have the same experience of technological development and therefore do not share the same level of "digitalization" of business activities.

On industry specificities, Malecki and Moriset (2008, p. 6) use the metaphor of the "pyramid of the digital economy" (see Figure 2) to help identify four distinct groups of industries, that vary in terms of ICT diffusion. Their scheme has the limit of not considering the important phenomenon of industrial convergence, which could reduce the significance of the proposed industry classification. In the new economic paradigm of the digital economy, in fact, industry boundaries are reshaped

and become open to new competitors from previously separate industries. When similar production processes and technologies—in this case, digital technologies—are applied to different industries, the division between these industries tends to fade (Ames & Rosenberg, 1977). New competitive dynamics occur because competitors from other industries arise who satisfy the customer needs in different ways. Furthermore, the concept of product substitution and complementarity are also deeply questioned (Greenstain & Khanna, 1997). As a consequence, it becomes more and more difficult to define the borders between two sectors and to which sector a firm belongs.

Despite these limitations, Malecki and Moriset's pyramid is suitable for our purpose, because it allows for a clear representation of the different extent of ICT diffusion in specific industries and supports a contextualization of the healthcare industry within the digital economy.

Malecki and Moriset represent the set of economic industries as a pyramid and first consider what they call the "spearhead" of the pyramid, that is, the chips and processors industry which produce the basic components of all digital technologies. Below this lies the "core," including

Figure 2. The pyramid of the digital economy

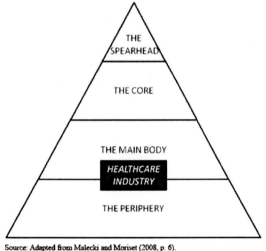

Source: Adapted from Malecki and Moriset (2008, p. 6).

the computer and telecommunication industries, which we define as ICT in a narrow sense. The third level, the "main body," includes all fully ICT-enabled industries, that is, those manufacturing and service industries which rely heavily on ICT; we can cite here the great majority of the most relevant industries in the contemporary economy: automobile making, high-tech mechanics, media and entertainment, business and financial services, and so on. The last group—at the base of the pyramid—is the "periphery," which comprises those sectors not yet or only partially, ICT-enabled or, in other words, where the use of ICT is still limited and not critical. Sectors traditionally included in this group are usually "old economy" ones, such as farming, fishing, mining, forestry or basic consumer and public services. However, examples of intense ICT use are present in these sectors as well, forerunners of a more widespread adoption still in progress. This explains why the boundary between the "main body" and the "periphery" is continuously moving down, as more and more industries reconfigure themselves through greater use of ICT in processes and in organizations.

Those industries belonging to the "spearhead" and the "core" are part of the "engine" of the ICT revolution, as they are the "main actors" of the revolution and drive the process. On the contrary, industries in the "main body" and the "periphery" perceive the ICT revolution as an exogenous factor influencing their general and competitive environment, being, in a way, "victims" of these forces.

In our opinion, the healthcare industry, is progressively entering the "main body" of the pyramid, due to the great changes caused by the pervasive application of ICT: the structure of the organizations in this industry is being fundamentally re-shaped; new ways of taking care of the patients are becoming possible; public and private institutions are looking for new and more efficient ways to cooperate; the "consumer" (be her the patient or a friend or relative) is becoming more and more informed and therefore more active and demanding—in terms of convenience, control and choice (Ball & Lillis, 2001)—in their relationship with the healthcare system.

As we are showing in this chapter, the more innovative components of the industry have already been experiencing such an evolving process: "ICT has already modified medical practice patterns extensively while facilitating coordination and close cooperation between health care professionals to improve patient management; it is already providing some solutions to the growing need for information and knowledge sharing" (Fieschi, 2002, p. 87). However, the more traditional components too—which are still in the "periphery" of the pyramid—will get soon to a new, more ICT-based, configuration. Such a profound phenomenon is consequently well worth of being analyzed and interpreted in the light of a theoretical model which helps to systematize the several and sometimes confused signals that the empirical reality throws up.

THE FRAMEWORK OF THE DIGITAL ECONOMY

The theoretical tool we are going to use to assess the impact of the ICT revolution on healthcare services is a framework developed by Spinelli (2008) and devoted to the identification of the foundations of the digital economy, which are the main drivers shaping the new economic paradigm. The purpose of the model is to explain the macro phenomena at the root of the evolution of the economic system, so as to make feasible a complete understanding of the structure of the new economic paradigm and the consequences that its advent has on the different industries and on the activity of the firms.

The framework proposed by Spinelli (2008) consists of the following six elements, that we call the "building blocks" of the digital economy:

1. the Internet standard, open and universal communication protocol;

2. the dematerialization of the economy;
3. the electronic interconnection of people, physical goods, institutions and countries;
4. the separation between the "economics of things" and the "economics of information";
5. the overcoming of the trade-off between reach and richness in information economics;
6. the shift from ownership to access in the economy.

The framework represents an evolution of the contribution of Valdani (2000), who designed an explanatory model of the digital economy including four building blocks. In comparison with the original structure, the new version by Spinelli (2008) adds two building blocks (blocks 2 and 6) and repositions all six blocks in a hierarchical way, showing cause-effect relations between the elements.

With respect to the applicability of the framework to healthcare services, it should be noted that it was built with a broad, non industry-specific approach in mind, because it aimed to stimulate reflection o the new economic paradigm in general. This was also consistent with the very nature of a framework, which, as Michael Porter stated, "tries to capture the full richness of a phenomenon with the most limited number of dimensions" (as cited in Argyres & McGahan, 2002, p. 46). Nevertheless, industry-specific elements can be retrieved in the framework when it is applied to a specific field of activity, as we do with healthcare services in this chapter.

In the next paragraphs, we first discuss the framework, which is then applied to healthcare services. Our aim is not to encompass the whole world of e-health—as its extreme articulation makes this unattainable—but to show the relationships and mutual dependences between the development of e-health and the advent of the digital economy. We consequently present some reflections on how the drivers which have shaped the paradigm of the digital economy directly impact on the actual development of healthcare services; to do that, we deconstruct some e-health applications and isolate the impact of the underlying drivers on their structure and on the way they are performed.

The Building Blocks

The first element of the model is the Internet standard, open, and universal communication protocol (block 1).

The functioning of the Internet is based on a number of communication protocols (TCP/IP, SMTP, FTP, WAP, HTTP, and the more recent XML and SOAP) which are standardized on a global scale, open and non-proprietary (Ruefli, Whinston, & Wiggins, 2001; Laudon & Laudon, 2010). Indeed, these protocols are developed and managed by international nonprofit organizations—such as the Internet Society (ISOC), the World Wide Web Consortium (W3C), the Internet Corporation for Assigned Names and Numbers (ICANN), the WiMAX Forum (WMF), or the Institute of Electrical and Electronics Engineers (IEEE)—who count, amongst their members, experts and delegates from firms, public entities and research centers.

Because of their very nature, these organizations have the authority to recommend and set the standards in the Internet for the whole ICT industry. Moreover, the adoption of non-proprietary standards allows the maximum interoperability among different systems, because protocols are "third party" compared to the different proprietary hardware and software architectures. Finally, as no firm "owns" the Internet protocols, no firm has exclusive rights over them.

The presence of globally accepted open standards and the lack of relevance of hardware and software configuration have consequently made the expansion of the Internet and the advent of the digital economy much quicker and simpler, because of the ease of connection for new users, even when geographically widespread or without latest generation ICT systems (Rayport & Jaworski, 2001).

The second block of the framework is the dematerialization of the economy (block 2), namely the complex evolution from material to immaterial, from the preeminence of physical transformation to the prominence of information creation. A new information-based immaterial economy is emerging for at least two reasons, contributing to the development of a new economic paradigm.

First, the importance of services in modern economies is increasing, due to so-called tertiarization: the core of production and consumption is moving from goods to services, in what is becoming a "weightless economy" (Rifkin, 2000). In this sense, the GDP of most countries is growing in value but at the same time is getting "lighter," as a growing and already majority part of the production is "weightless." In some cases, what used to be a physical product or activity has become an intangible service. Consider, for instance, the answering machine; this is a tangible device, which has been replaced by a service, offered by the telephone companies, that the customer can access through her phone, with no extra devices needed.

Second, the content of information in physical goods is becoming more relevant and critical to gaining a sustainable competitive advantage (Porter & Millar, 1985). In other words, the importance of the tangible component of physical goods is decreasing, while the intangible component is gaining significance: goods are becoming the material interface to "move" immateriality (Aldrich & Masera, 1999); furthermore, the value of the product is less and less connected to its physical attributes and increasingly depends on its intangible dimensions (ideas, meanings, emotions, flexibility, quickness, etc.).

The availability of a widespread and standardized infrastructure of communication leads to the third building block of the model, an unprecedented global electronic interconnection of people, physical goods, institutions and countries (block 3).

As confirmed by the growing data on ICT adoption, we live in an ever connected world, where people, institutions, firms and even machines can exchange information in real time at virtually no cost, thanks to specific communication protocols (Conti, 2006; Chang, et al., 2011). The World Wide Web is wrapping up "physical" reality in the "virtual" cyberspace (Rifkin, 2000), creating electronic networks which are intrinsically cross-border.

This process has relevant and potentially destabilizing effects on the existing economic paradigm, for it questions basic elements such as firm's borders, organizational structures, consumer behavior, logistic chains, production and supply methods, etc. (Vicari, 2001b). Most of these elements, indeed, have been shaped by limited connectivity. This imposed, for example, the adoption of strongly hierarchical firm structures, in order to configure top-bottom communication on multiple levels, or the creation of widespread distribution and logistics networks, to reach remote customers. Universal connectivity, on the contrary, puts everyone "within reach" and makes it feasible to overcome many limits of the consolidated industrial economic paradigm. In particular, the global interconnection creates a platform for multiple forms of collaboration within a universal workforce of people and computers (Friedman, 2006), dramatically increasing the possibility of creating networks of firms which can extend on a worldwide scale (Vicari, 2001b).

The fourth pillar of the foundations of the digital economy is the separation between the economics of things and the economics of information (block 4).

In the traditional economy, most information is transmitted using a physical device, like goods (for instance, a book carries the information about its content), specialized devices (like a DVD which carries a movie), or individuals (e.g., an insurance broker who explains the policy to a customer): in all these cases, information is constrained by the flow of the physical device, with all the limitations and costs that this implies.

ICT digitalize information and separates it from the physical device, allowing it to flow along telecommunication networks very quickly and cheaply. "Information is the glue that holds value chains and supply chain together. But that glue is now melting," state Evans and Wurster (2000, p.13). When information and physical flows are divided, each one is free to follow its own economic rules and their related economic activities are free to disaggregate and re-aggregate in new and more efficient ways. The inseparability of information and goods has lead to sub-efficient configurations in many economic activities, which now can and should be redesigned in new forms (Shapiro & Varian, 1999). Publishers, for example, are involved in an information-intensive production, but at the same time, they traditionally face costs and issues typical of manufacturing production, such as printing costs and distribution choices. When information is separated from its physical support, this duplicity can be overcome, and publishers can publish online, dramatically reducing the relevance of manufacturing issues in their activity, or they can outsource the printing and distribution of their products to an external partner, enabling them to focus on the creation and the electronic delivery of contents. Both solutions are not viable in a traditional economy where information has to flow together with its physical support. That explains why newspapers used to be traditionally written and printed in the same location, and then distributed with significant logistic costs (Chen, 2001; Mandelli & Parolini, 2003).

The fifth constituent of the digital economy is the overcoming of the trade-off between reach and richness in information economics (block 4).

As long as information flows together with a physical device, its transmission is strictly limited and it is necessary to choose between a wide audience for poor content and a narrow one for rich content. In the context of education, for example, when a traditional lecture is given before a large class, its contents are obviously not tailored around each student's specific needs and the level of instructor-student interaction is limited; in contrast, a one-to-one session is much more personalized and interactive, and its price "per capita" is consequently much higher. Given a limited budget of time and resources, it is not possible to both reach a wide audience and deliver rich, personalized, and interactive contents.

In other words, costs and logistics create a trade-off between reach and richness in information economics (Evans & Wurster, 2000), whose overcoming represents the fourth building block of the digital economy. In fact, ICT, as mentioned above, allows the separation of information from the physical device and consequently make it feasible to transmit a rich message to a wide audience, with no significant extra-costs, leading to unprecedented levels of interactivity between individuals and organizations (Kumar & Venkatesan, 2005; Prandelli & Verona, 2011). In marketing, this makes it feasible to perform actions more focused on very specific targets, all the way to the limit case of "segment of one" marketing, which Winger and Edelman (1989) and Pine (1993) were the first to anticipate.

The last building block is the shift from ownership to the access economy (block 6). This is the shift from a paradigm where ownership of resources is critical for value creation to a new one, where it is important to be able to access resources, which are no longer bought by firms (exclusive ownership) but supplied as services for the time strictly necessary for production (access). As stated by Rifkin (2000), networks are progressively displacing markets, and the economic power which used to be in the hands of those owning the resources is moving towards those who access the resources they need through a network. This is especially true for complementary assets (Teece, 1986), which support the critical assets that contribute directly to a firm's competitive advantage.

In a network information-based economy, market exchange is not always the most efficient way for procuring resources, which can be temporarily accessed in a client-server relation; in fact, the most suitable way to trade knowledge—the key resource in the digital economy—is not to sell it in a market, but to make it available by allowing temporary access in exchange for economic compensation. Economic power, which, in the past, used to be in the hands of land owners and capitalists during the second half of the XX century belonged to those who owned the knowledge resources; in the new economy, new business models are evolving, in which power belongs to those who can place themselves at the core of the management of a resource network (Sawhney & Parikh, 2001; Tapscott, 2001; Vicari, 2001a).

The more services become relevant in the economic systems, the more information becomes the critical resource to firms' activity, and the more access is preferred over ownership (Rullani, 2001).

Similarly, the way of using physical goods is increasingly changing, because new forms of "rent" are taking place, which are nothing more than access modes. Nowadays most firms assets—such as machineries, buildings, software and computing power (in the form of ASP, Saas, and grid/cloud computing)—are available not only by purchasing them, but on a leasing (or pay-per-use) basis too. In other words, exclusive ownership is losing importance and elements once considered assets now tend to be viewed as liabilities; in fact, in an ever-changing economic landscape, assets—especially the physical ones—are burdens reducing the firm's readiness to respond to the evolution of the competitive environment. On the contrary, access-based forms of usage of those assets are much more flexible and reversible in the short-term.

This tendency definitely contributes to the advent of the new paradigm, since the way to the "age of access" (Rifkin, 2000) necessary passes through the Internet and the digital networks, which provide firms with the instruments and the environment to share and access their resources.

The Complete Framework

As previously stated, the blocks of the framework are now arranged in a hierarchical way, to support the identification of mutual relations and temporal sequences between the six elements (see Figure 3).

The identification of a hierarchical structural among the building blocks makes it possible to

Figure 3. The hierarchical structure of the framework of the digital economy

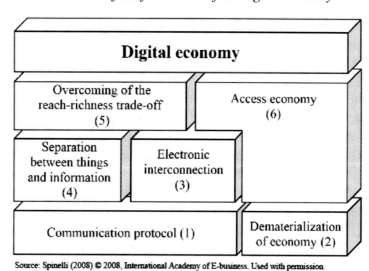

Figure 4. The flat layout of the framework of the digital economy

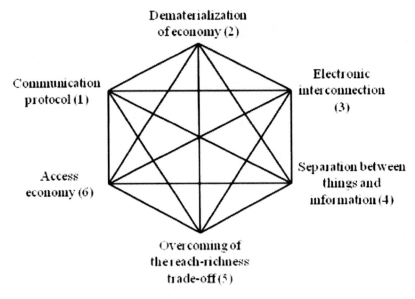

Source: Constructed by the authors.

draw two development paths, which explain the sequence of steps, which led to the final configuration of the new economic paradigm. These two paths can be traced back, respectively, to the supply and the demand side of the economic system. It is not surprising that such a complex occurrence as the advent of the digital economy finds its origins in the converging action of long-term dynamics from both the supply and demand side; it is also worth emphasizing that only the interaction of originally independent events has made it possible to subvert a long-standing economic paradigm and promote not only a new way of doing business but also a new economic environment.

On the supply side, the creation of the Internet protocol represents the starting point of the process: this—together with the possibility of digitalizing information from several different sources—made it possible to connect electronically all the elements of the global network and, at the same time, separate information from physical flows and overcome the reach-richness trade-off.

On the demand side, a crucial role must be ascribed to the dematerialization of the economy.

This prevailing tendency—jointly with the electronic interconnection on the supply side—has, as a consequence, seen a shift from ownership to the access economy. Even if the dematerialization concerns both supply and demand, in the framework it is located in the demand side, because the focus is on the evolution of the consumers' needs towards new forms of immaterial and service-based consumption. Indeed, this trend dates back to much earlier than the advent of the ICT revolution; the progressive substitution of services for material goods has historical roots, even if it gained new momentum when ICT made it much easier and opened previously unexplored tertiarization paths.

The chosen layout is probably not the only one feasible, but it is, in our opinion, the most adequate; nevertheless, this does not rule out that other equally consistent and justifiable configurations are possible. As previously noted, the relations among the blocks are complex, deep, and sometimes mutual.

For this reason, we propose a "flat layout" as well of all six elements (see Figure 4) as valuable in emphasizing the mutual connections, which link all the elements.

Indeed—as it emerged during the description of each of them—the six drivers of the digital economy are dependent on each other and the development of one of them was often enforced by the contemporary development of another one.

Furthermore—in a perspective view—ongoing processes such as the aforementioned convergence are leading to stronger connections between the blocks, which are getting more and more dependent from and related to each other.

THE IMPACT OF THE DIGITAL ECONOMY ON HEALTHCARE SERVICES

After presenting the paradigm of the digital economy, we introduce some reflections about its impact on healthcare services. As aforementioned, to this purpose we are going to deconstruct some e-health practices into their basic constituents, showing how those essential elements are a consequence of the drivers, which shape the paradigm of the digital economy. In other words, we show that e-health activities derive their structure and even their *raison d'être* from those fundamental underlying drivers we call the "the building blocks."

A proper application of the framework to healthcare services requires firstly overcoming the difficulty that healthcare services are not an homogeneous group, as they comprises activities which are very diverse from each other. To overcome the limitations related with the structural complexity of healthcare services, we make reference to service management literature (Thomas, 1978; Lovelock, 1983).

First of all, we note that a service is not a physical good, but the output of an economic activity which is characterized by a high degree of intangibility. The distinctive characteristics of services are: intangibility; simultaneous delivery and consumption; contact and interaction between

producer and user; perishability; variability; social innovation (Chase, 1978; Normann, 1984; Eiglier & Langeard, 1987; Grönroos, 1990; Lovelock, 1996; Zeithaml & Bitner, 2000). These characteristics are common to all services, but present in differing intensities according to the kind of service and delivery mode adopted. In the healthcare industry, for instance, public hospitals adopt a different mode of managing and delivering service compared to private hospitals.

Furthermore, service firms, even within the same industry, may differ for several reasons: the service package they offer; the hierarchy between core service and ancillary services; the degree of standardization; the degree of externalization; the delivery mode; the extent of the contact during the delivery, etc. A home-care service, for example, can present various degrees of completeness and personalization, according to the services which are provided, the frequency of the interventions, the kind of staff involved, etc.

Consequently, we need to focus our attention on those factors, which most help us in defining and analyzing the impact and the implications of the digital economy on healthcare services.

To this purpose, we refer to a model developed by Benevolo and Spinelli (2011). The model firstly shows "how a service firm may become international, according to the characteristics of the services it offers and the supply system it sets up" and then "the impact of the application of internet-based technologies to service delivery by showing the implications for the internationalisation processes and, consequently, for the model" (p. 252). We consider it useful to adopt the service taxonomy proposed by the authors when evaluating the impact of ICT on the service delivery. This part of the model is therefore considered—without any reference to the elements more strictly related to the internationalization processes—and applied with some adaptations to healthcare services.

The aim of the model is to show the relationship between the characteristics of the service and of its delivery modes, and the way in which the application of Internet-related technologies impact on the service delivery itself. The authors focus their attention on a specific group of ICT, which includes those informatics solutions and application platforms based on network technologies: corporate website, marketplaces, intranet and extranet, e-commerce, live chat, corporate blogs, EDI and databases via the Internet, computer reservation systems, etc. Thanks to these technologies, it is feasible to create and manage in a more functional way the business processes involving customers, providers, employees, etc. Part of the Internet-based technologies (for example, corporate websites or marketplaces) are also Web-based—as they are supported by the system of interlinked hypertext documents which constitutes the World Wide Web—while others (for instance Voice Over IP systems or machine-to-machine communication systems) can do without the Web interface. Internet-based technologies overcome the limitations, develop the potential and re-define the applicability of the service delivery, reshaping the way in which many services are actually performed and made available to the recepients.

To start, it is necessary to divide services into clusters, designed around two key dimensions. The first dimension is the need of physical co-presence or interaction between producer and user in service delivery. As regards this dimension, the aim is to identify those services in which delivery requires co-presence and interaction (even if from a distance) or a high degree of personalization, which necessarily implies a level of relationship directly related to the need for co-presence (Sung-Eui, 2005). Some services require the physical presence of both producer and consumer, such as most of the personal services. Some others do not: consider, for instance, long-distance services where the contact is not present (such in telecommunications) or is virtual; or service-embodied goods, where the delivery is mediated by a good (for instance a movie in a DVD) (Bhagwati, 1987). As regards healthcare services, most medical and nurse treatments belong to the first group of services, while other information-intensive services—such as communication, education, and administrative services—belong to the latter group.

The second dimension evaluates the possibility, opportunity, and convenience of performing the service delivery through the Internet, that is, replacing the traditional service delivery with Internet-based technologies.

When jointly considered, these two dimensions generate four groups of services, as in Table 1.

Those groups are now introduced and healthcare-related examples are given for each of them; furthermore, the evolution from the traditional delivery to the Internet-based one is analyzed with reference to the digital economy framework, to show the contribution of each block as a driver for such a process.

Digital Goods and Services [A]

Digital goods and services are services where the physical co-presence is not required and the service delivery can be performed through the Internet.

Table 1. Service delivery and internet-related technologies

Physical co-presence or interaction / personalization	Service delivery	
	can be performed through the Internet	*cannot be performed through the Internet*
necessary	virtual relationship or reality [C]	unavoidable "physical-ness" or humanisation [D]
unnecessary	digital goods and services [A] on-line delivery [B]	

Source: Adapted from Benevolo and Spinelli (2011) © 2011, Interscience Publishers. Used with permission.

They often represent the evolution from service-embodied goods, or services, which used to need the support of a physical good to be delivered. Here, technological innovation has acted in two seemingly conflicting ways: firstly, it has supported the "materialization" of services into transferable and tradable goods (for example, recording music on a digital device); later, it has increased the immateriality of services, separating them from physical evidence through digitalization and new Internet-based transferability (Evans & Wurster, 2000; Sung-Eui, 2005). In this sense, transferability has been made more pervasive by the possibility of digitalizing and transmitting data, archives, sounds, images, codified knowledge, and anything, which can be considered "information" (Shapiro & Varian, 1999). Consequently, information-based services are separated from their physical evidence and their delivery can be easily processed through the Internet.

As regards health care systems, a widely recognized source of inefficiencies is the fragmentation of the care delivery process and the poor transfer of information along the various steps (OECD, 2010, p. 32). The efficient sharing of health information is, however, indispensable for the effective delivery of care (IOM, 2001). To this aim, a major example of innovative health digital services is the so-called Electronic Health Record (EHR), the digital storage of all the health information of a patient generated by one or more encounters in any care delivery setting. This information includes patient demographics, progress notes, problems, medications, vital signs, past medical history, immunizations, laboratory data and radiology reports, etc. (HIMSS, 2011). "Before the advent of Internet technology, there was no way to escape the inefficiencies of a paper-based system: the piles of prescriptions, forms, and charts, the frustration associated with registering and filling in medical histories more than once, the high cost of such inefficiencies" (Ball & Lillis, 2001, p. 5). The electronic health records, on the contrary, carry great advantages compared to traditional paper, the main one being that it has evolved from a physical construct into pure information. First, this means that multimedia data can easily be stored in digital archives, something that previously was only true for written data; second, data can be embedded in a portable device the patient can easily carry with her or can be digitally transmitted anywhere at no cost. This allows for quick and inexpensive communications between doctors or medical centers. A specialist, for instance, can be asked for consultancy by colleagues in a distant location to study a patient's file, thus expanding the potential market of her activity virtually to the whole world. The use of EHR significantly and positively impacts on a wide array of variables: from treatments effectiveness and safety to healthcare quality, to decision support, to increased knowledge transfer capability and continuous training opportunities for practitioners (Osservatorio ICT in Sanità, 2011).

Exploiting the same principle, the results of an exam—for instance an ECG or a radiograph—can be remotely transmitted for analysis by a doctor who is not physically present with the patient. Picture Archiving and Communication Systems (PACS), for example, are computer systems that "replace conventional x-ray film, and greatly improves access to patient information by making it possible for referring clinicians to review their patient's images on PCs from their own offices" (OECD, 2010, p. 36). This is a typical example of telemedicine, which, in some cases, can lead to cost savings through the international outsourcing of medical activities (Orava, 2002): a radiograph taken in the US could be sent electronically to a doctor in India or in another "low-cost" country to be examined, with the doctor referring back to the host medical center via electronic networks (Friedman, 2006).

We can now deconstruct these applications and analyze them using the digital economy framework. The first step consists of the digitalization of a patient's history (or of the results of an exam), which is consequently separated from any physical support, typically a paper file (block 2 and 4); then, it becomes feasible to overcome the limitation of paper files, by enriching the collected data with multimedia elements without extra costs (block 5) and transmitting it through electronic networks (block 1 and 3). Once the patient's history has turned into an immaterial product, a doctor no longer needs to "own" (or have in her hands) a patient's file but can simply "access" it from where it is stored (block 6). As regards the storage of digital information, the earliest solutions were based on saving the data on a specific PC, sometimes accessible remotely within a local network, or on a physically portable device. Nowadays, remote storing services and cloud computing open innovative opportunities, progressively reducing the need for proximity between the user and the place where information is stored: information is available from the cloud provider from any location (or device) with an Internet connection.

On-Line Delivery [B]

The second group too includes services where the delivery can be performed through the Internet and co-presence is not necessary. In this case, we focus on the evolution of long-distance services—where delivery system is non-transportable but can work from a distance, and the co-presence of both producer and consumer is unnecessary (such as in telecommunications); these services can be delivered via remote communication and strongly benefit from Internet-based technologies.

Some of these services originated as digital services to satisfy on-line market needs, which were not, or not fully, satisfied by existing firms (on-line search engines, "wiki" encyclopedias, or tourist guides). Others have fundamentally changed their core service and delivery system (on-line insurance companies and banks, live chat services, on-line news and trading). Others have taken advantage of the greater transmission and communication capability and pervasiveness of

the new technologies, their lower usage costs, and the opportunity to enrich the service offer with new additional services (digital TV, Web radio, multimedia dictionaries, VOIP) (Benevolo & Spinelli, 2011).

With respect to healthcare activities, online services are widespread in the support processes. In this field, many services can already be fully delivered through the Internet: consider the booking of visits, the delivery of exam results, the billing and payment cycle, etc. Even if not strictly related with the "main" caretaking process, these services are crucial for health organizations, especially in terms of administrative costs and service quality; their impact on the overall efficiency and effectiveness is consequently very strong. Once more, the possibility of delivering those services through the Internet is the result of the action of all the building blocks of the framework: health organizations and their customers are connected (blocks 1 and 3) and can interact exchanging rich information flows (block 5) which substitute for paper files and personal interaction (block 2 and 4). Furthermore, these systems (for example the reservation systems) are quite often shared by several hospitals and other healthcare organizations which operate in the same geographic area; in this way, a common platform is accessed (block 6) by all the users, without having to build an own system and significantly reducing the operating costs for implementation, maintenance, updating, etc.

On-line delivery can be extremely useful in the diagnosis step too of the caretaking process. Consider, for instance, Internet-based on-demand clinical case analysis services, such as those developed by MEDgle©. MEDgle is a case analysis engine with a wide range of real-time, predictive health uses. The MEDgle platform is built on top of a large database of relationships between symptoms, diagnoses, drugs, tests, procedures, and associated statistical information (MEDgle Inc., 2011). Even if still at the experimental stage, this service could potentially bring valuable support to the medical staff in decision taking. As in digital goods and services, such a service originates from the possibility of codifying and digitalize a great amount of knowledge and information which was long available only in physical devices (such as books) or which was tacit and "embedded" in the practitioners' experience (block 2 and 4). Then each element of this huge knowledge base is combined in unprecedented ways, which enriches its value and create a new corpus of augmented knowledge (block 4). Finally, this new enriched knowledge base is made available through the Internet to every user (block 1 and 3). The user is even excused from the need of acquiring any ICT device or advance infrastructure, as the service is totally web-based and can be accessed from everywhere and by using any kind of Internet-capable device (block 6). This last feature is particularly interesting, because it allows for the possibility of using the platform even in extreme situations, such as in a rescue service, when the medical staff is outside the hospital facilities but can access the Internet with portable tools such as an IPad or similar. MEDgle belongs to the family of the Clinical Decision Support Systems (CDSS), a large group of stand-alone or Web-based systems, which aim to support the decision-making process of medical staff with inference engines or artificial intelligence software (Garg, et al., 2005). The reliability of CDSS is still questioned by the medical community, due to the limit that these technologies face in properly interpreting the whole clinical picture of a patient; nevertheless, the value of the business idea is certainly high and it is probable that, once refined and completely implemented, MEDgle and its competitors will become a useful and reliable support tool for medical staff.

A further research and diagnostic service which is delivered though the Web are bibliographic databases such as MEDLINE© (Medical Literature Analysis and Retrieval System Online), which includes bibliographic information for articles from academic journals covering most of medical science fields. The value added of such a service does not

lie only in that the articles are digitalized and knowledge is separated from the physical device (block 2 and 4); more important is the aspect related to the accurate ways in which this knowledge base can be explored, thanks to the connections which are created between the single piece of information and all the rest. In other words, the value lies in the enrichment of the collected knowledge, which overcomes any trade-off between reach and richness in information broadcasting (block 5). As usual, Internet technologies make possible the delivery of a world-wide service to every potential user (block 1 and 3) who, again, is both physical and economically separated from the resources accessed (block 6); physical separation means that it is no longer necessary to have the journal in one's hand, while economic separation refers to the shift from exclusive ownership to access of a shared resource.

Virtual Relationship or Reality [C]

In this third group of services, the co-presence and interaction of the producer and the consumer of the service is necessary, but this co-presence can be made virtual by performing the service delivery through the Internet. The feasibility of this process is a consequence of the degree of contact required for delivery and of how much this can be replaced by a simulation or an Internet-based relationship. In personal services, a partial replacement for a physical presence and a Web contact is sometimes possible, where a relationship is unnecessary or not critical for service quality. This is the case of some healthcare services, such as diagnostics, which have traditionally meant local services with high levels of contact and interaction between supplier (the doctor and his team) and consumer (the patient and her family).

Thanks to the advent of the digital economy, the delivery of these services can be completely redesigned, with consequences for both service performance and patient life quality.

413

We have especially in mind the mobile real time monitoring of patient vital signs, when patients are continually monitored on health-related parameters with wireless sensors, irrespective of where they happen to be (Van Halteren, et al., 2004). Sensors can be embedded on the patient (for instance, in small monitoring devices or in her clothes) and mobile phones or Personal Digital Assistants (PDAs) with wireless networking capabilities may serve as gateways that process, store, and transfer data to clinicians for further analysis or diagnosis (Bardram, Mihailidis, & Wan, 2006). The monitoring device could have multimedia capabilities—allowing for the transmission of audio and video too—or even be coupled with an operating device (for example an insulin pump) which performs a remotely controlled therapy on the patient (Haux, Ammenwerth, Herzog, & Knaup, 2002, p. 13).

These solutions offer great benefits because they free the patient from the need of being always "within reach" of the doctor, that is, of being physically present when the monitoring is performed. Furthermore, it allows for continuous monitoring (and, in some cases, intervention), which would be much more difficult to achieve in the traditional way. Finally, it can be a tremendous innovation in situations of limited mobility of the patients, such as with remote communities, or in developing countries, since they lack both expert practitioners and health structures on the territory and distances can be significant between patients and hospitals. In this case, patients can be monitored by doctors who are very far away, with a great benefit to the population of disadvantaged countries (Gerber, 2009). Similar considerations could be made as regards specific situations in which continuous monitoring is needed but the presence of a doctor or nurse is unfeasible: we have in mind, for instance, post-partum home recovery, post-discharge home treatments, long-term and chronic home care, etc.

Sometimes, the interconnection is on a machine-to-machine basis, which means that the first recipient of the transmitted information is not a person but another device, which is programmed to react in a certain way when receiving specific data.

These sensors forward their collected data to an M2M device (e.g., a patient's cell phone) that acts as an information aggregator and forwards the data to the M2M application server [...]. The M2M server responds to the collected data by sending alerts and appropriate medical records to medical providers. In emergency situations, an M2M device can directly provide the medical status of a patient en route to the hospital (e.g., in the ambulance), allowing physicians to prepare for treatment in advance of the patient's arrival" (Wu, et al., 2011, p. 38).

With reference to the building blocks of the framework, the crucial aspect is that the patient is out of the reach of the doctor (who does not "own" the patient any longer but can "access" her (block 6); nevertheless, the physical contact turns into a virtual relationship, as the patient is continuously connected with the medical center (block 1 and 3) and transmits to the doctors relevant and rich information about her health in a digital format (block 2, 4, and 5).

The last frontier in this virtual relationship regards the treatment step and is represented by tele-surgery via virtual reality 3D systems: in fact, they allow the surgeon to perform the operation from a distance, through an Internet connection by means of a robot-surgeon (Slack, 2007; Zhijiang, Zhiheng, & Minxiu, 2006). In this case, the main innovation is the capability of translating the physical act of surgery into a rich information flow (block 2, 4, and 5), which is able to include a very large set of multimedia data; then, the information is transmitted to the location where the surgery is actually performed (block 1 and 3); finally, the flow is converted back into actual movements, which are performed by the robot. As the information flow is bidirectional, the surgeon receives back all the information about the patient (data, images, simulation of the response of the patient's body to the surgeon's actions), without being close to her. In this kind of activity, the shift from ownership to access is double, because, on the one side, the surgeon has remote access to all the relevant information about the patient and, on the other side, the physical action on the patient is performed using a device (the robot) that the surgeon does not have in her hands but only "accesses" from a distance (block 6). This opens the way to a virtual relationship between doctor and patient, with promising consequences for the development of long-distance surgery, which can now be performed regardless of geographical separation; some visionary authors are even imaging space surgery, to support quality of life and medical care in human outposts on the Moon or Mars (Haidegger, Sándor, & Benyo, 2011)!

Unavoidable "Physical-Ness" or Humanization [D]

In this last group, services are included, which need co-presence and whose delivery cannot be performed through the Internet. As a consequence, for these services it is not possible to substitute an Internet-based delivery for a traditional one and the direct impact of the digital economy on them is thus indirect. Nevertheless, ICT can play a major role in the delivery of the additional services, which precede, follow, or accompany the delivery of the core service, thus enriching the traditional service and generating more value for the user (Benevolo & Spinelli, 2011). Consider, for instance, those services assisting the potential consumer in the information-gathering process or in the evaluation of possible options (pre-delivery); those services supporting the sale; the assistance and customer services (post-delivery); those specific additional services helping the customer during off-line delivery.

As regards healthcare, a great part of the medical and nursing activity is subject to these limitations. As previously seen, part of the traditional

set of medical and surgical activities have been moved to the Internet in some pioneering experiences, but in the vast majority of cases it still has to face the need of a real physical contact with the patient who is going to receive the service. This is certainly relevant for medical activity but may be even more significant for nursing, which in some cases requires a closer contact between the nurse and the patient than the doctor-patient relationship. So long as technological development does not introduce really break-through innovations, it is quite difficult to imagine an Internet-based delivery for nursing services which support the patient in her everyday activities—such as cleaning or feeding—or which relate to applying a medication or dressing a wound.

Nevertheless, the development of the digital economy can have a strong indirect impact on this group of healthcare activities as well, if we consider the additional services, which always complement the physical performance of the core service. Indeed, several of those e-health applications we included in the former three groups of services are often part of a complex service-system, which has at its core an unavoidably physical service; however, these non-core elements are critical with respect to value creation and customer satisfaction, as they can dramatically improve the performance of the medical staff. Electronic health records, together with on-line resources and services, are for instance a powerful tool for constantly accessing and updating the patient's history, so ensuring that the most effective therapy is determined and provided. Similarly, mobile real time monitoring of the patient can limit physical contact to circumstances where it is strictly needed, so allowing the medical staff to concentrate on higher-value creating activities. A doctor who does not have to look for medical examination results but finds them always available on a portable tool, can concentrate on diagnosis without losing time; similarly, a nurse who always has access to the prescribed therapies in the patient's file is much less likely to make mistakes or to misinterpret the doctor's instructions (Bates, et al., 2001).

FUTURE TRENDS

In this chapter, we have tried to highlight the impact of the advent of a new economic paradigm, - the digital economy- on healthcare services. To this purpose, we have shown how e-health applications can be deconstructed in the light of an interpretative framework, which traces them back to the main drivers of the paradigm evolution.

With specific reference to healthcare, the digital economy has not yet revealed all its potential. As reported by Kennedy and Berk (2011), the health care industry "despite being arguably the most information-intensive industry in the world, has been slow to join the digital revolution" and "the transition will be a sea change" (p. 1). Indeed the innumerable cases of innovative adoption of ICT—both in the intangible and tangible components of healthcare activities—suggest to us that the evolution of healthcare activities towards new digital configurations is a structural process already in progress, even if still far from reaching full deployment.

Indeed, a significant part of healthcare services are by their nature "high-touch services," due to the need for physical contact and relation, and they are consequently slow in evolving from "low-tech" to "high-tech" configurations, where the use of automatic systems, ICT and other physical supports is more and more significant (Salomann, Kolbe, & Brenner, 2006). The progress is not easy, due to cultural, organizational, and budget constraints, but the cases we have proposed suggest that innovation horizons in healthcare are broad and promising.

Coming back to the Malecki and Moriset (2008) classification which was presented in the "Background" paragraph, we confirm that the healthcare industry is going to increasingly join the pyramid's "main body," as more and more of its activities will require extensive use of ICT to be performed in innovative and more effective ways, with great benefits for patients, medical staff and national budgets too.

More broadly, this trend is stronger when we consider that medical activities in the strict sense of the word are only a part of the complex healthcare industry. Indeed, it includes several service-providing and manufacturing sectors—such as research companies, information providers, and diagnostic equipment manufacturers—which are already heavily ICT-enabled and consequently push the "medical core" of the industry towards new digital configurations.

While at the beginning of the century the Institute of Medicine (IOM, 2001) could state that the healthcare service delivery remained "relatively untouched by the revolution in information technology that [had] swept nearly every other aspect of society" (p. 15), nowadays the situation has radically evolved and the "revolution" is absolutely in progress.

Nevertheless, the process towards a widespread implementation of e-health practices has to face several obstacles, most of which do not strictly relate to technical matters. With respect to technical difficulties, it is very often just "a matter of time," as continuous innovation is able to progressively overcome them. We are more interested in non-technical questions and—even though a full examination of them is beyond the aim of this chapter—some references cannot be omitted.

A first major barrier concerns the financing of e-health initiatives; purchasing and implementation costs for these projects usually require a significant amount of financing with an uncertain (at least in the short term) assessment of the extent of the achievable benefits and of who is actually benefitting from the gains in efficiency and effectiveness:

one significant barrier to investment in ICTs is the widely recognized fact that any resulting cost savings may not always accrue to the implementer, but may be passed on to a third party. Benefits may appear at one site and in one budget; while a large share of the cost commitments appear at another site and in another budget (OECD, 2010, p. 46).

Furthermore, there may be lags between ICT investments and benefit realization (Devaraj & Kohli, 2000); quite commonly, the financial benefits are not realized until a level of functionality is reached—a kind of "critical mass"—that allows systems to truly serve the needs of clinicians and system planners. "Until IT investment reaches a threshold, total operating expenses increase in hospitals that have little IT" (PricewaterhouseCoopers, 2007, p. 18). In a time of shrinking public budget for healthcare, this limitation can be decisive in discouraging investments in health information technology. Moreover, poorer countries could be excluded from the innovation process, due to their limited budget to allocate to e-health initiatives.

In addition, there are no incentives, and may even be disincentives for care providers to be the first to adopt ICTs (Taylor, et al., 2005), as commonly happens with radical innovations. All the same, the development of a strong business case is crucial, because—as in Dixon (2007)—it "lowers the risk of adoption, implementation, and use of e-health" (p. 11) and is the first step of an effective roadmap for e-health adoption.

A second important barrier is associated with organizational factors, both between and within healthcare organizations.

As regards the first aspect, we have to keep in mind that several e-health services involve a plurality of organizations: healthcare systems, indeed, are usually very fragmented, with a multiplicity of public and private providers and payers. This constitutes a significant barrier to the adoption of e-health services, as this implies connecting systems managed by different organizations and with relevant differences as regards the standard

and content of the collected data, the transmission protocol, etc. (Kaye, et al., 2010). For this reason, a crucial role is played by the organizations for standardization—such as the International Organization for Standardization (ISO) or the Comité Européen de Normalisation (CEN)—which are working, in particular, for the definition of common standards for the Electronic Health Records (Moruzzi, 2009). Kennedy and Berk (2011) report about the US experience, where "a host of standards – Including Logical Observation Identifiers Names and Codes (LOINC), Digital Imaging and Communications in Medicine (DICOM), Health Level Seven International (HL7), and Systematized Nomenclature of Medicine Clinical Terms (SNOMED CT)—are allowing for rich information interchange across care settings and are being used by regional health-information organizations [...] to coordinate care across regions, with impressive results" (p. 5). The developmental work on standards is surely critical, but when standards are refined and become more commonplace, the ability to exchange, aggregate, and analyze health care data will increase dramatically.

The barrier associated with organizational factors internal to the healthcare organization represents an aspect not yet adequately studied in the literature (Shekelle & Goldzweig, 2009); nevertheless, this topic is crucial as the implementation of an health information system represents a strong organizational discontinuity and questions consolidated procedures, routines and habits (Gagnon, et al., 2005). This opens the door to a vast discussion about leadership and governance for ICT projects (Bernstein, McCreless, & Côté, 2007; Fickenscher & Bakerman, 2011); about technical education and training for doctors and nurses who are asked to use new technologies (Masys, 1998; Ball & Lillis, 2001); about how to increase the actual adoption of new systems and overcome the organizational and individual inertia (England, Steward, & Walker, 2000; Gaggioli, Di Carlo, Mantovani, Castelnuovo, & Riva, 2005). Furthermore, we should not forget that high technology cannot do without human skills and capabilities, which must remain absolutely central in the service delivery (Demattè, Biffi, Mandelli, & Parolini, 2007; Freeman, Vatz, & Demaerschalk, 2010).

Another big problem is related to privacy, security and legal issues in sharing sensitive patient data in a large and heterogeneous environment through the use of web-based applications (Berner, 2008; Moruzzi, 2009; Lateef, 2011). Several surveys and studies highlight the concern about the privacy of patients' health information. This concern is well motivated because, "as the contents of electronic health records are shared more widely, the risk increases that stigmatizing disclosures could affect areas such as employment status, access to health insurance and other forms of insurance, and participation in community activities" (OECD, 2010, p. 106).

This is certainly a major issue, which has to be addressed from both the legal and the technical side: from the legal side, to build a regulatory framework (better if on an international scale) for information gathering, storing and sharing; from the technical side to develop those standards and applications which make possible to match the application of e-health practices with the protection of individual rights.

Finally, another issue is also the degree of acceptance of e-health practices by the recipients, that is, the patients or their family. With respect to this, both cultural predisposition and technology acceptance are relevant, especially in older patients (see, among others, Eikelboom & Atlas, 2005; Whitten & Love, 2005); the patient have to accept the substitution of a technology-mediated relationship with the medical staff for physical contact and also have to develop such minimum skills which allow them to interact with the devices, such as in the mobile real time monitoring of vital signs. This is a subject that deserves much more attention and could be of major interest not only for medical practitioners but also for engineers

and software developers, who have to design those devices.

In spite of all these obstacles, the future of e-health is nevertheless very promising and this will certainly lead to interesting developments in research. New applications are constantly developed and the adoption of ICT in healthcare is increasingly pervasive, rich, and deep. It is consequently of undoubted interest to analyze and deconstruct these innovative activities to place them within the wider picture of the digital economy.

CONCLUSION

Our reflection about the impact of the digital economy on healthcare services has shown how the innovative e-health applications find their origins in the major drivers we have described as the building blocks of the new economic paradigm. As theorized in the model, the joint action of both technological innovation and evolution on the demand side has deeply influenced this crucial industry, opening the way to a fundamental reshaping of its structure and of the way in which services are performed by healthcare organizations and firms.

In essence, the adoption of ICT triggers a virtuous cycle of innovation: the new opportunities enabled by digital technologies stimulate the creation of original practices and the reconfiguration of the processes; this, in turn, supports the research for latest technologies—maybe "borrowed" from other sectors as a consequence of the industry convergence we aforementioned—to apply to healthcare, and so on.

Physical limitations—mostly due to the undoubted importance of the physical co-presence of producer (healthcare staff) and user (patient) in many healthcare services—are still present and central, but it is very probable that in the medium and long term, they will be gradually overcome and the application of ICT to healthcare will become widespread and pervasive.

REFERENCES

Aldrich, D., & Masera, P. (1999). *Mastering the digital market place*. New York, NY: John Wiley & Sons.

Ames, E., & Rosenberg, N. (1977). Technological change in the machine tool industry: 1840-1910. In Rosenberg, N. (Ed.), *Perspectives on Technology* (pp. 9–31). Cambridge, UK: Cambridge University Press.

Argyres, N., & McGahan, A. M. (2002). An interview with Michael Porter. *The Academy of Management Executive*, *16*(2), 43–52. doi:10.5465/AME.2002.7173495

Atkinson, R. D., & McKay, A. S. (2007). *Digital prosperity – Understanding the economic benefits of the information technology revolution*. Retrieved July 7, 2011 from http://www.itif.org/index.php?id=34.

Ball, M. J., & Lillis, J. (2001). E-health: Transforming the physician-patient relationship. *International Journal of Medical Informatics*, *61*, 1–10. doi:10.1016/S1386-5056(00)00130-1

Bardram, J. E., Mihailidis, A., & Wan, D. (Eds.). (2006). *Pervasive computing in healthcare*. Boca Raton, FL: CRC.

Bates, D. W., Cohen, M., Leape, L. L., Overhage, J. M., Shabot, M. M., & Sheridan, T. (2001). Reducing the frequency of errors in medicine using information technology. *Journal of the American Medical Informatics Association*, *8*(4), 299–308. doi:10.1136/jamia.2001.0080299

Benevolo, C., & Spinelli, R. (2011). International service delivery and Internet-based technologies. *International Journal of Services. Economics and Management*, *3*(3), 251–266.

Berner, E. S. (2008). Ethical and legal issues in the use of health information technology to improve patient safety. *HEC Forum*, *20*(39), 243–258. doi:10.1007/s10730-008-9074-5

Bernstein, M. L., McCreless, T., & Côté, M. J. (2007). Five constants of information technology adoption in healthcare. *Hospital Topics*, *85*(1), 17–25. doi:10.3200/HTPS.85.1.17-26

Bhagwati, J. (1987). International trade in services and its relevance for economic development. In Giarini, O. (Ed.), *The Emerging Service Economy* (pp. 3–57). Oxford, UK: Pergamon Press.

Burman, E. (2003). *Shift! The unfolding internet: Hype, hope and history*. Chichester, UK: John Wiley & Sons.

Castells, M. (2000). *The rise of the network society*. Oxford, UK: Blackwell Publishers.

Chang, K., Soong, A., Tseng, M., & Xiang, Z. (2011). Global wireless machine-to-machine standardization. *IEEE Internet Computing*, *15*(2), 64–69. doi:10.1109/MIC.2011.41

Chase, R. B. (1978). Where does the customer fit in a service operation. *Harvard Business Review*, *56*(5), 137–142.

Chen, S. (2001). *Strategic management of e-business*. Chichester, UK: John Wiley & Sons.

Commission of the European Communities. (2004). *e-Health - Making healthcare better for European citizens: An action plan for a European e-Health area*. Luxembourg: Commission of the European Communities.

Conti, J. P. (2006). The internet of things. *IET Communications Engineer*, *4*(6), 20–25. doi:10.1049/ce:20060603

Demattè, C., Biffi, A., Mandelli, A., & Parolini, C. (2007). Firms and the digital technology in Italy: The network moves forward. In Apte, U., & Karmarkar, U. (Eds.), *Managing in the Information Economy* (pp. 429–471). New York, NY: Springer. doi:10.1007/978-0-387-36892-4_18

Devaraj, S., & Kohli, R. (2000). Information technology payoff in the healthcare industry: A longitudinal study. *Journal of Management Information Systems, 16*(4), 41–67.

Dixon, B. E. (2007). A roadmap for the adoption of e-. *The Health Service Journal, 5*(3), 3–13.

Eiglier, P., & Langeard, E. (1987). *Servuction: Le marketing des services.* Paris, France: McGraw-Hill.

Eikelboom, R. H., & Atlas, M. D. (2005). Attitude to telemedicine, and willingness to use it, in audiology patients. *Journal of Telemedicine and Telecare, 11*, S22–S25. doi:10.1258/135763305775124920

England, I., Steward, D., & Walker, S. (2000). Information technology adoption in health care: When organizations and technology collide. *Australian Health Review, 23*(3), 176–185. doi:10.1071/AH000176

Evans, P., & Wurster, T. S. (2000). *Blown to bits: How the new economics of information transforms strategy.* Boston, MA: Harvard Business School Press.

Eysenbach, G. (2001). What is e-health? *Journal of Medical Internet Research, 3*(2), e20. doi:10.2196/jmir.3.2.e20

Fickenscher, K., & Bakerman, M. (2011). Leadership and governance for IT projects. *Physician Executive, 37*(1), 72–76.

Fieschi, M. (2002). Information technology is changing the way society sees health care delivery. *International Journal of Medical Informatics, 66*, 85–93. doi:10.1016/S1386-5056(02)00040-0

Freeman, W. D., Vatz, K. A., & Demaerschalk, B. M. (2010). Telemedicine in 2010: Robotic caveats. *The Lancet Neurology, 9*(11), 1046. doi:10.1016/S1474-4422(10)70261-1

Friedman, T. L. (2006). *The world is flat: A brief history of the twenty-first century.* New York, NY: Farrar Straus Giroux.

Frisse, M. E. (2009). Health information technology: One step at a time. *Health Affairs, n.d.,* 379–w384. doi:10.1377/hlthaff.28.2.w379

Gaggioli, A., Di Carlo, S., Mantovani, F., Castelnuovo, G., & Riva, G. (2005). A telemedicine survey among Milan doctors. *Journal of Telemedicine and Telecare, 11*(1), 29–34. doi:10.1258/1357633053430476

Gagnon, M.-P., Lamothe, L., Fortin, J.-P., Cloutier, A., Godin, G., Gagné, C., & Reinharz, D. (2005). Telehealth adoption in hospitals: An organisational perspective. *Journal of Health Organization and Management, 19*(1), 32–56. doi:10.1108/14777260510592121

Garg, A. X., Adhikari, N. K. J., McDonald, H., Rosas-Arellano, M. P., Devereaux, P. J., & Beyene, J. (2005). Effects of computerized clinical decision support systems on practitioner performance and patient outcomes: A systematic review. *Journal of the American Medical Association, 293*(10), 1223–1238. doi:10.1001/jama.293.10.1223

Gerber, T. (2009). Health information technology: Dispatches from the revolution. *Health Affairs, n.d.,* 390–w391. doi:10.1377/hlthaff.28.2.w390

Greenstain, S., & Khanna, T. (1997). What does industry convergence mean. In Yoffie, D. B. (Ed.), *Competing in the Age of Digital Convergence* (pp. 201–226). Boston, MA: Harvard Business School Press.

Grönroos, C. (1990). *Service management and marketing: Managing the moments of truth in service competition.* New Britian, CT: Lexington Books.

Haidegger, T., Sándor, J., & Benyo, Z. (2011). Surgery in space: The future of robotic telesurgery. *Surgical Endoscopy, 25*(3), 681–690. doi:10.1007/s00464-010-1243-3

Haux, R., Ammenwerth, E., Herzog, W., & Knaup, P. (2002). Health care in the information society: A prognosis for the year 2013. *International Journal of Medical Informatics, 66*, 3–21. doi:10.1016/S1386-5056(02)00030-8

HIMSS. (2011). *Electronic health record (HER)*. Retrieved on June 16, 2011 from http://www.himss.org/ASP/topics_ehr.asp.

IOM. (2001). *Crossing the quality chasm: A new health system for the 21st century*. Washington, DC: National Academy Press.

Javalgi, R. G., Martin, C. L., & Todd, P. R. (2004). The export of e-services in the age of technology transformation: Challenges and implications for international service providers. *Journal of Services Marketing, 18*(7), 560–573. doi:10.1108/08876040410561884

Kaye, R., Kokia, E., Shalev, V., Idar, D., & Chinitz, D. (2010). Barriers and success factors in health information technology: A practitioner's perspective. *Journal of Management & Marketing in Healthcare, 3*(2), 163–175. doi:10.1179/175330310X12736577732764

Kennedy, S., & Berk, B. (2011). Enabling e-health: A revolution for informatics in health care. *BCG Perspectives*. Retrieved on June 17, 2011 from www.bcgperspectives.com.

Kumar, V., & Venkatesan, R. (2005). Who are the multichannel shoppers and how do they perform? Correlates of multichannel shopping behavior. *Journal of Interactive Marketing, 19*(2), 44–62. doi:10.1002/dir.20034

Lateef, F. (2011). The practice of telemedicine: Medicolegal and ethical issues. *Ethics & Medicine, 27*(1), 17–25.

Laudon, K., & Laudon, J. (2010). *Management information systems* (11th ed.). Upper Saddle River, NJ: Prentice Hall.

Lovelock, C. H. (1983). Classifying services to gain strategic marketing insights. *Journal of Marketing, 47*(3), 9–20. doi:10.2307/1251193

Lovelock, C. H. (1996). *Service marketing* (3rd ed.). London, UK: Prentice Hall International.

Malecki, E. J., & Moriset, B. (2008). *The digital economy: Business organization, production processes, and regional developments*. Oxon, UK: Routledge.

Mandelli, A., & Parolini, C. (2003). Imprese e tecnologie digitali: La rete avanza. In Biffi, A., & Dematté, C. (Eds.), *L'araba Fenice: Economia Digitale Alla Prova Dei Fatti* (pp. 3–62). Milano, Italy: Etas.

Masys, D. (1998). Advances in information technology: Implications for medical education. *The Western Journal of Medicine, 168*(5), 341–347.

MEDgle Inc. (2011). *The details*. Retrieved on June 15, 2011 from http://www.medgle.com/front.jsp?task=technology&section=details.

Moruzzi, M. (2009). *E-health e fascicolo sanitario elettronico*. Milano, Italy: Il Sole 24 Ore.

Normann, R. (1984). *Service management strategy and leadership in service business*. Chichester, UK: John Wiley & Sons.

OECD. (2010). *Improving health sector efficiency: The role of information and communication technologies*. Paris, France: OECD.

Oh, H., Rizo, C., Enkin, M., & Jadad, A. (2005). What is eHealth: A systematic review of published definitions. *Journal of Medical Internet Research, 7*(1), e1. doi:10.2196/jmir.7.1.e1

Orava, M. (2002). Globalising medical services: Operational modes in the internationalization of medical service firms. *International Journal of Medical Marketing, 2*(3), 232–240. doi:10.1057/palgrave.jmm.5040081

Osservatorio ICT in Sanità. (2008). *ICT e innovazione in sanità: Nuove sfide e opportunità per i CIO*. Milano, Italy: Politecnico di Milano, Dipartimento di Ingegneria gestionale.

Osservatorio ICT in Sanità. (2011). *ICT in sanità: L'innovazione in cerca di autore*. Milano, Italy: Politecnico di Milano, Dipartimento di Ingegneria gestionale.

Pagliari, C., Sloan, D., Gregor, P., Sullivan, F., Detmer, D., & Kahan, J. P. (2005). What is eHealth: A scoping exercise to map the field. *Journal of Medical Internet Research, 7*(1), e9. doi:10.2196/jmir.7.1.e9

Pine, J. (1993). Mass customizing products and services. *Planning Review, 22*(4), 7–55.

Porter, M., & Millar, V. E. (1985). How information gives you competitive advantage. *Harvard Business Review, 63*(4), 149–160.

Porter, M. E. (2001). Strategy and the internet. *Harvard Business Review, 79*(2), 63–78.

Prandelli, E., & Verona, G. (2011). *Vantaggio competitivo in rete: Dal Web 2.0 al cloud computing*. Milano, Italy: McGraw Hill.

PricewaterhouseCoopers. (2007). *The economics of IT and hospital performance*. Retrieved July 14, 2011 from http://www.pwc.com/us/en/healthcare/publications/the-economics-of-it-and-hospital-performance.jhtml.

Rahman, Z. (2004). E-commerce solution for services. *European Business Review, 16*(6), 564–576. doi:10.1108/09555340410565396

Rayport, J. F., & Jaworski, B. J. (2001). *E-commerce*. New York, NY: McGraw Hill.

Rifkin, J. (2000). *The age of access: The new culture of hypercapitalism, where all of life is a paid-for experience*. New York, NY: Tarcher/Putnam.

Ruefli, T. W., Whinston, A., & Wiggins, R. R. (2001). The digital technological environment. In Wind, J., & Mahajan, V. (Eds.), *Digital Marketing* (pp. 26–58). New York, NY: John Wiley & Sons.

Rullani, E. (2001). New/net/knowledge economy: Le molte facce del postfordismo. *Economia e Politica Industriale, 110*, 6–31.

Salomann, H., Kolbe, L., & Brenner, W. (2006). Self-services in customer relationships: Balancing high-tech and high-touch today and tomorrow. *E-Service Journal, 4*(2), 65–84. doi:10.2979/ESJ.2006.4.2.65

Sawhney, M., & Parikh, D. (2001). Where value lives in a networked world. *Harvard Business Review, 79*(1), 79–86.

Shapiro, C., & Varian, H. R. (1999). *Information rules: A strategic guide to the network economy*. Boston, MA: Harvard Business School Press.

Shekelle, P., & Goldzweig, C. L. (2009). *Costs and benefits of health information technology: An updated systematic review*. London, UK: The Health Foundation.

Slack, C. (2007). The robot surgeon. *Proto Magazine*. Retrieved June 17, 2011 from http://www.protomag.com/assets/the-robot-surgeon?page=1.

Spinelli, R. (2008). The digital economy: A conceptual framework for a new economic paradigm. *The Journal of Business, 8*(1/2), 53–59.

Stroetmann, K. A., Jones, T., Dobrev, A., & Stroetmann, V. N. (2006). *eHealth is worth it: The economic benefits of implemented eHealth solutions at ten European sites*. Luxembourg: Commission of the European Communities.

Sung-Eui, C. (2005). Developing new frameworks for operations strategy and service system design in electronic commerce. *International Journal of Service Industry Management, 16*(3), 294–314. doi:10.1108/09564230510601413

Tapscott, D. (2001). Rethinking strategy in a networked world. *Strategy + Business, 24,* 1-8.

Taylor, R., Bower, A., Girosi, F., Bigelow, J., Fonkych, K., & Hillestad, R. (2005). Promoting health information technology: Is there a case for more-aggressive government action? *Health Affairs, 24*(5), 1234–1345. doi:10.1377/hlthaff.24.5.1234

Teece, D. J. (1986). Profiting from technological innovation: Implications for integration, collaboration, licensing and public policy. *Research Policy, 15*(6), 285–305. doi:10.1016/0048-7333(86)90027-2

Thomas, D. R. E. (1978). Strategy is different in service businesses. *Harvard Business Review, 56*(4), 158–165.

Tocci, R. (1988). *Digital system- Principles and applications* (4th ed.). Englewood Cliffs, CA: Prentice-Hall International.

Valdani, E. (2000). I quattro fondamenti dell'economia digitale. *Economia & Management, 3,* 51–67.

Van Halteren, A., Bults, R., Wac, K., Konstantas, D., Widya, I., & Dokovsky, N. (2004). Mobile patient monitoring: The MobiHealth system. *The Journal on Information Technology in Healthcare, 2*(5), 365–373.

Vicari, S. (2001a). Il management della virtualità. In Vicari, S. (Ed.), *Economia Della Virtualità* (pp. 5–59). Milano, Italy: Egea.

Vicari, S. (2001b). Dalla catena alla rete virtuale del valore. In Vicari, S. (Ed.), *Il Management Nell'era Della Connessione* (pp. 3–50). Milano, Italy: Egea.

Whitten, P., & Love, B. (2005). Patient and provider satisfaction with the use of telemedicine: Overview and rationale for cautious enthusiasm. *Journal of Postgraduate Medicine, 51*(4), 294–299.

WHO. (2006a). *eHealth tools and services: Needs of the member states.* Geneva, Switzerland: WHO.

WHO. (2006b). *Building foundations for eHealth: Progress of member states.* Geneva, Switzerland: WHO.

Winger, R., & Edelman, D. (1989). *The segment-of-one-marketing.* Boston, MA: The Boston Consulting Group.

Wu, G., Talwar, S., Johnsson, K., Himayat, N., & Johnson, K. D. (2011). M2M: From mobile to embedded internet. *IEEE Communications Magazine, 49*(4), 36–43. doi:10.1109/MCOM.2011.5741144

Zeithaml, V. A., & Bitner, M. J. (2000). *Service marketing: Integrating customer focus across the firm.* New York, NY: McGraw Hill.

Zhijiang, D., Zhiheng, J., & Minxiu, K. (2006). Virtual reality-based telesurgery via teleprogramming scheme combined with semi-autonomous control. In *Proceedings of the 27th Annual International Conference, Engineering in Medicine and Biology Society,* (pp. 2153-2156). Shanghai, China: IEEE.

Chapter 16
Clinical–Pull Approach to Telemedicine Implementation Policies using Health Informatics in the Developing World

Maria J. Treurnicht
Stellenbosch University, South Africa

Liezl van Dyk
Stellenbosch University, South Africa

ABSTRACT

Telemedicine could effectively aid hospital referral systems in bringing specialized care to rural communities. South Africa has identified telemedicine as part of its primary health care strategic plan, but similar to many other developing countries, the successful implementation of telemedicine programs is a daunting challenge. One of the contributing factors is the insufficient evidence that telemedicine is a cost-effective alternative. Furthermore, many telemedicine services are implemented without a thorough needs assessment. Throughout this chapter, the authors investigate the use of medical informatics in quantitative telemedicine needs assessments. A framework is introduced to direct implementation policies towards a proven clinical need rather than pushing technology into practise. This clinical-pull strategy aims to reduce the amount of failed projects, by providing decision support to implement appropriate technologies that have the potential to contribute towards better quality healthcare.

INTRODUCTION

A primary goal for public health systems is to provide equal quality health services to the entire population. Most developing countries consider this to be a fundamental challenge. One of the largest constraints in developing countries' public health sectors is the acute shortage of financial resources that inevitably leads to a shortage of medical expertise. Referral systems aim to utilise scarce resources more effectively by ranking

DOI: 10.4018/978-1-4666-0888-7.ch016

hospital services according to different levels of speciality and allocating resources accordingly. Patients are referred between the different levels, to have access to higher levels of care when needed. These referrals are expensive and contribute to the over utilisation of high-level care hospitals, which inevitably causes poor service delivery.

Telemedicine is identified as a possible solution to reducing patient transfer between hospitals. However, the success rate of telemedicine projects in developing countries is disappointingly low. A further concern is the fact that telemedicine is a complex field to evaluate due to its multi-disciplinary nature. Since evaluation plays a critical role in obtaining criteria for policy making, the result of inadequate evaluation has a ripple effect, threatening its sustainability.

A telemedicine project should be continuously evaluated throughout its lifecycle. Nevertheless, many projects are approached on a pilot basis, without the support of needs assessment and evaluation frameworks. At the other end of the spectrum, telemedicine systems are often designed from a technological point of view with too little consideration of the clinical needs. Wyatt (1996) refers to this phenomenon by suggesting that the primary objective is to put technology on the market as a 'technology-push' strategy. A 'clinical-pull' strategy is defined as the opposite of technology-push, being a practice that draws technology towards a proven clinical need. It is expected that systems that are developed and based on a proven need, have a better chance of being successful and sustainable than those without it (Wyatt, 1996).

'Evidence-based management,' is a term commonly used in healthcare policy making. It refers to the practice where decision-making is based on facts rather than opinions. Concrete data are used, together with analysis tools and frameworks, to gain evidence as a foundation for decisions. Literature studies have revealed that there is a lack of evidence that telemedicine is a cost-effective and beneficial alternative to patient referrals (Hailey, Ohinmaa, & Roine, 2004). To follow a clinical-pull approach in telemedicine projects, evidence can be gathered prior to implementation by conducting a needs assessment. Telemedicine systems that are implemented on the foundation of a thorough needs assessment will have the potential to benefit the health system. Although there is no guarantee of utilisation, if there is a proven need for a system, it does, however, validate the capital spent on implementation, since other issues preventing utilisation can be solved after implementation.

Most healthcare facilities that are enrolled in e-health start with the implementation of a patient record system. Hence medical informatics can be considered a predecessor of telemedicine. These information systems are capable of storing valuable data relating to telemedicine. However, few studies have been done where medical informatics are used to contribute to telemedicine needs assessments. Since data are crucial in making evidence-based decisions, the clinical-pull approach should draw upon relevant data to determine whether telemedicine would have the potential to be beneficial at a given facility or region.

South Africa is one of many developing countries that has identified telemedicine as an important new development in the health system. The first telemedicine pilot projects were initiated in 1997, but little success has been reported since. The South African Minister of Health reported in 2010 that of the 86 telemedicine sites in South Africa, only 32 were functional. He attributed the poor performance to a severe lack of leadership, inefficient use of funds and a lack of critical skills at provincial offices. The current poor performance of telemedicine systems indicates a desperate need for evidence that telemedicine can be beneficial (Sabinet, 2010). This chapter is therefore, dedicated to providing policy makers, in South Africa as well as in other developing countries, with a measurement tool to assess the needs and potential benefits of telemedicine systems, prior to implementation.

This chapter argues the case for using medical informatics in needs assessments, towards evidence-based telemedicine management and clinical-pull approaches for implementation. The aim is to reduce telemedicine projects that employ unnecessary systems and equipment, by providing them with an alternative for better planning, prior to implementation. The objectives of this chapter are 1) to identify and describe the potential benefits of telemedicine as an alternative to conventional hospital referrals in public healthcare, 2) discuss the need for clinical-pull strategies with their various dimensions, 3) define health informatics attributes applicable to a telemedicine needs assessment, and 4) provide a needs assessment framework for future use. The chapter is sub-divided into an introduction, a literature review component, a framework for needs assessments, conclusions and suggestions for future work.

BACKGROUND

The innovative application of Information and Communication Technologies (ICTs) in healthcare service delivery has evolved dramatically over the past 30 years. The use of ICTs in healthcare can be traced back to as early as the mid-19th century, where telegraphy was used during the American Civil War to signal medical information between sites (Field, 1996). ICTs have seen a radical development since then, even to the extent that complicated surgeries can now be performed in remote locations, using robots, manipulated by surgeons. This is just one of many groundbreaking innovations in healthcare technology. However, various challenges still remain in the sustainable and effective use of diagnostic telemedicine systems, which use simple technologies such as telephones, cellular phones and email (Craig & Patterson, 2005; Ferguson, 2006).

During the 1960's and continuing until the early 1980's, several telemedicine projects were initiated in the developed world, but most of these projects failed due to a lack of funding. ICTs were expensive and technologies were, for the most part, difficult to use. Many telemedicine projects were driven merely as pilot projects, without a business plan or a program that requires results (Bashshur, 2002). Many of the challenges faced by the developed world during the early stages of implementation are still applicable today in the developing world. However with the rapid development of ICTs, the cost has dropped, enabling significant growth in the applications of telemedicine (Field, 1996).

Defining Telemedicine

There are many different definitions of telemedicine given in the literature. Each definition highlights a combination of the different characteristics of this multi-disciplinary field. Sood *et al.* (2007) researched 104 peer-reviewed definitions of telemedicine from a literature review and combined it to form one universal definition for modern telemedicine:

Telemedicine, being a subset of telehealth, uses communications networks for delivery of health care services and medical education from one geographical location to another, primarily to address challenges like uneven distribution and shortage of infrastructure and human resources (Sood, et al., 2007, p. 576).

Telemedicine consultations are primarily classified according to the type of interaction that takes place between the patient and the health practitioner. 'Synchronous telemedicine' (also called real-time telemedicine) refers to real-time interaction between the sender and the receiver of the data. During such a teleconsultation, there are insignificant time delays between the sending, receiving and collection of data. The most widely used means of synchronous telemedicine is videoconferencing. Synchronous telemedicine is sometimes preferred by practitioners, since it enables the practitioner to have a conversation with the patient. However, this type of interaction requires high bandwidth, which is often either unavailable or unreliable in the rural areas of developing countries. Moreover, some scheduling difficulties may also occur because the patient and practitioner have to be available at the same time (Craig & Patterson, 2005; Ferguson, 2006).

'Asynchronous telemedicine' (also called store-and-forward or pre-recorded telemedicine) allows data to be sent regardless of the receiver's availability at the time of sending. Unfortunately, this type of interaction causes time delays between the sending, receiving and collection of data. A typical method of asynchronous telemedicine is email consultations between health practitioners. In spite of the fact that this form of telemedicine generally requires lower bandwidth than synchronous telemedicine, the direct interaction between specialist and patient is lost. This is of concern to many practitioners, but could be overcome through good communication from the sender (Craig & Patterson, 2005; Ferguson, 2006).

Evidence for Telemedicine Benefits

The growing global awareness of telemedicine led to a substantial growth in published articles concerning telemedicine. Many studies have been done to evaluate the effectiveness and benefits of telemedicine systems. However systematic reviews done by Roine *et al.* (2001), Clarke and Thiyagarajan (2008), Hailey *et al.* (2004), and Curioso and Mechael (2010) agree that there are not sufficient studies done that scientifically and rigorously assess the benefits of telemedicine systems. Scientific evidence of the clinical effectiveness and cost-effectiveness of telemedicine remains lacking (Clarke & Thiyagarajan, 2008; Curioso & Mechael, 2010; Roine, Ohinmaa, & Hailey, 2001). Hence the evident need for "hard evidence produced by rigorous scientific studies

that evaluate its benefits and costs" (Bashshur, Shannon, & Sapci, 2005, p. 296).

Towards Policy Making

Healthcare evaluation often unites scientific studies and political drivers that could have conflicting outcomes. Scientific studies place an emphasis on methodologies and research design to provide factual evidence through reliable measurements using data collection and analysis (Stevens, Fitzpatrick, Abrams, Brazier, & Lilford, 2001). Political motivators are driven by priorities related to public policies, funding parties and allocation of funds (Bashshur, Shannon, & Sapci, 2005). Sensible policies are however based on factual information such as the costs and benefits of the program (Roine, Ohinmaa, & Hailey, 2001). Therefore scientific studies and political motivations share a common goal to gather evidence rather than speculations.

The evaluation of programs is typically driven by political concerns regarding the performance of the health program. Telemedicine, especially in the developing world, was introduced to address political and public concerns regarding quality and equity in healthcare. Telemedicine program evaluation therefore assesses the extent to which telemedicine programs addresses issues such as equity of quality care and reducing costs in healthcare (Bashshur, Shannon, & Sapci, 2005).

Program evaluation is directed towards providing decision support for policy makers to determine the current status of the program, identify better alternatives, assess the effects and provide decision support on actions to be taken (Bashshur, Shannon, & Sapci, 2005). Evaluation that is built on scientific evidence promotes acceptance among clinicians and provides policy makers with confidence towards achieving defined goals and objectives.

The scope of telemedicine is continuing to evolve as new telemedicine technologies emerge and more applications become feasible (Roine,

Ohinmaa, & Hailey, 2001). The wide range of telemedicine applications, technologies and perspectives complicates the evaluation of telemedicine as a fixed entity (Stevens, Fitzpatrick, Abrams, Brazier, & Lilford, 2001). Telemedicine programs can differ between people, settings and times. However when assessing telemedicine programs for policy purposes a more general assessment of telemedicine with respect to the health system is required. Policy making within the health system would not require details regarding the different applications of telemedicine but rather the overall benefits of the telemedicine (Bashshur, Shannon, & Sapci, 2005).

Telemedicine Services vs. Systems

Taylor (1998) surveyed publications in telemedicine and distinguished between telemedicine systems and services. According to Taylor (1998) studies on telemedicine systems were technically focused and included equipment specifications, safety and effectiveness. The majority of these studies were concerned about the technical performance of systems relating to the diagnostic accuracy of decision making supported by telemedicine equipment. Telemedicine services however are not only concerned with whether the technology works, but rather in the effectiveness of care and benefits that can be obtained using the technology (Taylor, 1998).

Wyatt (1996) defines the development of telemedicine systems without a concern for a need of the technology as 'technology-push' and argues that a 'clinical-pull' approach, where a needs assessment is done prior to development, serves as a better foundation for successful implementation. Hebert (2001) describes program evaluation as examining technology use to "provide a service or deliver a program" (p. 1145). Program evaluation, with the emphasis on usage of technology and service provision, could be considered to be the evaluation complimenting a clinical-pull approach.

Dimensions for Telemedicine Assessment and Evaluation

Bashshur *et al.* (2005) adapted a model for evaluation approaches as shown in Figure 1. The model identifies three different dimensions for telemedicine evaluation. The first dimension separates the applications by grouping them in three speciality areas; public health, education and clinical. The second dimension takes into account that evaluation can be done from different perspectives. The perspectives of the society, provider and client are of importance in telemedicine evaluation. The third dimension divides telemedicine programs by technology usage. A telemedicine program using asynchronous technology will differ from a program using synchronous technology. Bandwidth and peripheral devices will also have a noteworthy impact on the program characteristics (Bashshur, Shannon, & Sapci, 2005).

The focus of this chapter is on asynchronous technology from a provider's perspective in the public health application of telemedicine. It is generally accepted that it is not yet feasible to use synchronous technologies in the public health sector of South Africa. Many hospitals, especially in the rural areas, do not have reliable internet connections. Low bandwidth also limits the connectivity for real-time consultations. Another significant constraint is that the nature of practitioners' schedules currently do not allow for reliable continuous real-time telemedicine consultation. It is expected that in the future, when ICT implementations and bandwidth capacity increase, it will become feasible to expand to synchronous telemedicine.

Later in this chapter, a health needs assessment framework is discussed to consider the potential benefits of asynchronous telemedicine systems in public healthcare from a policy perspective. Once the need for a telemedicine program has been proven and systems are implemented, the potential of telemedicine from the needs assessment can be used to serve as a benchmark for evaluation.

Figure 1. Three dimensions for telemedicine evaluation (adapted from Bashshur, Shannon, & Sapci, 2005)

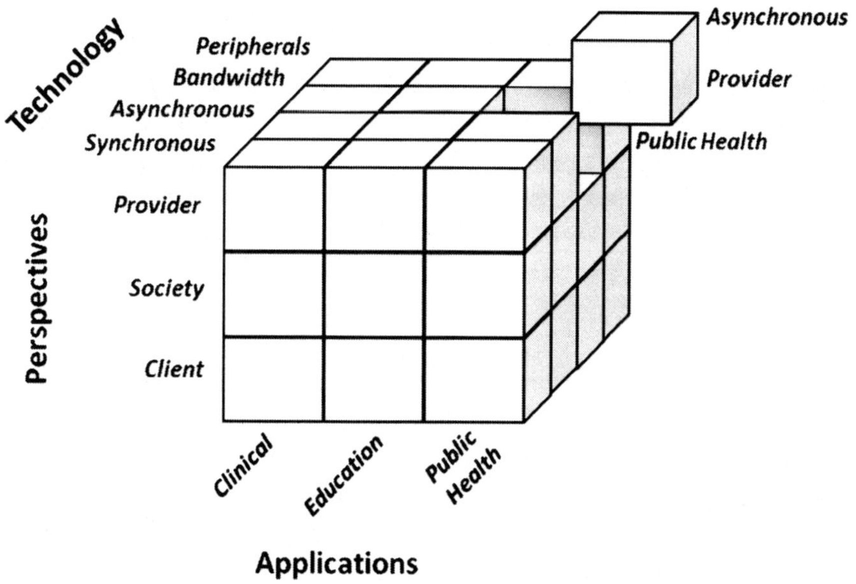

Evaluation Typology

Taylor (1998) identified that evaluation regarding services should consider the stages of the implementation life cycle as each phase has unique measurements and outcomes. The implementation life cycle in short consists of a feasibility study, pilot project, program and outcome. The typology of program evaluation as suggested by Bashshur *et al.* (2005) closely corresponds to the implementation life cycle mentioned by Taylor (1998). The typology of program evaluation according to Bashshur *et al.* (2005) is as follows: (1) evaluability assessment, (2) documentation evaluation, (3) process evaluation, and (4) summative or outcome evaluation.

Evaluability assessment takes place during the planning phase of telemedicine programs. During this stage the aim is to assess what should be evaluated in the program and to develop tools for evaluation. The goals and objectives of the program are defined and used as a benchmark for further evaluation. Evaluability of the program is assessed prior to implementation, since tools for evaluation are likely to be included into the program design (Bashshur, Shannon, & Sapci, 2005).

Documentation evaluation includes the sequential description of the implementation of the program. The aim is to contribute towards improving the implementation of telemedicine projects, by documenting pitfalls, tips and guidelines for future projects. *Process evaluation* is performed after the program is implemented and is continued throughout the life-cycle of the program. This evaluation phase is directed towards measuring the process variables that influence the performance of the program (Bashshur, Shannon, & Sapci, 2005).

Summative or outcome evaluation determines the extent to which the system satisfies the intended effects of the system. Scientific methodologies such as cost-benefit and cost-effectiveness analyses are used to evaluate the performance of the system. Evaluation tools that were developed in the evaluability assessment phase are used to evaluate the performance of the program in relation to the previously defined goals and objectives (Bashshur, Shannon, & Sapci, 2005).

Evaluability assessments, builds the foundation for further evaluation and could play an integral role in implementation policies, because it defines the goals and objectives for the program and develop tools to evaluate performance. Documentation, process and outcome evaluation are all introduced after implementation, and are therefore of less importance to implementation policy making. Nevertheless implementation policies should be evaluated throughout the entire life cycle of the program.

Later in this chapter, a framework is introduced to assess the needs of telemedicine by calculating the quantitative benefits of telemedicine programs. Evaluability assessment is included in this framework, using the results from the needs assessment to develop tools and goals for the telemedicine program to be implemented. Before the framework is introduced, some perspectives and tools are explained that will contribute towards the assessment framework.

Hospital Referrals and Telemedicine

A universal goal of Primary Health Care (PHC) is to provide quality healthcare for the entire population. However, limited resources, among other constraints in developing countries, prevent health sectors from reaching this goal. Treating patients as close as possible to their homes, at the lowest possible cost but still providing quality care with the necessary expertise, is a daunting challenge, especially in developing countries. To this end, referral systems contribute to the deliberate distribution of expertise by distinguishing between different levels of care. In this way, scarce resources are allocated to higher level health facilities, resulting in a cost-effective practice where patients arriving at low-level care facilities, are referred to higher-level facilities if they need more specialised treatment. In such a way, resources are restricted to those who need it (Hensher, Price, & Adomakoh, 2006).

The Referral System: Definitions and Characteristics

All healthcare facilities, on all levels of care, send and receive patients to and from other facilities. It is to be expected that higher-level hospitals would likely receive more referrals than they send, whereas hospitals on a lower-level would probably send more referrals than they receive. Hensher *et al.* (2006) defined a referral as:

Any process in which healthcare providers at lower levels of the health system, who lack the skills, the facilities, or both, to manage a given clinical condition, seek the assistance of providers who are better equipped or specially trained to guide them in managing or, to take over responsibility for a particular episode of a clinical condition in a patient (Hensher, Price, & Adomakoh, 2006, p. 1230).

The definition for a referral does not exclude the use of ICTs and therefore, includes telemedicine practices. According to the definition of telemedicine, the delivery of any healthcare service using an ICT can be regarded as telemedicine. ICTs are moreover, commonly used to assist in referrals, for example, a simple telephone call between practitioners during patient referrals could be argued as being a form of telemedicine.

Since the overlapping of definitions could be the cause of some confusion, for the purposes of this chapter, the following definitions will be used:

A *telemedicine referral* is a referral during which a patient is diagnosed, treated, or both using an ICT, to prevent having to transport the patient to another facility.

A *transfer referral* is a referral during which a patient is physically transferred to another health practitioner or facility.

The referral system distinguishes between the three levels of care according to the availability of specialised personnel and the sophistication of diagnostic and therapeutic technologies.

Table 1. Standard definitions of hospital levels

Disease Control Priorities Project: Terminology and definitions	Alternative terms
Primary-level hospital: **Few specialties – mainly internal medicine, obstetrics, gynae-cology, paediatrics, general surgery, general practice, limited laboratory services for general analysis**	*District hospital* *Rural hospital* *Community hospital* *General hospital*
Secondary-level hospital: **Highly differentiated by functions with 5-10 specialties** **Sizes range from 200 – 800 beds**	*Regional hospital* *Provincial hospital* *General hospital*
Tertiary-level hospital **Highly specialized staff and technical equipment- for example cardiology, intensive care unit, and specialized imaging units, clinical services highly differentiated by function.** **Could have teaching activities** **Sizes range from 300 – 1500 beds**	*National hospital* *Central hospital* *Academic, Teaching or University hospital*
Specialised hospital **Specialise in specific diseases or conditions such as tuber-culosis, psychiatry, substance abuse, infectious diseases and rehabilitation**	

Adapted from sources: (Hensher, Price, & Adomakoh, 2006; World Health Organization, 2003),

Table 1 lists and describes the functions of the three levels of care in hospitals. A fourth type of healthcare facility, the specialised hospitals, also plays an integral role in the referral system and is also mentioned in Table 1 (Hensher, Price, & Adomakoh, 2006). Specialised hospitals perform different functions from other hospitals, in the sense that patients are referred to these facilities for specialised treatment, rather than for diagnostic purposes. Asynchronous telemedicine would therefore, not be a feasible alternative for the majority of referrals to specialised hospitals.

The hierarchy of referrals between the hospitals in South Africa, as described in Table 1, are illustrated in Figure 2. As can be seen, in South Africa, there are few selected tertiary hospitals nationwide that provide specialised services (National referral services) as an add-on to the usual services of a tertiary hospital. One of these national referral tertiary hospitals also provides a highly specialised service and is called the Central Referral Unit. Although regional and tertiary hospitals treat a high percentage of referral patients, these hospitals are not restricted to referred patients. However, the amount of 'non-referred' patients in

tertiary hospitals is restricted by limiting the emergency ambulance services at these hospitals (National Department of Health, 2003).

Benefits of using Telemedicine as an Aid to Referrals

Transfer referrals between the different health facilities serve as a crucial link so that all patients have access to higher levels of care. Unfortunately, there are risks involved in patient referrals and they are not always feasible. Transportation of patients between facilities also has high cost implications (Hensher, Price, & Adomakoh, 2006). Telemedicine could aid referral systems by reducing the negative aspects (Bashshur, Reardon, & Shannon, 2000). Currently, asynchronous telemedicine referrals are not considered to be an absolute replacement for transfer referrals since not all diagnoses and treatments can be performed using asynchronous telemedicine (Della Mea, 2005). Yet, transfer referrals could serve as a control case for telemedicine referral evaluation studies, in those consultations where telemedicine is effective in eliminating the need to travel.

Figure 2. Referral hierarchy in South Africa (adapted from National Department of Health, 2003)

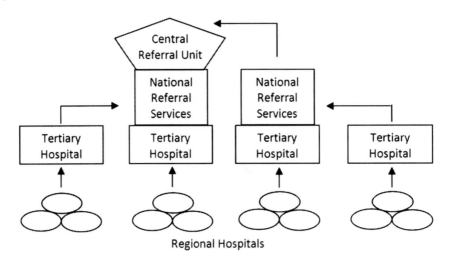

Regional Hospitals

Consistency and Quality of Healthcare

In statistical analysis, a type I error is defined as the false detection of a fault. During type I errors, unnecessary action is taken, while type II errors occur from failing to detect an error and thus, neglecting to take the necessary action (Gitlow, Oppenheim, Oppenheim, & Levine, 2005). In terms of medical referrals, type I errors occur when patients are unnecessarily referred. In contrast, type II errors occur when patients who should have been referred, were not. Table 2 illustrates the referral errors and their consequences.

There are few medical risks in type I errors, because if the initial diagnosis is correct, it would be confirmed by the second consultation. The cost of referring a patient during a type I error could be considered a waste, because it does not add any value to the service. Type I errors also result in patients being admitted to hospitals further away from home and occupying beds in

high-care hospitals, with a limited number of available beds.

On the other hand, type II errors result in high medical risks for the patient because of failure to refer them. Costs are perhaps reduced by not referring a patient, but the quality of care would certainly be compromised. Furthermore, in the healthcare environment, equity of care and the safety of the patient are considered more important than marginal savings. Cautious practitioners would therefore be more likely to 'play it safe' by referring more cases than necessary. This would, in turn lead to a pattern of type I errors occurring more frequently than type II errors.

According to Craig and Patterson (2005), the consistency of quality care could be improved through telemedicine. Telemedicine provides practitioners with an easier and more effective means to obtain a second opinion than would otherwise have been possible. Second opinions

Table 2. Referral errors

	Patient Referred	**Patient Not Referred**
Referral Not Necessary	Type I Error (Unnecessary Cost)	No Error
Referral Necessary	No Error	Type II (Medical Risk)

can serve as a quality control measurement, limiting the chances of misdiagnosis. When a practitioner is in doubt about a patient's diagnosis, a telemedicine referral can greatly reduce the amount of possibly unnecessary, referrals thereby reducing costs. More importantly, through regular use of telemedicine systems, a practitioner can afford to refer more patients at lower costs and therefore double-check even if he/she is relatively sure of the diagnosis. Hence, by reducing the amount of type II errors, the medical risks also decrease.

Telemedicine referrals allow a local doctor to remain involved in the diagnosis of the patient by simultaneously collaborating with a specialist who has a higher level of knowledge (Hjelm, 2005). This holds many benefits, especially in smaller districts where respective practitioners sometimes have a long-standing relationship with the patient and are more familiar with a patient's medical history than the specialist. Therefore, this collaboration between the local doctor and the specialist, affords the patient the best possible treatment.

Reduced Information Loss

Good communication between hospitals is essential in ensuring that information, regarding the current condition and medical history of a patient, does not get lost. The fact that different hospitals' information systems are not synchronised in South Africa, complicates the transfer of patient information. In this country, patients are required to take a booklet, containing their medical history, with them when they are referred to another hospital. However, patients sometimes lose these booklets, forcing specialists to prescribe treatment without any knowledge of a patient's medical history or a letter of referral. Until hospital information systems are linked and synchronised, patient information will continue to get lost, contributing to the risks associated with referrals (Nakahara, et al., 2010).

A further explanation for documentation, concerning a patient's medical history, getting lost is caused by stress suffered by patients being transferred from one hospital to another. Telemedicine referrals can reduce this type of human error during a referral. In the case of a telemedicine referral, all the appropriate information is sent together in a bundle, thereby reducing the risk of information being lost. In circumstances where the receiver requires additional information about the patient, this can be requested from the sender, thus improving communication between the sender and the receiver in the referral.

Equity and Improved Access to Specialists

Hensher *et al.* (2006) found that specialists prefer to practice at tertiary hospitals rather than hospitals offering lower levels of care. One of the main reasons for this is that tertiary hospitals are almost always located in metropolitan areas. Another reason is that tertiary hospitals have access to better resources that allows for valuable professional experience and opportunities for private practice. Typically, patients in remote and rural areas only have direct access to primary health care. Telemedicine could assist in providing equity of care between these patients and the patients living in urban areas, where secondary and tertiary care is more accessible. In this way, rural patients can have faster access to specialists by saving time on referral administration and travelling (Hensher, Price, & Adomakoh, 2006).

The phenomenon mentioned above, where practitioners migrate away from rural areas, leaves these areas with a critical shortage of highly trained health practitioners (Ferguson, 2006). Telemedicine referrals could, therefore, serve as an outsourcing mechanism to utilise specialists' time more effectively. The use of telemedicine could also reduce the effect of staff shortages, by training general healthcare practitioners, for example, nurses, to indirectly deliver medical services and treatment that were previously restricted to specialists. Support, provided by appropriate doctors and specialists, via information and communications technology, could empower nurses to be an integral part of service delivery in the South African healthcare system. In addition, this would reduce the amount of valuable time spent by doctors by consigning time-consuming tasks to nurses, therefore ensuring better utilisation of resources (Ferguson, 2006).

Practitioner Support

The trend of skilled professionals moving away from rural areas often leave those left behind feeling isolated. Professionals with little experience in rural areas are therefore in need of guidance and support from specialists and professionals in tertiary hospitals with more experience. The referrals system ideally meets this need through the collaboration of professionals between the different levels of care (Hensher, Price, & Adomakoh, 2006; Wootton, 1998).

Education

Telemedicine can be used as an educational tool for undergraduate and postgraduate studies but also continuing training of health professionals. Information and communication technologies are suitable to provide support networks through which students can remain connected to their professors while being away from campus during practical training. This allows professors to be involved in the training of the student even though they are not present at the facility. The students can collaborate with professors and fellow students and therefore are not isolated in a remote or rural area (Ferguson, 2006; Hjelm, 2005). Some telemedicine systems have been developed specifically for training purposes. An example of this is the virtual patient that is used by students and practitioners to create a safe environment for the development of consultative skills (Hjelm, 2005).

Hospital Utilisation

In most developing countries, the number of available beds in many high-level care facilities is severely constrained. Furthermore many of these hospitals do not have the resources to sustain good quality care during high occupation seasons. Therefore high utilisation of these hospitals inevitably leads to low quality of care in these hospitals. The number of patients admitted to tertiary hospitals can be reduced, by referring more patients through telemedicine, hence treating more patients in district hospitals, clinics or even at home. Telemedicine would therefore reduce the utilisation of tertiary hospitals allocating resources more effectively (Hjelm, 2005).

Reduction in Transport

One of the most obvious advantages of telemedicine is that, in remote or rural areas, patients no longer need to travel from one health facility to another (Hjelm, 2005). Predominantly, patients in rural areas are in the extreme, low income group and cannot afford to travel far distances to receive specialised treatment. Furthermore, some special populations such as the elderly, pregnant women, disabled and acute sick patients can avoid taking health risks normally accompanied by travelling (Alverson, Holtz, D'Iorio, DeVany, Simmons, & Poropatich, 2008; Craig & Patterson, 2005; Jahn & De Brouwere, 2001).

Reduces Cost

Telemedicine has the potential to fundamentally restructure the way in which healthcare is delivered. If restructuring is done in such a way that service processes are more efficient, specialist time spent per patient, transport and hospital stay can be reduced. In the long term, these reductions will ultimately contribute towards overall cost savings (Hjelm, 2005). Telemedicine services are expected to have financial benefits, but various sources have stated that there is not efficient evidence to confirm this (Craig & Patterson, 2005;

Hjelm, 2005; Hailey, Ohinmaa, & Roine, 2004; Roine, Ohinmaa, & Hailey, 2001)

Health Informatics

The health informatics discipline has grown remarkably with the evolvement of ICTs. Health informatics has been playing a crucial role in delivering healthcare for many decades, contributing in the development of tools for the collection, analysis and sharing of medical data (Imhoff, Webb, & Goldschmidt, 2001). Providing quality healthcare involves the interaction of many different processes and disciplines. Health informatics spread across various processes such as communication, decision making, educational etc. The different viewpoints from which health informatics are approached would deliver different perspectives on how it influences healthcare (Hasman, Haux, & Albert, 1996).

The variation of perspectives on health informatics is apparent in literature from the many different definitions for this discipline. There are also inconsistencies in literature and between different cultures as to what the differences are between `health informatics` and `medical informatics` (Imhoff, Webb, & Goldschmidt, 2001; Hasman, Haux, & Albert, 1996). However for the purposes of this chapter we will adopt the general definition of health informatics from Imhoff *et al.* (2001):

Health informatics is not only the application of computer technology to problems in healthcare but covers all aspects of the generation, handling, communication, storage, retrieval, management, analysis, discovery and synthesis of data, information and knowledge in the entire scope of healthcare (p. 180).

Health informatics can play a number of different roles in healthcare, but ultimately all these roles have the universal goal to improve healthcare quality. The roles of health informatics can be divided into the following categories of application:

- Clinical decision support
- Hospital administration
- Higher-level decision making
- Educational, training and research

Traditionally the largest overlap between the telemedicine and health informatics fields is in the area of *clinical decision support* (Hasman, Haux, & Albert, 1996). Through telemedicine, clinical decision support is provided over a distance through the transfer of information between practitioners (Nannings & Abu-Hanna, 2006). These two fields are both included under the e-health definition and could complement each other superbly. However due to the complexity of integrating information systems, telemedicine systems often make use of their own information systems. Hence, these telemedicine systems do not have direct access to the general Hospital Information System (HIS).

Hospital administration, billing and other accounting processes are critical for the business management of a hospital. Health informatics plays an essential role in patient billing calculations, hospital accounting, resource allocation, information management, the evaluation of cost-effectiveness and other information intensive management processes (Hasman, Haux, & Albert, 1996). Management information systems often use simulation and other tools to optimise operations, effectively allocate resources and ultimately reduce costs for healthcare delivery without the loss of quality care (Imhoff, Webb, & Goldschmidt, 2001).

Higher-level decision making are concerned with performance indicators and policy making for a district, including a number of hospitals. Health informatics for higher-level management, would therefore address issues such as district resource allocation, equity between healthcare facilities, district performance, disease burden, *etc*. Health informatics on higher management levels does not involve information of individual patients, but rather information of a population. Trends and statistics from the population equips policy makers and other decision makers to more accurately allocate resources and intervene where necessary (Williamson, Stoops, & Heywood, 2001).

The use of real patient information in *education, training and research* assures that it is relevant to the needs of the patients. An effective method of teaching is through the use of case studies, simulating the conditions, history, treatment and care processes of the patients. However there are many ethical issues in using real data for education and research. It is crucial that the privacy of the patients is protected and that research studies are designed in such a way to accurately reflect reality (Hasman, Haux, & Albert, 1996).

Health Informatics in South Africa

The growing awareness in developing countries of ICTs potential to improve healthcare delivery has led to the evolvement and implementation of various health information systems in South Africa. However due to the complex nature of developing health information systems for primary health care together with ICT implementation challenges, initial results from these systems failed to reach its desired potential (Walsham & Sahay, 2006). Typical characteristics of primary health care in developing countries such as culture, lack of infrastructure and a lack of skills complicated the implementation of information systems (Byrne & Sahay, 2003; Williamson, Stoops, & Heywood, 2001).

Information Systems for Management

The District Health Information System (DHIS) and the Electronic Tuberculosis (TB) Register are examples of well-established health information systems in South Africa. The DHIS was designed for collecting data from health facilities and sharing aggregated data to higher levels in the public health system (Williamson, Stoops, & Heywood, 2001). The District Health Barometer (DHB) uses a selected set of data from the DHIS to monitor performance in terms of socio-economic and other healthcare indicators. Annual reports are compiled using data from the DHIS, Electronic TB Register, Statistics South Africa and the National Treasury. Data are analysed and interpreted in such a way to highlight disparities regarding the equity of services, health resource allocation and efficiency of healthcare processes between districts (Mars & Seebregts, 2008).

The issue of inadequate training and support for ICTs in healthcare applications is widely covered (Byrne & Sahay, 2003; Mars & Seebregts, 2008; Walsham & Sahay, 2006; Williamson, Stoops, & Heywood, 2001). The need for training and support spans from the data entry-level to high-level management, using information for decision making. Williamson *et al.* (2001) highlighted the issue that managers pay inadequate attention to data entry processes, leading to poor quality data. An underlying reason for this is that managers do not appreciate that software is merely a tool aiding in collecting and storing data, leading to many human errors in the data collection process.

The use of the DHIS is separated into three levels for assessment. The first level includes data collection, validation and combining data into sets for transmission to higher levels during an acceptable time limit. At the second level, trends, profiles and indicators are compiled and combined in reports. These monthly reports are available to managers and decision makers, who discussed trends and performances at regular meetings. The third level is for decision making and higher level management. Information is used for monitoring health success using performance indicators as well as higher-level policy making such as the DHB (Mars & Seebregts, 2008; Williamson, Stoops, & Heywood, 2001).

The market for health information systems is rapidly growing in South Africa and as a result many international and local companies are becoming involved. This necessitated the consideration of interoperability between information systems. To address the issues and promote interoperability, several standards were accepted, including standards from the International Organization for

Standardization (ISO). The ICD-10 coding standard has been adopted as South Africa's national diagnosis coding standard for both the public and private sectors. There are still no agreed standards for procedures, pharmaceuticals, surgeries, pathology, radiology and clinical terms. Procedural standards such as the National Health Reference Price List (NHPRL) and the related Uniform Patient Fee Schedule (UPFS) are used in the public sector. The National Pharmaceutical Product Interface (NAPPI) is used for coding new medical devices and medicines (Bah, 2009). The adoption of Logical Observation Identifiers Names and Codes (LOINC) are being considered for Electronic Health Records (EHR) as there are currently no national standards for this purpose (Mars & Seebregts, 2008).

Electronic Health Records

The South African Electronic Health Record (EHR) initiative started in 2003 in the form of a planning workshop to standardise the concept of implementing EHR on a national level. This workshop provided a foundation from where the National Strategic Framework for EHR's in South Africa was compiled. The National Strategic Framework defined an EHR as "a longitudinal collection of personal health information of a single individual, entered or accepted by healthcare providers, and stored electronically" (National Department of Health, 2007, p. 8).

The implementation of EHR applications in South Africa are growing rapidly. In 2008 more than a third of the provincial hospitals, nationwide, have implemented computerized systems (Mars & Seebregts, 2008). It is expected that the percentage of hospitals using EHR's have increased significantly since 2008, because the use of computerized systems offers many benefits to the health system and management, in these hospitals.

Although the South African National EHR Strategy has a vision to integrate health record systems throughout the country, currently, a number of different commercial EHR systems are implemented throughout South Africa. The ideal that the strategy is aiming towards is that all South African citizens' records can be accessed, whenever or wherever the patients seek medical attention. Furthermore, the ideal of the National Department of Health (2007) is to merge telemedicine records with EHR. This ideal is still far from reality and substantial growth is necessary before it will realize. However, the standardisation of data between telemedicine and EHR systems, can already be integrated that will simplify future system merging.

The integration of telemedicine with EHR's would be more favourable after the integration of all EHR's throughout the country. If EHR's are stored on a central data warehouse, with practitioner access, the need to send data between hospitals will be reduced. However the storage of images and video files would require much more storage space than mere text files. Telemedicine cost calculations and performance evaluation could also benefit from integration with financial patient data, referral patterns, diagnostic data and procedure data that are included in EHR's.

EHR data play an integral part in financial calculations of medical procedures. Likewise this data can also be used to calculate some of the benefits of telemedicine. Ultimately, if telemedicine systems can be integrated with EHR's, these calculations can be done automatically by a decision support system. Table 3 lists all the different data attributes of a typical EHR. Some of these attributes can be useful for telemedicine assessment. In the next section a framework is suggested to use the data in needs and evaluability assessments, for telemedicine program planning.

TELEMEDICINE NEEDS AND EVALUABILITY ASSESSMENTS USING HEALTH INFORMATICS

Medical practitioners are trained to assess the needs of individual patients before starting a

Table 3. Contents of the South African EHR (adapted from National Department of Health, 2007)

Personal Details	Demographic data	Past Medical History
Name (First name and surname)	Names	Diagnosis
Physical + Postal Address	DOB/Age	Treatments and procedures
Postal Code	Gender	Medications
Telephone numbers	Nationality	Free text field
ID number	Address	Institutions (Hospital / clinic etc.)
Next of kin details	Telephone contact(s)	Practitioner
Guardian details	Family linkage	Dates (treatment/entry/exit/death)
Date of birth		Encounter outcomes
Insurer / med aid – number	Major Medical Events	Categorisations
Insurer / med aid – name	Parity / Gravidity	Previous blood results – history
Employment	Genetic markers	Test results
Level of education	Pre-dispositions to illness	Vaccinations
Gender	Current treatment	Confidentiality indicator
Religion	Blood group	
Marital Status	Allergies	
Number of children	Donor status	
Unique patient identifier (ID)	Episode history	
Nationality	- Facility or institution ID	
Blood groups	- Care provider ID	
Allergies	- ICD-10 diagnoses	
Current chronic conditions	- Procedures (CPT-4 or other standard)	
Current medication	- Discharge summary (Free text)	
Current medical conditions	- Medication (prescribed vs. dispensed)	
Current practitioner /GP	- Lab Results	
Immunisation Status	- Imaging results (storage currently out of scope)	
Disability status		
Pregnancy status		
Smoking indicator		

treatment. Most practitioners are accustomed to following a systematic approach that they were taught during training and later refined through clinical experience. However, this systematic approach is based on the needs of an individual patient and is unlikely to reflect the needs of an entire population. Furthermore, it is unlikely that different communities would have exactly the same healthcare needs. The importance of assessing the needs of each community separately is often neglected. Too many high-level decisions are based on what some people perceive to be the needs of the population, resulting that many health services are ineffective and waste scarce resources (Wright, Williams, & Wilkinson, 1998).

Prior to performing needs assessments it is important to clarify what is meant by the term 'need,' since different disciplines mostly do not have the same perceptions of what needs are. The concepts of needs, demands and supply are com-

Figure 3. Relation between needs, demands, and supply (adapted from Wright, Williams, & Wilkinson, 1998)

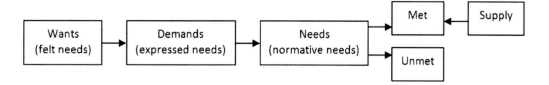

monly mistaken for each other, as these concepts overlap (Wright, Williams, & Wilkinson, 1998). Wright *et al.* (1998) differentiate between need, demand, and supply as illustrated in Figure 3.

In the healthcare discipline, the definition of need is commonly accepted to be 'the capacity to benefit.' Medical practitioners are likely to experience 'demand' as the needs of the patients, but in reality these demands can reflect what patients believe they need, rather than what their true needs are. Demand can be influenced by the media, creating an interest among patients for a service. Supply can also play a large role in demand, for example, the number of beds available in a hospital, might cause that it is more popular among patients. 'Supply' is the care that is provided by health professionals. This is largely dependent upon policies and the resources available in terms of money, specialists and technology (Wright, Williams, & Wilkinson, 1998).

A needs assessment for telemedicine programs is a form of health needs assessment. Wright *et al.* (1998) define a health needs assessment as "the systematic approach to ensuring that the health service uses its resources to improve the health of the population in the most efficient way" (p. 1310). Telemedicine, being a health service, will therefore conform to the same principles that apply to health needs assessments.

Many telemedicine evaluation frameworks and techniques can be cited, but telemedicine needs assessments are still considered to be almost an art form, requiring creative solutions to determine the need for telemedicine in a given setting (Harrop, 2002). There is no universal and quick-fix recipe, as different areas of assessment will require different approaches. Quantitative, qualitative, or a combination of both research methods can be used for assessments (Wright, Williams, & Wilkinson, 1998).

There are a variety of formal and informal approaches to assessing needs. Steadham (1980) argues that selecting the appropriate research method is of critical importance to assure that the results reflect the true need that is being determined. Figure 4 illustrates the process of a needs assessment. Steadham (1980) argues that, pre-assessment is important to consider the situation and select appropriate methods. Data collection and analysis are more often than not time-consuming tasks, hence the need to be sure that the correct methods are followed.

A Decision Support Framework for Using Health Informatics in Telemedicine Needs Assessments

The decision support framework illustrated in Figure 5 and discussed throughout this section is specifically adapted to assist decision makers in telemedicine implementation planning. The aim is to equip decision makers with tools to assess the needs for telemedicine (prior to implementation) and hereby promoting clinical-pull strategies to telemedicine implementation.

Implementation policies and decision making requires assessment from clinical, economic and social perspectives. The suggested decision support framework has a primary focus on the quantitative assessment of benefits for telemedicine implementation. The clinical and social perspectives of telemedicine implementation should also

Figure 4. the needs assessment process (adapted from Steadham, 1980)

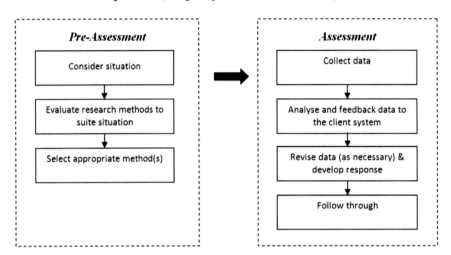

be included in thorough needs assessments. However, since this study examines the use of health informatics for the quantitative assessment, clinical and social perspectives are not directly included in this chapter.

The needs assessment process from Steadham (1980) was combined with decision support system frameworks by Turban, Aronson and Liang (2005) and data warehouse design frameworks by Kimball and Ross (2002) as well as evaluability assessment guidelines by Bashshur, Shannon and Sapci (2005) to form the framework for needs and evaluability assessment, illustrated in Figure 5. This framework can be expanded to include clinical and social perspectives, as well as quantitative research methods and relevant data analysis tools.

The framework consists of three sections, as indicated on the top of this framework. The first section is the pre-assessment phase. During this phase the benefits (potential) of telemedicine is considered, simultaneously taking the data sources available into account and the research methods that should be followed to assess the magnitude of the benefits. The second section of the framework

Figure 5. Framework for using health informatics in telemedicine needs assessments

Pre-Assessment			Needs Assessment			Implementation planning	
Consider Telemedicine Potential	Data Sources	Research Method(s)	Extract Transform Load	Data Warehouse	Data Analysis	Decisions	Evaluability Assessment
• Reduce Transport • Hospital Utilization • Cost Savings • Improve quality by reducing referral errors	DHIS EHR Reports	Literature Reviews Records & Reports Ethical Guidelines Privacy Protection	**Extract:** Physical data collection **Transform:** Cleaning & Classification **Load:** Relational Database	Referral Data Mart Technology Data Mart Health Indicator Data Mart	*Trends analyses* *Mathematical Models* Stochastic Modeling Economic Analysis Linear Programming	1. Implementation Yes / No 2. Synchronous / Asynchronous 3. Which hospitals 4. For what departments 5. Infrastructure requirements 6. Bandwidth 7. Telemedicine equipment	1. Clarify goals and objective of program 2. Identify variables of interest 3. Develop data collection schemes 4. Develop measurement tools for variables 5. Specify analytical and statistical methods to interpret findings

contains the essence of the needs assessment, including data collection methods, warehousing and analysis. The aim of the third section is to use the results from the needs assessment to direct decision makers towards evidence based decision making. The implementation decisions are followed by an evaluability assessment that uses the results from the needs assessment to assess and guide the evaluability of the program.

Pre-Assessment

The pre-assessment section of the framework is concerned with choosing the appropriate methods and data sources to direct the needs assessment towards the required benefit analysis. The pre-assessment serves as the planning phase of the needs assessment. Decision makers play an integral role in this phase, through directing the needs assessment towards analysing the benefits that would be of most value in the intended telemedicine program.

Consider Telemedicine Potential

Ideally, all the benefits of telemedicine should be assessed prior to the implementation of a telemedicine program. However, assessing these benefits requires the use of different research methods and data sources. As discussed previously, this study has a focus on asynchronous technology from a provider's perspective in the public health application of telemedicine. Measurements that could quantitatively assess the need for telemedicine and thus aid decision making for implementation are included in the framework and are listed below.

- Hospital utilisation
- Reduction in transport
- Reduces cost
- Quality improvements by reducing referral errors

An estimate of the potential number of referrals, that could have been avoided when using telemedicine, is measured using the framework. By determining the potential number of referrals, the maximum potential utilisation of the telemedicine system is estimated. The utilisation of the telemedicine system has an influence on the benefits of telemedicine, as listed above. The potential utilisation of the systems is combined with other needs assessment methods to determine the extent to which this telemedicine system will offer the quantitative benefits.

The quantitative measurement of quality and reliability of telemedicine systems is a very complex and diverse task. There are little data available from health information systems that can be used to thoroughly audit the quality of care a patient receives, with or without telemedicine. However, as discussed earlier, telemedicine could reduce type I and type II errors. Type I errors could be detected in some cases by matching reasons for referral (from the sending hospitals) with the treatment diagnosis (from the receiving hospital). In this way it could be determined whether patients were referred unnecessarily. Type II errors are less likely to be detected, but could be found by calculating the number of return visits for a specific condition of a patient, before being referred. Unfortunately, it is challenging to compare patient data between different hospitals when the hospital information systems are not integrated.

Other benefits that are not easily measured using EHR are listed below. Data to quantify these benefits are not readily available in EHR, and are therefore not included in the proposed framework. Nevertheless, these benefits are relevant to telemedicine needs assessments. The assumption can be made that after implementation and effective utilisation, the telemedicine system could be managed to include the following benefits.

- Reduced information loss
- Equity and improved access to specialists
- Practitioner support
- Education

Identify Data Sources

Finding the appropriate data for telemedicine needs assessments is often a formidable challenge. Trends from successful telemedicine programs are used and applied to other regions where the possibility of a new telemedicine program is investigated. This is not the ideal approach, as health needs can be rather different depending on the different regions and healthcare settings.

Data sources should provide the assessment framework with the opportunity for determining the extent to which a telemedicine program would change the existing program of healthcare service delivery. The primary goal of telemedicine programs is to deliver a service to patients, by referring the information of these patients and hereby reducing the need to transfer the patient to another facility. Therefore, by examining the referral processes in hospitals (prior to telemedicine implementation) the potential of telemedicine to change existing referral processes are assessed.

Electronic Health Records

The South African National Strategy for EHR made provision that the discharge status of each patient release from a hospital should be recorded on the EHR, refer to Table 3. Delta 9™ UniCare, the EHR system of the Eastern Cape Province, makes further provision for four different types of patient discharges. One of these discharge types is referrals. For each patient discharge the following information is captured:

- Reason for referral (free-text)
- ICD-10 codes (optional)
- Ward referred from (free-text)
- Date and time of hospital admission
- Date and time of discharge (referral)
- Name of hospital referred to (free-text)

Referral discharge reports offer information valuable to telemedicine assessment, because it records information of referrals that might not have been necessary, if telemedicine were an option. The reason for referral is linked to the probability that transfer referrals could have been avoided, using telemedicine. All the referral discharge reports for a given time period and hospital are extracted to give an estimate of possible telemedicine referrals for a time period.

District Health Information Systems (DHIS)

Telemedicine could possibly improve indicators of district health, such as hospital utilisation, patient referral transport and health expenditure. The DHIS captures data regarding these indicators. Data are analysed by each hospital separately before it is transmitted to district offices for further analysis of the entire region.

Possible telemedicine referrals are expected to have an effect on district health indicators. The estimated number of telemedicine referrals are therefore used to determine the effect that telemedicine has on district health indicators. To assess this, district health data are used to assess the effect of telemedicine on a district.

Choose Appropriate Research Methods

Literature Reviews

Published literature is a valuable source of information, and can include any literature from professional journals to notes and in-house publications. Telemedicine needs assessments could benefit extensively from literature reviews that might provide some perspective and proof from other similar telemedicine programs. Literature reviews can also be used to identify data sources and tools necessary for analysis and decision making.

Records and Reports

Records and reports provide valuable, unbiased data that can be used for a variety of assessments. Any reports such as planning documents, strategic documents, evaluation reports, audits and budget reports can be used to assess needs. The assessment of health records is essential in determining healthcare needs of individual patients, practitioners and the population as an entity. Records are mostly not created for assessment purposes and therefore provide objective evidence as it is not influenced by personal opinions. Nevertheless the technical analysis of raw data is considered to be a skill and could easily result in infeasible solutions (Shaw, 2001; Steadham, 1980). The use of records and reports is a rewarding but time consuming and difficult process. The methods relating to records and reports are applicable when using EHR and DHIS data.

Ethical Guidelines and Patient Privacy Protection

Collecting data from EHR requires extensive consideration to ethical guidelines and standards for protecting the privacy of the patients. Standards may vary between different countries. In South Africa it is required that research studies have ethical clearance from a health ethics committee, registered with the South African Department of Health's National Health Research Ethics Council (NHREC). Furthermore, approval from the Department of Health is a prerequisite, prior to collecting data from hospital information systems.

Needs Assessment

Analysing data can be a difficult task. In this section of the framework, some tools are explained that are compatible with the type of data found in health informatics. Data collection methods are specifically chosen to collect data that are relevant to telemedicine needs assessments. Analysis tools are then discussed with the data in mind, aiming towards the goal, to support decision making for telemedicine implementation.

Data Collection

To analyse the data for the needs assessment, the data have to be in a form that would allow the use of mathematical models and other analysis tools. Data are extracted, transformed and loaded into a data warehouse from where analysis is performed.

Extract

Data are extracted from the EHR system in a format that can be imported into the assessment database. Another set of data from the DHIS and health reports are also extracted to require relevant information for decision making.

Transform

Currently the standards for EHR in South Africa allow that discharge reports could contain a large amount of free-text. Free-text entries that are intuitive and not structured or categorised, complicates data analysis, because data have to be cleaned in a way that does not compromise the validity and integrity of the data. The reason for referral is mostly related to the diagnosis of the patient. At some hospitals, ICD-10 codes are used to record the reason for referral, but in most cases free-text is used. In cases where free-text is used, the 'reason for referral' attribute can be transformed into an ICD-10 code, in the majority cases by a person with knowledge of the healthcare environment. The transformation from free-text to standard fields and codes is essential to enable quantitative data analysis.

As part of the data transformation process, data are cleaned in order to eliminate ambiguity and incomplete or incorrect entries. Furthermore, to protect the anonymity of patients, data that could reveal the identity of patients are removed. It is of utmost importance to transform the data in such a way that the study complies with ethical guidelines.

Load

Data are stored after the extraction and transformation of the data. A relational database is developed to contain the referral and technology data marts. The relationships between referrals,

Figure 6. Database relationship diagram to store referral data

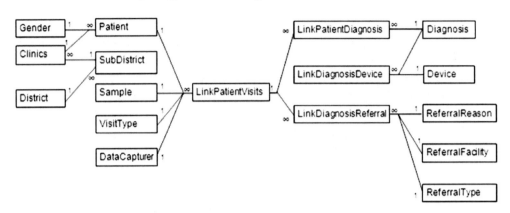

diagnoses, telemedicine technologies, referral hospitals and different districts are used effectively to draw reports for analyses relating to specific health indicators. Figure 6 illustrates an example of a database in MS-Access that can be used to store the data.

It should be noted that the format in which data are extracted should be compatible with the format of the software used for the relational database. Data are then imported into the database, and stored for analysis.

Data Warehouse

The data warehouse comprises of three data marts, namely the *Referrals Data Mart, Technology Data Mart* and *Health Indicator Data Mart*. Information stored in these data marts are relevant for telemedicine needs assessment and are stored in such a way that the data can be analysed and used in mathematical models for decision making.

Referrals Data Mart

The referrals data mart is populated using data from the discharge reports. The reason for referral, discharge dates and hospital names are the data entities that are extracted, transformed into standard codes and loaded into the referrals data mart of the database. Aggregate data contributing to referral patterns at the healthcare facilities

are also contained in the referral data mart. The referral data mart will ultimately contain generic lists of ICD-10 codes and names of hospitals within a region.

Technology Data Mart

The technology data mart is a repository of medical equipment and subcomponents that can potentially make up a telemedicine workstation. Component, assembly, operational and maintenance costs are typically included in this data mart. The devices used for different telemedicine applications are then used together with the diagnosis data to determine what devices would be used in the different facilities.

Health Indicator Data Mart

Data revealing current trends in health indicators are also stored in a separate data mart. The indicator data will be used during analysis to calculate the extent to which telemedicine programs will influence current trends in healthcare.

Data Analysis

Specific tools for data analysis together with some mathematical models are chosen to effectively analyse the data collected in delivering the required output for decision making. Table 4 provides an outline of the inputs, calculations, and outputs of the analysis.

Table 4. Data management and analysis for a telemedicine needs assessment

Data Management and Analysis			
Input Data ⇒	Warehouse ⇒	Analyse ⇒	Output
Electronic Patient Records • **Reason for referral** • **Name of hospital admitted** • **Name of hospital referred to** • Length of stay	• Referral Data Mart	• Trends analysis • Referral pattern modelling • Calculations and comparisons between different hospitals • Type I / Type II error calculations	• Trend graphs • Travel distances • Referral patterns • Average length of stay • Procedures done for referred patients • Quality Improvement potential
Technology Data • **Telemedicine systems** • **Peripheral devices** • Technologies	• Technology Data Mart		
DHIS Data • **Hospital utilisation** • **Patient day equivalent** • **Average length of stay** • Transport distances	• Health Indicator Data Mart	• Hospital utilisation calculation • Reduced utilisation calculation • Patient throughput	• Hospital utilisation reduction • Transport reduction
Financial data • **Transport costs** • **Procedure costs** • Hospital patient day cost		• Linear Programming • Cost analysis	• Cost savings

Trends Analysis

Firstly, data from the referral data mart are analysed to determine trends in referral patterns among hospitals in the chosen region. The referral patterns are used to determine between which hospitals patients are normally referred. Distances between these hospitals are consequently calculated and included in the health indicator data mart, from where potential transport reduction is calculated.

Pareto analysis is used to determine the relative 'popularity' of reasons for referrals. The Pareto principle states that approximately 20% of the effort or cost accounts for approximately 80% of the benefit of a program (Gitlow, Oppenheim, Oppenheim, & Levine, 2005). Following this principle, it is expected that approximately 80% of referred cases would be because of 20% of the reasons for referrals. The Pareto distributions are subsequently used to assign a probability for specific reasons for referrals to occur in a specific region.

Mathematical Models

Stochastic process modelling could map the probabilities of referrals between the hospitals. Using existing data, predictions are made as to the potential benefits of telemedicine. These probabilities are necessary for financial analysis. The operational performance metrics are expanded by adding cost rates of the different resources used in the system. The financial and capacity utilisation feasibilities of the implementation of the telemedicine system are delivered as outputs for decision making.

Linear programming is a deterministic mathematical modelling technique that is used for the optimization of a linear objective function. The linear programming model yields an optimal solution, guided by the mathematical model. This model contains an objective function in terms of maximised profit or minimized cost that is subject to given constraints represented as linear equations (Winston & Goldberg, 2004). The Fixed Charge Mixed Integer Programming problem is a specific linear programming application that is suitable to support decisions with respect to the selection of equipment. The selection of telemedicine technologies and equipment is supported through the combination of economic, stochastic and linear programming techniques.

Implementation Planning

The needs assessment provides quantitative results on the benefits of telemedicine. The needs assessment may portray that telemedicine would have several benefits, but still decisions need to be made regarding the implementation. Telemedicine implementation planning is considerably more complex than making a single decision whether to implement or not. Choosing the appropriate systems for a specific region, while at the same time standardising systems for an entire district, might be a challenge. The results from the needs assessment will assist in the following implementation decisions:

- Implementation or Not
- Synchronous / Asynchronous telemedicine systems
- Bandwidth
- Implement at which hospitals
- For which departments
- Infrastructure requirements
- Telemedicine equipment

Evaluability Assessments

Clarify Goals and Objectives of Program

To implement a successful telemedicine program, the goals and objectives of the programs should be clearly defined. Results from the needs assessment will guide decision makers to set realistic goals. It might be wise to structure the program in such a way to leave opportunities for improvement. For example, when a telemedicine program is introduced for the first time at a facility it might not be necessary to implement telemedicine at all the departments of the hospital. A department that proved to have the most potential should be targeted first after which the program can be expanded into other departments as well.

Identify Variables of Interest

The continuous assessment of programs is essential to promote continuous improvement. Variables of interest in program evaluation should be defined before the program is formally implemented. This will enable evaluation to take place from the start of the program. Evaluation could play an integral role in change management, ensuring that the program is driven towards tangible results. The variables of interest are likely to include quantitative variables used in the needs assessment.

Develop Data Collection Schemes and Measurement Tools

Similar to the needs assessment, evidence based evaluation depends on scientific analysis of relevant data. Qualitative and quantitative data can be used for evaluation. The data collection and measurement tools that were used in the needs assessment can be modified and applied to evaluation studies. The data warehouse developed for the needs assessment is designed in such a way to be modified for continuous assessment. The results from the needs assessment serve as a benchmark for further evaluation and are therefore kept separate from evaluation studies.

Specify Analytical and Statistical Methods to Interpret Findings

Analytical and statistical methods such as trends analysis are used to evaluate the performance of the telemedicine program. During evaluability assessment, prior to implementation, the analytical and statistical methods that will be used during process and outcome evaluation are specified and developed. Hence, a toolbox for evaluation is created to evaluate the performance of the telemedicine program.

FUTURE WORK

The quantitative needs assessment should be supported by qualitative studies, assessing social and clinical perspectives of telemedicine implementation needs. The extent to which telemedicine improve aspects such as quality of care, equity of care, practitioner support and education, should be assessed using appropriate research methods. It is advised that implementation policy making should use results from the framework suggested in this chapter combined with the other benefits of telemedicine.

Health informatics has proved to be a valuable source of data for decision making. There are however still many improvements necessary in health information systems to be integrated with telemedicine. Ideally, the strategy for EHR's should be improved by restricting the information systems not to allow free-text in the discharge reports. If the reason for referral were not a free-text field, reports could have been drawn; indicating why patients are being referred. The relationship of telemedicine to ICD-10 codes can then be linked to the reasons for referral, allowing for telemedicine assessments to be been integrated into the system, allowing calculation to be done automatically by the information system.

The framework for needs assessments as presented in the chapter requires an in-depth study to determine the relationship between conventional reason for referrals (ICD-10 codes) and telemedicine referrals. To calculate the probability that a telemedicine referral could be an alternative to a transfer referral, it is necessary to assign a probability that a telemedicine technology or device could prevent the transfer for each reason of referral (ICD-10 code). It is critical to the accuracy of the analysis, to have an accurate probability assigned between different technologies and reasons for referrals. However there is a severe lack of published studies that investigate these relationships. It is therefore recommended that a relation between diagnoses and telemedicine services are established prior to implementing the framework.

It is envisaged that the framework will be applied and validated in the Eastern Cape and Western Cape Provinces of South Africa. Detailed studies regarding the accuracy of referral data, relationships between ICD-10 codes and telemedicine devices, financial measurements in telemedicine programs and the development of a prototype relational database are to follow in the validation study.

CONCLUSION

Decision making across the entire healthcare field rely heavily on the use of health informatics. Telemedicine should also use secondary data from health informatics to improve decision making for telemedicine implementation and evaluation for the purpose of continuous improvement. The improvements of EHR systems in terms of standardisation of data fields could path the way for integration between telemedicine and health informatics. This would ultimately improve healthcare systems and promote equity and quality care.

There is no generic quick-fix recipe to perform a telemedicine needs assessment. The framework presented in this chapter is not a universal method that can be followed to the letter, but rather a guide to assist decision makers in systematically approaching the needs assessment process, using health informatics. The methods and tools discussed in this chapter are merely examples of what can be used. There are several other appropriate tools that can also be used to assess the benefits of telemedicine. Following a clinical-pull approach in the implementation of telemedicine programs, the services implemented will be appropriate. By implementing telemedicine systems for which there is a proven need, capital will not be wasted in equipment that is seldom used. Ultimately through policy making that allocate resources effectively, developing countries are better equipped to provide quality healthcare for all.

ACKNOWLEDGMENT

The authors would like to thank the South African National Research Foundation, South African

Eastern Cape Department of Health and the South African Medical Research Council for their support in this research.

REFERENCES

Alverson, D. C., Holtz, B., D'Iorio, J., DeVany, M., Simmons, S., & Poropatich, R. K. (2008). One size doesn't fit all: Bringing telehealth services to special populations. *Telemedicine and e-Health, 14*(9), 957-963.

Bah, S. (2009). Strategies for managing the change from ICD-9 to ICD-10 in developing countries: The case of South Africa. *Journal of Health Informatics in Developing Countries, 3*(2), 44–49.

Bashshur, R., Shannon, G., & Sapci, H. (2005). Telemedicine evaluation. *Telemedicine and e-Health, 11*(3), 296-317.

Bashshur, R. L. (2002). Telemedicine and health care. *Telemedicine Journal and e-Health, 8*(1), 5–12. doi:10.1089/15305620252933365

Bashshur, R. L., Reardon, T. G., & Shannon, G. W. (2000). Telemedicine: A new health care delivery system. *Annual Review of Public Health, 21*, 613–637. doi:10.1146/annurev.publhealth.21.1.613

Byrne, E., & Sahay, S. (2003). Health information systems for primary health care: Thinking about participation. In M. Korpela, R. Montealegre, & A. Poulymenakou (Eds.), *Proceedings of the International Federation of Information Processing, IFIP 9.4 and 8.2 Joint Conference on Organizational Information Systems in the Context of Globalization,* (pp. 237-249). Dordrecht, The Netherlands: Kluwer.

Clarke, M., & Thiyagarajan, C. A. (2008). A systematic review of technical evaluation in telemedicine systems. *Journal of Telemedicine and e-Health, 14*(2), 170-183.

Craig, J., & Patterson, V. (2005). Introduction to the practice of telemedicine. *Journal of Telemedicine and Telecare, 11*(1), 3–9. doi:10.1258/1357633053430494

Curioso, W. H., & Mechael, P. N. (2010). Enhancing 'm-health' with south-to-south collaborations. *Health Affairs, 29*(2), 264–267. doi:10.1377/hlthaff.2009.1057

Della Mea, V. (2005). Prerecorded telemedicine. *Journal of Telemedicine and Telecare, 11*(6), 276–284. doi:10.1258/1357633054893382

Ferguson, J. (2006). How to do a telemedical consultation. *Journal of Telemedicine and Telecare, 12*(5), 220–227. doi:10.1258/135763306777889037

Field, M. J. (1996). *Telemedicine: A guide to assessing telecommunications in health care.* Washington, DC: National Academy Press.

Gitlow, H. S., Oppenheim, A. J., Oppenheim, R., & Levine, D. M. (2005). *Quality management* (3rd ed.). Singapore: McGraw-Hill.

Hailey, D., Ohinmaa, A., & Roine, R. (2004). Study quality and evidence of benefit in recent assessments of telemedicine. *Journal of Telemedicine and Telecare, 10*(6), 318–324. doi:10.1258/1357633042602053

Harrop, V. M. (2002). *Digital diffusion in the clinical trenches: Findings from a telemedicine needs assessment.* Cambridge, MA: MIT Press. Retrieved from http://mit.dspace.org/handle/1721.1/8315.

Hasman, A., Haux, R., & Albert, A. (1996). A systematic view on medical informatics. *Computer Methods and Programs in Biomedicine, 51*(3), 131–139. doi:10.1016/S0169-2607(96)01769-5

Hebert, M. (2001). Telehealth success: Evaluation framework development. In Patel, V. L., Rogers, R., & Haux, R. (Eds.), *MEDINFO 2001* (pp. 1145–1149). Amsterdam, The Netherlands: IOS Press.

Hensher, M., Price, M., & Adomakoh, S. (2006). Referral hospitals. In Jamison, D., Breman, J., Measham, A., Alleyne, G., Claeson, M., & Evans, D. (Eds.), *Disease Control Priorities in Developing Countries* (2nd ed., pp. 1229–1244). New York, NY: Oxford University Press.

Hjelm, N. (2005). Benefits and drawbacks of telemedicine. *Journal of Telemedicine and Telecare, 11*(2), 60–70. doi:10.1258/1357633053499886

Imhoff, M., Webb, A., & Goldschmidt, A. (2001). Health informatics. *Intensive Care Medicine, 27*(1), 179–186.

Jahn, A., & De Brouwere, V. (2001). Referral in pregnancy and childbirth: Concepts and strategies. In De Brouwere, V., & Van Lerberghe, W. (Eds.), *Studies in Health Services Organisation & Policy 17* (pp. 229–246). Antwerp, Belgium: ITG Press.

Kimball, R., & Ross, M. (2002). *The data warehouse toolkit: The complete guide to dimensional modeling* (2nd ed.). New York, NY: John Wiley & Sons Inc.

Mars, M., & Seebregts, C. (2008). *Country case study for ehealth South Africa*. Retrieved from http://www.ehealth-connection.org/content/country-case-studies.

Nakahara, S., Saint, S., Sann, S., Ichikawa, M., Kimura, A., & Eng, L. (2010). Exploring referral systems for injured patients in low-income countries: A case study from Cambodia. *Health Policy and Planning, 25*(4), 319–327. doi:10.1093/heapol/czp063

Nannings, B., & Abu-Hanna, A. (2006). Characterizing decision support telemedicine systems. *Methods of Information in Medicine, 45*(5), 523–527.

National Department of Health. (2003). *Strategic framework for the modernisation of tertiary hospital services*. Retrieved from http://www.doh.gov.za/mts/docs/framework.html.

National Department of Health. (2007). *The national strategic framework for eHR implementation in South Africa*. Pretoria, South Africa: South African National Department of Health. Retrieved from http://www.pnc.gov.za/images/stories/focus_area/report/ehr_fm.pdf.

Roine, R., Ohinmaa, A., & Hailey, D. (2001). Assessing telemedicine: A systematic review of the literature. *Canadian Medical Association Journal, 165*(6), 765–771.

Sabinet. (2010). *Minister of health calls for national telemedicine strategy*. Retrieved November 19, 2010, from http://www.sabinetlaw.co.za/health/articles/minister-health-calls-national-telemedicine-strategy.

Shaw, M. (2001). Finding and using secondary data on the health and health care of populations. In Stevens, A., Fitzpatrick, R., Abrams, K., Brazier, J., & Lilford, R. (Eds.), *The Advanced Handbook of Methods in Evidence Based Healthcare* (pp. 164–189). London, UK: SAGE Publications.

Sood, S., Mbarika, V., Jugoo, S., Dookhy, R., Doarn, C. R., Prakash, N., et al. (2007). What is telemedicine? A collection of 104 peer-reviewed perspectives and theoretical underpinnings. *Telemedicine and e-Health, 13*(5), 573-590.

Steadham, S. V. (1980). Learning to select a needs assessment strategy. *Training and Development Journal, 34*(1), 56–61.

Stevens, A., Fitzpatrick, R., Abrams, K., Brazier, J., & Lilford, R. (2001). Methods in evidence based healthcare and health technology assessment: An overview. In Stevens, A., Fitzpatrick, R., Abrams, K., Brazier, J., & Lilford, R. (Eds.), *The Advanced Handbook of Methods in Evidence Based Healthcare* (pp. 1–5). London, UK: SAGE Publications.

Taylor, P. (1998). A survey of research in telemedicine: Telemedicine services. *Journal of Telemedicine and Telecare, 4*(2), 63–71. doi:10.1258/1357633981931948

Turban, E., Aronson, J., & Liang, T. (2005). *Decision support systems and intelligent systems* (7th ed.). Upper Saddle River, NJ: Prentice Hall.

Walsham, G., & Sahay, S. (2006). Research on information systems in developing countries: Current landscape and future prospects. *Information Technology for Development, 12*(1), 7–24. doi:10.1002/itdj.20020

Williamson, L., Stoops, N., & Heywood, A. (2001). Developing a district health information system in South Africa: A social process of technical solution? In Patel, V. L., Rogers, R., & Haux, R. (Eds.), *MEDINFO 2001* (pp. 773–777). Amsterdam, The Netherlands: IOS Press.

Winston, W., & Goldberg, J. (2004). *Operations research: Applications and algorithms.* Ottawa, Canada: Duxbury Press.

Wootton, R. (1998). Telemedicine in the national health service. *Journal of the Royal Society of Medicine, 91*(12), 614–621.

World Health Organization. (2003). *Unit costs for patient services.* Retrieved from http://www.who.int/choice/costs/unit_costs/en/index.html.

Wright, J., Williams, R., & Wilkinson, J. R. (1998). Health needs assessment: Development and importance of health needs assessment. *British Medical Journal, 316*, 1310–1313. doi:10.1136/bmj.316.7140.1310

Wyatt, J. C. (1996). Commentary: Telemedicine trials—Clinical pull or technology push? *British Medical Journal, 313*, 1380. doi:10.1136/bmj.313.7069.1380

KEY TERMS AND DEFINITIONS

Telemedicine: The use of Information and Communications Technologies (ICT) to deliver or support healthcare services over a distance.

Health Informatics: A discipline concerned with creating, storing and managing health information through the use and development of ICT.

e-Health: An umbrella term for the development and application of ICT in healthcare.

Needs Assessment: It is a process to determine the needs of a population through data collection and analysis. Needs assessments are typically used in creating design specifications, strategic program planning and gap analysis.

Clinical-Pull: An approach that directs technology implementation decisions toward meeting a proven clinical need.

Developing Countries: A term used to define countries with low income and a lower level of development with respect to countries with a high level of development.

Public Health: A term used for health issues and services applicable to the entire population.

Chapter 17

Bridging the Abridged:
The Diffusion of Telemedicine in Europe and China

Xiaohong W. Gao
Middlesex University, UK

Martin Loomes
Middlesex University, UK

Richard Comley
Middlesex University, UK

ABSTRACT

In this chapter, a comprehensive review of the development of telemedicine in China, with the focus on the establishment of PACS (Picture Archiving and Communications Systems) and image-guided tele-surgery, will be accounted for together with a comparative study in reference to the counterparts in Europe, leading to a framework of a sustainable, scalable, and flexible e-health infrastructure for the future global digital (paper-less) hospital. The study is drawn from the first-hand knowledge gained through the conduction of a 3-year networking project on Telemedicine: Tele-Imaging in Medicine (TIME, 2005-2007) funded by the European Commission under the Asia-link programme. It is the authors' hope that this chapter resonates with the future prospect of telemedicine by providing the right contents, at the right time and to the right extent, especially when the implementations taking place are in countries with disparate economic development.

INTRODUCTION

Over the last twenty years, China has achieved unprecedented economic growth, with an accompanying growth of the wealthy and middle classes, which has led to the building of a well-off society in a comprehensive way. To this end, China is currently in the process of reforming its health care systems by equipping its hospitals with many modern medical systems, such as, medical imaging scanners, as well as building its own. Because of the size of its territory and

DOI: 10.4018/978-1-4666-0888-7.ch017

the number of its population coupled with the uneven development of the economy across the country, the distribution of the facility of modern medicine mainly resides in the major cities, such as Beijing and Shanghai. In order to reach to remote areas, China has begun the development telemedicine techniques in the late 1980s. In the first decade (~1990-2000), the main focus was on the implementation of communication networks with a faster and wider bandwidth, such as ISDN (Integrated Services Digital Network), in the hope to connect far and wide. Within this digital network service, tele-education, tele-conferencing, and tele-consultation have flourished. However, these activities mainly serve as demonstrations to showcase the feasibility of the communications networks and the advances of computer technology. With the advent of World Wide Web, many internet-based services are made available and more importantly free, such as Skype, making the services of tele-conferencing/tele-consultation not only affordable but also flexible and mobile, i.e., a network connection being able to set up in an operation room instead of in a conference room, bringing hopes of practical applications at the point of care, such as tele-surgery, a reality. The first case of tele-neurosurgery took place in 2005 between Beijing and Yan'an with a distance of 1300 kilometres.

By contrast, Europe is well advanced in many of these fields. Firstly, Europe originated imaging field when the first Nobel laureate, physicist Wilhelm Roentgen, discovered X-rays that led eventually to the birth of radiology, and thereafter the medical imaging industry. With the application of advanced computer techniques in the 1970s, Computerised Tomography (CT) and Magnetic Resonance Imaging (MRI) were invented, prompting another Nobel Prize award shared between the UK and the USA. With typically 80,000 2D images (e.g., in Geneva Hospital) generated per day, *Picture Archiving and Communications Systems* (PACS) have been developed to manage them. Up to 2005, most European countries have installed PACS in their hospitals with Norway topping the chart with 100% hospitals equipped with PACS. Elsewhere more than 70% hospitals in the countries of United Kingdom, Germany and Italy are implemented with PACS, whereas in China up to 2005, only 1% hospitals managed to install miniPACS, a stand-alone version of PACS.

On the other hand, PACS is not penicillin taking care of any type of images. In its current form, it can only archive radiologic images. Hence, a plethora of effort has been put into it to entail PACS with the ability of managing the other images. Unfortunately, it has been proven that the model of 'one size fits all' is not sustainable in the e-health domain.

This chapter will give a detailed account on the latest development of telemedicine and PACS systems with a focus on China. In comparison with their counterparts in Europe, the results are drawn from the completed TIME project funded by EU and the initial work conducted from the newly funded FP7 project WIDTH on *Infrastructure for the Digital Hospital*. The novelty of this chapter lies in the fact that it might be the first of the kind since most of existing literature reviews tend to be in comparison with the USA or Japan who has more presence in China than in Europe, aiming at exploring the breadth of innovations in the field of telemedicine and keeping abreast of the new developments, leading to a roadmap for the future global digital hospital.

It starts with a background study on the standards and terminologies that are currently adopted in telemedicine, including PACS, DICOM, HL7, RIS, HIS, and EU Asia ICT programme, in particular, the TIME project. This is then followed by the introduction of telemedicine activities that have been conducted or are on-going in Europe, specifically, in the United Kingdom, Switzerland, Italy, Norway and Poland. Although not comprehensive, it is representative of the range of recent advances. Preceding the Section on Lessons Learned, *Telemedicine in China* is detailed, spanning from *Hospital Infrastructure*, *Tele-communications*

Infrastructure and *Telemedicine Infrastructure* to the *Diffusion of PACS* and *Tele-surgery* in China. Future trends are later discussed before the Conclusion is drawn. The chapter ends with the Acknowledgement and References.

BACKGROUND

Generally speaking, telemedicine refers to the use of *communications* and *information technologies* for the delivery of clinical care remotely. In reality, the means to be applied to access any type of medical care has to be physical, such as telephone, internet or any other communication network. Therefore the development of telemedicine, to a certain extent, follows the advances of Information Communications Technology (ICT). Telemedicine is therefore defined by the American Telemedicine Association (ATA, 2011) as the use of medical information exchanged from one site to another via electronic communications to improve patients' health status. *Closely associated with telemedicine is the term Telehealth, which is often used to encompass a broader definition of remote healthcare that does not always involve clinical services* (http://en.wikipedia.org/wiki/Talk%3ATelehealth). To this end, video-conferencing, transmission of still images, e-health including patient portals, remote monitoring of vital signs, continuing medical education and nursing call centres are all considered part of telemedicine and telehealth.

Starting out in the 1960s with demonstrations of hospitals that provided extended care to patients in the remote regions, the use of telemedicine has spread rapidly and is now becoming integrated into the ongoing operations of hospitals, specialty departments, home health agencies, private physician offices as well as consumers' homes and workplaces. In its early days, telemedicine was employed as a communication channel between the user and the medical industry. For example, at the UK, a person can dial 999 for help in the event of a medical emergency and, at present can call NHS Direct for advice on any suspicious symptoms or simply asking for health recommendations. The specialities of telemedicine can cover nearly every medical domain, for example:

- Home Care
- Emergency Care
- Pre-hospital Care
- Out-patient Care
- Surgery
- Dermatology
- Psychiatry
- Oncology
- Pathology
- Ophthalmology
- Cardiology
- Radiology

PACS

One of the most important advances of computer technology brings to medical field for the last 30 years is the emerging array of medical imaging scanners, e.g., Computerised Tomography (CT), Magnetic Resonance (MR), Positron Emission Tomography (PET), or CT/PET and MR/PET, which have revolutionised the way we obtain detailed information from inside the human body. Since these medical images are acquired in digital forms as opposed to 'films', a systematic way has to be in place to store, manage, retrieval, or transmit them either locally or over a network. *Picture Archiving and Communications Systems*, more commonly known as PACS, has therefore emerged. It enables images, such as X-ray scans, to be stored electronically and viewed on video screens, so that doctors and other health professionals can access the information and compare it with previous images at the touch of a button. The arrival of PACS has since replaced large numbers of radiological films, the medium that had been around for over 100 years and had been almost the exclusive way for capturing, storing,

Figure 1. The implementation of PACS in a number of European countries (Bergstrøm, 2006)

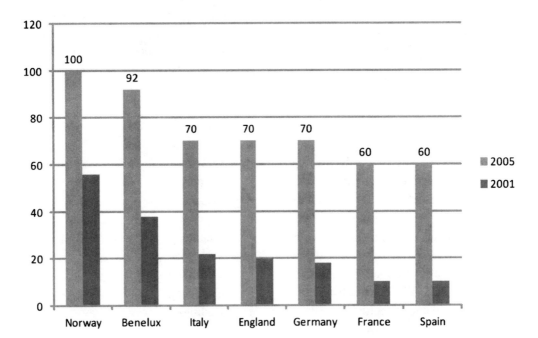

and displaying radiographic pictures. By then, film had been a relatively fixed medium with usually only one set of images available for each scan. By contrast, PACS technology permits a near filmless process, with all of the flexibility that a digital system can offer. PACS also removes all the costs associated with hard films and releases valuable space currently used for storage. Most importantly, PACS has the potential to transform patients' experience of the care they receive across an array of networked hospitals, for example, NHS network in the UK. By this way, if a patient has relocated from one place to another, his/her medical records can be easily retrieved from the system as if from the same hospital.

The first generation of the software of PACS was developed in the mid-1980s in the USA and Europe (Huang & Taira, 1992) when modules of PACS were programmed and were implemented independently in the departments of different domains, e.g., paediatric, coronary, or neuro-radiology.

Because of its potential benefit of going 'filmless,' in 1982, a series of annual meetings, Euro-

PACS (http://www.europacs.org/), was funded in Europe, to establish a scientific reference circle of reputable experts in the field of imaging informatics and PACS. Nearing its 30th anniversary, Euro-PACS had gained its credentials at the time when the deployment of PACS was still at its frontier with regard to technical innovations in medicine. Before this, there had not been any commercial system nor had vendor solution available, the annual meetings of EuroPACS provided a unique platform to interface the pioneers in the field with the technical innovations and developments, paving the way to its currently near-mature status. As of 2005, most European countries had installed PACS across many of their hospitals. Figure 1 illustrates such a development (Bergstrøm, 2006).

In terms of telemedicine, one particular technical issue of concern for PACS is the speed of data flow. Due to the fact that most of radiologic images are of higher resolutions and are going to higher dimensions (>2), in the late 1980s, a network with a typical capacity of 10 MByte per second such as IEEE 802.3 Ethernet was discovered inadequate for PACS to transmit integrated data of audio, video, and text forms in one stream. A high-speed fibre optic network with rate upto 200 MByte/ps has since then been in place (Schmiedl, Rowberg, 1990) to replace the copper wire network, which slowly but surely pushed the further refinement of PACS in the 1990s.

DICOM Images

In principle, PACS can take an image of any format, such as TIFF (Tagged Image File Format), or lossy compression format JPEG, created by Joint Photographic Expert Group, as well as home grown formats built into an image scanner. In practice, in order to communicate images with each other to ensure an image acquired from one radiology department can be readable by the others, a standard format is required to prevent the repetitive work on converters translating formats from one to another. DICOM, also known as (aka) *Digital Imaging and Communications in Medicine*, was initiated in 1992 in the USA by ACR (*the American College of Radiology*) and NEMA (the National Electrical Manufacturers Association). Since then it has been developed in liaison with other Standardization Organizations in both Europe and Japan (NEMA, 2004), and currently has been widely utilised in medical imaging field, in an attempt to facilitate standard communications of medical images. A DICOM image contains multiple parts providing a means for expansion and updating. The advantages of using DICOM images include among many others that DICOM standard has been widely applied in the medical field, and that DICOM has a header file of fixed format and an image dataset, leading to a fixed size of vocabulary in terms of representation of pathology. For instance, a typical DICOM image comprises a textual header file containing around 700 lines detailing imaging time, modality, and manufacturer of the scanning, etc., together with an image data file. To most radiologists and clinicians, the context of around 100 lines can

provide enough information for a patient. This standard has been continuously extended to meet the demands of practical applications. Recently in 2000, DICOM has been added *Structure Reporting* (SR) (Clunie, 2000) classes, *Supplement 23* that is employed for transmission and storage of clinical documents. The SR classes fully support both conventional free-text reports and structured information, thus enhancing the precision, clarity, and value of clinical documentation. In addition, the SR standard provides the capability to link text and other data (e.g., blood test results) with a group of particular images or waveforms, arriving at storing the parameters of findings and bridging the traditional gap between imaging systems and information systems. In addition, SR also plays an essential role in *Integrating the Healthcare Enterprise* (IHE) by providing healthcare practitioners with an effective tool that encompasses a variety of clinical contexts.

HL7

Health Level Seven (HL7) is an all-volunteer, non-profit organization involved in the development of international healthcare standards (http://www.hl7.org/about/index.cfm), one of several ANSI-accredited (*American National Standards Institute*) *Standards Developing Organizations* (SDOs) (ANSI) operating in the healthcare arena. Most SDOs produce standards (aka specifications or protocols) for a particular healthcare domain such as pharmacy, medical devices, imaging or insurance (claims processing) transactions. '*Level Seven*' refers to the seventh level of the *International Organization for Standardization* (ISO), i.e., the seven-layer communications model for *Open Systems Interconnection* (OSI). This application level (layer) that is independent of lower layers interfaces directly to and performs common application services for the application processes. Although other protocols have largely superseded it, the OSI model remains valuable as a starting point to begin the study of network architecture.

HL7's domain is clinical and administrative data and is dedicated to offering a comprehensive framework and related standards for the exchange, integration, sharing, and retrieval of electronic health information that supports clinical practice and the management, as well as delivery and evaluation of health services. Specifically, it aims to create flexible, cost effective approaches, standards, guidelines, methodologies, and related services for interoperability between healthcare information systems. At present, HL7 has more than 2,300 members, including approximately 500 corporate members, from 55 countries, who represent more than 90% of the information systems vendors serving healthcare.

One of the HL7 standards is *Electronic Health Record / Personal Health Record* (HER/PHR), within which the *System Functional Model* that provides a reference list of functions may be present in an EHR System (EHR-S). Described from a user perspective, the function list has the intention to enable consistent expression of system functionalities, allowing a set of standardized descriptions and common understanding of functions in a given setting, e.g. intensive care, cardiology, office practice in one country or primary care in another country, etc..

HIS and RIS

A *Hospital Information System* (HIS), aka *Clinical Information System* (CIS), is a comprehensive, integrated information system designed to manage the administrative, financial and clinical data of a hospital. This encloses both paper-based and machine-based information processing. CISs are sometimes separated from HISs in that the former concentrates on patient-related and clinical-state-related data (i.e., Electronic Patient Record [EPR]) whereas the latter keeps track of administrative issues. However, the distinction is not always clear and there is contradictory evidence against a consistent use of both terms.

The aim of an HIS is to achieve the best possible support for patient care and administration by the application of electronic data processing. Because of the variations in size and in specialty at each hospital, usually, each hospital has their own tailored in-house HIS. Specifically, it can be either composed of or independent of one or more software components with specialty-oriented extensions, such as a *Laboratory Information System* (LIS), or a *Radiology Information System* (RIS).

A RIS is a computerized database used by radiology departments to store, manipulate and distribute patient radiological data and imagery data (RIS, 2011). The system generally consists of capabilities of patient tracking, scheduling, result reporting and image tracking, and is critical to efficient workflow to radiology practices. Although RIS complements HIS, it can be substantially different in many ways from HIS, with many components being independent between the two. Furthermore, attention should be paid to the fact that the data structures in HIS and RIS are usually different. This is because that the retrieval system of HIS is centred around clinicians' notes, whereas RIS is based on the 'checklist' of a scanning procedure. In order to interface them with each other, a converter, i.e., a look-up table, usually, should be in place.

Figure 2 illustrates a typical relationship between HIS, RIS, and PACS. On the one hand, HIS deals with patients' check-in/check-out and scheduling for examinations. On the other, PACS manages patients' image data. Whereas RIS interfaces the two systems with each other by connecting a patient's personal records with his/her imagery data. Thus to ensure that HIS and RIS communicate with each other smoothly, five aspects should be taken into consideration (Guo, Huang, Gan, Yang, Jing, 2006):

a. **Patient information** – RIS must identify all the patients that are registered in HIS, i.e., to avoid repetitive entries or even

Figure 2. A typical relationship between HIS, RIS, and PACS

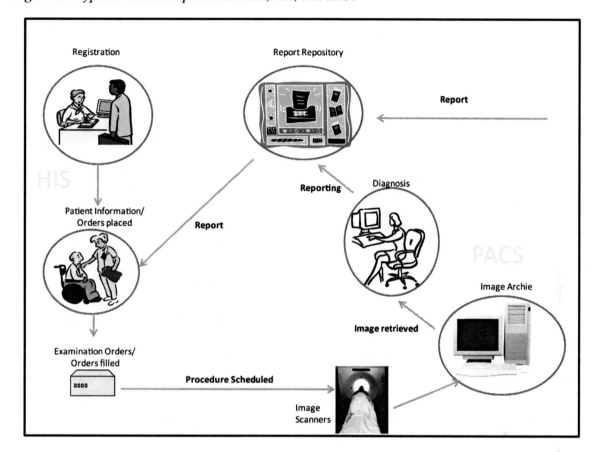

worse, wrong entries, RIS should be able to read all the information from HIS.

b. **Sharing the same clinical and management dictionary** – In order to process scheduling and billing information from HIS correctly, RIS should employ the same check list, materials and clinical management terms as in HIS. For the benefit of HIS, RIS should also adhere to the same information on facility and personnel that are allocated to the patent by HIS.

c. **Diagnostic information** – Usually, there are two ways to accept clinicians' diagnostic reports. One is for out-patents and another is for the in-patients. For those out-patients, the notes written on papers are accepted that later can be input into the system. Whilst for the in-patients,

HIS is employed for clinicians to input patients' diagnostic/checking information, which can be obtained from RIS, including next checking time, follow-ups, reports, etc.

d. **Billing** – RIS needs to be able to give a price list, detailing the checklist for a patient who undergoes one or more scans. It should take into account of the categories that a patient belongs to, i.e., free, on-benefit, etc.

e. **Clinical report** – RIS should have the ability of checking a patient's information, whereas radiologists can write reports based on the patient's scanned images. Clinicians from different departments should be able to read them through HIS via a hospital network.

IHE

Integrating the Healthcare Enterprise (IHE, 2011) is a global initiative that creates the framework for passing vital health information seamlessly—from application to application, system to system, and setting to setting—across multiple healthcare enterprises. It might not create any new standard, but it is the nature of its proven process of collaboration, demonstration and real-world implementation of interoperable solutions that puts IHE in a unique position to significantly accelerate the process for defining, testing and implementing standards-based interoperability among digital health record systems by driving the adoption of standards to address specific clinical needs. For example, the IHE *Technical Framework* identifies functional components of a distributed healthcare environment solely from the point of view of their interactions in the healthcare enterprise. At its current level of development, it defines a coordinated set of transactions based on the HL7 and DICOM standards. IHE encourages implementers to ensure that any product that is implemented in accordance with the IHE Technical Framework also meet the full requirements of the standards underlying the IHE (Fu Fu, Jin, Dai, Chen, Wang, Li, Gao, 2003).

EuropeAid Programme: TIME Project

In the European Commission, EuropeAid (http://ec.europa.eu/) has been a major player on the external assistance scene and up to 2005 has committed €7 billion to more than 150 countries and territories in a bid to meet the daily challenge of improving lives worldwide and to build long-term partnerships.

Since the release of World Wide Web in 1990 by Tim Berners-Lee in Europe, the way people live has been changed forever by the emerging ICT (*Information Communications Technology*), in a good way. From then on, European Commission (EC) has initiated dialogues with Asia with the aim of helping the development of ICT in Asia and to strengthen the economic links between the two continents.

As a result, the first ASEM (Asia Europe Meeting) meeting took place in 1996 in Bangkok. Subsequently, second ASEM II was held in London in 1998 and the third ASEM III in Seoul in 2000. At the first meeting, it was stressed that intensified cross-flows between Asia and Europe in ICT were central to strengthening the economic links between the two continents. Moreover, an extensive survey in both Europe and Asia indicated that the potential and desire to co-operate existed on both sides. With this in mind, in 1999, EC launched *Asia IT&C Programme Phase One*, and thereafter, in 2004, *Asia IT&C Programme Programme Phase Two*.

The programme of EU-Asia IT&C had the aims of (http://cordis.europa.eu/fp7/home_en.html):

- Stimulating an open dialogue between governments, citizens and key players in the ICT sector, professional associations, chambers of commerce, NGOs (Non-Governmental Organisations), regulators, standardisation bodies, and the private sector of both regions;
- Improving co-operation in ICT between Europe and Asia (and within Asia), particularly in the least developed countries (LDC's);
- The formation of long lasting ICT partnerships;
- Further integration of Asian countries into the Information Society;
- The strengthening of ICT mutual trade and investment flows between the regions; and
- Increasing the European ICT presence in Asia.

Five components of the EU-Asia IT&C programme were in place, including:

- Get-in-Touch & Keep-in-Touch Activities;

Figure 3. The TIME webpage funded under the scheme of European Commission Asia ICT programme

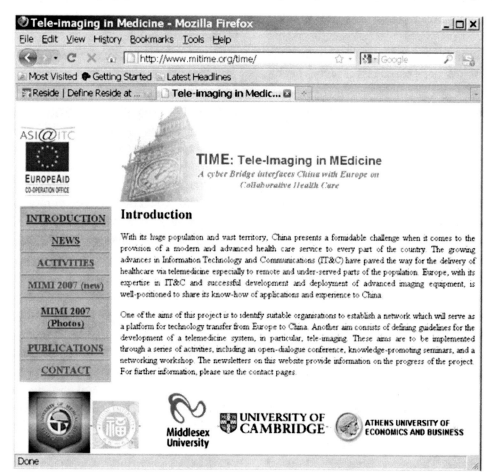

- Short Courses (university or technical level);
- Liaison with European ICT Initiatives and Programmes;
- Understanding European and Asian Regulatory and Legislative Organisation Structures;
- Practical Demonstration Actions.

The project TIME (http://www.mitime.org/time/), acronym for *Tele-Imaging in Medicine: A Cyber Bridge Interfaces China with Europe on Collaborative Health Care*, received funding of €200,000 in January 2005 under the strand of Asia IT&C Phase II with the component of *Get-in-Touch & Keep-in-Touch*. It was coordinated by

Gao, the first author of this Chapter, at Middlesex University, UK, with partners including University of Cambridge in the UK, Athens University of Economics and Business in Greece, Fuzhou University in China and Capital University of Medical Sciences in China. TIME strived to form a network for technology transfer from Europe to China; and to set up guidelines for the development of telemedicine systems (in particular for tele-imaging), in which it had succeeded, as will be described later. Figure 3 shows the TIME webpage.

The main motivation for running this project was that there was a mismatch of the levels of IT&C applications between developed and developing countries, and such a mismatch would affect global economic growth. For examples, in

Asia, mainly China, the first case of Severe Acute Respiratory Syndrome (SARS) appeared in 2003, whereas Avian influenza (bird flu) was discovered in both Asia and Europe. Due to their infectious nature, these diseases could affect global health if not being treated in a timely manner.

The methodology that the TIME project employed was to organise international conferences/workshops, opening up dialogues in a hope to form collaborative research between two continents. Figure 4 demonstrates the first conference MIT2005 (Medical Imaging and Telemedicine) organized in China in August 2005 with delegates coming from 9 countries. Taking into consideration the short space of 6 months spent from preparing to completion of the conference, the conference was a success. During the TIME project, Fuzhou partner, led by Prof. Qiang Lin, developed a LEJ-2 Omni-directional M-mode echocardiography system (Figure 4, bottom-left) that was awarded the top price for technology innovation in China in 2007.

The second conference, on MIMI2007 (*Medical Imaging and Informatics*, http://www.mitime.org/time/mimi07.html) took place on August 14-16, 2007 in Beijing, as yet another element of the TIME activities. Delegates from 18 countries/regions (China, Japan, Korea, Pakistan, Singapore, Malaysia, Libya, Taiwan, Hong Kong, Macao, UK, Finland, Italy, Switzerland, Norway, Greece, USA, Canada) attended this event. Figure 5 illustrates two snapshots from the conference (top) and a visit to observe image-guided neurosurgery (bottom) during the conference. Significantly, these activities have borne fruit in a number of publications (Gao, et al., 2005; Gao, et al., 2008; Müller, et al., 2006; Müller, et al., 2008).

As part of the project, a framework of e-PACS, i.e., an online imaging system was developed to transfer and communicate medical images for research purpose, forming a collaborative platform as illustrated in Figure 6 (http://image.mdx.ac.uk). With server located at Middlesex University in the UK, the system at present accommodates over 100,000 2D and 3D images. Built on the

open source GNU Image Finding Tool (GIFT) that was initially developed at the University of Geneva, the online database offers a facility of Content-Based Image Retrieval (CBIR). It is based on the Query-By-Example (QBE) paradigm whereby images from a collection that most closely resemble a query image in appearance (i.e., the content that an image is carrying) are retrieved from the server. The GIFT software is installed on the server side only.

On the client side, a web page based interface is given. The client-server communication is achieved using the XML-based Multimedia Retrieval Markup Language (MRML). All client-server communication, including queries from the client or results returned by the server, is realised using message passing. As a result, the client can be implemented in any programming language. The current TIME client is implemented using PHP (Personal Home Programming) language to generate dynamic web pages for the client web browser.

During the project, this system enabled the sharing of data among the project partners, with data including ultrasound images and digital human being transmitted from China, and Image-CLEF (ImageCLEF) data from Europe. Two main extensions to further enrich the system have since been conduced, one of a technical nature implemented during the TIME project and the other a pedagogical character that has been carried out after the completion of TIME.

The first extension involved contribution to the online interpretation of PET images. The brain PET collection contains images of a functional nature. As such they provide little structural information. A digit anatomic atlas is therefore provided by pressing the 'Map' button in Figure 6(b). This leads to a new window depicting slices of a standard template of the human brain with anatomic labels that can be displayed by clicking on the relevant locations of the slice. The second extension is concerned with teaching students undertaking a Biomedical Modelling and Informatics masters programme at Middlesex University using the da-

Figure 4. The webpage of MIT2005 (top-left) and the delegates in the conference from 9 countries (top-right). Bottom-left: LEJ-2 Omni-directional M-mode echocardiography system devloped during TIME project by Fuzhou parter team. Bottom-right: TIME team visited Fuzhou University where Prof. Lin (3rd from left) is from.

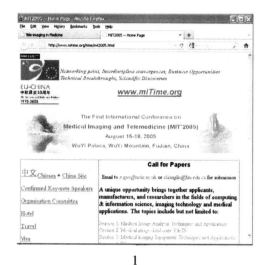

1

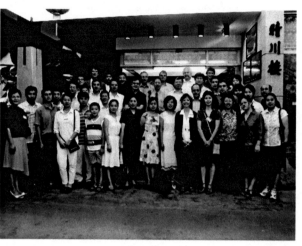

2

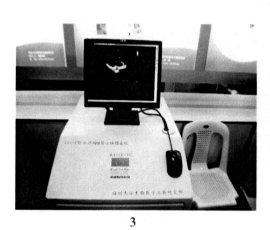

3

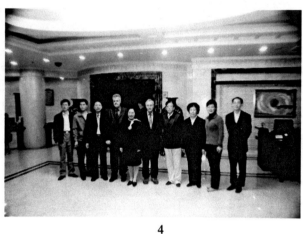

4

tabase, which is further funded by UK JISC (JISC) under Repository programme Phase 1 and Phase 2 respectively. The Phase 1 project MIRAGE (2009-2010) (aka *Middlesex University medical Image Repository with CBIR ArchivinG Environment*) involved digesting more images into the server by including 3D images (Gao, et al., 2010; Qian, et al., 2011), especially in the brain domain, the data that are collected from the Chinese partner from Navy General Hospital. MIRAGE 2011 has just started and will be focusing on the development of an interface for visualization of 3D images and will be completed at the end of 2011.

TELEMEDICINE ACTIVITIES IN EUROPE

To a certain extent, it can be said that the advances in Information and Communication Technologies

Figure 5. MIMI2007 conference, (top left) Prof. Maryellen Giger, University of Chicago, USA, delivering a keynote speech that was enjoyed by the audience (top right). Conference delegates visited General Navy Hospital at Beijing while they were performing image-guided tumour removal surgery (bottom left). Patient (60-year-old female) was back to normal in 20 minutes after the operation (bottom right). © Courtesy of Prof. Tian at NGH, China.

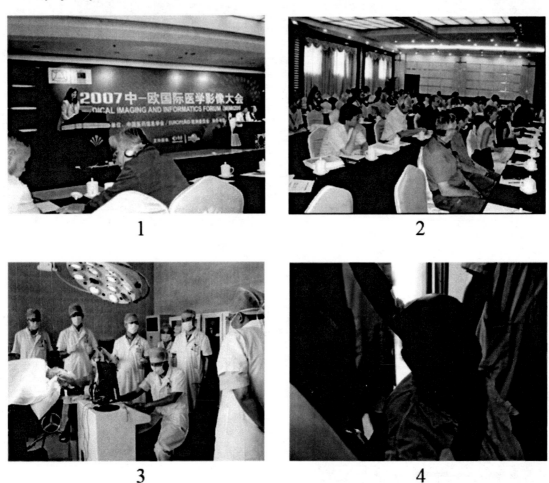

(ICT) have brought forth telemedicine, the service that is able to provide health care, to perform clinical surgery and to present consultation to the patients remotely via ICT devices. Built on the advances of ICT emerged in the 1980s, especially in the hardware domain, many countries have initiated the application of ICT to health departments and formed telemedicine services.

Europe has led the way in many aspects in both medical imaging and ICT. As early as in 1895, the first Nobel laureate, physicist Wilhelm Roentgen, discovered X-rays that led eventually to the birth of a new medical speciality, radiology, and thereafter the medical imaging industry. Since the 1970s, advances in imaging techniques, and in particular the uses of the computer, have revolutionised the application of radiographic imaging techniques in medical diagnosis. In 1979, Professor Allan Cormack at Tufts University, USA, and Sir. Godfrey Hounsfield at EMI Limited, UK, shared the Nobel Prize in Physiology or Medicine for their work on Computerised Tomography

Figure 6. TIME image retrieval database with CBIR facility. (a) (b) The interface and the login; (c) Select a group of images by clicking 'Random' button; (d) One or more images can be chosen as query (queries) by select 'Rel' (aka Relevant) of the pull-down menu under each image with the similar images returned when the button 'Query' being clicked; and (e) the template brain images for PET.

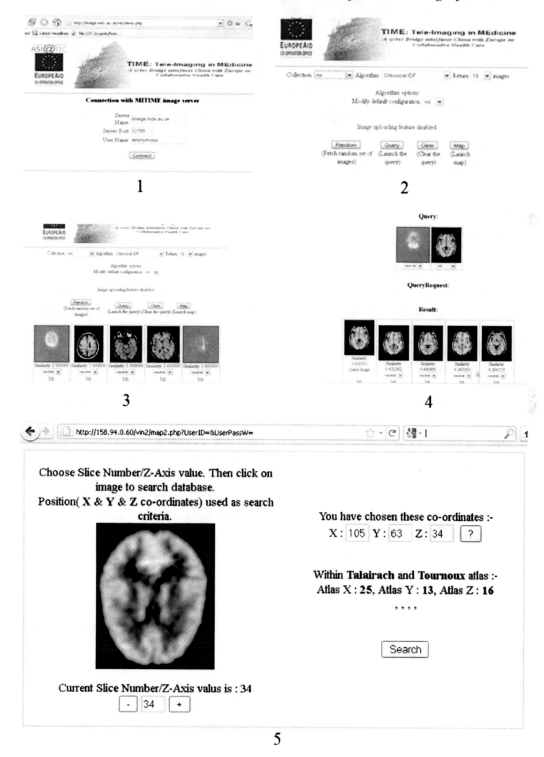

Figure 7. 3D brain images for the same subject acquired from CT(left), MR (middle), and PET (FDG-tracer) scanners. © Courtsey of Prof. John Clark at Wolfson Brain Imaging Centre of University of Cambridge.

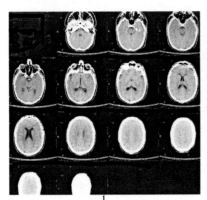 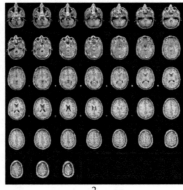 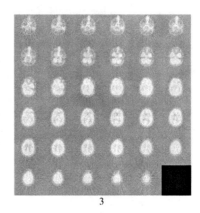

(CT). In the same field, more recently, in 2003, Sir Peter Mansfield from Nottingham University, UK, together with Professor Paul Lauterbur from the USA, was jointly awarded the Nobel Prize for their discoveries in Magnetic Resonance Imaging (MRI). Figure 7 illustrates a set of 3D brain images for the same subject from each of the three imaging modalities of CT (left), MR (middle), and PET (right).

In addition, Europe has also been a major player in the field of IT&C. It was British physicist Tim Berners-Lee who invented the World Wide Web (WWW) while working at CERN in Switzerland in December 1990, allowing computers to talk to each other through a new language HTML (Hyper-Text Markup Language). Since he wrote the first browser, the WWW has changed the world, ushering in a new era that makes information more accessible than ever before.

Furthermore, in 2009, Charles Kao, aka the *Godfather of Broadband*, was awarded half of Nobel Prize in Physics (Nobel Foundation, 2009) for his groundbreaking achievements concerning the transmission of light in fibres for optical communication while working at Standard Telecommunication Laboratories, at the UK, revolutionised the telecommunications industry and paved the way to the advent of today's *information age* by

replacing the copper wire-based network that had been the main materials before the 1960s with optical fibres that can achieve a capacity of 2.56 Terabit/second. As of 2010, submarine cables that are laid beneath the sea have linked all the world's continents except Antarctica (Wiki, 2010), connecting the world into one.

In terms of the application of ICT to medicine, Europe has been very actively involved, which will be described in the following sections by listing a number of projects in telemedicine, the activities that the TIME project actively interacted with during 2005 to 2007. Although it is not intended to be a completed account nor a conclusive one, it is in the hope that the following description resonates with the latest diffusion of telemedicine in both Europe and Asia.

United Kingdom (NHS)

In United Kingdom (UK), the National Health Service (NHS) has established a unique national healthcare system providing *free health for all* since 1948 (Istepanian, 1999). However, at the advent of the new century, thanks to the accumulated funding constraints and the increased aging populations, the NHS faced fundamental changes in its operational structures and the quality of medical services it provided, reflected on long patient and operation waiting lists, shortages in hospital beds and community care, and inadequate medical facilities in intensive care and emergency units as well as nursing staff. One solution was to make healthcare more productive, technologically efficient by the application of the advances of ICT.

Telemedicine therefore has gained a rapid growth since 1998 (TeleMed, 1997; TeleMed, 1998). Large number of research and application programs on telemedicine/telehealth flourished in different universities, hospitals, and health institutes, with a significant increase in funding from the national funding research councils including EPSRC (www.epsrc.ac.uk), ESRC (www.esrc.ac.uk), BBSRC (www.bbsrc.ac.uk), and MRC (www.mrc.ac.uk). At the mean time, the UK Telemedicine and E-Health Information Service (TEIS, http://www.teis.nhs.uk/about/TEIS.htm) was established in 1998 running by the University of Portsmouth and was formally launched in January 2004 with a goal to provide a background source of information to anyone researching the field or proposing a trial or planning a larger scale implementation of telemedicine. The service gives access to information about all aspects of telemedicine from telemedicine activities, contact information for the people or organisations involved, to publications and equipment that are currently available for telemedicine.

The UK's largest e-health project is NHS Direct, which has been in operation since 2000. It is a 24-hour nurse led telephone help line supported by a website @ http://www.nhsdirect.nhs.uk, covering England and Wales. A separate service, NHS24 @ http://www.nhs24.com, covers Scotland. It aimed to '*provide people at home with easier and faster advice and information about health, illness, and the NHS, so that they are better able to care for themselves and their families.*' Because of the huge impact it has made to society, NHS Direct has been acclaimed as *the largest and most successful healthcare provider of its kind, anywhere in the world* (Department of Health, 2011).

As a core service, a call to NHS Direct can often be the starting point of a patient's treatment process. It currently handles more than half a million telephone calls per day with over 3 millions web transactions each month. Users of the service, through whichever channel, are asked questions about their symptoms or problem. Common problems are often given simple self care advice, by which people can follow so as to avoid an expensive visit to a health care professional. More complex problems are assessed by a nurse and can then be given treatment advice or referred on to another service within the NHS. In addition, NHS Direct provides a number of commissioned services throughout the NHS, such as specialised support for patients with long term conditions, access to General Practitioner (GP) and dental healthcare out of hours, and a professional response system for times of public health anxiety.

In terms of collaboration with Asia on telemedicine, between 2005 and 2007, the TIME project was conducted between Europe and China as explained in the above Section. In 2011, a new FP7 project has been funded to continue the work of the TIME project, which will be coordinated by the author, Gao, in the UK. As a follow-up project, WIDTH (*Warehousing images in the digital Hospital [WIDTH], interpretation, infrastructure, and integration*) is under the FP7 People Marie Curie Programme with a total funding of €411,600. It comprises 6 European partners and 5 Chinese as listed at Table 1. It is expected that this three-year collaboration between Europe and China will not only promote the close tie that has been established between the two regions, but also contribute in a great deal to the global development of the digital hospital, while gaining perspective of future sustainable, flexible, and integrated health care systems in the digital hospital.

It is anticipated that the findings from the WIDTH project will be published in due course to inform researchers the lessons and experiences learned.

Table 1. The list of partners for the forthcoming project WIDTH

No	Full Name	City/Country	Coordinator
P1	School of Engineering and Information Sciences, Middlesex University	London/United Kingdom	Dr. Xiaohong Gao (Project Coordinator)
P2	University of Applied Sciences Western Switzerland	Sierra/Switzerland	Prof. Henning Müller
P3	Department of Medical Informatics Aachen University of Technology	Aachen/Germany	Prof. Thomas Deserno
P4	School of Informatics, Athens University of Economics and Business	Athens/Greece	Prof. Theodore Kalamboukis
P5	Department of Oncology, University of Pisa	Pisa/Italy	Prof. Davide Caramella
P6	Norwegian Centre for Informatics in Health and Social Care	Trondheim/Norway	Dr. Roald Bergstrom
P7	Biomedical Engineering Institute, Fuzhou University	Fuzhou/China	Prof. Chiang Lin
P8	Department of Neurosurgery, General Navy Hospital	Beijing/China	Prof. (Dr) Zengmin Tian
P9	Centre of Biomedical Engineering, Fudan University, China	Shanghai/China	Prof. Yuanyuan Wang
P10	Capital University of Medical Sciences, Beijing, China	Beijing/China	Prof. Shuqian Luo
F11	First Hospital of Tsinghua University, Beijing, China	Beijing/China	Prof. (Dr) Lianyi Wang

Switzerland (RAFT Project)

In 2001, the University Hospitals of Geneva in Switzerland and French-speaking countries in Africa initiated the RAFT project (Réseau en Afrique Fancophone pour la Télémédecine) by building a multinational telemedicine communication network in order to facilitate distance learning and tele-consultations through the internet-based platform (Bagayoko, et al., 2006). In 2001, the project started with the establishment of connections to Mali with four sites in Namako, including three regional hospitals and one rural hospital. Whilst in 2002, Mauritania was linked to the network with 7 sites in Nouakchott, together with 8 regional hospitals and 1 rural telecentre. Later between 2003 to 2004, Morocco was bridged when Burkina-Faso, Senegal, and Tunisia were connected. By 2005, the network grid had been extended to Cameroon, Ivory Coast, Madagascar, and

Djibouti (RAFT). As a direct result, through ustilising the internet-based technologies, distance learning and teleconsultation were facilitated via various communication schemes. For example, there were programmes of North-South, South-South, and South-North distance learning and tele-consultation respectively as illustrated in Figure 8, where top-left showing the South-North distance learning and top-right the IT infrastructure implemented in Africa. Several other countries are currently in the process of joining this network. So far, this network has connected 18 Africain countries, extending its activities from French-speaking to English-speaking countries. Later in 2009, RAFT became a partner of the e-Diabetes programme (e-Diabetes Programme, 2009) developed by the World French-speaking Digital University (UNFM). The bottom row in Figure 8 illustrates the encounters between two RAFT team and the TIME team.

Figure 8. The meeting between RAFT and TIME projects. **Top-left**: *South-North of Africa distance learning;* **top-right**: *IT infrastructure in the RAFT.* © *Courtsey of Prof. Henning Müller from University of Applied Sciences Western Switzerland.* **Bottom-left**: *discussion of IT infrastructure between two teams of TIME and RAFT;* **bottom-right**: *RAFT team Prof. Muller (left) and Prof. Geissbuhler (middle), and TIME team Dr. Gao (2ⁿᵈ left, UK), Prof. Clark (2ⁿᵈ right, UK), and Dr. Stumbris (right, Latvia).*

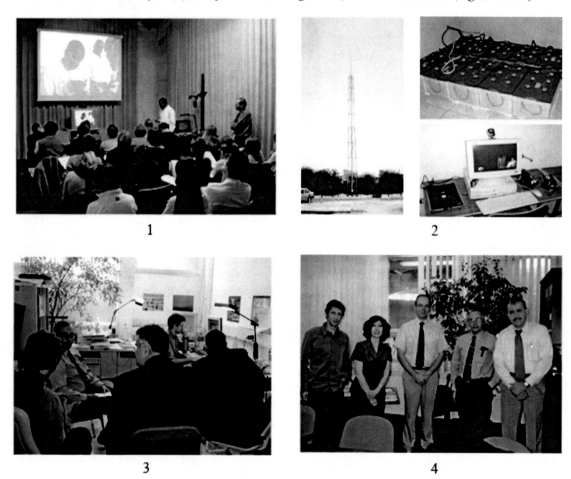

Italy

In 2004, Italy, Trieste University hosted an international conference on *EuroPACS-2004 in the Enlarged Europe*. During the conference, innovative and organizational solutions for the ICT-based integration of the health systems in the enlarged Europe were discussed and proposed by about 400 people from 47 Countries (Inchingolo, 2005). The key motifs of the conference focused on the '*Integrating the Healthcare Enterprise*' (IHE) of world-wide projects and the integral solutions offered by Trieste. Figure 9 demonstrates the Trieste PACS system (left) and the virtual multi-regional Alpe-Adria PACS booth at the '*EuroPACS-MIR 2004 in the enlarged Europe.*'

From 1991 to 1995, Trieste University led a project on Open-PACS, with the aim to distribute PACS services and to pioneer a surgical PACS by releasing the AT&T Commview PACS that had been installed in 1988 in Trieste (Inchingolo, 2008). Subsequently, in 1995, Trieste started project DPACS (aka data PACS) in an attempt to initiate an open, scalable, cheap and universal system

*Figure 9. Tele-imaging system at Trieste University, Italy (**left**) and the virtual multi-regional Alpe-Adria PACS booth (**right**) at the 'EuroPACS-MIR 2004 in the enlarged Europe' (© Courtsey of late Prof. Paolo Inchingolo from Italy).*

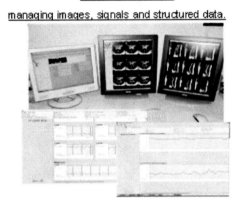

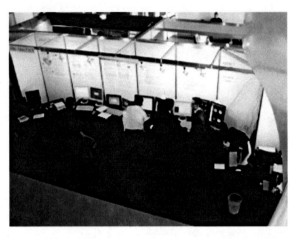

1   2

with accompanying tools to store, exchange and retrieve all health information (Fioravanti, et al., 1997). It was anticipated to offer an integrated virtual health card to the European Citizen, prompting the latest development of PACS that can be traced in a number of projects funded by the European Union's 7th Framework Programme (EU FP7) (http://cordis.europa.eu/fp7/home_en.html).

The other development in Italy comes from the University of Pisa, Division of Diagnostic and Interventional Radiology (www.rad.unipi.it). Since 1994, the division has been actively involved in the field of IT applications to Radiology, with EU funded projects including among many others:

- PARCS – The project carried out design and implementation of a PACS based on a parallel architecture;
- HIM (High-performance information Infrastructure in Medicine) – the project included experimental use of ATM (Asynchronous Transfer Mode) networks for the transmission of radiological images;

- Tip-TV (LIVE, Lifetime Investment in Vocational Education) – the project prepared training courses for radiology technicians in the field of CT post-processing; and
- Europe-MMM – to prepare a multimedia course accessible from the internet or a CD-ROM for radiology students.

In particular, the project *E-learning @ University of Pisa* has developed a niche interactive system for uploading and consulting teaching materials that can be applied to performing self-evaluation tests and exams, targeting at medical students. Further more, they have co-funded ENDOCAS (Centre for Computer Assisted Surgery) as shown in Figure 10 (ENDOCAS, 2011), with a goal of implementing an Imaging Assisted Surgery (IAS) systems to provide *information help, action help,* and *training help,* which can be achieved by offering assistance on planning surgical intervention, integrating mechanic components of the robots, and simulating complex environment for surgical training respectively. At the European Conferences of Radiology 2007 and 2008, Professor Caramella from Pisa and

Figure 10. ENDOCAS webpage (top-left) and virtual patient at ENDOCAS (top-right). © Courtsey of Prof. Davide Caramella from University of Pisa, 2007. Bottom left: Prof. Caramella was delivering a speech to the TIME team. Bottom right, TIME team practicing virtual reality (VR) tools by wearing VR goggles in order to view the simulated details inside a body.

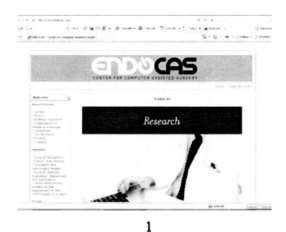

1

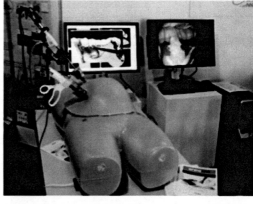

2

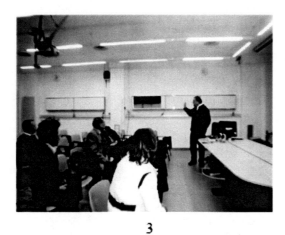

3

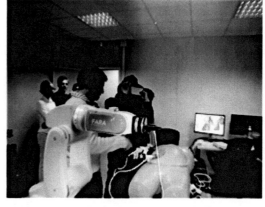

4

Professor Pokieser from Vienna delivered ePACS courses on Cardio CT and Breast Imaging. The concept of ePACS offers a new way of learning that is built on a modified web-based PACS system and the basis of original radiological reports. Students can either learn by themselves or be guided to train in a simulated radiological working environment as demonstrates in Figure 10, where top-left shows a webpage of ENDO-CAS and top-right the IAS. At bottom-left, Prof. Caramella gave an introduction to the TIME team and the TIME team was practicing IAS robotic system at bottom-right.

Norway

Although the hospitals in Norway are state owned, they work as private health enterprises. Distributed in regions with separate boards, each region is managed by a dedicated director and is connected to the other regions using intra-regional broadband communications.

Norway has a long history of the development of telemedicine thanks to the nature of national geography with an elongated shape, forming one of the longest and most rugged coastlines in the world. Within this geography, there are around

50,000 islands off the much indented coastline, home to one of the most sparsely populated countries in Europe with a population of only 4.9 million. With this in mind, telemedicine provides a niche solution and has been eagerly promoted in Norway. As early as in the 1990s, Norway pioneered projects with Teleradiology-services, which had been in great demand when it comes to consultation in the situations of emergencies, seeking for second opinion and information retrieval between hospitals and the primary health care units. Within which, Teleradiology-services are carried out in 2 ways. One is to perform communications from RIS/PACS to RIS/PACS, and the other is to interface Teleradiology-services with the use of IHE and the new services with XDS-profiles (extended data services). By the end of 2005 nearly all the hospitals in Norway had digital x-ray scanners with RIS and PACS installed. Moreover, all the *Regional Health Network* could communicate with the National Health Network (Bergstrøm, 2005).

In 2006, Norway, Trondheim organised the 24th EuroPACS conference. The TIME project team jointed in and delivered a China-EU-workshop, which was a great success with around 100 del-

egates attended. Figure 11 illustrates the Call for Papers.

During the conference, two live operations were demonstrated as displayed in Figure 12 (top-row) taking place at Oslo University, and visit to St. Lovas Hospital by the TIME team (bottom-left). The bottom right reflects the meeting with Norwegian team during the conference.

During the meeting, the TIME and Norwegian teams had an inspiring discussion on the future opportunities to collaborate in the field of telemedicine, which has attributed to the success of the forthcoming FP7 project WIDTH to start in 2011.

Poland

Despite the fast development of telemedicine as a scientific and practical discipline it was still considered a novelty in a global scale. That is because telemedicine in nature is a strictly interdisciplinary field, combining together medicine, computer science, telecommunications, multimedia technology, biomedical engineering, psychology, electronics as well as certain branches of physics (e.g. acoustics and optics)

Figure 11. The 24th EuroPACS webpage with TIME workshop (in red box)

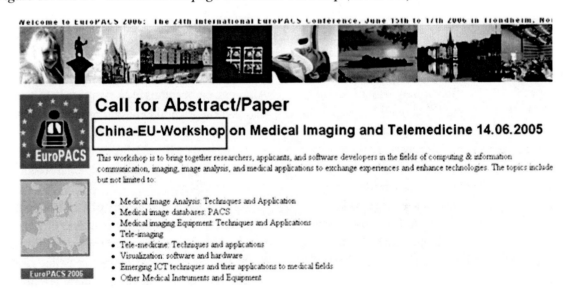

Figure 12. Live operations (top row) shown at EuroPACS 2006 via video conferencing links. Bottom left, visit to St. Lovas Hospital by the TIME team, whereas on the bottom-right meeting between the two teams of the TIME and Norwegian.

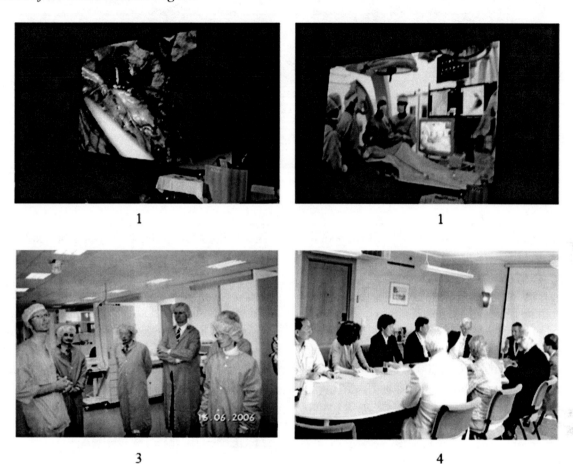

1   1

3   4

and mathematics (data analysis techniques) (Telemedicine, 2005). To this end, in 2005, the Third International Conference on Telemedicine and Multimedia Communications was held in the modern health care centre in Kajetany, near Warsaw in Poland. The conference was held jointly with counterparts in both USA and Germany via their video-consultation rooms, in an effort to showcase the advantages and the huge benefit of tele-communications, such as reducing the cost and time of travelling as demonstrated in Figure 13. On the left, a tele-conferencing session was in place whilst on the right, the delegates who attended the conference.

With focuses on Tele-medicine, PACS and multimedia, the conference gave an opportunity for the TIME project to stay abreast of the current developments in the field. In particular, the project on *Tele-Pathology in the Developing Countries in South East Asia* brought more attention and similarity to the TIME team, the work that was carried out between Germany, Switzerland, and Southeast Asia including Thailand, Vietnam and Cambodia (Stauch, et al., 2005). In Asia, there has been very limited number of experienced doctors and fewer experts. For example, in Cambodia, up to 2000 there were only 6 qualified pathologists who were running a morphological service by providing

*Figure 13. Teleconferencing with USA (**left**) and all the attendees at the conference (**right**)*

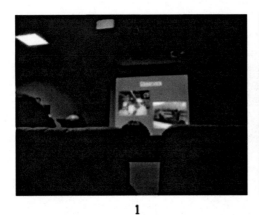

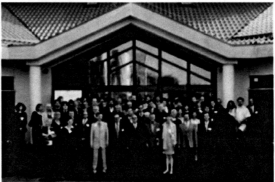

1

2

medical advice and diagnosis to 13 million people. As a result, there was a huge backlog of microscopic samples waiting to be analysed. With the advent of telemedicine, not only distance diagnosis can be achieved but also distance learning and training can be offered to local trainees. Subsequently, the project was initiated in 1996 between Thai and Germany. By 2000, it had established a central service system, DIAGAID and iPath (http://telepath.patho.unibas.ch/ipath/) as an internet-based platform for communication of specimen samples and experts' diagnosis, served by the University of Basel at Switzerland. It was expected that by training local participants, the numbers of specimen sending to the central service, i.e., the server, could be reduced from 100% to 60% for pathological diagnosis. From 2002 to 2003, there were still 100% cases sending to the server located at the University of Basel, whereas 80%, 60% and 50% cases were recorded in the years of 2004, 2005, and 2007, respectively (Chhut, 2008), suggesting the tele-training programmes to the local doctors had made significant impact.

More activities in many other European countries are being carried out. For example, the project, Regional Telemedicine Forum (http://regional-telemedicine.eu/project), started in late 2010. between countries of **Denmark, Estonia, France, Italy, Norway, Poland, Spain, Sweden,** **and United Kingdom** is working on exploring alternative models of telemedicine related policies and in addition, from practical implementation of telemedicine services already provided by other European regions. Another Telemedicine Forum is conducted between Norway and Portugal (http://www.innovasjonnorge.no/portugal) to address the status and opportunities of Telemedicine and Health ICT in both Portugal and Norway, and beyond.

TELEMEDICINE IN CHINA

With its huge population and vast territory China presents a great challenge in supplying modern advanced health care services to all parts of the country. On the other hand, continuing IT&C advances in the delivery of healthcare via telemedicine can help in providing healthcare to remote and under-served populations. In this Section, the development of telemedicine in China is addressed with emphasis on the infrastructures in hospitals, tele-communications, and telemedicine.

Hospital Infrastructure

In many ways, the situation in China is quite different from the other countries. Being the most populated country in the world, China also enjoys

Table 2. Infrastructure data in China as of 2008 in comparison with their counterparts in the UK (Wiki-2, 2011)

	Population (million)	Areas (km²)	People/ area	Hospitals	Beds/per hospital (average)	Doctors	Doctor/1000 people	Hospital with PACS
China	1,330	9,600,000	138	19,246	130	2,000,000	1.4	**6.1%**
UK	60.6	243,820	248	775	250	138,000	2.3	**70%**
ratio	23.10	39.37	**0.55**	24.83	**0.52**	14.49	**0.60**	**0.087**

having the 3rd largest area. Table 2 lists a number of key demographic data in both China and the UK for the purpose of comparison, whereas the classification of hospitals in China is given in Table 3.

By accommodating more than 1.33 billion people, China represents 20% of the world population. In comparison with the UK, the population density in China is only half that of the UK with a ratio of 0.55 between the two countries. However, in terms of bed numbers in hospitals, China has only half as many beds as in the UK with 1.4 doctors per 1000 people, whilst the UK has 2.3 per 1000 people. With only 6.1% hospitals (Grade 3) in China that have been equipped with PACS in comparison with 70% in the UK, China is far behind when it comes to the implementation of modern advanced medical equipment with a ratio of 0.087 between the two countries.

Hospitals in China are categorized into three grades with four levels of each grade consented by the Chinese Ministry of Health who conducted the classification according to the facility, equipment, and staffing that each hospital can offer. The grades as shown in Table 3 include Grades

1, 2, and 3 with the highest grade being 3A+, standing at an international leading position with only two hospitals (i.e., Beijing Union and PLA 301 General Hospital), whereas Grade 3A is expected to be the leaders nationally. In total, as of 2008, there are 19,246 classfied hospitals (including both in-patient and no-bed hospitals) and 2 millions doctors in service in China (Fu, et al., 2006; Grade, 2011). Within these hospitals, there are 2.2 million beds with 149 (1%) hospitals having beds over 800 (Grade 3A/3A+), whilst 1930 hospitals (12%) offer beds between 300- to 800 (Grade 2A/3B).

Within Grade 3 hospitals, radiology departments are in place to be responsible for acquiring medical images from modern medical image scanners, including CT, MR, and/or PET as well as from film digitisers to digitise X-ray films and many other forms of pictures/images.

Figure 14 illustrates the official statistical data on the number of hospital beds and doctors distributed in both urban and rural regions from 1952 to 2000 in China (China Statistical Yearbook, 2003).

It can be seen from Figure 14 that there is a big gap between rural (green patterns) and urban

Table 3. The number of in-patient hospitals in China classified by the ministry of health (Grade, 2011)

Level	3					2				1			
		3A+	3A	3B	3C		2A	2B	2C		1A	1B	1C
Number of hospitals	1192					6780				4989			
			2										
			772										

Figure 14. The number of hospital beds and doctors (in 10,000) in cities and countries in China between 1952 and 2002 (http://www.china-profile.com/data/fig_health_1.htm) (China Statistical Yearbook, 2003)

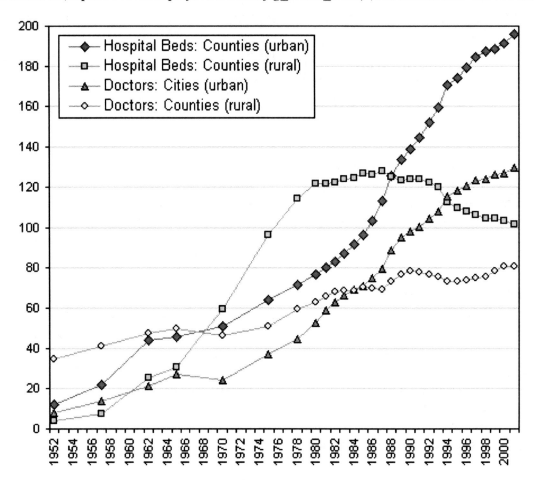

(in red) regions. In terms of the number of beds, the numbers in the rural areas, in particular from the 1980s, have decreased, whereas in the cities, the number has doubled since the 1980s. On the other hand, the gap between the numbers of doctors are increasing with more and more doctors are in place at city hospitals. At the mean time, the number of medical doctors and physicians in the counties stagnated or even declined since 1988.

The Diffusion of PACS in China

When the EuroPACS conference series started in 1984, China had just begun its initial stage of economy reform. In 2006, two decades later, the first Symposium of China-PACS-RIS was held in Beijing, reflecting the latest development of PACS in China. Although a number of advanced imaging scanners are brought in after the economic reform in several high grade hospitals (3A+/3A), such as CT, MR and PET, the majority of hospitals mainly house the following scanners due to their lower cost:

- X-ray
- US – ultrasonic scanner
- DR – document scanner
- DSA – Digital Subtraction Angiography
- DF– digital Film scanner
- CR – Computer Radiography scanner

- VE – Virtual Endoscopy
- VR – Volume Rendering
- VA – Virtual Analysis

Technically, two types of PACS are in service, named whole hospital PACS (usually called PACS) and miniPACS respectively. While whole hospital PACS provides a system of image management over one or multiple networks, miniPACS offers an off-line archiving service with a facility of external online archiving on-demand. In this way, miniPACS is available at limited cost in comparison with whole-PACS. As a result, In China, the implementation of PACS started with miniPACS. In 1994, the first system of miniPACS was installed at Beijing Union Medical College Hospital (Fu, et al., 1995) based on a UNIX platform. The features included an image reviewing workstation, an image archiving server and a soft reporting workstation, whereas a long-term archiving device in the *module file format* (MOD) was developed in-house. In 1996 (Fu, et al., 2006), the first DI-COM 3.0 compatible miniPACS was purchased from Siemens at Sichuan Province. At the same year, research projects on the topic started to take interests within China with the establishment of many domestic companies. However, in the two years that followed, i.e., from 1997 to 1998, the development on PACS went less progressive. The main barrier at the time was that PACS could only function well on UNIX systems that were then considerably expensive in China, due to the face that only UNIX systems could deliver high enough processing speed at the time to display images smoothly, whereas the then PCs with Win95/Intel Pentium architecture could only compete with lower specifications. On the other hand, at the time DICOM was only available for UNIX and offered fewer image modalities. To further exacerbate the situation, Asia was mired in a financial crisis during that time, triggering less spending. Most importantly, China was lagging behind at the development of technologies. The complete concept of digital imaging, storage and communicate had just started to be appreciated within hospital sectors. In the following two years, i.e., from 1999 to 2001, miniPACS took China by storm with many hospitals directly ordering the systems from abroad, giving rising to the second tide of implementation of miniPACS in China. Table 4 gives a list of majority hospitals that implemented the solutions of miniPACS in China from 1999-2001 together with a few between 2003 and 2005.

A typical miniPACS offers the services of *Soft Reporting*, *Image Reviewing*, *Image Archiving*, and *Jukebox/Tape Library* (Based on CD-R, DVD-ROM, MOD, or DLT), the four features however that somehow appeared not functioning completely. This is due to the following factors:

- Lack of local research and development team to maintain the system in relation to localization, integration, and service to ensure that miniPACS can be properly configured.
- Differences in the workflow and management between the radiology department in China and overseas, and also differences among the hospitals in China resulting in the less efficient use of PACS, i.e., a PACS that works perfectly in one hospital may not work well in another.
- High performance coming from high cost. Because of the relatively low cost of miniPACS in comparison with whole PACS, limited performance should be expected.
- Scarce experiences in using UNIX platform applications in hospitals, arriving at a less performed PACS with little communications with the other parts of hospital systems (such as HIS, RIS) since most people were accustomed to Personal Computers (PCs) running Windows systems.

After three years' effort, the miniPACS supplied by ROGAN could be run successfully on the

Table 4. MiniPACS solutions in China from 1999 to 2005

Hospital	Year of Installation	Beds	Supplier
Beijing Tumour Hospital, Beijing	February 1999	300	SIEMENS
The first Affiliated Hospital of Medical College of Zhejiang University Zhejiang Province	March 1999	1100	AGFA
Beijing Red Cross Chaoyang Affiliated Hospital of Capital University of Medical Sciences, Beijing	March 1999	900	GE Hangwei Medical System
Shanghai First People's Hospital, Shanghai	October 1999	1000	ROGAN
Beijing Xuanwu Hospital Capital University of Medical Sciences, Beijing	August 2000	900	SIEMENS
The First Affiliated Hospital of China Medical University, Liaoning Province	September 2000	1000	NEUSOFT
Beijing General Navy Hospital Beijing	October 2000	800	SMIT
Zhejiang Taizhou Central Hospital Zhejiang Province	October 2000	400	SIEMENS
Yunnan Provincial Hospital, Yunnan Province	December 2000	1000	SIEMENS
Shanghai Ruijin Hospital, Shanghai	June 2001	1500	EBM
The Affiliated Hospital of Guiyang Medical College Guizhou Province	October 2001	800	GE
The first affiliated hospital, Kunming Medical University, Yunnan Province	2003	1500	
Wuhan Asia Heart Hospital, Hunan Province	2005	500	KONICA

platform Intel/Windows at Shanghai First People's Hospital (Tao, Miao, 2002), while integrating with the Chinese RIS, showcasing the performance and impact of the whole hospital PACS. Although a miniPACS starts with a relatively lower price, more components have to be purchased when it comes to integration with the other systems in the hospital, such as RIS or HIS. In many cases, a brand new whole hospital PACS had to be brought in order to fill the gap of missing components from a particular vendor. As a direct result, starting from 2001, many hospitals in China tended to invest in whole hospital PACS solutions and sometimes together with RIS, which can be seen from the list in Table 5.

In each hospital at China, HIS was established first before RIS. So when PACS was installed, the issue of compatibility between the three systems becomes dominant as it sometimes does not go down well with the other two. To ensure that they interface with each other, hospitals have to make choices as to which product from which provider should be purchased. Different companies have different views on the relationship between PACS and RIS. Some think they are independent, whereas the others consider them as one, depending on the functionalities each system can offer. For a PACS, it mainly manages image data flow, scanner connections, image storage, compression, retrieval, quering, all boilinig down to the point of

Table 5. List of hospitals with full PACS solution in China from 2001 to 2005

Hospital	Year of Installation	Systems Installed	Beds	Supplier
Beijing Tiantan Hospital Beijing	2001	PACS	960	NEUSOFT
Shanghai Ruijin Hospital Shanghai	2001	PACS	1500	EBM
Fuzhou Dongfang Hospital (Fujian Province)	2001	PACS	1200	TIANJIAN
The Affiliated Hospital of Qingdao Medical College (Shandong Province)	2002	PACS	900	GE
Beijing Xuan Wu Hospital Capital University of Medical Sciences Beijing	2002	PACS	900	GE
Beijing Tumour Hospital Beijing	2002	PACS	300	HUAHAI
Chong Qing South-west Hospital, Sichuan Province	2002	PACS	1000	TIANJIAN
Taiwan New Building Hospital, Taiwan	2002	PACS/HIS	2000	
Cancer Institute and Hospital, Chinese Academy of Sciences Beijing	2005	PACS/RIS	1198	
Nanjing Medical University, First Affiliated Hospital Jiangsu Province	2005	PACS/RIS	2200	SONY
Beijing General Army Hospital, Beijing	2002-2005	PACS/RIS/HIS	4000	GE
The first Affiliated Hospital of China Medicine University, Liaoning Province	2005	PACS	1300	IBM
The third affiliated hospital, Zhongshan University, Guangdong Province	2003	PACS/RIS	1000	GE
Zhunyi Medical College, Guizhou Province	2003	PACS/RIS	1500	SIEMENS

images and focusing on techniques with emphasis on secrurity and sustainbility. As for RIS, it takes care of work flow or clinical flow and centres at patients, i.e., RIS is for comunication and compromising, reflecting on flexibility and agility. In a way, it can be said that RIS is part of HIS. So it is very reasonable to consider that PACS and RIS are separate, giving rising to the importance of which brand of systems should be employed.

On the other hand, in term of communications, PACS and RIS share one local network, residing in the radiology departments and being seperated from HIS that utilises a global network, in a bid to ensure that the data flow goes smoothly. The interface between the local and global networks can be bridged using the internet service i.e., the Internet Explorer (IE). In this way, the huge flow of image volumns within radiology departments will not affect the whole hospital data flow running using HIS with reasonably wide bandwidth. Thus, the e-patient record can be formed through IE by obtaining both an image-based report and a textual report.

The Infrastructure of Tele-Communication in China

Telemedicine stems from technologies of communications and computer information, within which the clinical care is delivered via a line-telephone, wireless mobile phone, video-conferencing equipment, or internet between medical specialists (and patients) in two or more different locations (e.g., countries) for the purpose of conducting consulting, remote medical procedures or examinations. Hence to provide any kind of tele-service, a tele-communication facility has to be in place first.

Lined Network

The people in China live geographically in 22 provinces, five autonomous regions and four metropolitan municipalities. Such a vast population and territory sets a correspondingly vast challenge to keep people in touch with each other. Starting from the late 1990s, China has established more than 2 million kilometres (Wiki-3, 2011) nationwide optical cable network, built on Asynchronous Transfer Mode (ATM), in which data are encoded into small, fixed-sized cells, Synchronous Digital Hierarchy (SDH) and Dense Wavelength Division Multiplexing (DWDM) technologies, laying a lasting foundation for tele-communications through lined telephones. In addition, several submarine cables (i.e., the cables that are laid beneath the sea), have been installed. As of 2008, there are around 362 million land-line users (of both private and business) in China, equivalent to 81% households/business suites on the assumption that an average household accommodating 3 people.

In terms of networks that are employed for the purpose of telemedicine, three major routes (Wang, Gu, 2009) have been connected, including the Golden Health Network (GHN), the International MedioNet of China (IMNC) network, and the Peoples' Liberation Army (PLA) telemedicine network. Since the implementation in 1997, IMNC has been widely applied to telecommunications between medical specialists within around 300 hospitals (1.5% of all hospitals) that have registered on this line cross China. As the network is primarily a telephone line employing a low bandwidth, the major activities between these hospitals have been limited to communications with textual data, being analogous to an internal telephone line.

On the other hand, merely providing cables is not sufficient. With the advent of internet service, large numbers of video image data are called for in addition to audio signals. Faster transmission is therefore in demand, not only for just viewing still pictures but also for visualising moving videos together with accompanying sound simultaneously. Technically, this requirement has led to the establishment of a set of communications standards, i.e., Integrated Services Digital Network (ISDN) (Wiki-4, 2011) in 1988. The key feature of ISDN is that it integrates speech and data on the same lines, adding features that were not available in the classic telephone system. ISDN is a circuit-switched telephone network system and can typically provide up to 128 kbit/s. In the event of transmission speed, when the same telephone line is converted to a non-loaded twisted-pair wire (i.e., without filtering out any bandwidth by increasing the inductance by the inserting of a loading coil), it becomes hundreds of kilohertz wide (i.e., broadband) and can carry several megabits per second, coined the name *broadband* since 1996.

Teleconferencing Systems

In order to make the presence of telemedicine felt, many hospitals in China, such as Peking Union Medical College Hospital, have acquired video-based teleconferencing systems in an attempt to deliver telemedical services. Because of the high cost of proprietary video conferencing systems, the hospitals that can afford to install them in China are more likely to be the last ones that are in need of advice due to their own rich supply of expertise and resources. Furthermore, although China has a small number of telemedicine systems in many of these leading hospitals, they hardly communicate with each other because of different standards of hardware and software that are employed in China, yielding these systems are essentially stand-alone.

To access rural and regional medical centres, connections have to draw from the existing resources that are in considerably less quantity for many hospitals in the rural regions.

Wireless Network

Because of the wealth that China has grown since the 1980s, China has tapped into a fashion-conscious market, with specially interest in those high-tech gadgets. As a result, mobile phones are a must-have accessory among young generations. Unprecedentedly, China has around 833 million (62%) mobile phone users (Wiki-3, 2011), thanks to the satellite network systems. The primary service of a mobile phone at present is to transfer voice data although other services have been deployed gradually, including email reading, web accessing, and messaging, admittedly at a higher cost since internet surfing involves downloading a number of pictures, taking longer to complete, in comparison with landline services. However, with such large army of mobile users, personal health system can be exploited in the future, offering services based on the wireless network.

Internet Network

By 2010, China has 420 million internet users (31.6% of its population) (China Daily, 2010) with 277 million accessing web pages via cell phones. Since broadband is the most popular way to access the internet with a wired connection, with 98.1% of wired Internet users choosing broadband, a total of 364 million people are now online in China, leading China being the second largest market of internet users after USA (Zhu, Wang, 2005) with

major activities covering online chat, gaming, and internet surfing. Because of the very low cost of internet via land lines, web-based practices of telemedicine is much feasible in China, especially when many online meeting applications, such as Skype, are at the moment free available. In comparison, Europe has 475 million internet users, amounting to 58.4% of its population.

Telemedicine Infrastructure

To a certain extent, the first generation of telemedicine in China (Zhao, et al., 1998; Chen, Xia, 2009) started from a famous event. In 1995, a case of text-based consultation via emails had been reported, when the email was sent from Beijing to the U.S. and later the whole world, concerning a patient with heavy metal poisoning, by which a prescription of medicine was recommended and obtained that eventually cured the patient. Considering the high cost to setup a teleconferencing suite, internet based applications flourished in China in the late 1990s. It took off in 1998 when a much publicised activity of tele-consultation based on Internet took place (http://michaelfuchs.org/china/, http://telemed.stanford.edu/), whereby doctors from both China at Xi'an Medical University Hospital and the USA, Stanford University Health Care, conducted a conferring and reviewing session discussing the cases of two critically ill children, by the application of audio, video, and whiteboard, the emerging facilities at the time. Although feasible, much of the event was to prove the viability of webcast architecture, leading to a number of subsequent applications all with the same intention of showcasing. The similar view is shared by Hsieh et al (Hsieh, et al., 2001). In addition, much of the effort still focused on tele-consultation and tele-education as detailed in (Zhao, et al., 2010; Wang, Gu, 2009).

The real turning point of telemedicine came in 2005 when a series of operations via tele-manipulation/tele-neurosurgery were concerted to removal brain tumours using image-guided key-hole surgery technique (Tian, et al., 2008). The operation distance is 1300 kilometres away in Yan'an, a mountainous region, whereas the tele-manipulation was conducted from Beijing, with a home-made frameless stereotactic surgical robotic system CAS-BH5. The transmission of neuro-navigation data, planning, monitoring and manipulating was carried out through a digital network with a speed of 2 MByte/s on the platform of Internet. In total, 10 patients were operated on that year with 90% of patients improved neurologically with no complications, the conclusions being drawing from a 12-month post-operation check. When compared with local operations where a 93.3% improvement is achieved (Tian, et al., 2008a) based on the results of over 1000 cases, the accuracy of tele-surgery is very much similar to the conventional operation although not conclusive. The details of this activity will be adressed in the Section of *Tele-neurosurgery in China* given below.

TELE-NEUROSURGERY IN CHINA

With the advances of information and imaging technology, application of robotic systems to the health sector is a burgeoning field in assisting surgeons manipulating, monitoring, and/or guiding operations, with the advantages of being higher precision of targeting, persistence of longer duration, and having the ability of pre-operation planning drawing from patients' images. As of 2001, there are around 270,000 cases of image-guided robotic operations conducted every year worldwide (MedMarket Diligence, 2002).

Unlike keyhole approaches applied on many other organs (e.g. in the abdomen as shown in Figure 12 [top-left]), where a micro-camera can be inserted inside to provide an augmented view, for a brain that is a compact organ and extremely of high value, there is simply no 'room' to accommodate any extra instruments as every tissue in a brain plays an important role to ascertain

a person's normal life. Minimal invasion and sacrifice of healthy tissues are hence the prerequisite for a brain intervention. Therefore, only recently, the first case of robotic image-guided neuro-surgery took place in the USA in 1985 (Kwoh, et al., 1988) for the procedure of biopsy using robotic stereotactic technique, i.e., to probe the tumour with a tip through a small burr hole (~3 mm) drilled on the skull. In order to 'see' inside a brain while performing keyhole surgery, surgeons relied on a CT scanner that performs scanning in real time while the robotic system was mounted on the gantry of the CT. Although this system was applied only for biopsy at the time, it implied potentials of applications to the other procedures. Also, because it is a robotic system, i.e., controlled by a computer, it is well suitable for being operated 'remotely,' leading to a tele-robotic system when coupled with the advances of computer communications techniques.

Frame and Frameless Stereotactic

Before modern imaging tomographiers were invented, many approaches had been developed in order to locate the exact position inside a brain. Among them, stereotaxis was the most popular one and was conceived by Horsley and Clark (Horsley, Clarke, 1908). The method employs an external three-dimensional frame as a reference to locate a position in the brain and was applied to animals as early as in the 20th century (Kandel, 1972). The frame is a mechanical apparatus attached to an animal's head and incorporates a Cartesian coordinate system. In this way, the movement of a probe to be inserted into the brain can be monitored.

Wearing a frame is cumbersome in both a scanning suite for acquiring images and in an operation room during surgery, hence frameless stereotaxis has gradually replaced the frames. By which, landmarks, i.e., fiducial marks, on a skull have to be defined in advance to assist geometric registrations. Significantly, with the

Figure 15. The comparison between frame (left column) and frameless with markers (right column) robotic systems. © Courtsey of Prof. Zengmin Tian, NGH, China.

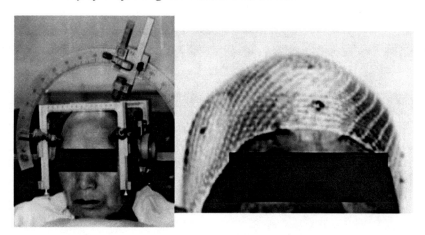

benefit of advances of computer hardware and software, frameless stereotactic can achieve the same precision as that with a frame. China began this kind of procedure in the late 1990s. Figure 15 illustrates the approach using both frame (left) and frameless (right) stereotactic neurosurgery. In total, between 1998 and 2005, about 4,000 operations with frame and 1,500 with frameless stereotactic have been performed at the Navy General Hospital (NGH) (Yu, et al., 2000; Gao, et al., 2009) at Beijing China, led by Professor Zengmin Tian, vice president of NGH.

Due to its high success rate of near 100%, Prof Tian's work on frameless stereotactic operation has elicited considerable interest in China in the non-medical press. The television programme *Approaches to Science* explained the procedure as illustrated in Figure 16. In the figure, it shows (a) the logo of the TV programme; (b) a team led by Prof. Tian (second from right) studying the MR images from a patient; (c) the planed route to target the tumour; and (d) computer graphics illustrating the registration between images and the patient's brain.

Robots

With the help of a frame or frameless stereotactic system, minimally invasive techniques can be performed on tumour removal or biopsy from a brain by locating a precise position on a skull (and thence the target in the brain). The procedure normally involves the drill of a burr hole (1-10 mm), which usually is done manually. During an operation, surgical dexterity can be limited to a certain extent by surgeons' physiological tremor. Therefore, robotic hands or robots have been introduced into operation theatres in the late 1980s (Kwoh, et al., 1988; Kelly, 2000), which could replace stereotactic frame and accomplish precise position location, and precision bone drilling.

In China, the building of robotic system for neuro-surgery began a decade later and mainly confined to tumour resection in order to achieve minimally invasive operations. Thanks to the expensive cost of buying a commercial Robot, such as RoboDoc, China began building its own. From 1997 to 2007, in collaborating with Beijing University of Aeronautics and Astronautics, Navy General Hospital developed their own robotic systems from CAS-R-1 (Computer Assistant Surgery-Robot, Type 1), and CAS-R-2 to CAS-BH5 as depicted in Figure 17. The robotic system employs a six-jointed server-controlled (or called a Programmable Logic Controller [PLC]) and motorised robotic arm (Figure 17[a]) and a software system responsible for location calcula-

Figure 16. China TV programme explaining the frameless operations performed in Navy General Hospitals in China. (a) the logo of the TV programme; (b) a team led by Prof. Tian (second from right) studying the MR images from a patient; (c) the planed route to target the tumour when the probe (top yellow line) moving closer to the planned route (yellow line inside the brain image); and (d) a computer graphics showing the registration between images and the patient's brain. © Courtsey of Prof. Tian from NGH, China.

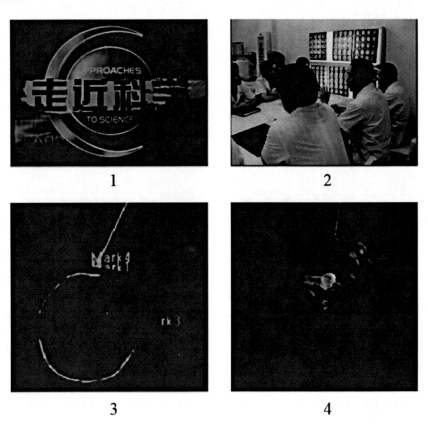

tion, markers recognition, surgical planning, and intra-operative navigation.

In operation, the system allows for identification of the intended target defined by CT or MR images, delineating boundaries, planning optimised route, opening burr holes, and incising tumours.

The first operation took place in 1997 (Tian, et al., 1998) by CAS-R-2 for assisting tumour removal. In the following 10 years of its service, over 2000 cases of operations have been carried out with total effect rate of 93.3% (Tian, et al., 2008a). Formal consents were complied prior to any operation in those cases.

Tele-Neurosurgery

In general, the advent of robotics in an operation room provides the ability to position the probe-directing system rapidly, to compute the necessary trajectory and target coordinates in an error-free manner, and to remove tumour more completely. On top of these benefits, it also offers the possibility of being controlled remotely, i.e., to conduct tele-neurosurgery.

Subsequently, in 2005, the CAS-R-2 robotic system was modified into CAS-R-BH5 (Figure 17[b]) that was employed in performing the first series of tele-neurosurgery in China, exclusively

Figure 17. The development of a home-made robotic system for neurosurgery in China (a) CAS-R-2 for local operation and (b) CAS-BH5 for tele-surgery; (c) drilling the hole by the robotic arm supervised by Prof. Tian; and (d) probe introduction using robotic hand. © Courtsey of Prof. Tian.

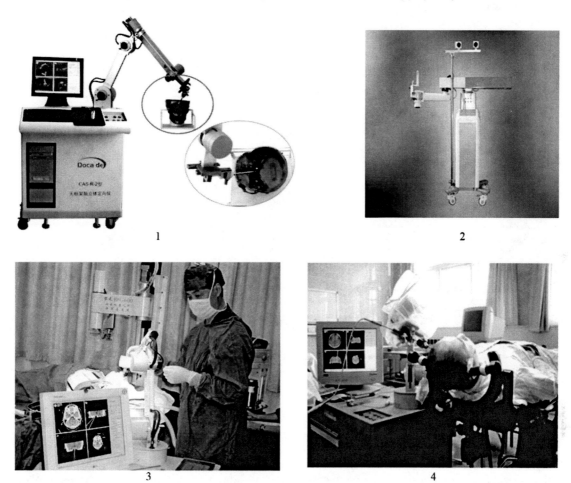

for removal of tumours and taking place between Beijing and Yan'an as shown on the map in Figure 18. The distance is 1300 km between Beijing where Navy General Hospital resides and Yan'an, a mountainous city.

CAS-R-BH5 has five degrees of freedom (i.e., 6 joints) and weighs about 40kg with dimensions of $280 \times 800 \times 1100$ mm^3. The system runs three modules that are responsible for conducting surgical planning, target directing and tele-manipulation operations. The system of surgical planning (Module 1) provides surgeons with expedient tools to store, retrieve and analyse relevant data,

to study collectively the case history, to visualise resonstructed 3D images in order to define the boundary of a target for more complete removal, and to locate centrally the brain tumours by the safest and least invasive route possible. The module for target directing (Module 2) is concerned with the robotic arm in arriving at the precise position of the skull in order to perform the openning and in pointing to the direction of the route defined by module 1. Via a rapid and accurate measurement and calcualtion, the length of the probe (or catheter) is determinted in order to minimisie the trauma to normal tussues. The

Figure 18. The map showing the distance (arrow) between Beijing (*), the control centre guiding the operation, and Yan'an (the red box) where the operation took place. © Courtsey of Prof. Tian.

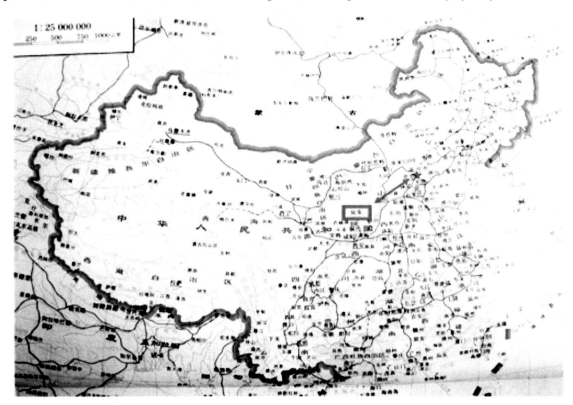

module 3 focuses on telemanimulation systems, which spans from network communication, video transmission, graphics simulation, to human-machine interaction, providing technical supports for surgeons who are performing the tele-operation procedures. The system comprises two terminals, one being the master to conduct the remote controlling locating at Beijing and another, the operation terminal, i.e., the slave one, residing at the same room as the patient, to be employed to carry out the resection of physical tumour. Figure 19 schematically illustrates the relationship between the two (Tian, et al., 2008).

The platform of telecommunication is the Internet with the speed of transmission being 2 Mbytes/s. Although it is lower than the current standard of broadband with a typical speed of 20 Mbyte/s, the transmission was good enough to allow real-time online visualization and com-munications. The following procedures are then required to complete a tele-surgery successfully.

- Slave to master – Firstly the patient's data (e.g., MR/CT scan, history record and the live view of patient in the operation room) from slave computer were transmitted to the master computer;
- Master to slave – The experts sent back the surgical plan and confirmations of surgical procedures, including the precise movement the robot arm should comply in order to arrive at the exact location pre-defined from Module 1 on the skull of the patent.
- Slave to master – the registration data between robotic arm and the fiducial markers on the patient's skull to ensure the error was below the pre-defined threshold. Otherwise, the following step repeated.

Figure 19. The structure of tele-manipulation system. Experts at the remote control terminal (left) get on-line real-time view of the surgical scene via the camera (right) that provides a panoramic view and remote control the robot at the operation room (Tian, et al., 2008).

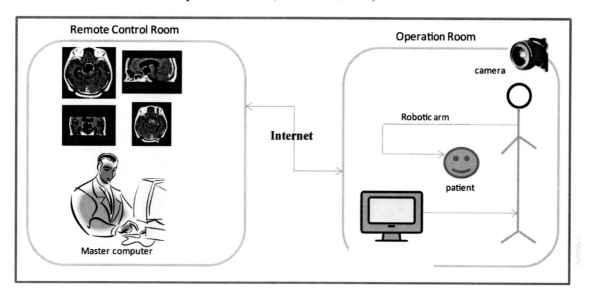

- Master to slave – A series commands that the arm should following in the light of six joints instructed from master to slave then to the robot, e.g., forward/backward, left/right, up/down, side tilting, anterior/posterior tilting of the supporting device itself, and forward/backward of the probe (Tian, et al., 2008).

The speed of the movement of robotic arm was at 8 mm/s. Figure 20 demonstrates the whole process of the tele-operation, where (a) shows the master computer where surgical planning is drawn on; (b) the computer screen showing the activities in the remote operation room; (c) tele-mentoring and tele-manipulation; and (d) activities in the operation room.

The clincal outcome is then graded based on the Glasgow Outcome Scale (GOS, http://www.nervous-system-diseases.com/glasgow-outcome-scale.html), the measurement of a 5-point score given to victims of traumatic brain injury at some point in their recovery as shown in Table 6.

GOS is a very general assessment of the general functioning of a person who has suffered a head injury. Based on the data of 10 patients who were operated on using tele-neurosurgery procedure in 2005, four patients recovered nearly completely with 5 points on the GOS scale, whereas three with 4 GOS scores. Two patients are with GOS score of 3 and one with 2. These results are obtained from the follow-ups for each patient that took place between 3 to 14 months after surgery, with the average of 12 months.

Between 2005 and 2006, thirty-two patients underwent surgery of tumour removal at Yan'an with the technique of tele-surgery and were all successfully recovered without any complication with the average GOS point of 4. The mean accuracy of remote fiducial registration is within the range of 1.50 mm, whilst the standard deviation is 0.32 mm between the planned and actual target (Tian, et al., 2008a).

LESSONS LEARNED

China is still in the developing stage and in the process of reform of its health care systems. Due

Figure 20. Remote control of operations. (a) The master computer where surgical planning takes place; (b) The computer screen showing the activities in the remote operation room; (c) tele-mentoring and tele-manipulation; and (d) activities in the operation room. © Courtsey of Prof. Tian.

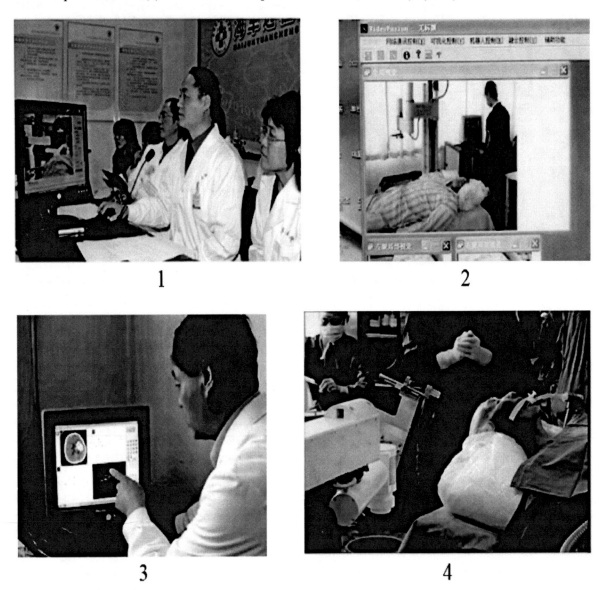

Table 6. GOS scale of 5 points

GOS point	Description
1	Dead
2	Vegetative State (meaning the patient is unresponsive, but alive; a "vegetable" in lay language)
3	Severely Disabled (conscious but the patient requires others for daily support due to disability)
4	Moderately Disabled (the patient is independent but disabled)
5	Good Recovery (the patient has resumed most normal activities but may have minor residual problems)

to its unique situation, i.e., large populations distributed in a vast area, China should opt for the solutions that fit her best. During the analysis of recent studies, the following recommendations should be considered in the future.

In light of the installation of PACS in China, the following suggestions are made:

a. **Strategic plan with incremental realisation**: The assurance for PACS to live up to its full potentials is to update PACS incrementally when needed. For example, if a hospital only has CT scanners at the time, PACS should mainly work for CT and can be updated when the other imaging modalities arrive, e.g., MR, or PET, leading to a lower cost, lower mantainence, and less training time. Many hospitals in China install a miniPACS in the first instance, and later find out that the existing PACS is lacking in capability of expansion when they need to grow. Consquently, they face a dilemma as to whether to re-purchase a whole PACS at an expensive cost that they might not be able to offord or to buy another mini-PACS at a lower cost as a tempoary solution that however might not be compatible with the exisiting one, causing information seperation.

b. **Substainable software providers are the key to success of implementation of PACS:** Because of the modular structure of PACS, system surpliers should be able to provide updated modulars when they are available as well as substainable maitainence, especially when the curcumstances of a hospital change, i.e., extension or updating computer operation systems. Therefore, frenquent communication between the technical support team from the software provider and the hospital is improtant.

c. **Good management of PACS**: Since a PACS as well as RIS stores valuable medical images, carrying key information related to both patients and hospitals. Its safty is paramount.

On the other hand, the seamlessly clinical flow together with PACS information flow can improve a patient's clincal outcome significantly. Therefore, a team of techical personnel should be in place to make sure PACS is functioning effectively and efficiently.

d. **Connnections**: Some PACS systems have interfaces with DICOM and some not, especially when a specific scanner has its own image format. Another connection issue should be considered is the link with RIS, to which a number of miniPACS systems have encountered difficulties.

e. **Integration**: Integration is still behind the high-end requirements. Although there are several applications that have been extended to the clinical department, from a strict definition point of view, the whole hospital integration of PACS has not been in place in China yet per se. In terms of techniques, the necessary hardware components and the technology for system integration with a successful PACS installation are now readily available in China. However, in the event of integration, software development in order to interface with each other is still far behind the requirements of hospital customers. For example, it is not sufficient for PACS software to act alone to store, communicate, and display images, acting like a warehouse. A PACS should work together with RIS/HIS by offering efficient support to radiologists and physicians in many aspects, including routine conferencing, consultation, interpreting, communication of image findings through hospital information networks and doctors' workstations, workflow management, integration with RIS/HIS, and computer-assisted diagnosis. The advantages of digitalization and integration of PACS, HIS and RIS will be, apart from reduction of film cost and space, the optimised workflow with the access to digital images from everywhere at any time seamlessly for the benefit of patients.

f. **Updating with the newly evolving technologies**: In principle, a PACS can be updated whenever it is necessary thanks to its modular nature. In practice however, it is far from ideal. In China, a PACS has been constrained in unpredictable ways by contingencies that arise in the field, e.g., a new arrival of an emerging technology. For instance, the current installed systems have difficulties to cope with large amount of slices produced by modern Multi-Detector-CT and 3.0T MR studies. Multi-slice CT and 3.0T MRI scanners generate large quantities of image data flow with a typical dataset up to thousands of 2D slices, far beyond the capacity of the system that a PACS is installed can offer. The alternative would be to print them all on films with more than 10 sheets (even 50 sheets) per dataset in order to analyse/visualise. In addition, a dedicated image processing system is also in demand that can not only store these up to thousands of images for per dataset, but also can manipulate and deliver them to multiple remote clients, without putting too much strain on the host processor of server itself. Therefore a serve with a powerful processing speed for images of 2D/3D/4D should be in place on which to install PACS, with the hope that it will be able to face the challenges coming from the evolving new technology.

g. **Standard architecture**: The most important issue for the Chinese Ministry of Health is to establish the State Drug and Device Admittance System (SDA approval) (Fu, et al., 2006). Two types of certification systems can be adapted for independent modality and integrated system respectively, i.e., modality licence (Type 1) and system licence (Type 2). Furthermore, adoption to the current international standards should take place as soon as possible, especially in the field of information system standard (DICOM, HL7, HIPAA, IHE, etc.) for the sake of application, certification, security, management, and integration, as well as in the area of standard for the *State Medical Insurance Information Exchange*.

h. **Quality control/assurance**: In China, the procedure of routinely quality control and assurance is very relaxed as a PACS does not provide a check to the quality of a monitor for image viewer. As a result, the verification of acquired images is normally neglected. On the other hand, because of the high cost of a high-resolution monitor for viewing medical images, the soft reporting of CR/DR images is conducted on the normal colour monitor. Although this is strongly discouraged in hospitals, it is the reality in China since there is not any coherent rule for digital diagnosis, partly due to the newness of the emerging imaging scanners in China.

i. **Conformation with HL7 and IHE**: Conformation with HL7 and IHE is another issue on the agenda towards the establishment of the future digital hospital. Although it has a long way to go, especially in the case of China, it should be taken into consideration as early as possible not only to avoid huge capital investment in the future but also to be able to contribute to the process of clinical decision making.

j. **Showcases in need**: In China, as of 2002, only two hospitals have implemented whole-scale PACS while the others are still in the process of deploying miniPACS. Within these two hospitals, i.e., Shanghai Ruijin Hospital and Beijing Tiantan Hospital, those large-scale PACS systems have been slowly defused and integrated. It is therefore essential that more model hospitals should be established to showcase the deployment of PACS, pointing to a cost-effective solution to be exploited in the other hospitals in the future.

During the Execution of the TIME Project, Attention was drawn to the Problem of Language Barrier

a. Increasing specialisation within disciplines is one of the difficulties when interfacing with other fields, especially when it comes to the translation between two languages. This was exactly what happened in some sessions at the MIT2005 conference. Some Chinese speakers could not explain their work in details in English to the audience (e.g. in the area of insulin), whereas the people who knew both English and Chinese well did not have sufficient medical background to translate this information precisely. With this in mind, in the 2nd conference organised by the TIME project, MIMI2007, simultaneous translation was in place to overcome this barrier. Although this simultaneous-translation only facilitated key-note speakers in the preliminary session, precaution was taken to select chair persons in each Session to ensure that every session was equipped with the necessary expertise in both English and Chinese, leading to the success of the MIMI2007 conference.

b. The language barrier has always been an issue in any collaborative work involving Chinese (or any Asian country) and Europeans. Although many leading Chinese scientists have been studying/visiting in an English-speaking country for a certain period, there still exist a number of communication problems.

c. The TIME project was aimed at ordinary Chinese people, reflecting at the selection of the first conference of MIT2005 being held in a remote area in China. Every delegate enjoyed the conference and its beautiful scenery. However, some facilities were not up to the standard in those remote areas in China. For example, although the conference venue was located at a 4* hotel, the hotel neither accepted credit cards nor other means of payment apart from cash. Surprisingly, there was not a single person in the hotel who could speak English.

China Telemedicine

a. Due to the disparity of economic development in both Europe and China, China has to develop telemedicine systems that fit its purpose instead of simply copying the systems that work well in the other countries. For instance, at the UK, the success of NHS Direct owes much to the fact that everyone in the UK (and many other developed countries) is connected with 100% of households having land line telephones and 122% people have mobiles (many users have more than one handset), which proffers advices to anyone who has any doubt on their health. Whereas in China, because of the huge number of the population, large number of knowledgeable nurses has to be required to provide the service, which is highly unlikely. In addition, many peasants who live remotely do not have any means of communications (more than 30% households without land lined phones) nor electricity. Centralised local or regional medical centres are therefore a way forward and can facilitate telemedicine services.

b. In the light of digital divide between rural areas and big cities, it is very unlikely in the short period for China to go to paper-less (digital) hospital. Region-based medical centres or hospitals are still in demand to provide basic health care and advice to the local people.

c. The nature of relatively independence of hospitals in China has made hospitals as competitors as well as collaborators, hampering the development of telemedicine. This because each hospital is relatively finance independent. A typical example appears to be in the purchase of PACS. On the one hand, the main purpose of PACS is to allow communications between each other. Whereas on the other, some hospitals install PACS with the intention to prevent the data flow going to the other sites, albeit for the benefit of security. Therefore a centralised management system with top-down architecture should be promoted to share and communicate.

d. Since over 60% population own a mobile phone, wireless applications could be considered in providing a reliable, day-to-day modern medical service to any location and in any environment. This approach should be treated as a strategic means of meeting the priority of providing medical care to everyone. Further more, any new gadget can appeal to huge number of followers in China, the trend could be exploited towards the application of telemedicine.

e. Similar to the other developing countries (Androuchko, 2010), Chinese Government is promoting eHealth vigorously, which can be evidenced by the way of implementation of communications networks. However, due to each medical staff's busy schedule, extra training of ICT and eHealth is not on the agenda yet, leaving telemedicine is practiced mainly on individual basis.

f. On the other hand, since most of medical insurance only covers 80% of medical cost, even for many medical staff, each individual has to cover the remaining cost, which results in a degree of competation between hospitals and in a way might hamper the development of eHealth systems. Top-down policy is in need to ensure the collaboration and co-existing, especially between unban and rural hospitals..

FUTURE TRENDS

In the developing countries it is certain that telemedicine is a way forward to allow health care services being accessed evenly by the people. To this end, collaboration with the developed countries is one of the future trends to acquire expertise, knowledge, and experience with less cost and in a short time period.

IHE is a useful system framework that has the capability to solve the interactive problem in the integration of healthcare systems. The sophisticated HIS/PACS/RIS/LIS workflow and environment supported by various vendors employ different interfaces that should interact. For instance, HL7 would be the choice to provide a common framework for interfacing and exchanging data (not only for DICOM images, but also for transaction of information) between disparate vendors. Significantly the lack of process conformity within healthcare delivery environments that experience continuously changing and transforming healthcare requirements demands continuous '*negotiation*' between users and vendors. In this case, IHE would be the answer to integrate disparate HIS/PACS/RIS/LIS systems together as an integrated, scalable 'plug-in' Healthcare Solution. The ultimate aim of integrated Healthcare solutions is to implement not only the operational management control systems, but also the systems for strategic decision support.

Medical images are highly heterogeneous with a variety of domains (brain, abdominal, cardiac, etc.), modalities (MR, CT, X-ray, microscopy, photography, ultrasound), formats (DICOM, TIFF, JPEG), and dimensions (2D [retinal], 3D [brain], 4D [e.g, a 3D heart over a period of time], and even 5D [e.g, a functional 4D at a specific anatomic location]). Thus it is impractical to standardise these data into a 'one size for all' model. To exploit such data or other demographic data effectively requires a novel architecture to ensure accessing not only from data sources of distributed collections, but also without prior standardisation of the original data, entailing each database with scope, scale, and the necessary flexibility. Therefore, incremental approach is appealing.

With over 800 million mobile users in China, it certainly has got momentum. Telemedicine services, in particular the services that focus on well-being and health care, should aim at mobile phone applications.

The advances of technology should make greater impacts to the poorer people who are still in poverty in the underdeveloped countries in helping them weather the storm. From personal point of view, this helping hand should be ushered by a number of developed countries, like the project RAFT. In this way, benifits can be felt not only in a short period, but also with less cost. Likewise, to reinforce the effort, a top-down policy should be opted for with a certain degree of governmental involvement. On the other hand, with the implementation of telemedicine, those people can profit not only in relation to health issues, but also in terms of education by bringing up their literacy rate, for underdeveloped countries have lower literacy rate, e.g., Ethiopia has 35.9% of Literacy rate whereas 99% occurs in most of the developed countries (http://en.wikipedia.org/wiki/List_of_countries_by_literacy_rate), and are in need of means for accessing and learning.

CONCLUSION

Although the techniques of telemedicine/tele-surgery are available, the calls for employing them vary from country to country. In the UK, medical resources are evenly distributed across the whole country and are provided by the National Health Service (NHS), coupled with adequate emergency systems that are equipped with fast means of transportations. In this way, a patient can be located to an intended hospital within required time. In contrast, China has a very different geographic pattern. Many places, e.g., mountainous regions, are difficult to locate even with several means of transportations. Significantly, China is still in the developing stage and has a long and bumpy way to go in order to allow everyone access their much

needed health care, especially for those 70% peasants who live in the remote areas, far afield from those big cities where modern medical equipment are concentrated. In this case, China should be in favour of the services allowing telemedicine/teleservices to be provided over the Internet. By this way, it can save time, personnel and money substantially without compromising patients' safety. Considering over 300 million people are with land telephone line and over 800 million are with mobile phones, tele-services in medicine have huge potentials in China. One of the promising areas is tele-surgery like the one pioneered by the Navy General Hospital in Beijing. The strength of the approach lies in the knowledge transfer. Due to the limited number of experts in the field, performing remote surgery retains its positive features. In particular, it has the ability that one expert team can supervise several tele-surgeries that are operated at different locations at the same time, reducing patients' waiting list, prolonged suffering, and the cost of experts' time.

ACKNOWLEDGMENT

The TIME project is financially funded by EC under Asia IC&T programme. Their support is gratefully acknowledged. JISC in the UK has provided funding to further refine the online image repository. Their financially support is gratefully received. The authors also would like to thank many colleagues who not only shared their valuable experience on the running of their telemedicine projects, but also showed their warm hospitality while receiving the TIME team to their institutes, in particular, Prof. Henning Müller from Switzerland, Prof. Davide Caramella from Italy, Dr. Roald Bergstrøm from Norway, and Prof. Andrzej Czyżewksi from Poland. The author is in Prof. Zengmin Tian's debt for his kindly demonstration of image-guided neurosurgery showcased to the TIME team and for many of his images given to the author, some of them being displayed in this Chapter. The subsequent project, WIDTH (2011-2014), is financially funded by EC under FP7-people programme.

REFERENCES

Androuchko, L. (2010). *Improving access to healthcare services by using information and telecommunication technologies, ITU SG2, Q12-3/2*. Retrieved from www.itu.int/ITU-D/study_groups/.../SG2/SG2-index.html.

ANSI. (2011). *Website*. Retrieved from http://webstore.ansi.org/FindStandards.aspx?Action=displaydept&DeptID=3104&Acro=HL7&DpName=HL7:%20Health%20Level%20Seven/.

ATA. (2011). *Website*. Retrieved from http://www.americantelemed.org/.

Bagayoko, C. O., Müller, H., & Geissbuhler, A. (2006). Assessment of internet-based tele-medicine in Africa (the RAFT project). *Computerized Medical Imaging and Graphics, 30*, 407–416. doi:10.1016/j.compmedimag.2006.09.014

Bergstrøm, R. (2005). Norway PACS. In *Proceedings of MIT 2005 International Conference on Medical Imaging and Telemedicine*, (pp. 52-56). China: MIT.

Bergstrøm, R. (2006). PACS, teleradiology, telemedicine and eHealth in Norway. In *Proceedings of First Symposium of ChinaPACS-RIS*, (pp. 6-17). ChinaPACS.

Chen, J., & Xia, Z. (2009). Telehealth in China: Opportunity and challenges. In *Telehealth in the Developing World*. London, UK: Royal Society of Medicine Press/IDRC.

Chhut, S. V. (2008). *Need, feasibility and sustainability in two projects of telepathology in developing countries, Africa and South East Asia*. Retrieved from http://www.seapcongresos.com/telepathology2008/pages/video2.html#SV.

China Daily. (2010). *China internet population hits 420m*. Retrieved from http://www.chinadaily.com.cn/china/2010-07/15/content_10112957.htm.

China Statistical Yearbook. (2003). *Table 21-36*. Beijin, China: Government of China.

Clunie, D. A. (2000). *DICOM structured reporting*. Bangor, ME: Pixel Medical Publishing.

Department of Health. (2011). *Website*. Retrieved from http://www.dh.gov.uk/en/Publicationsandstatistics/Publications/PublicationsPolicyAndGuidance/Browsable/DH_4920815.

e-Diabetes Programme. (2009). *Website*. Retrieved from http://www.e-diabete.org/index.php?page=fr_anglais.

ENDOCAS. (2011). *Website*. Retrieved from http://www.endocas.org.

Fioravanti, F., Inchingolo, P., Valenzin, G., & Dalla Palma, L. (1997). The DPACS project at the University of Trieste. *International Journal of Medical Informatics, 22*(4), 301–314. doi:10.3109/14639239709010902

Fu, H., et al. (2006). The retrospective of PACS development in China. In *Proceedings of the 1st China Symposium of PACS-RIS*, (pp. 22-29). Beijing, China: PACS-RIS.

Fu, H., Chen, Z., & Dai, X. (1995). The research on MiniPACS: Abstract. In *Proceedings of the 7th Annual Meeting of Chinese Society of Radiology*, (pp. 585-586). Beijing, China: Chinese Society of Radiology.

Fu, H., Jin, Z., Dai, J., Chen, K., Wang, T., Li, T., & Gao, P. (2003). Picture archiving and communication system in China: The development, problem, and integrating strategy with IHE. *International Congress Series, 1256*, 915–923. doi:10.1016/S0531-5131(03)00246-2

Gao, X., Qian, Y., Hui, R., Loomes, M., Comley, R., Barn, B., et al. (2010). Texture-based 3D image retrieval for medical applications. In *IADIS e-Health2010*, (pp. 101-108). IADIS.

Gao, X. W., Hui, R., Tian, Z., & White, A. (2009). A new approach to estimation of non-isotropic scale factors for correction of MR distortions. *International Journal of Computer Assisted Radiology and Surgery, 4*(1), 349–350.

Gao, X. W., Lin, C., & Tully, C. (Eds.). (2005). *Proceedings of medical imaging and telemedicine (MIT 2005)*. Wuyi, China: MIT.

Gao, X. W., Müller, H., Loomes, M., Comley, R., & Luo, S. (Eds.). (2008). *Lecture notes in computer science,* (vol 4987). Berlin, Germany: Springer.

GIFT. (2011). *Website.* Retrieved from http://www.gnu.org/software/gift/.

Grade. (2011). *Website.* Retrieved from http://www.4panda.com/chinamedtreat/chinahospitals/grade.htm.

Guo, L., Huang, Z. L., Gan, L. Y., Yang, J., & Jing, Q. (2006). Introduction to HIS/RIS at Beijing general army hospital (in Chinese). In *Proceedings of First Symposium of ChinaPACS-RIS.* ChinaPACS-RIS.

HER/PHR. (2011). *Website.* Retrieved from http://www.hl7.org/implement/standards/ehrphr.cfm.

Horsley, V., & Clarke, R. H. (1908). The structure and functions of the cerebellum examined by a new method. *Brain, 31,* 45–125. doi:10.1093/brain/31.1.45

Hsieh, R. K. C., Hjelm, N. M., Lee, J. C. K., & Aldis, J. W. (2001). Telemedicine in China. *International Journal of Medical Informatics, 61*(2), 139–146. doi:10.1016/S1386-5056(01)00136-8

Huang, H. K., & Taira, R. K. (1992). Infrastructure design of a picture archiving and communication system. *AJR. American Journal of Roentgenology, 158,* 743–749.

IHE. (2011). *Website.* Retrieved from http://www.ihe.net.

Image, C. L. E. F. (2011). *Website.* Retrieved from http://www.imageclef.org/.

Inchingolo, P. (2005). Synergy of bioengineering, organizational and economical methodologies for the success of the e-health integration at wide national and international levels. In X. Gao, et al. (Eds.), *Proceedings of MIT 2005 International Conference on Medical Imaging and Telemedicine.* Beijing, China: MIT.

Inchingolo, P. (2008). The open three consortium: An open-source initiative at the service of healthcare and inclusion. *Lecture Notes in Computer Science, 4987,* 5–11. doi:10.1007/978-3-540-79490-5_2

Istepanian, R. (1999). Telemedicine in the United Kingdom: Current status and future prospects. *IEEE Transactions on Information Technology in Biomedicine, 3*(2), 158–159. doi:10.1109/4233.767091

JISC. (2011). *Website.* Retrieved from http://www.jisc.ac.uk/.

Kandel, E. I. (1972). Stereotaxic apparatus and operations in Russia in the 19th century. *Journal of Neurosurgery, 37,* 407–411. doi:10.3171/jns.1972.37.4.0407

Kelly, P. J. (2000). Stereotactic surgery: What is past is prologue. *Neurosurgery, 46*(1), 16–27. doi:10.1097/00006123-200001000-00005

Kwoh, Y. S., Hou, J., Jonckheere, E. A., & Hayathi, S. (1988). A robot with improved absolute positioning accuracy for stereotactic brain surgery. *IEEE Transactions on Bio-Medical Engineering, 35,* 153–160. doi:10.1109/10.1354

MedMarket Diligence. (2002). *Report #S150.* Retrieved from http://mediligence.com/web-files/prod01.htm.

Müller, H., Gao, X. W., & Lin, C. (Eds.). (2006). Special issue. *Computerised Medical Imaging and Graphics, 30*(6-7).

Müller, H., Gao, X. W., & Luo, S. (Eds.). (2008). *Computer Methods and Programs in Biomedicine, 92*(3). doi:10.1016/j.cmpb.2008.07.004

NEMA. (2004). *Digital imaging and communications in medicine (DICOM).* Fredericksburg, VA: NEMA.

Nobel Foundation. (2009). *The nobel prize in physics 2009.* Retrieved from http://nobelprize.org/nobel_prizes/physics/laureates/2009/index.html.

Qian, Y., Gao, X. W., Loomes, M., Comley, R., Barn, B., Hui, R., & Tian, Z. (2011). *Content-based retrieval of 3D medical images.* Paper presented at the Third International Conference on eHealth, Telemedicine, and Social Medicine, eTELEMED 2011. Guadeloupe, France.

RAFT. (2011). *Website.* Retrieved from http://raft.hcuge.ch.

RIS. (2011). *Website.* Retrieved from http://en.wikipedia.org/wiki/Radiology_information_system.

Schmiedl, U. P., & Rowberg, A. H. (1990). Literature review: Picture archiving and communication systems. *Journal of Digital Imaging, 3*(3), 178–194. doi:10.1007/BF03167608

Stauch, G., Oberholzer, M., Kuakpaetoon, T., & Schattka, S. (2005). *Telepathology in developing countries in south east Asia: Results, limits, future Phnom Penh project.* Paper presented at the 3rd International Conference on Telemedicine & Multimedia Communication. Poland.

Tao, Y., & Miao, J. (2002). The management and realizing of image data flow in PACS. *Chinese Journal of Radiology, 36*(10), 171–173.

TeleMed. (1997). Proceedings of International Conference on Telemedicienne and Telecare (Telemed'96). *Journal of Telemedicine and Telecare, 3,* 1–120.

TeleMed. (1998). Proceedings of international conference on telemedicienne and telecare (Telemed 1997). *Journal of Telemedicine and Telecare, 4,* 1–112.

Telemedicine. (2005). *Website.* Retrieved from http://www.kpk.gov.pl/pliki/2493/Telemedicine_Conference%20in%20Poland.pdf.

Tian, Z., Lu, W., Wang, T., Ma, B., Zhao, Q., & Zhang, G. (2008). Application of a robotic telemanipulation system in stereotactic surgery. *Stereotactic and Functional Neurosurgery, 86,* 54–61. doi:10.1159/000110742

Tian, Z., Lu, W., Zhao, Q., Yu, X., Qi, S., & Wang, R. (2008a). From frame to frameless stereotactic operation—Clinical application of 2011 cases. *Lecture Notes in Computer Science, 4987,* 18–24. doi:10.1007/978-3-540-79490-5_4

Tian, Z., Wang, T., Liu, Z., Zhao, Q., Du, J., & Liu, D. (1998). Robot assisted system in stereotactic neurosurgery. *Academic Journal of PLA Postgraduate Medicine School, 1,* 4–5.

Wang, Z., & Gu, H. (2009). A review of Tele-Medicine in China. *Journal of Telemedicine and Telecare, 15,* 23–27. doi:10.1258/jtt.2008.080508

Wiki-2. (2011). *Website.* Retrieved from http://en.wikipedia.org/wiki.

Wiki. (2010). *Website.* Retrieved from http://en.wikipedia.org/wiki/Submarine_communications_cable.

Wiki-3. (2011). *Website.* Retrieved from http://en.wikipedia.org/wiki/Telecommunications_industry_in_China.

Wiki-4. (2011). *Website.* Retrieved from http://en.wikipedia.org/wiki/Integrated_Services_Digital_Network.

Yu, X., Liu, Z., Tian, Z., Li, S., Huang, H., Xiu, B., & Zhao, Q. (2000). Stereotactic biopsy for intracranial space-occupying lesions: Clinical analysis of 550 cases. *Stereotactic and Functional Neurosurgery, 75,* 103–208. doi:10.1159/000048390

Zhao, J., Zhang, Z., Guo, H., Ren, L., & Chen, S. (2010). Development and recent achievements of telemedicine in China. *Telemedicine and e-Health, 16*(5), 634-638.

Zhao, J. A., Xu, Y. X., & Chen, J. (1998). The implementation of telemedicine network group. *China Hospital Management, 18,* 27–28.

Zhu, J. H., & Wang, W. (2005). Diffusion, use, and effect of the internet in China. *Communications of the ACM, 48*(4), 49–53. doi:10.1145/1053291.1053317

KEY TERMS AND DEFINITIONS

Digital hospital: paper-less hospital

e-Health: healthcare services provided via electric systems or devices.

HIS: Hopstial Information Systems

IHE: Integrated Healthcare Enterprise

PACS: Picture Archiving and Communications Systems

RIS: Radiology Information System

Telemedicine: Practicing medicine remotely via tele-communication systems, e.g., telephone, internet, etc.

TIME Project: Telemedicine in Medicine: a cyber bridge interfaces China with Europe on collaborative health care.

Compilation of References

3 gdoctor. (2010). *mHealth is the leverage of mobile, the newest mass media, to improve health*. Retrieved January 30, 2010, from http://3gdoctor.wordpress.com/2010/03/22/the-definition-of-mHealth/.

Aanensen, D. M., Huntley, D. M., Feil, E. J., al-Own, F., & Spratt, B. G. (2009). EpiCollect: Linking smartphones to web applications for epidemiology, ecology and community data collection. *PLoS ONE, 4*(9), 6968. doi:10.1371/journal.pone.0006968

Abhaya, G. (2008). *Measurement scales used in elderly care*. New York, NY: Radclife Publishing.

Abid, Z., Chabridon, S., & Conan, D. (2009). A framework for quality of context management. In Proceedings of the 1st International Conference on Quality of Context, (pp. 120 – 131). Stuttgart, Germany: Springer.

Aboobakur, M., Latheef, A., Mohamed, A. J., Moosa, S., Pandey, R. M., & Prabhakaran, D. (2010). Surveillance for non-communicable disease risk factors in Maldives: Results from the first STEPS survey in male. *International Journal of Public Health, 55*(5), 489–496. doi:10.1007/s00038-009-0114-y

Adami, A. M., Hayes, T. L., & Pavel, M. (2003). Unobtrusive monitoring of sleep patterns. In *Proceedings of the 25th Annual International Conference of the IEEE Engineering in Medicine and Biology Society*, (pp. 17 – 21). Cancun, Mexico: IEEE Press.

Adams, A., Dale, J., Griffiths, F., Martin, S., Powell, J., Sturt, J., & Sutcliffe, P. (2011). Systematic review of communication technologies to promote access and engagement of young people with diabetes into healthcare. *BMC Endocrine Disorders, 11*(1).

Adams, D. L., & Leath, B. A. (2008). A role for health informatics and information technology (HIIT): Shaping a global research agenda to eliminate health disparities. In Wallace, B. C. (Ed.), *Toward Equity in Health: A New Global Approach to Health Disparities* (pp. 297–321). New York, NY: Springer Publications.

Afonso, V. X., Tompkins, W. J., Nguyen, T. Q., & Shen, L. (1999). ECG detection using filter banks. *IEEE Transactions on Bio-Medical Engineering, 46*(2), 192–202. doi:10.1109/10.740882

Albert, M. S., Cates, G. D., & Driehuys, B. (1994). Biological magnetic resonance imaging using laser-polarized ^{129}Xe. *Nature, 370*, 199–201. doi:10.1038/370199a0

Aldrich, D., & Masera, P. (1999). *Mastering the digital market place*. New York, NY: John Wiley & Sons.

Allen, C., Manyika, P., Jazayeri, D., Rich, M., Lesh, N., & Fraser, H. (2006). Rapid deployment of electronic medical records for ARV rollout in rural Rwanda. In *Proceedings of the AMIA Annual Symposium*, (p. 840). AMIA.

Allen, C., Jazayeri, D., Miranda, J., Biondich, P. G., Mamlin, B. W., & Wolfe, B. A. (2007). Experience in implementing the OpenMRS medical record system to support HIV treatment in Rwanda. *Studies in Health Technology and Informatics, 129*(1), 382–386.

Allen, M., Sargeant, J., Mann, K., Fleming, M., & Premi, J. (2003). Videoconferencing for practice-based small-group continuing medical education: Feasibility, acceptability, effectiveness, and cost. *The Journal of Continuing Education in the Health Professions, 23*(1), 38–47. doi:10.1002/chp.1340230107

Alonso, L., Agusti, R., & Sallent, O. (2000). A near-optimum MAC protocol based on the distributed queuing random access protocol (DQRAP) for a CDMA mobile communication system. *IEEE Journal on Selected Areas in Communications, 18,* 1701–1718. doi:10.1109/49.872957

Alonso, L., Ferrús, R., & Agustí, R. (2005). WLAN throughput improvement via distributed queuing MAC. *IEEE Communications Letters, 9*(4), 310–312. doi:10.1109/LCOMM.2005.1413617

Alonso-Zárate, J., Kartsakli, E., Alonso, L., & Verikoukis, C. (2010). Performance analysis of a cluster-based MAC protocol for wireless ad hoc networks. *EURASIP Journal on Wireless Communications and Networking, n.d.,* 16.

Alpay, L., Verhoef, J., Xie, B., Te'eni, D., & Zwetsloot-Schonk, J. (2009). Current challenge in consumer health informatics: Bridging the gap between access to information and information understanding. *Biomedical informatics insights, 2*(1), 1.

Alverson, D. C., Holtz, B., D'Iorio, J., DeVany, M., Simmons, S., & Poropatich, R. K. (2008). One size doesn't fit all: Bringing telehealth services to special populations. *Telemedicine and e-Health, 14*(9), 957-963.

American Institute for Medical and Biological Engineering. (2011). *Website.* Retrieved from http://www.aimbe.org.

American Lung Association. (2011). *More protective air quality standard would reduce pollution in NY.* Retrieved March 28, 2011, from http://www.lungusa.org/associations/states/new-york/pressroom/news-releases/2010-2011/tighter-no2-standard.html.

Ames, E., & Rosenberg, N. (1977). Technological change in the machine tool industry: 1840-1910. In Rosenberg, N. (Ed.), *Perspectives on Technology* (pp. 9–31). Cambridge, UK: Cambridge University Press.

Amft, O., Troster, G., Lukowicz, P., & Schuster, C. (2006). Sensing muscle activities with body-worn sensors. In *Proceedings of the International Workshop on Wearable and Implantable Body Sensor Networks (BSN 2006),* (pp. 138-141). Washington, DC: IEEE Computer Society.

Aminian, K., De Andres, E., Rezakhanlou, K., Fritch, C., Schutz, Y., & Depairon, M. ... Robert, P. (1998). *Motion analysis in clinical practice using ambulatory accelerometry, modelling and motion capture techniques for virtual environments.* Berlin, Germany: Springer.

Analog Devices. (2007). *Small, low power, 3-axis 3g MEMS accelerometer.* Technical Report. Retrieved from www.analog.com.

Anandkumar, A., Meng, W., Lang, T., & Swami, A. (2009). Prize-collecting data fusion for cost-performance tradeoff in distributed inference. In *Proceedings of IEEE INFOCOM* (pp. 2150–2158). Rio de Janeiro, Brazil: IEEE Press. doi:10.1109/INFCOM.2009.5062139

Androuchko, L. (2010). *Improving access to healthcare services by using information and telecommunication technologies, ITU SG2, Q12-3/2.* Retrieved from www.itu.int/ITU-D/study_groups/.../SG2/SG2-index.html.

Anliker, U., Ward, J. A., Lukowicz, P., Tröster, G., Dolveck, F., & Baer, M. (2004). AMON: A wearable multi-parameter medical monitoring ans alert system. *IEEE Transactions on Information Technology in Biomedicine, 8*(4), 415–427. doi:10.1109/TITB.2004.837888

ANSI. (2011). *Website.* Retrieved from http://webstore.ansi.org/FindStandards.aspx?Action=displaydept&DeptID=3104&Acro=HL7&DpName=HL7:%20Health%20Level%20Seven/.

Apple Inc. (2011). *iPhone provides vital link to medical records.* Retrieved February 16, 2011, from http://www.apple.com/iphone/business/profiles/mt-sinai/.

Apple. (2011). *Apple's app store downloads top 10 billion.* Retrieved February 16, 2011, from http://www.apple.com/pr/library/2011/01/22appstore.html.

Arasu, A., Babcock, B., Babu, S., Cieslewicz, J., Datar, M., & Ito, K. (2004). *STREAM: The Stanford data stream management system.* Technical Report. Palo Alto, CA: Stanford InfoLab.

Argyres, N., & McGahan, A. M. (2002). An interview with Michael Porter. *The Academy of Management Executive, 16*(2), 43–52. doi:10.5465/AME.2002.7173495

Arnrich, B., Mayora, O., Bardram, J., & Tröster, G. (2010). Pervasive healthcare: Paving the way for a pervasive, user-centered and preventive healthcare model. *Methods of Information in Medicine, 49*(1), 67–73.

Arroyo-Valles, R., Marques, A. G., & Cid-Sueiro, J. (2011). Optimal selective forwarding for energy saving in wireless sensor networks. *IEEE Transactions on Wireless Communications, 10*(1), 164–175. doi:10.1109/TWC.2010.102810.100014

Arsand, E., Tufano, J., Ralston, J., & Hjortdahl, P. (2008). Designing mobile dietary management support technologies for people with diabetes. *Journal of Telemedicine and Telecare, 14*(7), 329. doi:10.1258/jtt.2008.007001

Assisted Living Computing and Telecommunications Laboratory. (2010). *ALLab @ instituto de telecomunicações.* Retrieved 7 April 2011, from http://allab.it.ubi.pt.

Association for the Advancement of Medical Instrumentation (AAMI). (2011). *Website.* Retrieved from http://www.aami.org.

ATA. (2011). *Website.* Retrieved from http://www.americantelemed.org/.

Atallah, L., Elhelw, M., Pansiot, J., et al. (2007). Behavior profiling with ambient and wearable sensing. In *Proceedings of the 4th International Workshop on Wearable and Implantable Body Sensor Networks,* (pp. 133-138). Berlin, Germany: Springer.

Atkinson, R. D., & McKay, A. S. (2007). *Digital prosperity – Understanding the economic benefits of the information technology revolution.* Retrieved July 7, 2011 from http://www.itif.org/index.php?id=34.

Bacon, D. T. (2007). *An internet evaluation of "DIVAS": A website designed to prevent human immunodeficiency virus and other sexually transmitted infections (STIs) among young black women.* Unpublished Doctoral Dissertation. New York, NY: Columbia University.

Bagayoko, C. O., Müller, H., & Geissbuhler, A. (2006). Assessment of internet-based tele-medicine in Africa (the RAFT project). *Computerized Medical Imaging and Graphics, 30,* 407–416. doi:10.1016/j.compmedimag.2006.09.014

Bahillo, A., Prieto, J., Mazuelas, S., Lorenzo, R. M., Fernández, P., & Abril, E. J. (2010). E-field assessment errors caused by the human body on localization systems. In *Proceedings of the IEEE 71th Vehicular Technology Conference,* (pp. 1-5). Taipei, Taiwan: IEEE Press.

Bah, S. (2009). Strategies for managing the change from ICD-9 to ICD-10 in developing countries: The case of South Africa. *Journal of Health Informatics in Developing Countries, 3*(2), 44–49.

Bai, Y., & Lu, C. (2005). Web-based remote digital stethoscope. In *Proceedings EuroIMSA,* (423-428). Springer.

Balanis, C. A. (2005). *Antenna theory analysis and design.* New York, NY: John Wiley & Sons Inc.

Ball, M. J., & Lillis, J. (2001). E-health: Transforming the physician-patient relationship. *International Journal of Medical Informatics, 61,* 1–10. doi:10.1016/S1386-5056(00)00130-1

Bandettini, P. A., Wong, E. C., Hinks, R. S., Tikofsky, R. S., & Hyde, J. S. (1992). Time course EPI of human brain function during task activation. *Magnetic Resonance in Medicine, 25,* 390–397. doi:10.1002/mrm.1910250220

Bankman, I. (2000). *Handbook of medical imaging: Processing and analysis management.* San Diego, CA: Academic Press.

Bar-Dayan, Y. (2008). International collaboration in disaster medicine—It is time for the "big step" in disaster preparedness. *Prehospital and Disaster Medicine, 23,* 280–281.

Bardram, J. E., & Bossen, C. (2003). Moving to get ahead: Local mobility and collaborative work. In *Proceedings of the Eighth European Conference on Computer Supported Cooperative Work.* Helsinki, Finland: Kluwer Academic Publishers.

Bardram, J. E., Mihailidis, A., & Wan, D. (Eds.). (2006). *Pervasive computing in healthcare.* Boca Raton, FL: CRC.

Bashshur, R., Shannon, G., & Sapci, H. (2005). Telemedicine evaluation. *Telemedicine and e-Health, 11*(3), 296-317.

Bashshur, R. L. (2002). Telemedicine and health care. *Telemedicine Journal and e-Health, 8*(1), 5–12. doi:10.1089/15305620252933365

Bashshur, R. L., Reardon, T. G., & Shannon, G. W. (2000). Telemedicine: A new health care delivery system. *Annual Review of Public Health, 21*, 613–637. doi:10.1146/annurev.publhealth.21.1.613

BASUMA Project. (2006). *Webpage.* Retrieved from http://www.basuma.de/.

Bates, D. W., Cohen, M., Leape, L. L., Overhage, J. M., Shabot, M. M., & Sheridan, T. (2001). Reducing the frequency of errors in medicine using information technology. *Journal of the American Medical Informatics Association, 8*(4), 299–308. doi:10.1136/jamia.2001.0080299

Batini, C., Cappiello, C., Francalanci, C., & Maurino, A. (2009). Methodologies for data quality assessment and improvement. *ACM Computing Surveys, 41*(3), 1–52. doi:10.1145/1541880.1541883

Beale, T. (2002). *Archetypes: Constraint-based domain models for future-proof information systems.* Paper presented at the Eleventh OOPSLA Workshop on Behavioral Semantics: Serving the Customer. Seattle, WA.

Becker, E., Metsis, V., Arora, R., Vinjumur, J., Xu, Y., & Makedon, F. (2009). SmartDrawer: RFID-based smart medicine drawer for assistive environments. In *Proceedings of the 2nd international Conference on Pervsive Technologies Related To Assistive Environments (PETRA 2009)*, (pp. 1-8). New York, NY: ACM Press.

Belbachir, A. N., Drobics, M., & Marschitz, W. (2010). Ambient assisted living for ageing well – An overview. *E&I Elektrotechnik und Informationstechnik, 127*(7-8), 200–205. doi:10.1007/s00502-010-0747-9

Bellotti, V., & Bly, S. (1996). Walking away from the desktop computer: Distributed collaboration and mobility in a product design team. In *Proceedings of ACM 1996 Conference on Computer Supported Cooperative Work.* ACM Press.

Benabou, C. (1999). Polychronicity and temporal dimensions of work in learning organizations. *Journal of Managerial Psychology, 14*(3/4), 257–268. doi:10.1108/02683949910263792

Benevolo, C., & Spinelli, R. (2011). International service delivery and Internet-based technologies. *International Journal of Services. Economics and Management, 3*(3), 251–266.

Benjak, T. (2011). *Report on disabled persons in Croatia.* Retrieved March 26, 2011, from http://www.hzjz.hr/epidemiologija/kron_mas/invalidi10.pdf.

Bergstrøm, R. (2005). Norway PACS. In *Proceedings of MIT 2005 International Conference on Medical Imaging and Telemedicine*, (pp. 52-56). China: MIT.

Bergstrøm, R. (2006). PACS, teleradiology, telemedicine and eHealth in Norway. In *Proceedings of First Symposium of ChinaPACS-RIS*, (pp. 6-17). ChinaPACS.

Bern, C., Maguire, J. H., & Alvar, J. (2008). Complexities of assessing the disease burden attributable to Leishmaniasis. *PLoS Neglected Tropical Diseases, 2*(10), 313. doi:10.1371/journal.pntd.0000313

Berner, E. S. (2008). Ethical and legal issues in the use of health information technology to improve patient safety. *HEC Forum, 20*(39), 243–258. doi:10.1007/s10730-008-9074-5

Bernstein, M. L., McCreless, T., & Côté, M. J. (2007). Five constants of information technology adoption in healthcare. *Hospital Topics, 85*(1), 17–25. doi:10.3200/HTPS.85.1.17-26

Bhagwati, J. (1987). International trade in services and its relevance for economic development. In Giarini, O. (Ed.), *The Emerging Service Economy* (pp. 3–57). Oxford, UK: Pergamon Press.

Bianchi, G. (2000). Performance analysis of the IEEE 802.11 distributed coordination function. *IEEE Journal on Selected Areas in Communications, 18*(3), 535–547. doi:10.1109/49.840210

Bidargaddi, N., Klingbeil, L., Sarela, A., Boyle, J., Cheung, V., & Yelland, C. ... Gray, L. (2007). Wavelet based approach for posture transition estimation using a waist worn accelerometer. In *Proceedings*, (pp. 1884-1887). IEEE Press.

Biodevices, S. A. (2010). *Biodevices.* Retrieved 7 April 2011, from http://www.biodevices.pt.

Biomedical Engineering Society (BMES). (2011). *Website.* Retrieved from http://www.bmes.org/aws/BMES/pt/sp/home_page.

Biomedical Engineering Society. (1996). *Planning a career in biomedical engineering.* Retrieved from http://www.bmes.org/aws/BMES/pt/sp/be_faqs.

Biondich, P. G., Anand, V., Downs, S. M., & McDonald, C. J. (2003). Using adaptive turnaround documents to electronically acquire structured data in clinical settings. In *Proceedings of the AMIA Annual Symposium*, (pp. 86-90). AMIA.

BIRT. (2010). *Web page*. Retrieved December 14, 2010, from http://www.eclipse.org/birt/phoenix.

Bluedorn, A. C., & Denhardt, R. B. (1988). Time and organizations. *Journal of Management, 14*(2), 299–320. doi:10.1177/014920638801400209

Bluedorn, A. C., Kalliath, T. J., Strube, M. J., & Martin, G. D. (1999). Polychronicity and the inventory of polychronic values (IPV): The development of an instrument to measure a fundamental dimension in organizational culture. *Journal of Managerial Psychology, 14*(3/4), 205–230. doi:10.1108/02683949910263747

Blumenthal, D., & Tavenner, M. (2010). The "meaningful use" regulation for electronic health records. *The New England Journal of Medicine, 363*(6), 501–504. doi:10.1056/NEJMp1006114

Boerma, T., Zahr, C. A., Bos, E., Hansen, P., Addai, E., & Beer, D. L. (2010). *Monitoring and evaluation of health systems strengthening: An operational framework*. Retrieved October 20, 2011, from http://www.who.int/entity/healthinfo/HSS_MandE_framework_Oct_2010.pdf.

Bonato, P. (2005). Advances in wearable technology and applications in physical medicine and rehabilitation. *Journal of Neuroengineering and Rehabilitation, 2*(2).

Borycki, E. M., Lemieux-Charles, L., Nagle, L., & Eysenbach, G. (2009a). Evaluating the impact of hybrid electronic-paper environments upon novice nurse information seeking. *Methods of Information in Medicine, 48*(2), 137–143. Retrieved from http://dx.doi.org/10.3414/ME9222

Borycki, E. M., Lemieux-Charles, L., Nagle, L., & Eysenbach, G. (2009b). Novice nurse information needs in paper and hybrid electronic-paper environments: A qualitative analysis. *Studies in Health Technology and Informatics, 150*, 913–917.

Bottazzi, D., Corradi, A., & Montanari, R. (2006). Context-aware middleware solutions for anytime and anywhere emergency assistance to elderly people. *IEEE Communications Magazine, 44*(4), 82–90. doi:10.1109/MCOM.2006.1632653

Bourgard, B., Catthoor, F., Daly, D. C., Chandrakasam, A., & Dehaene, W. (2005). Energy efficiency of the IEEE 802.15.4 standard in dense wireless microsensor networks: modeling and improvement perspectives. In *Proceedings of the Design, Automation and Test in Europe*, (Vol. 1), (pp. 196 - 201). IEEE Press.

Branch, J., Szymanski, B., Giannella, C., Wolff, R., & Kargupta, H. (2006). In-network outlier detection in wireless sensor networks. In *Proceedings of ICDCS 2006*. Lisboa, Portugal: ICDCS.

Brengelmann, G. L. (2000). Body surface temperature: Manifestation of complex anatomy and physiology of the cutaneous vasculature. In *Proceedings of the 22nd Annual International Conference of the IEEE*, (pp. 1927-1930). IEEE Press.

Brgulja, N., Kusber, R., David, K., & Baumgarten, M. (2009). Measuring the probability of correctness of contextual information in context aware systems. In *Proceedings of the IEEE International Symposium on Dependable, Autonomous and Secure Computing*, (pp. 246 – 253). Chengdu, China: IEEE Press.

Bronzino, J. D. (2000). Clinical engineering: Evolution of a discipline. In Bronzino, J. D. (Ed.), *The Biomedical Engineering Handbook* (2nd ed.). Boca Raton, FL: CRC Press LLC.

Brown, J. H. U. (1975). The biomedical engineer and the health care system. *IEEE Transactions on Bio-Medical Engineering, 22*, 95–99. doi:10.1109/TBME.1975.324425

Bu, Y., Gu, T., Tao, X., Li, J., Chen, S., & Lu, J. (2006). Managing quality of context in pervasive computing. In *Proceedings of the Sixth International Conference on Quality Software*, (pp. 193 – 200). IEEE Press.

Buchholz, T., Krause, M., Linnhoff-Popien, C., & Schiffers, M. (2004). CoCo: Dynamic composition of context information. In *Proceedings of the Annual International Conference on Mobile and Ubiquitous Systems*, (pp. 335 – 343). IEEE Press.

Buchholz, T., Küpper, A., & Schiffers, M. (2003). Quality of context: What it is and why we need it. In *Proceedings of the 10th International Workshop of the HP OpenView University Association (HPOVUA)*. Geneva, Switzerland: ACM Press.

Burman, E. (2003). *Shift! The unfolding internet: Hype, hope and history.* Chichester, UK: John Wiley & Sons.

Burr-Brown. (1996). *Dual, low power, G-10, 100 instrumentation amplifier.* Technical Report. Retrieved from http://focus.ti.com.cn.

Bustillo, M. (2010, July 23). Wal-Mart radio tags to track clothing. *Wall Street Journal.* Retrieved Feb. 18, 2011, from http://online.wsj.com/article/SB100014240527487 04421304575383213061198090.html.

Byrne, E., & Sahay, S. (2003). Health information systems for primary health care: Thinking about participation. In M. Korpela, R. Montealegre, & A. Poulymenakou (Eds.), *Proceedings of the International Federation of Information Processing, IFIP 9.4 and 8.2 Joint Conference on Organizational Information Systems in the Context of Globalization,* (pp. 237-249). Dordrecht, The Netherlands: Kluwer.

California, EMF Program. (2001). *An evaluation of the possible risks from electric and magnetic fields (EMFs) from power lines, internal wiring, electrical occupations and appliances.* Draft 3. Oakland, CA: California Department of Health Services.

Campbell, I. (2008). Body temperature and its regulation. *Anaesthesia and Intensive Care Medicine, 9,* 259–263. doi:10.1016/j.mpaic.2008.04.009

Canadian Health Informatics Association. (2011). *COACH definition of health informatics: Health informatics (HI) is the intersection of clinical, IM/IT and management practices to achieve better health.* Retrieved January 30, 2011, from http://coachorg.com/health_informatics.

Cangialosi, A., Monaly, J. E., & Yang, S. C. (2007). Leveraging RFID in hospitals: Patient life cycle and mobility perspectives. *IEEE Communications Magazine, 45*(9), 18–23. doi:10.1109/MCOM.2007.4342874

Castells, M. (1996). The information age: Economy, society and culture: *Vol. I. The rise of the network society.* Oxford, UK: Blackwell Publisher.

Castells, M. (2000). *The rise of the network society.* Oxford, UK: Blackwell Publishers.

Castillo-Salgado, C. (2010). Trends and directions of global public health surveillance. *Epidemiologic Reviews, 32,* 93–109. doi:10.1093/epirev/mxq008

Catrysse, M., Puers, R., Hertleer, C., Langenhove, L. V., Egmond, H. V., & Matthys, D. (2011). Towards the integration of textile sensors in a wireless monitoring suit. *Sensors and Actuators. A, Physical, 113*(2-3), 302–311.

Cavalcanti, D., Schmitt, R., & Soomro, A. (2007). *Performance analysis of 802.15.4 and 802.11e for body sensor network applications.* Paper presented at the 4th International Workshop on Wearable and Implantable Body Sensor Networks (BSN 2007). Aachen, Germany.

Central Intelligence Agency. (2011). *The world factbook.* Washington, DC: CIA. Retrieved January 28, 2011, from https://www.cia.gov/library/publications/the-world-factbook/index.html.

Cerutti, S., Baselli, G., & Bianchi, A. (2011). Biomedical signal and image processing. *IEEE Pulse, 2*(3), 41–54. doi:10.1109/MPUL.2011.941522

Chaczko, Z., Klempous, R., Nikodem, J., et al. (2008). Applications of cooperative WSN in homecare systems. In *Proceedings of the 3rd International Conference on Broadband Communications, Information Technology & Biomedical Applications,* (pp. 215-220). Washington, DC: IEEE Press.

Chang, K., Soong, A., Tseng, M., & Xiang, Z. (2011). Global wireless machine-to-machine standardization. *IEEE Internet Computing, 15*(2), 64–69. doi:10.1109/MIC.2011.41

Chang, L., Kagaayi, J., Nakigozi, G., Packer, A., Serwadda, D., & Quinn, T. (2008). Responding to the human resource crisis: Peer health workers, mobile phones, and HIV care in Rakai, Uganda. *AIDS Patient Care and STDs, 22*(3), 173. doi:10.1089/apc.2007.0234

Chapman, B., Turner, R., & Ordidge, R. J. (1987). Readl-time movie imaging from a single cardiac cycle by NMR. *Magnetic Resonance in Medicine, 5,* 246–254. doi:10.1002/mrm.1910050305

Charny, B., & Cheng, R. (2009). Palm's pre to access itunes. *The Wall Street Journal.* Retrieved February 16, 2011, from http://online.wsj.com/article/SB124353594043063537.html?mod=googlewsj.

Chase, R. B. (1978). Where does the customer fit in a service operation. *Harvard Business Review, 56*(5), 137–142.

Che, S. S. (2011). *Country health systems surveillance: Improving data availability, quality and use for better performance*. Retrieved February 11, 2011, from http://www.internationalhealthpartnership.net/en/working_groups/monitoring_and_evaluation.

Chen, H., Zeng, D., & Yan, P. (2010). *Infectious disease informatics: Syndromic surveillance for public health and BioDefense*. New York, NY: Springer Science+Business Media, LLC.

Chen, L., Yu, C., Sun, T., Chen, Y., & Chu, H. (2006). Hybrid routing approach for opportunistic networks. In *Proceedings of the ACM SIGCOMM Workshop on Challenged Networks (CHANTS)*, (pp. 213-220). ACM Press.

Chen, S., Lee, H., Chen, C., et al. (2007). A wireless body sensor network system for healthcare monitoring application. In *Proceedings of IEEE Biomedical Circuits and Systems Conference (BIOCAS)*, (pp. 243-246). Washington, DC: IEEE Press.

Chen, E. S., Mednonca, E., McKnight, L., Stetson, P., Lei, J., & Cimino, J. (2003). PalmCIS: A wireless handheld application for satisfying clinician information needs. *Journal of the American Medical Informatics Association, 11*(1), 19–28. doi:10.1197/jamia.M1387

Chen, H., & Zeng, D. (2009). AI for global disease surveillance: Trends & controversies. *IEEE Intelligent Systems, 24*(6), 66–69. doi:10.1109/MIS.2009.126

Chen, J., & Xia, Z. (2009). Telehealth in China: Opportunity and challenges. In *Telehealth in the Developing World*. London, UK: Royal Society of Medicine Press/IDRC.

Chen, L. K., & Shieh, Y. A. (2011). Jackknife prevention for articulated vehicles using model reference adaptive control. *Journal of Automobile Engineering, 225*(1), 28–42. doi:10.1243/09544070JAUTO1513

Chen, M., Gonzalez, S., Leung, V., Zhang, Q., & Li, M. A. (2010). 2G-RFID-based e-healthcare system. *IEEE Wireless Communications, 17*(1), 37–43. doi:10.1109/MWC.2010.5416348

Chen, S. (2001). *Strategic management of e-business*. Chichester, UK: John Wiley & Sons.

Chevrollier, N., & Golmie, N. (2005). *On the use of wireless network technologies in healthcare environments*. Paper presented at the 5th Workshop on Applications and Services in Wireless Networks (ASWN 2005). Paris, France.

Chhut, S. V. (2008). *Need, feasibility and sustainability in two projects of telepathology in developing countries, Africa and South East Asia*. Retrieved from http://www.seapcongresos.com/telepathology2008/pages/video2.html#SV.

China Daily. (2010). *China internet population hits 420m*. Retrieved from http://www.chinadaily.com.cn/china/2010-07/15/content_10112957.htm.

China Statistical Yearbook. (2003). *Table 21-36*. Beijin, China: Government of China.

Chipcon, A. S. (2004). *SmartRF. CC2420 - 2.4 GHz IEEE802.15.4/Zigbee RF transceiver, CC2420 data sheet*. Retrieved from http://inst.eecs.berkeley.edu/~cs150/Documents/CC2420.pdf.

Choubert, J. M., Martin Ruel, S., Esperanza, M., Budzinski, H., Miège, C., Lagarrigue, C., & Coquery, M. (2011). Limiting the emissions of micro-pollutants: What efficiency can we expect from wastewater treatment plants? *Water Science and Technology, 63*, 57–65. doi:10.2166/wst.2011.009

Chui, M., Miller, A., & Roberts, R. (2009). Six ways to make web 2.0 work. *The McKinsey Quarterly, n.d.*, 1–7.

Clarke, M., & Thiyagarajan, C. A. (2008). A systematic review of technical evaluation in telemedicine systems. *Journal of Telemedicine and e-Health, 14*(2), 170-183.

ClearHealth. (2011). *Web page*. Retrieved May 12, 2011, http://en.wikipedia.org/wiki/ClearHealth.

Clunie, D. A. (2000). *DICOM structured reporting*. Bangor, ME: Pixel Medical Publishing.

Commission of the European Communities. (2004). *e-Health - Making healthcare better for European citizens: An action plan for a European e-Health area*. Luxembourg: Commission of the European Communities.

Community Health Information Tracking System. (2011). *Web page*. Retrieved May 12, 2011, from http://www.chits.ph/web.

Consumer Electronic Show. (2011). *2011 international CES wows world with innovation and optimism*. Retrieved February 5, 2011, from http://www.cesweb.org/news/rssNews.asp.

Contandriopoulos, A. P., Denis, J. L., Touati, N., & Rodriguez, C. (2003). *The integration of health care: Dimensions and implementation.* Working Paper (N04-01). Montreal, Canada: Universite de Montreal.

Conti, J. P. (2006). The internet of things. *IET Communications Engineer, 4*(6), 20–25. doi:10.1049/ce:20060603

Cook, A. M., & Hussey, S. M. (2002). *Assistive technology: Principles and practice* (2nd ed.). St. Louis, MO: Mosby.

Cooper, R. A., Ohnabe, H., & Hobson, D. A. (2006). *An introduction to rehabilitation engineering.* Boca Raton, FL: CRC Press Taylor & Francis.

Couto, R. G., & Garcia, N. M. (2001). *CE marking - A synthesis of the conformance CE marking on medical devices.* White Paper. Covilhã, Portugal: Instituto de Telecomunicações.

Cox, A. (2010). *mHealth: What scope is there in the remote monitoring market for chronic diseases?* Retrieved February 14, 2011, from http://www.juniperresearch.com/analyst-xpress-blog/2010/08/23/mHealth-what-scope-is-there-in-the-remote-monitoring-market-for-chronic-diseases/.

Cox, J. R. Jr, Pfeiffer, R. R., & Pickard, W. F. (1975). Experience with a training program in technology in health care. *IEEE Transactions on Bio-Medical Engineering, 22,* 129–134. doi:10.1109/TBME.1975.324432

Craig, J., & Patterson, V. (2005). Introduction to the practice of telemedicine. *Journal of Telemedicine and Telecare, 11*(1), 3–9. doi:10.1258/1357633053430494

Crilly, J. F., Keefe, R. H., & Volpe, F. (2011). Use of electronic technologies to promote community and personal health for individuals unconnected to health care systems. *American Journal of Public Health, 101*(7), 1163–1167. doi:10.2105/AJPH.2010.300003

Cristov, I. I. (2004). *Real time electrocardiogram QRS detection using combined adaptative threshold.* Retrieved 7 April 2011, from http://www.biomedical-engineering-online.com/content/3/1/28.

Curioso, W. H., & Mechael, P. N. (2010). Enhancing 'm-health' with south-to-south collaborations. *Health Affairs, 29*(2), 264–267. doi:10.1377/hlthaff.2009.1057

Dadvand, P., Rankin, J., Rushton, S., & Pless-Mulloli, T. (2011). Ambient air pollution and congenital heart disease: A register-based study. *Environmental Research, 111*(3), 435–441. doi:10.1016/j.envres.2011.01.022

Dall'Acqua, L., Tonin, C., Peila, R., Ferrero, F., & Catellani, M. (2004). Performances and properties of intrinsic conductive cellulose–polypyrrole textiles. *Synthetic Materials, 146,* 213–221.

Damadian, R. (1971). Tumor detection by nuclear magnetic resonance. *Science, 171,* 1151. doi:10.1126/science.171.3976.1151

De Lombaerde, P., & Van Langenhouve, L. (2011). Monitoring and evaluating the provision of (donor-funded) regional public goods. *Regions & Cohesion, 1,* 101–123. doi:10.3167/reco.2011.010107

de Vries, W., Veltink, P. H., Koper, M. P., & Koopman, B. F. J. M. (1994). Calculation of segment and joint angles of the lower extremities during gait using accelerometers. In *Proceedings of the Second World Congress of Biomechanics on Dynamic Analysis Using Body Fixed Sensors.* Amsterdam, The Netherlands: McRoberts.

Declich, S., & Carter, A. O. (1994). Public health surveillance: Historical origins, methods and evaluation. *Bulletin of the World Health Organization, 72,* 285–304.

Deligianni, F., Chung, A., & Yang, G. (2004). Decoupling of respiratory motion with wavelet and principal component analysis. In *Proceedings of Medical Image Understanding and Analysis (MIUA04)* (pp. 13–16). London, UK: Springer.

Delin, K. A., & Jackson, S. P. (2001). *The sensor web: A new instrument concept.* Paper presented at SPIE's Symposium on Integrated Optics. San Jose, CA.

Delin, K. A. (2002). The sensor web: A macro-instrument for coordinated sensing. *Sensors Journal, 2*(7), 270–285. doi:10.3390/s20700270

Della Mea, V. (2005). Prerecorded telemedicine. *Journal of Telemedicine and Telecare, 11*(6), 276–284. doi:10.1258/1357633054893382

Demattè, C., Biffi, A., Mandelli, A., & Parolini, C. (2007). Firms and the digital technology in Italy: The network moves forward. In Apte, U., & Karmarkar, U. (Eds.), *Managing in the Information Economy* (pp. 429–471). New York, NY: Springer. doi:10.1007/978-0-387-36892-4_18

Demmer, M., Brewer, E., Fall, K., Jain, S., Ho, M., & Patra, R. (2004). *Implementing delay tolerant networking*. IRB-TR-04-020. Retrieved from http://www.dtnrg.org/docs/papers/demmer-irb-tr-04-020.pdf.

Dengler, S., Awad, A., & Dressler, F. (2007). Sensor/actuator networks in smart homes for supporting elderly and handicapped people. In *Proceedings of the 21st International Conference on Advanced Information Networking and Applications Workshops*, (pp. 863–868). IEEE Press.

Denning, P. J. (2006). Hastily formed networks. *Communications of the ACM, 49*(4), 15–20. doi:10.1145/1121949.1121966

Department of Defense. (2006). *National industrial security program operating manual*. Washington, DC: Department of Defense.

Department of Health. (2011). *Website*. Retrieved from http://www.dh.gov.uk/en/Publicationsandstatistics/Publications/PublicationsPolicyAndGuidance/Browsable/DH_4920815.

Department of Veterans Affairs. (2011). *Web page*. Retrieved January 15, 2011, from http://www.va.gov/vista_monograph.

Detwiler, J. S., Sanderson, A. C., & Vas, R. (1975). A clinically oriented bioengineering program for undergraduates. *IEEE Transactions on Bio-Medical Engineering, 22*, 140–145. doi:10.1109/TBME.1975.324434

Devaraj, S., & Kohli, R. (2000). Information technology payoff in the healthcare industry: A longitudinal study. *Journal of Management Information Systems, 16*(4), 41–67.

Dey, A. K., & Abowd, G. D. (1999). The context toolkit: Aiding the development of context-aware applications. In *Proceedings of the Workshop on Software Engineering for Wearable and Pervasive Computing*, (pp. 434–441). ACM Press.

Diero, L., Rotich, J. K., Bii, J., Mamlin, B. W., Einterz, R. M., Kalamai, I. Z., & Tierney, W. M. (2006). A computer-based medical record system and personal digital assistants to assess and follow patients with respiratory tract infections visiting a rural Kenyan health centre. *BMC Medical Informatics and Decision Making, 6*, 21. doi:10.1186/1472-6947-6-21

Dix, A. (2000). Exploiting space and location as a design framework for interactive mobile systems. *ACM Transactions on Computer-Human Interaction, 7*(3), 285–321. doi:10.1145/355324.355325

Dixon, B. E. (2007). A roadmap for the adoption of e-. *The Health Service Journal, 5*(3), 3–13.

Dolan, B. (2009). *ReachMD: 60,000+ downloads for CME app*. Retrieved February 21, 2011, from http://mobihealthnews.com/2990/reachmd-60000-downloads-for-cme-app/.

Dolan, B. (2009). *WebMD: Medscape mobile, 200,000+ downloads*. Retrieved February 21, 2011, from http://mobihealthnews.com/5307/webmd-medcape-mobile-has-200000-downloads/.

Dongsoo, H., Sungjoon, P., & Minkyu, L. (2009). The-muss: Mobile u-health service system. *Communications in Computer and Information Science, 25*(4), 377–389.

Draft, IEEE. 802.15.4b™/D2. (2005). *Draft revision for standard for information technology part 15.4b: Wireless medium access control (MAC) and physical layer (PHY) specifications for low-rate wireless personal area networks (WPANs)*. New York, NY: IEEE Press.

Dumoulin, C. L., Souza, S. P., & Hart, H. R. (1987). Rapid scan magnetic resonance angiography. *Magnetic Resonance in Medicine, 5*, 238–245. doi:10.1002/mrm.1910050304

DuoFertility. (2009). *Website*. Retrieved from http://www.duofertility.com.

Durand, D. M. (2007). What is neural engineering? In *Journal Of Neural Engineering* (Vol. 4). Dordrecht, The Netherlands: IOP Publishing.

Durresi, A., Durresi, M., & Barolli, L. (2008). Secure ubiquitous health monitoring system. *Lecture Notes in Computer Science, 5186*(1), 273–282. doi:10.1007/978-3-540-85693-1_29

Dyntex Korea. (2011). *Dyntex Korea web site*. Retrieved 14 February 2011, from http://www.dyntex.co.kr.

Economist. (2011). *Mobile services in poor countries: Not just talk*. Retrieved January 30, 2011, from http://www.economist.com/node/18008202.

e-Diabetes Programme. (2009). *Website.* Retrieved from http://www.e-diabete.org/index.php?page=fr_anglais.

eHealthServer. (2010). *UPMC brings key patient records to the bedside using blackberry smart phones.* Retrieved February 23, 2011, from http://www.ehealthserver.com/research-and-development/442-upmc-brings-key-patient-records-to-the-bedside-using-blackberry-smartphones.

Eiglier, P., & Langeard, E. (1987). *Servuction: Le marketing des services.* Paris, France: McGraw-Hill.

Eikelboom, R. H., & Atlas, M. D. (2005). Attitude to telemedicine, and willingness to use it, in audiology patients. *Journal of Telemedicine and Telecare, 11,* S22–S25. doi:10.1258/135763305775124920

Eklund, J. M., Hansen, T. R., Sprinkle, J., & Sastry, S. (2005). *Information technology for assisted living at home: Building a wireless infrastructure for assisted living.* Paper presented at the 27th Annual International Conference of the IEEE Engineering in Medicine and Biology Society. Shanghai, China.

El-Bassel, N., Witte, S. S., & Gilbert, L. (2008). HIV/AIDS risk reduction with couples: Implications for reducing health disparities in HIV/AIDS prevention. In Wallace, B. C. (Ed.), *Toward Equity in Health: A New Global Approach to Health Disparities* (pp. 253–274). New York, NY: Springer Publications.

Elemental Clinic. (2011). *Web page.* Retrieved May 12, 2011, from http://directory.fsf.org/project/elemental_clinc.

EMF. (2010). *Eclipse modeling framework project.* Retrieved Mach 05, 2011, from http://www.eclipse.org/modeling/emf/.

Emmerich, W. (2000). *Engineering distributed objects.* New York, NY: John Wiley & Sons.

Enderle, J., Blanchard, S. M., & Bronzino, J. (2005). *Introduction to biomedical engineering* (2nd ed.). New York, NY: Academic Press.

ENDOCAS. (2011). *Website.* Retrieved from http://www.endocas.org.

England, I., Steward, D., & Walker, S. (2000). Information technology adoption in health care: When organizations and technology collide. *Australian Health Review, 23*(3), 176–185. doi:10.1071/AH000176

EPCGlobal Inc. (2008). *EPC™ radio-frequency identity protocols class-1 generation-2 UHF RFID protocol for communications at 860 MHz – 960 MHz version 1.2.0.* New York, NY: EPCGlobal, Inc.

Epocrates. (2011). *Website.* Retrieved February 9, 2011, from http://itunes.apple.com/us/app/epocrates/id281935788?mt=8#.

Esbjörnsson, M., & Vesterlind, D. (2002). *Mobility and social spatiality.* Paper presented at the Workshop Transforming Spaces: The Topological Turn in Technology Studies. Darmstadt, Germany.

Escobar, A. (2001). Culture sits in places: Reflections on globalism and subaltern strategies of localization. *Political Geography, 20,* 139–174. doi:10.1016/S0962-6298(00)00064-0

Eudon, K. K. (2008). *Video streaming over 802.11b in the presence of fading due to human traffic and Bluetooth interference.* MSc Thesis. New Brunswick, Canada: University of New Brunswick.

European Commission. (1999a). *Directive 1999/5/EC of the European parliament and of the council on radio equipment and telecommunications terminal equipment and the mutual recognition of their conformity.* Geneva, Switzerland: Official Journal of the European Communities.

European Commission. (1999b). *Council recommendation 1999/519/EC on the limitation of exposure of the general public to electromagnetic fields (0 Hz to 300 GHz).* Geneva, Switzerland: Official Journal of the European Communities.

Evans, P., & Wurster, T. S. (2000). *Blown to bits: How the new economics of information transforms strategy.* Boston, MA: Harvard Business School Press.

Eysenbach, G. (2001). What is e-health? *Journal of Medical Internet Research, 3*(2), 20. Retrieved from http://www.jmir.org/2001/2/e20/; doi: 10.2196/jmir.3.2.e20; PMID, 11720962.

Eysenbach, G. (2006). Infodemiology: Tracking flu-related searches on the web for syndromic surveillance. In *Proceedings of the AMIA Annual Symposium,* (pp. 244-248). AMIA. Retrieved from http://www.pubmedcentral.nih.gov/articlerender.fcgi?tool=pubmed&pubmedid=17238340.

Eysenbach, G. (2000). Recent advances: Consumer health informatics. *British Medical Journal, 320*(7251), 1713. doi:10.1136/bmj.320.7251.1713

Eysenbach, G. (2001). What is e-health? *Journal of Medical Internet Research, 3*(2), e20. doi:10.2196/jmir.3.2.e20

Faridi, Z., Liberti, L., Shuval, K., Northrup, V., Ali, A., & Katz, D. (2008). Evaluating the impact of mobile telephone technology on type 2 diabetic patients' self-management: The NICHE pilot study. *Journal of Evaluation in Clinical Practice, 14*(3), 465–469. doi:10.1111/j.1365-2753.2007.00881.x

FCC. (1997). *Evaluating compliance with FCC-specified guidelines for human exposure to radiofrequency electromagnetic fields. OET Bulletin 65.* Washington, DC: FCC.

FCC. (2010). *Federal communications commission – FCC - 10-129.* Retrieved March 05, 2011, from http://www.fcc.gov/Daily_Releases/Daily_Business/2010/db0720/FCC-10-129A1.pdf.

Felizardo, V. (2010). *Validação do acelerómetro xyzplux para estimação do gasto energético com aquisição de dados de diversos parâmetros fisiológicos.* MSc Thesis. Covilhã, Portugal: University of Beira Interior. Retrieved from http://allab.it.ubi.pt/images/documents/disertacao_%20virginie.pdf.

Felshin, N. (Ed.). (1995). *But is it art? The spirit of art as activism.* Seattle, WA: Bay Press.

Ferguson, J. (2006). How to do a telemedical consultation. *Journal of Telemedicine and Telecare, 12*(5), 220–227. doi:10.1258/135763306777889037

FFEHR. (2011). *Web page.* Retrieved May 12, 2011, from http://trac.afterfivetech.com/ffehr.

Fickenscher, K., & Bakerman, M. (2011). Leadership and governance for IT projects. *Physician Executive, 37*(1), 72–76.

Field, M. J. (1996). *Telemedicine: A guide to assessing telecommunications in health care.* Washington, DC: National Academy Press.

Fieschi, M. (2002). Information technology is changing the way society sees health care delivery. *International Journal of Medical Informatics, 66,* 85–93. doi:10.1016/S1386-5056(02)00040-0

Filho, J. B., Miron, A. D., Satoh, I., Gensel, J., & Martin, H. (2010). Modeling and measuring quality of context information in pervasive environments. In *Proceedings of the 24th IEEE International Conference on Advanced Information Networking and Applications,* (pp. 690–697). Perth, Australia: IEEE Press.

Finley, S. (2008). Arts-based inquiry: Performing revolutionary pedagogy. In Denzin, N. K., & Lincoln, Y. S. (Eds.), *Collecting and Interpreting Qualitative Materials* (pp. 75–113). Los Angeles, CA: Sage Publications, Inc.

Fioravanti, F., Inchingolo, P., Valenzin, G., & Dalla Palma, L. (1997). The DPACS project at the University of Trieste. *International Journal of Medical Informatics, 22*(4), 301–314. doi:10.3109/14639239709010902

Fjeldsoe, B. S., Marshall, A. L., & Miller, Y. D. (2009). Behavior change interventions delivered by mobile telephone short-message service. *American Journal of Preventive Medicine, 36*(2), 165–173. doi:10.1016/j.amepre.2008.09.040

Fjeldsoe, B., Marshall, A., & Miller, Y. (2009). Behavior change interventions delivered by mobile telephone short-message service. *American Journal of Preventive Medicine, 36*(2), 165–173. doi:10.1016/j.amepre.2008.09.040

Flexman, J. (2007). Alternative careers for biomedical engineers. *IEEE Engineering in Medicine and Biology Magazine, 26*(5), 10–11. doi:10.1109/EMB.2007.906029

Folea, S., Avram, C., Vidican, S., & Astilean, A. (2010). Telemonitoring system of neurological signs in a health telematique network. *International Journal of E-Health and Medical Communications, 1*(4), 14–33. doi:10.4018/jehmc.2010100102

Folea, S., & Ghercioiu, M. (2010). Tag4M, a Wi-Fi RFID active tag optimized for sensor measurements. In Turcu, C. (Ed.), *Radio Frequency Identification Fundamentals and Applications Design Methods and Solutions* (pp. 287–310). PA, Austria: InTech Education and Publishing.

Folea, S., Ghercioiu, M., & Ursuţiu, D. (2010). cloud instrument powered by solar cell sends data to pachube. *International Journal of Online Engineering, 6*(4), 20–25.

Forslund, D. W., Joyce, E. L., Burr, T., Picard, R., Wokoun, D., & Umland, E. (2004). Setting standards for improved syndromic surveillance: The importance of using standard, distributed components for medical surveillance for discovering and managing a public health threat. *IEEE Engineering in Medicine and Biology Magazine, 24*(1), 65–70. doi:10.1109/MEMB.2004.1297176

Fox, S. (2010). Mobile health 2010. *Pew Internet and American Life Project*. Retrieved November, 2010 from http://pewinternet.org/~/media//Files/Reports/2010/PIP_Mobile_Health_2010.pdf.

Fox, S., & Jones, S. (2009). The social life of health information. *Pew Internet and American Life Project*. Retrieved November, 2010 from http://www.pewinternet.org/~/media//Files/Reports/2009/PIP_Health_2009.pdf.

Fox, M. (2009). A systematic review of the literature reporting on studies that examined the impact of interactive, computer-based patient education programs. *Patient Education and Counseling, 77*(1), 6–13. doi:10.1016/j.pec.2009.02.011

Fraser, H. S., Blaya, J., Choi, S. S., Bonilla, C., & Jazayeri, D. (2006). Evaluating the impact and costs of deploying an electronic medical record system to support TB treatment in Peru. In *Proceedings of the AMIA Annual Symposium,* (pp. 264–268). AMIA.

Fraser, H. S., Biondich, P., Moodley, D., Choi, S., Mamlin, B. W., & Szolovits, P. (2005). Implementing electronic medical record systems in developing countries. *Informatics in Primary Care, 13*(2), 83–95.

Fraser, H. S., Jazayeri, D., Nevil, P., Karacaoglu, Y., Farmer, P. E., & Lyon, E. (2004). An information system and medical record to support HIV treatment in rural Haiti. *British Medical Journal, 329*(7475), 1142–1146. doi:10.1136/bmj.329.7475.1142

Freeman, W. D., Vatz, K. A., & Demaerschalk, B. M. (2010). Telemedicine in 2010: Robotic caveats. *The Lancet Neurology, 9*(11), 1046. doi:10.1016/S1474-4422(10)70261-1

FreeMED. (2011). *Web page*. Retrieved May 12, 2011, from http://freemedsoftware.org.

FreeMedForms. (2011). *Web page*. Retrieved May 12, 2011, from http://www.freemedforms.com/en/start.

Freescale Semiconductor. (2009). *High temperature accuracy integrated silicon pressure sensor for measuring absolute pressure, on-chip signal conditioned, temperature compensated and calibrated.* Technical Report. Retrieved from www.freescale.com.

Frerichs, R. R. (1991). *Epidemiologic surveillance in developing countries. Annual Revision Public Health* (pp. 257–280). Los Angeles, CA: University of California.

Friedman, T. L. (2006). *The world is flat: A brief history of the twenty-first century*. New York, NY: Farrar Straus Giroux.

Frisse, M. E. (2009). Health information technology: One step at a time. *Health Affairs, n.d.*, 379–w384. doi:10.1377/hlthaff.28.2.w379

Frühwirth, T., Molwitz, J. R., & Brisset, P. (1996). Planning cordless business communication systems. *IEEE Expert Magazine. Special Track on Intelligent Telecommunications, 11*(1), 50–55.

Fry, E. A., & Lenert, L. A. (2005). MASCAL: RFID tracking of patients, staff and equipment to enhance hospital response to mass casualty events. In *Proceedings of the AMIA Annual Symposium Proceedings,* (pp. 261 – 265). San Diego, CA: AMIA.

Fu, H., Chen, Z., & Dai, X. (1995). The research on MiniPACS: Abstract. In *Proceedings of the 7th Annual Meeting of Chinese Society of Radiology,* (pp. 585-586). Beijing, China: Chinese Society of Radiology.

Fu, H., et al. (2006). The retrospective of PACS development in China. In *Proceedings of the 1st China Symposium of PACS-RIS,* (pp. 22-29). Beijing, China: PACS-RIS.

Fu, H., Jin, Z., Dai, J., Chen, K., Wang, T., Li, T., & Gao, P. (2003). Picture archiving and communication system in China: The development, problem, and integrating strategy with IHE. *International Congress Series, 1256*, 915–923. doi:10.1016/S0531-5131(03)00246-2

Fung, Y. C. (1996). *Biomechanics* (2nd ed.). New York, NY: Springer-Verlag.

Fuschini, F., Piersanti, C., Sydanheimo, L., Ukkonen, L., & Falciasecca, G. (2010). Electromagnetic analyses of near field UHF RFID systems. *IEEE Transactions on Antennas and Propagation, 58*(5), 1759–1770. doi:10.1109/TAP.2010.2044328

G2 Microsystems. (2008). *G2C547 SoC data sheet.* Technical Report. Retrieved from www.g2microsystems.com.

G2 Microsystems. (2008). *G2C547 software, example application.* Technical Report. Retrieved from www.g2microsystems.com.

G2 Microsystems. (2008). *G2M5477 wi-fi module data sheet.* Technical Report. Retrieved from www.g2microsystems.com.

Gaggioli, A., Di Carlo, S., Mantovani, F., Castelnuovo, G., & Riva, G. (2005). A telemedicine survey among Milan doctors. *Journal of Telemedicine and Telecare, 11*(1), 29–34. doi:10.1258/1357633053430476

Gagnon, M.-P., Lamothe, L., Fortin, J.-P., Cloutier, A., Godin, G., Gagné, C., & Reinharz, D. (2005). Telehealth adoption in hospitals: An organisational perspective. *Journal of Health Organization and Management, 19*(1), 32–56. doi:10.1108/14777260510592121

Gandhi, O. P., & Aslan, E. (1995). *Human equivalent antenna for electromagnetic fields.* US Patent no.5394164. Washington, DC: US Patent Office.

Gang, L., Krishnamachari, B., & Raghavendra, C. S. (2004). Performance evaluation of the IEEE 802.15.4 MAC for low-rate low-power wireless networks. In *Proceedings of the IEEE International Conference on Performance, Computing and Communications,* (pp. 701 - 706). Phoenix, AZ: IEEE Press.

Ganti, R. K., Jayachandran, P., Abdelzaher, T. F., & Stankovic, J. A. (2006). SATIRE: A software architecture for smart attire. In *Proceedings of MobiSys 2006.* Uppsala, Sweden: ACM Press.

Gao, X. W., Lin, C., & Tully, C. (Eds.). (2005). *Proceedings of medical imaging and telemedicine (MIT 2005).* Wuyi, China: MIT.

Gao, X. W., Müller, H., Loomes, M., Comley, R., & Luo, S. (Eds.). (2008). *Lecture notes in computer science,* (vol 4987). Berlin, Germany: Springer.

Gao, X., Qian, Y., Hui, R., Loomes, M., Comley, R., Barn, B., et al. (2010). Texture-based 3D image retrieval for medical applications. In *IADIS e-Health2010,* (pp. 101-108). IADIS.

Gao, X. W., Hui, R., Tian, Z., & White, A. (2009). A new approach to estimation of non-isotropic scale factors for correction of MR distortions. *International Journal of Computer Assisted Radiology and Surgery, 4*(1), 349–350.

Garcia, N. M., Tavares, P., Miguel, R., Trindade, I., Lucas, J., & Pereira, M. (2011). *Resilient heart-beat detection algorithm for signals captured by smart-textiles.* Paper presented at the AUTEX 2011 - 11th World Textile Conference. Mulhouse, France.

Garfield, E. (1987). Exploring the frontiers of biomedical-engineering - An overview of historical and current considerations. *Current Contents, 9*(10), 3–11.

Garg, A. X., Adhikari, N. K. J., McDonald, H., Rosas-Arellano, M. P., Devereaux, P. J., & Beyene, J. (2005). Effects of computerized clinical decision support systems on practitioner performance and patient outcomes: A systematic review. *Journal of the American Medical Association, 293*(10), 1223–1238. doi:10.1001/jama.293.10.1223

Garlan, D., Allen, R., & Ockerbloom, J. (1994). Exploiting style in architectural design environments. In *Proceedings of the SIGSOFT 1994 Symposium on the Foundations of Software Engineering,* (pp. 175 – 188). SIGSOFT.

Gauci, C., Melillo Fenech, T., Gilles, H., O'Brien, S., Mamo, J., & Stabile, I. (2007). Sentinel surveillance: An option for surveillance of infection intestinal diseases. *Eurosurveillance, 12,* 129–132.

George, J. M., & Jones, G. R. (2000). The role of time in theory and theory building. *Journal of Management, 26*(4), 657–684.

Gerber, T. (2009). Health information technology: Dispatches from the revolution. *Health Affairs, n.d.,* 390–w391. doi:10.1377/hlthaff.28.2.w390

German, R. R., & the CDC Guidelines Working Group. (2011). *Updated guidelines for evaluating public health surveillance system.* Retrieved March 18, 2011, from http://www.cdc.gov/mmwr/preview/mmwrhtml/rr5013a1.htm.

Ghista, D. N. (2000). Biomedical engineering: Yesterday, today, and tomorrow. *IEEE Engineering in Medicine and Biology Magazine, 19*(6), 23–28. doi:10.1109/51.887243

GHO. (2011). *Global health observatory.* Retrieved February 11, 2011, from http://apps.who.int/ghodata/.

Gholiha, A., Fransson, G., Fürst, C. J., Heedman, P. A., Lundström, S., & Axelsson, B. (2011). Big gaps in documentation of end-of-life care: Incomplete medical records reported to the Swedish registry of palliative care. *Lakartidningen, 108*(16-17), 918–921.

Gibbs, P., & Asada, H. H. (2005). Reducing motion artifact in wearable bio-sensors using MEMS accelerometers for active noise cancellation. *American Control Conference, 3*(1), 1581 – 1586.

Giddens, A. (1984). *The constitution of society*. Cambridge, UK: Polity Press.

Giddens, A. (1990). *The consequences of modernity*. Palo Alto, CA: Stanford University Press.

GIFT. (2011). *Website.* Retrieved from http://www.gnu.org/software/gift/.

Ginsberg, J., Mohebbi, M. H., Patel, R. S., Brammer, L., Smolinski, M. S., & Brilliant, L. (2009). Detecting influenza epidemics using search engine query data. *Nature, n.d.*, 457.

Gitlow, H. S., Oppenheim, A. J., Oppenheim, R., & Levine, D. M. (2005). *Quality management* (3rd ed.). Singapore: McGraw-Hill.

Giurgiutiu, V., & Yu, L. (2003). *Comparison of short-time Fourier transform and wavelet transform of transient and tone burst wave propagation signals for structural health monitoring*. Paper presented at the 4th International Workshop on Structural Health Monitoring. Palo Alto, CA.

GNUmed. (2011). *Web page.* Retrieved May 12, 2011, from http://wiki.gnumed.de/bin/view/Gnumed.

Goel, A., & Estrin, D. (2003). Simultaneous optimization for concave costs: Single sink aggregation or single source buy-at-bulk. In *Proceedings of ACM-SIAM Symposium on Discrete Algorithms,* (pp. 499-505). Baltimore, MD: ACM Press.

Gold, J., Lim, M. S., Hellard, M. E., Hocking, J. S., & Keogh, L. (2010). What's in a message? Delivering sexual health promotion to young people in Australia via text messaging. *BMC Public Health, 10*, 792. doi:10.1186/1471-2458-10-792

Golmie, N., Cypher, D., & Rebala, O. (2005). Performance analysis of low-rate wireless technologies for medical applications. *Elsevier Computer Communications, 28*(10), 1266–1275.

Gomes, A. T. A., Ziviani, A., Souza e Silva, N. A., & Feijóo, R. A. (2006). Towards a ubiquitous healthcare system for acute myocardial infarction patients in Brazil. In *Proceedings of the IEEE International Workshop on Pervasive and Ubiquitous Health Care – UbiCare 2006,* (pp. 585-589). IEEE Press.

Grade. (2011). *Website.* Retrieved from http://www.4panda.com/chinamedtreat/chinahospitals/grade.htm.

Graff, L. G., & Robinson, D. (2001). Abdominal pain and emergency department evaluation. *Emergency Medicine Clinics of North America, 19*(1), 123–136. doi:10.1016/S0733-8627(05)70171-1

Graham, L. (2008). Gestalt theory in interactive media design. *Gestalt Theory, 2*(1).

Graham, S. (1998). The end of geography or the explosion of place? Conceptualizing space, place and information technology. *Progress in Human Geography, 22*(2), 165–185. doi:10.1191/030913298671334137

Grayson, A. C. R., Shawgo, R. S., & Johnson, A. M. (2004). A biomems review: Mems technology for physiologically integrated devices. *Proceedings of the IEEE, 92*(1), 6–21. doi:10.1109/JPROC.2003.820534

Green, N. (2002). On the move: Technology, mobility, and the mediation of social time and space. *The Information Society, 18*, 281–292. doi:10.1080/01972240290075129

Greenstain, S., & Khanna, T. (1997). What does industry convergence mean. In Yoffie, D. B. (Ed.), *Competing in the Age of Digital Convergence* (pp. 201–226). Boston, MA: Harvard Business School Press.

Grigsby, J., & Sanders, J. H. (1998). Telemedicine: Where it is and where it's going. *Annals of Internal Medicine, 129*, 123–127.

Grimaldi, G., & Manto, M. (2010). Neurological tremor: Sensors, signal processing and emerging applications. *Sensors (Basel, Switzerland), 10*, 1399–1422. doi:10.3390/s100201399

Grimes, S. L. (2003). The future of clinical engineering: The challenge of change. *IEEE Engineering in Medicine and Biology Magazine, 22*(2), 91–99. doi:10.1109/MEMB.2003.1195702

Grimes, S. L. (2004a). Clinical notes: Opportunities and challenges in clinical engineering. *IEEE Engineering in Medicine and Biology Magazine, 23*(2), 94–95. doi:10.1109/MEMB.2004.1310991

Grimes, S. L. (2004b). Clinical engineers: Stewards of healthcare technologies. *IEEE Engineering in Medicine and Biology Magazine, 23*(3), 56–58. doi:10.1109/MEMB.2004.1317982

Grönroos, C. (1990). *Service management and marketing: Managing the moments of truth in service competition.* New Britian, CT: Lexington Books.

Grossmann, M., Hönle, N., Lübbe, C., & Weinschrott, H. (2009). An abstract processing model for the quality of context data. In *Proceedings of the 1st International Conference on Quality of Context*, (pp. 132–143). Berlin, Germany: Springer.

Grubb, A. (2010). Non-invasive estimation of glomerular filtration rate (GFR): The Lund model: Simultaneous use of cystatin C- and creatinine-based GFR-prediction equations, clinical data and an internal quality check. *Scandinavian Journal of Clinical and Laboratory Investigation, 70*(2), 65–70. doi:10.3109/00365511003642535

Guide to Career Education. (2011). *Website.* Retrieved from http://www.guidetocareereducation.com/careers/biomedical-engineering.

GuidelinesICNIRP (1998). Guidelines for limiting exposure to time-varying electric, magnetic, and electromagnetic fields. *Health Physics, 74*(4), 494–522.

Guo, L., Huang, Z. L., Gan, L. Y., Yang, J., & Jing, Q. (2006). Introduction to HIS/RIS at Beijing general army hospital (in Chinese). In *Proceedings of First Symposium of ChinaPACS-RIS*. ChinaPACS-RIS.

Gvozdanović, D., Koncar, M., Kojundzić, V., & Jezidzić, H. (2007). National healthcare information system in Croatian primary care: The foundation for improvement of quality and efficiency in patient care. *Journal of Informatics in Primary Care, 15,* 181–185.

Hadim, S., & Mohamed, N. (2006). Middleware challenges and approaches for wireless sensor networks. *IEEE Distributed Systems Online, 7*(3).

Hagler, S., Austin, D., Hayes, T. L., Kaye, J., & Pavel, M. (2010). Unobtrusive and ubiquitous in-home monitoring: a methodology for continuous assessment of gait velocity in elders. *IEEE Transactions on Bio-Medical Engineering, 57*(4), 813–820. doi:10.1109/TBME.2009.2036732

Haidegger, T., Sándor, J., & Benyo, Z. (2011). Surgery in space: The future of robotic telesurgery. *Surgical Endoscopy, 25*(3), 681–690. doi:10.1007/s00464-010-1243-3

Hailey, D., Ohinmaa, A., & Roine, R. (2004). Study quality and evidence of benefit in recent assessments of telemedicine. *Journal of Telemedicine and Telecare, 10*(6), 318–324. doi:10.1258/1357633042602053

Hailpern, B., & Tarr, P. (2006). Model-driven development: The good, the bad, and the ugly. *IBM Systems Journal, 45*(3), 451–461. doi:10.1147/sj.453.0451

Hall, E. T. (1983). *The dance of life: The other dimension of time.* Garden City, NY: Anchor Press.

Hansen, T. R., Bardram, J. E., & Soegaard, M. (2006). Moving out of the lab: Deploying pervasive technologies in a hospital. In *Proceedings of the IEEE Pervasive Computing*, (pp. 24–31). IEEE Press.

Hanser, F., Gruenerbl, A., Rodegast, C., & Lukowicz, P. (2008). Design and real life deployment of a pervasive monitoring system for dementia patients. In *Proceedings of the Second International Conference on Pervasive Computing Technologies for Healthcare*, (pp. 279-280). IEEE.

Hanson, J. (2005). *Event-driven services in SOA.* Javaworld.

Harmon, L. D. (1975). Biomedical engineering education: How to do what, with which, and to whom. *IEEE Transactions on Bio-Medical Engineering, 22,* 89–94. doi:10.1109/TBME.1975.324424

Harrington, L., Kennerly, D., & Johnson, C. (2011). Safety issues related to the electronic medical record (EMR): Synthesis of the literature from the last decade, 2000-2009. *Journal of Healthcare Management, 56*(1), 31–43.

Harris, M., & Habetha, J. (2007). The MyHeart project: A framework for personal healh care applications. *Computers in Cardiology, 34,* 137–140.

Harrison, S., & Dourish, P. (1996). Re-place-ing space: The roles of place and space in collaborative systems. In *Proceedings of CSCW 1996*. Cambridge, MA: ACM Press.

Harris, T. R., Bransford, J. D., & Brophy, S. P. (2002). Roles for learning sciences and learning technologies in biomedical engineering education: A review of recent advances. *Annual Review of Biomedical Engineering, 4*, 29–48. doi:10.1146/annurev.bioeng.4.091701.125502

Harrop, V. M. (2002). *Digital diffusion in the clinical trenches: Findings from a telemedicine needs assessment*. Cambridge, MA: MIT Press. Retrieved from http://mit.dspace.org/handle/1721.1/8315.

Harvey, D. (1989). *The Condition of postmodernity*. Oxford, UK: Blackwell.

Hashemi, H. (1993). The indoor radio propagation channel. *Proceedings of the IEEE, 81*(7), 943–968. doi:10.1109/5.231342

Hasman, A., Haux, R., & Albert, A. (1996). A systematic view on medical informatics. *Computer Methods and Programs in Biomedicine, 51*(3), 131–139. doi:10.1016/S0169-2607(96)01769-5

Haux, R. (2006). Health information systems - Past, present, future. *International Journal of Medical Informatics, 75*, 268–281. doi:10.1016/j.ijmedinf.2005.08.002

Haux, R., Ammenwerth, E., Herzog, W., & Knaup, P. (2002). Health care in the information society: A prognosis for the year 2013. *International Journal of Medical Informatics, 66*, 3–21. doi:10.1016/S1386-5056(02)00030-8

Hawrylak, P. J., Cain, J. T., & Mickle, M. H. (2008). RFID tags. In Yan, L., Zhang, Y., Yang, L. T., & Ning, H. (Eds.), *The Internet of Things: From RFID to Pervasive Networked Systems* (pp. 1–32). Boca Raton, FL: Auerbach Publications, Taylor & Francis Group. doi:10.1201/9781420052824.ch1

Hawrylak, P. J., & Mickle, M. H. (2010). EPC gen-2 standard for RFID. In Yan, L., Zhang, Y., Yang, L. T., & Chen, J. (Eds.), *RFID and Sensor Networks: Architectures, Protocols, Security, and Integrations* (pp. 97–123). Boca Raton, FL: Auerbach Publications, Taylor & Francis Group.

Haynes, K., Linkin, D. R., Fishman, N., Bilker, W. B., Strom, B. L., Pifer, E. A., & Hennessy, S. (2011). Effectiveness of an information technology intervention to improve prophylactic antibacterial use in the postoperative period. *Journal of the American Medical Informatics Association, 18*, 164–168. doi:10.1136/jamia.2009.002998

Häyrinen, K., Saranto, K., & Nykänen, P. (2008). Definition, structure, content, use and impacts of electronic health records: A review of the research literature. *International Journal of Medical Informatics, 77*(5), 291–304. doi:10.1016/j.ijmedinf.2007.09.001

HealthForge. (2011). *Web page*. Retrieved May 12, 2011, from http://healthforge.codeplex.com.

HealthService24 Project. (2009). *Website*. Retrieved from http://www.healthservice24.com/.

HeartWise Blood Pressure Tracker for iPad. (2010). *Website*. Retrieved February 22, 2011, from http://itunes.apple.com/us/app/heartwise-blood-pressure-tracker/id364899989?mt=8#.

Hebert, M. (2001). Telehealth success: Evaluation framework development. In Patel, V. L., Rogers, R., & Haux, R. (Eds.), *MEDINFO 2001* (pp. 1145–1149). Amsterdam, The Netherlands: IOS Press.

Heimbigner, D. (2011). A tamper-resistant programming language system. *IEEE Transactions on Dependable and Secure Computing, 8*(2), 194–206. doi:10.1109/TDSC.2010.51

Heinzelman, W. B., Chandrakasan, A. P., & Balakrishnan, H. (2002). An application-specific protocol architecture for wireless microsensor networks. *IEEE Transactions on Wireless Communications, 1*(4), 660–670. doi:10.1109/TWC.2002.804190

Hemming, L. H. (2002). *Electromagnetic anechoic chambers: A fundamental design and specification guide*. New York, NY: John Wiley & Sons Inc.

Hendee, W. R., Chien, S., Maynard, C. D., & Dean, D. J. (2002). The national institute of biomedical imaging and bioengineering: History, status, and potential impact. *Annals of Biomedical Engineering, 30*(1), 2–10. doi:10.1114/1.1433491

Henricksen, K., & Indulska, J. (2004). Modelling and using imperfect context information. In *Proceedings of the Conference on Pervasive Computing and Communications Workshops*, (pp. 33 – 37). IEEE.

Henricksen, K., Indulska, J., & Rakotonirainy, A. (2009). Modeling context information in pervasive computing systems. In *Proceedings of the First International Conference on Pervasive Computing*, (pp. 167 – 180). London, UK: IEEE Press.

Hensher, M., Price, M., & Adomakoh, S. (2006). Referral hospitals. In Jamison, D., Breman, J., Measham, A., Alleyne, G., Claeson, M., & Evans, D. (Eds.), *Disease Control Priorities in Developing Countries* (2nd ed., pp. 1229–1244). New York, NY: Oxford University Press.

HER/PHR. (2011). *Website.* Retrieved from http://www.hl7.org/implement/standards/ehrphr.cfm.

Hertleer, C., Troquo, A., Rogier, H., & Langenhove, L. V. (2008). The use of textile materials to design wearable microstrip patch antennas. *Textile Research Journal, 78*(8), 651–658. doi:10.1177/0040517507083726

Heymsfield, S. B., & Wang, Z. (1996). Human body composition: Conceptual advances. In *Progress in Obesity Research* (pp. 245–257). London, UK: John Libbey & Co.

Hibernate. (2010). *Web page.* Retrieved December 14, 2010, from http://www.hibernate.org.

HIMSS. (2011). *Electronic health record (HER).* Retrieved on June 16, 2011 from http://www.himss.org/ASP/topics_ehr.asp.

Hirata, A., Fujiwara, O., Nagaoka, T., & Watanabe, S. (2010). Estimation of whole-body average SAR in human models due to plane-wave exposure at resonance frequency. *IEEE Transactions on Electromagnetic Compatibility, 52*(1), 41–48. doi:10.1109/TEMC.2009.2035613

Hjelm, N. (2005). Benefits and drawbacks of telemedicine. *Journal of Telemedicine and Telecare, 11*(2), 60–70. doi:10.1258/1357633053499886

HL7. (2010). *Web page.* Retrieved December 14, 2010, from http://www.hl7.org.

HL7. (2011). *Health level seven international.* Retrieved January 28, 2011, from http://www.HL7.org.

HMN. (2008). *Framework and standards for country health information systems - Health metrics network.* Geneva, Switzerland: World Health Organization.

Honeybourne, C., Sutton, S., & Ward, L. (2006). Knowledge in palm of your hands: PDAs in the clinical setting. *Health Information Library Journal, 23*(1), 51-59. Retrieved from http://www.ncbi.nlm.nih.gov/pubmed/16466499.

Honeywell. (2010). *HIH 5030/5031 series, low voltage humidity sensors.* Technical Report. Retrieved from http://sensing.honeywell.com.

Hoque, E., Dickerson, R. F., & Stankovic, J. A. (2010). Monitoring body positions and movements during sleep using WISPs. In *Proceedings of Wireless Health, 2010*, 44–53.

Hornak, J. P. (2011). *The basics of MRI.* Retrieved from http://www.cis.rit.edu/htbooks/mri/.

Horsley, V., & Clarke, R. H. (1908). The structure and functions of the cerebellum examined by a new method. *Brain, 31*, 45–125. doi:10.1093/brain/31.1.45

Hospital, O. S. (2011). *Web page.* Retrieved May 12, 2011, from http://www.hospital-os.com/en.

HOSxP. (2011). *Web page.* Retrieved May 12, 2011, from http://hosxp.net.

Hounsfield, G. N. (1973). Computerized transverse axial scanning (tomography). *The British Journal of Radiology, 46*, 1016–1022. doi:10.1259/0007-1285-46-552-1016

Hsieh, R. K. C., Hjelm, N. M., Lee, J. C. K., & Aldis, J. W. (2001). Telemedicine in China. *International Journal of Medical Informatics, 61*(2), 139–146. doi:10.1016/S1386-5056(01)00136-8

HTML. (2010). *Web page.* Retrieved December 14, 2010, from http://www.w3.org/html.

Huang, H. K., & Taira, R. K. (1992). Infrastructure design of a picture archiving and communication system. *AJR. American Journal of Roentgenology, 158*, 743–749.

Hurford, R., Martin, A., & Larsen, P. (2006). *Designing wearables.* Paper presented at the 10th IEEE International Symposium on Wearable Computers. Montreaux, Canada.

iArthritis. (2009). *Website.* Retrieved February 22, 2011, from http://itunes.apple.com/us/app/iarthritis/id322993302?mt=8.

iAsthma in Control. (2010). *Website*. Retrieved February 22, 2011, from http://itunes.apple.com/us/app/iasthma-in-control/id329847125?mt=8#.

Ibis. (2011). *Evidence based public health practice*. Retrieved March 19, 2011, from http://ibis.health.state.nm.us/resources/EvidenceBased.html.

ICD. (2011). *International classification of diseases*. Retrieved January 20, 2011, from http://www.who.int/classifications/icd/en/.

ICF. (2011). *International classification of functioning, disability and health*. Retrieved January 20, 2011, from http://www.who.int/classifications/icf/en/.

IEEE. (1999). *IEEE C95.1-1991: Safety levels with respect to human exposure to radio frequency electromagnetic fields, 3 KHz to 300 GHz*. New York, NY: IEEE Press.

IEEE. (2003). *ANSI/IEEE standard 149-1965, revision of standard 149-1979 test procedures for antennas*. New York, NY: IEEE Press.

IEEE. 802.15.4 Std. (2003). *Wireless medium access control (MAC) and physical layer (PHY) specification for low-rate wireless personal area networks (LR-WPANs)*. New York, NY: IEEE Press.

IEEE. Engineering in Medicine and Biology Society. (2011). *Website*. Retrieved from http://www.embs.org.

iFirstAid. (2011). *Website*. Retrieved February 22, 2011, from http://itunes.apple.com/us/app/ifirstaid-lite/id295238909?mt=8#.

IHE. (2011). *Website*. Retrieved from http://www.ihe.net.

Image, C. L. E. F. (2011). *Website*. Retrieved from http://www.imageclef.org/.

Imhoff, M., Webb, A., & Goldschmidt, A. (2001). Health informatics. *Intensive Care Medicine*, 27(1), 179–186.

Inchingolo, P. (2005). Synergy of bioengineering, organizational and economical methodologies for the success of the e-health integration at wide national and international levels. In X. Gao, et al. (Eds.), *Proceedings of MIT 2005 International Conference on Medical Imaging and Telemedicine*. Beijing, China: MIT.

Inchingolo, P. (2008). The open three consortium: An open-source initiative at the service of healthcare and inclusion. *Lecture Notes in Computer Science, 4987*, 5–11. doi:10.1007/978-3-540-79490-5_2

Indivo. (2011). *Web page*. Retrieved May 12, 2011, from http://indivohealth.org.

Indulska, J., Robinson, R., Rakotonirainy, A., & Henricksen, K. (2003). Experiences in using CC/PP in context-aware systems. In *Proceedings of the 4th International Conference on Mobile Data Management*, (pp. 247–261). Springer.

Intanagonwiwat, C., Estrin, D., Govindan, R., & Heidemann, J. (2002). Impact of network density on data aggregation in wireless sensor networks. In *Proceedings of the 22nd International Conference on Distributed Systems*, (pp. 457-458). Vienna, Austria: IEEE.

International Society of Biomechanics (ISB). (2011). *Website*. Retrieved from http://isbweb.org.

IOM. (2001). *Crossing the quality chasm: A new health system for the 21st century*. Washington, DC: National Academy Press.

iRadiology. (2009). *Website*. Retrieved February 22, 2011, from http://itunes.apple.com/us/app/iradiology/id346440355?mt=8.

ISO. (2008). *ISO 13606 - Health informatics - Electronic health record communication*. Geneva, Switzerland: International Organization for Standardization (ISO).

ISO/IEC 18000-6. (2010). *Information technology -- Radio frequency identification for item management -- Part 6: Parameters for air interface communications at 860 MHz to 960 MHz*. Geneva, Switzerland: International Organization for Standardization.

ISO/IEC 18000-7. (2009). *Information technology — Radio frequency identification (RFID) for item management — Part 7: Parameters for active RFID air interface communications at 433 MHz*. Geneva, Switzerland: International Organization for Standardization.

Istepanian, R., & Lacal, J. (2003). Emerging mobile communication technologies for health: Some imperative notes on m-health. In *Proceedings of the 25th Silver 59 Anniversary International Conference of the IEEE Engineering in Medicine and Biology Society*. Cancun, Mexico: IEEE Press.

Istepanian, R. (1999). Telemedicine in the United Kingdom: Current status and future prospects. *IEEE Transactions on Information Technology in Biomedicine, 3*(2), 158–159. doi:10.1109/4233.767091

Istepanian, R., Laxminarayan, S., & Pattichis, C. S. (Eds.). (2006). *M-Health.* New York, NY: Springer. doi:10.1007/b137697

Ito, S., & Okuno, K. (2010). Visualization and motion analysis of swimming. In *Proceedings of the 8th Conference of the International Sports Engineering Association (ISEA).* London, UK: Elsevier.

Jacob, N., & Reddy, K. T. V. (2011). Smart hospital using RFID and ZigBee technology. In *Proceedings of the International Conference & Workshop on Emerging Trends in Technology (ICWET 2011),* (pp. 987-989). New York, NY: ACM Press.

Jacobs, J. E. (1975). The biomedical engineering quandary. *IEEE Transactions on Bio-Medical Engineering, 22,* 100–106. doi:10.1109/TBME.1975.324426

Jahn, A., & De Brouwere, V. (2001). Referral in pregnancy and childbirth: Concepts and strategies. In De Brouwere, V., & Van Lerberghe, W. (Eds.), *Studies in Health Services Organisation & Policy 17* (pp. 229–246). Antwerp, Belgium: ITG Press.

Jain, A., Wim, L., Martens, J., Mutz, G., Weiss, R. K., & Stephan, E. (1996). Towards a comprehensive technology for recording and analysis of multiple physiological parameters within their behavioral and environmental context. *Journal of Psychophysiology, 13*(13).

Janamanchi, B., Katsamakas, E., Raghupathi, W., & Gao, W. (2009). The state and profile of open source software projects in health and medical informatics. *International Journal of Medical Informatics, 78*(7), 457–472. doi:10.1016/j.ijmedinf.2009.02.006

Jantunen, I., Wang, X., Pekkola, M., & Korhonen, T. (2010). *Applying ethical guidelines to ubiquitous health care in China.* Paper presented at the 1st ETICA Conference. Tarragona, Spain.

Jara, A. J., Zamora, M. A., & Skarmeta, A. F. (2011). An internet of things--Based personal device for diabetes therapy management in ambient assisted living (AAL). *Personal and Ubiquitous Computing, 15*(4), 431–440. doi:10.1007/s00779-010-0353-1

Java. (2010). *Web page.* Retrieved December 14, 2010, from http://www.java.com/es.

Javalgi, R. G., Martin, C. L., & Todd, P. R. (2004). The export of e-services in the age of technology transformation: Challenges and implications for international service providers. *Journal of Services Marketing, 18*(7), 560–573. doi:10.1108/08876040410561884

Jeste, D. V., Dunn, L. B., Folsom, D. P., & Zisook, D. (2008). Multimedia educational aids for improving consumer knowledge about illness management and treatment decisions: A review of randomized controlled trials. *Journal of Psychiatric Research, 42*(1), 1–21. doi:10.1016/j.jpsychires.2006.10.004

Jeukendrup, A., & Diemen, A. V. (1998). Heart rate monitoring during training and competition in cyclists. *Journal of Sports Sciences, 16*(1), 91–99. doi:10.1080/026404198366722

JISC. (2011). *Website.* Retrieved from http://www.jisc.ac.uk/.

John, I. (2011). *Tablets steal the show in Las Vegas.* Retrieved February 5, 2011, from http://www.khaleejtimes.com/biz/inside.asp?xfile=/data/business/2011/January/business_January271.xml&section=business.

Johnson, C. R. (2000). Numerical methods for bioelectric field problems. In Bronzino, J. D. (Ed.), *The Biomedical Engineering Handbook* (2nd ed.). Boca Raton, FL: CRC Press LLC.

Johns, R. J. (1975). Current issues in biomedical engineering education. *IEEE Transactions on Bio-Medical Engineering, 22,* 107–110. doi:10.1109/TBME.1975.324427

Jones, W. D. (2006). Taking body temperature, inside out. *IEEE Spectrum, 43,* 13–15. doi:10.1109/MSPEC.2006.1572338

Jongho, L. (2009). Yasuhiro Kagamihara and Shinji Kakei: A new method for quantitative evaluation of neurological disorders based on eMG signals. In Naik, G. R. (Ed.), *Recent Advances in Biomedical Engineering.* Philadelphia, PA: InTech.

Joshi, R. (2006). *Biosensors.* India: Isha Book.

Journal, R. F. I. D. (2010). RFID news roundup – March 15, 2010. *RFID Journal.* Retrieved February 19, 2011, from http://www.rfidjournal.com/article/view/7492.

Jovanov, E., Milenkovic, A., & Otto, C. (2005). A wireless body area network of intelligent motion sensors for computer assisted physical rehabilitation. *Journal of Neurological Engineering and Rehabilitation, 2*(1), 1–10.

Jovanov, E., Milenkovic, A., Otto, C., & de Groen, P. C. (2005). A wireless body area network of intelligent motion sensors for computer assisted physical rehabilitation. *Journal of Neuroengineering and Rehabilitation, 2*(1), 6. doi:10.1186/1743-0003-2-6

Judd, G., & Steenkiste, P. (2003). Providing contextual information to pervasive computing applications. In *Proceedings of the 1st IEEE International Conference on Pervasive Computing and Communications*, (p. 133). IEEE Press.

Juels, A., & Brainard, J. (2004). Soft blocking: Flexible blocker tags on the cheap. In *Proceedings of the 2004 ACM Workshop on Privacy in the Electronic Society*, (pp. 1-7). ACM Press.

Juels, A., Rivest, R. L., & Szydlo, M. (2003). The blocker tag: Selective blocking of RFID tags for consumer privacy. In *Proceedings of the 10th ACM Conference on Computer and Communications Security*, (pp. 103-111). ACM Press.

Jur, J. S., Sweet, W. J. III, Oldham, C. J., & Parsons, G. N. (2011). Electronic textiles: Atomic layer deposition of conductive coatings on cotton, paper, and synthetic fibers: Conductivity analysis and functional chemical sensing using "all-fiber" capacitors. *Advanced Functional Materials, 21*(11), 1948. doi:10.1002/adfm.201190035

Kahn, A. R. (1975). Biomedical engineering education for employment by industry. *IEEE Transactions on Bio-Medical Engineering, 22*, 147–149. doi:10.1109/TBME.1975.324436

Kahn, J., Yang, J., & Kahn, J. (2010). 'Mobile' health needs and opportunities in developing countries. *Health Affairs, 29*(2), 252. doi:10.1377/hlthaff.2009.0965

Kakihara, M., & Sørensen, C. (2002). Mobility: An extended perspective. In *Proceedings of the Hawai's International Conference on System Sciences*. Big Island, Hawaii: IEEE Press.

Kalbach, J. (2006). "I'm feeling lucky": The role of emotions in seeking information on the web. *Journal of the American Society for Information Science and Technology, 57*(6), 813–818. doi:10.1002/asi.20299

Kalyuga, S., Chandler, P., & Sweller, J. (2000). Incorporating learner experience into the design of multimedia instruction. *Journal of Educational Psychology, 92*(1), 126–136. doi:10.1037/0022-0663.92.1.126

Kandel, E. I. (1972). Stereotaxic apparatus and operations in Russia in the 19th century. *Journal of Neurosurgery, 37*, 407–411. doi:10.3171/jns.1972.37.4.0407

Karigiannis, T., Eydt, B., Barber, B., Bunn, L., & Phillips, T. (2007). *Special publication 800-98 guidelines for securing radio frequency identification (RFID) systems*. Washington, DC: National Institute of Standards and Technology.

Karunarathna, M. A. A., & Dayawana, J. (2005). Human exposure to RF radiation in Sri Lanka. *Sri Lankan Journal of Physics, 6*, 19–32.

Katona, P. G. (2002). The Whitaker foundation: The end will be just the beginning. *IEEE Transactions on Medical Imaging, 21*(8), 845–849. doi:10.1109/TMI.2002.803606

Katona, P. G. (2006). Biomedical engineering and the Whitaker foundation: A thirty-year partnership. *Annals of Biomedical Engineering, 34*(6), 904–916. doi:10.1007/s10439-006-9087-7

Kaye, R., Kokia, E., Shalev, V., Idar, D., & Chinitz, D. (2010). Barriers and success factors in health information technology: A practitioner's perspective. *Journal of Management & Marketing in Healthcare, 3*(2), 163–175. doi:10.1179/175330310X12736577732764

Kelly, P. J. (2000). Stereotactic surgery: What is past is prologue. *Neurosurgery, 46*(1), 16–27. doi:10.1097/00006123-200001000-00005

Kelly, S. E. (2003). Bioethics and rural health: Theorizing place, space, and subjects. *Social Science & Medicine, 56*, 2277–2288. doi:10.1016/S0277-9536(02)00227-7

Kennedy, S., & Berk, B. (2011). Enabling e-health: A revolution for informatics in health care. *BCG Perspectives*. Retrieved on June 17, 2011 from www.bcgperspectives.com.

Kern, J. (2006). Standardization in health and medical informatics. In Lazakidou, A. A. (Ed.), *Handbook of Research on Informatics in Healthcare and Biomedicine* (pp. 44–50). Hershey, PA: IGI Global. doi:10.4018/978-1-59140-982-3.ch006

Khalatbari, S., Sardari, D., Mirzaee, A. A., & Sadafi, H. A. (2006). Calculating SAR in two models of the human head exposed to mobile phones radiations at 900 and 1800 MHz. *PIERS Online, 2*(1), 104–109. doi:10.2529/PIERS050905190653

Khan, A. S., Fleischauer, , Casani, J., & Groseclose, S. L. (2010). The next public health revolution: Public health information fusion and social networks. *American Journal of Public Health, 100*(7), 1237–1242. doi:10.2105/AJPH.2009.180489

Khandpur, R. S. (2004). *Biomedical instrumentation: Technology and applications.* New York, NY: McGraw-Hill Professional.

Kikuchi, M. (2007). Status and future prospects of biomedical engineering: A Japanese perspective. *Biomedical Imaging and Intervention Journal, 3*(3), 1–6. doi:10.2349/biij.3.3.e37

Kim, J., Choi, H., Wang, H., Agoulmine, N., Deerv, M. J., & Hong, J. W. (2010). Postech's u-health smart home for elderly monitoring and support. In *Proceedings of the IEEE International Symposium on a World of Wireless, Mobile and Multimedia Networks,* (pp. 1 – 6). Montreal, Canada: IEEE Press.

Kim, Y., & Jo, H. (2009). Patient information display system in hospital using RFID. In *Proceedings of the 2009 International Conference on Hybrid Information Technology,* (pp. 397-400). New York NY: ACM Press.

Kim, Y., & Lee, K. (2006). A quality measurement method of context information in ubiquitous environments. In *Proceedings of the International Conference on Convergence and Hybrid Information Technology,* (pp. 576 - 581). Washington, DC: IEEE Press.

Kimball, R., & Ross, M. (2002). *The data warehouse toolkit: The complete guide to dimensional modeling* (2nd ed.). New York, NY: John Wiley & Sons Inc.

Kim, K., & Chung, C. W. (2010). In/out status monitoring in mobile asset tracking with wireless sensor networks. *Sensors (Basel, Switzerland), 10*(4), 2709–2730. doi:10.3390/s100402709

Klein, N., & David, K. (2010). Time locality: A novel parameter for quality of context. In *Proceedings of the Seventh International Conference on Networked Sensing Systems,* (pp. 277 – 280). IEEE Press.

Knowledge for Health Organization. (2011). *What is mhealth?* Retrieved January 30, 2011, from http://www.k4health.org/toolkits/mHealth.

Kodner, D. L. (2002). Integrated care: Meaning, logic, applications, and implications – A discussion paper. *International Journal of Integrated Care, 2*, 12.

Kohatsu, N. D., Robinson, J. G., & Torner, J. C. (2004). Evidence-based public health: An evolving concept. *American Journal of Preventive Medicine, 27*, 417–421. doi:10.1016/S0749-3797(04)00196-5

Končar, M., & Gvozdanović, D. (2006). Primary healthcare information system—The cornerstone for the next generation healthcare sector in Republic of Croatia. *International Journal of Medical Informatics, 75*, 306–314. doi:10.1016/j.ijmedinf.2005.08.007

Koppel, R., Wetterneck, T., Telles, J. L., & Karsh, B. T. (2008). Workarounds to barcode medication administration systems: Their occurrences, causes and threats to patient safety. *Journal of the American Medical Informatics Association, 15*(4), 408–423. doi:10.1197/jamia.M2616

Krause, M., & Hochstatter, I. (2005). Challenges in modelling and using quality of context (QoC). In *Proceedings of the Mobility Aware Technologies and Applications,* (pp. 324 - 333). Heidelberg, Germany: Springer.

Kraus, J. D., & Marhefka, R. J. (2002). *Antennas for all applications* (3rd ed.). New York, NY: McGraw-Hill.

Kreps, G. L., & Neuhauser, L. (2010). New directions in ehealth communication: Opportunities and challenges. *Patient Education and Counseling, 78*(3), 329–336. doi:10.1016/j.pec.2010.01.013

Kress, G. R., & NetLibrary Inc. (2003). Literacy in the new media age. *Literaciespp, 13*, 186. Retrieved from http://www.columbia.edu/cgi-bin/cul/resolve?clio4255051.

Kress, G. R. (2003). *Literacy in the new media age literacies.* London, UK: Taylor & Francis. doi:10.4324/9780203164754

Kress, G. R., & Van Leeuwen, T. (1996). *Reading images: The grammar of visual design.* London, UK: Routledge.

Kress, G., & Van Leeuwen, T. (2001). *Multimodal discourse: The modes and media of contemporary communication.* New York, NY: Hodder Arnold.

Krishnamachari, B. (2002). The impact of data aggregation in wireless sensor networks. In *Proceedings of International Workshop on Distributed Event-Based Systems,* (pp. 575-578). IEEE.

Kristoffersen, S., & Ljungberg, F. (2000). Mobility: From stationary to mobile work. In Braa, K., Sørensen, C., & Dahlbom, B. (Eds.), *Planet Internet* (pp. 41–64). Lund, Sweden: Studentliteratur.

Krutz, R. L., & Vines, R. D. (2003). *The CISSP® prep guide: Gold edition.* Indianapolis, IN: Wiley Publishing, Inc.

Kubben, P. (2011). *Website.* Retrieved February 27, 2011, from http://blog.digitalneurosurgeon.com/?p=1116.

Kubler, S., Derigent, W., Thomas, A., & Rondeau, É. (2011). *Prototyping of a communicating textile.* Paper presented at the International Conference on Industrial Engineering and Systems Management - IESM 2011. Metz, France.

Kühn, S., & Kuster, N. (2006). *Development of procedures for the EMF exposure evaluation of wireless devices in home and office environments supplement 1: Close-to-body and base station wireless data communication devices.* Zurich, Switzerland: The Foundation for Research on Information Technologies in Society (IT'IS).

Kumar, A. D., Welti, D., & Ernst, R. R. (1975). NMR Fourier zeugmatography. *Journal of Magnetic Resonance (San Diego, Calif.), 18*(1), 69–83.

Kumar, V., & Venkatesan, R. (2005). Who are the multichannel shoppers and how do they perform? Correlates of multichannel shopping behavior. *Journal of Interactive Marketing, 19*(2), 44–62. doi:10.1002/dir.20034

Kushniruk, A. W., Triola, M. M., Borycki, E. M., Stein, B., & Kannry, J. L. (2005). Technology induced error and usability: The relationship between usability problems and prescription errors when using a handheld application. *International Journal of Medical Informatics, 74*(7-8), 519–526. doi:10.1016/j.ijmedinf.2005.01.003

Kushniruk, A., & Borycki, E. (2007). Human factors and usability of healthcare systems. In Bardram, J., Mihailidis, A., & Wan, D. (Eds.), *Pervasive Computing in Healthcare* (pp. 191–215). Boca Raton, FL: CRC Press. doi:10.1201/9781420005332.ch8

Kwoh, Y. S., Hou, J., Jonckheere, E. A., & Hayathi, S. (1988). A robot with improved absolute positioning accuracy for stereotactic brain surgery. *IEEE Transactions on Bio-Medical Engineering, 35,* 153–160. doi:10.1109/10.1354

Kyriacou, E. C., Pattichis, C. S., & Pattichis, M. S. (2009). An overview of recent health care supported systems for eemergency and mhealth applications. In *Proceedings from the IEEE English Medical Biological Society,* (pp. 1246-1249). IEEE Press.

Lahtela, A. (2009). A short overview of the RFID technology in healthcare. In *Proceedings of the Fourth International Conference on Systems and Networks Communications,* (pp.165-169). IEEE.

Lai, C.-H., Chien, S.-W., Chang, L.-H., Chen, S.-C., & Fang, K. (2007). Enhancing medication safety and healthcare for inpatients using RFID. In *Proceedings of the Portland International Center for Management of Engineering and Technology,* (pp. 2783-2790). Portland, OR: Portland International Center for Management of Engineering and Technology.

Lajoie, S. (Ed.). (2000). *Computers as cognitive tools: No more walls (Vol. 2).* Mahwah, NJ: Lawrence Erlbaum.

Landoll, J. R., & Caceres, C. A. (1969). Automation of data acquisition in patient testing. *Proceedings of the IEEE, 57*(11), 1941–1953. doi:10.1109/PROC.1969.7440

Landt, J. (2001). *Shrouds of time.* New York, NY: AIM Inc.

Landt, J. (2005). The history of RFID. *IEEE Potentials, 24*(4), 8–11. doi:10.1109/MP.2005.1549751

Lanza, R., Langer, R., & Vacanti, J. (2000). *Principles of tissue engineering.* San Diego, CA: Academic Press, Inc.

Lateef, F. (2011). The practice of telemedicine: Medicolegal and ethical issues. *Ethics & Medicine, 27*(1), 17–25.

Laudon, K., & Laudon, J. (2010). *Management information systems* (11th ed.). Upper Saddle River, NJ: Prentice Hall.

Lau, F., & Hayward, R. (2000). Building a virtual network in a community health research training program. *Journal of the American Medical Informatics Association, 7*(4), 361–377. Retrieved from http://www.ncbi.nlm.nih.gov/pmc/articles/PMC61441/doi:10.1136/jamia.2000.0070361

Lauterbur, P. C. (1973). Image formation by induced local interactions: examples employing nuclear magnetic resonance. *Nature, 242*, 190–191. doi:10.1038/242190a0

Lavine, G. (2008). RFID technology may improve contrast agent safety. *American Journal of Health-System Pharmacy, 65*(15), 1400–1403. doi:10.2146/news080064

Laxminarayan, S., & Istepanian, R. S. (2000). Unwired e-med: The next generation of wireless and internet telemedicine systems. *IEEE Transactions on Information Technology in Biomedicine, 4*(3), 189–193. doi:10.1109/TITB.2000.5956074

Layouni, M., Verslype, K., Sandıkkaya, M. T., Decker, B., & Vangheluwe, H. (2009). Privacy-preserving telemonitoring for ehealth. *Lecture Notes in Computer Science, 5645*(1). doi:10.1007/978-3-642-03007-9_7

Lee, S.-Y., & Cho, G.-S. (2007). A simulation study for the operations analysis of dynamic planning in container terminals considering RTLS. In *Proceedings of the Second International Conference on Innovative Computing, Information and Control (ICICIC 2007)*, (p. 116). IEEE.

Lee, H., & Liebenau, J. (1999). Time in organizational studies: Towards a new research direction. *Organization Studies, 20*(6), 1035–1058. doi:10.1177/0170840699206006

Lenhart, A., Purcell, K., Smith, A., & Zickuhr, K. (2010). Social media & mobile internet use among teens and young adults. *Pew Internet and American Life Project*. Retrieved February, 6, 2010 from http://www.pewinternet.org.

Lenzini, G. (2009). Trust-based and context-aware authentication in a software architecture for context and proximity-aware services. *Architecting Dependable Systems, 6*, 284–307.

Lesk, A. M. (2002). *Introduction to bioinformatics*. Oxford, UK: Oxford University Press.

Lester, P. M. (2003). *Visual communication: Images with messages* (3rd ed.). Belmont, CA: Thomson/Wadsworth.

Li, H., & Tan, J. (2005). An ultra-low-power medium access control protocol for body sensor network. In *Proceedings of the Engineering in Medicine and Biology Society Annual International Conference (IEEE-EMBS)*, (pp. 2451 – 2454). IEEE Press.

Liang, D., Wu, J., & Chen, X. (2007). Real-time physical activity monitoring by data fusion in body sensor networks. In *Proceedings of the 10th Internaional Conference on Information Fusion*, (pp. 1-7). Washington, DC: IEEE.

Lin, J. C. (2003). Biological bases of current guidelines for human exposure to radio-frequency radiation. *IEEE Antennas and Propagation Magazine, 45*(3).

Lin, J. C. (2003). Microwave cataracts and personal communication radiation. *IEEE Microwave, 4*, 26–32.

Lin, K., Lai, C., & Chen, M. (2011). Research on body sensor networks in cold region. In *Proceedings of IEEE ICC*. Kyoto, Japan: IEEE Press.

Lindberg, D. A. B., Humphreys, B. L., & McCray, A. T. (1993). The unified medical language system. *Methods of Information in Medicine, 32*, 281–291.

Lindemann, U., Hock, A., Stuber, M., Keck, W., & Becker, C. (2005). Evaluation of a fall detector based on accelerometers: A pilot study. *Medical & Biological Engineering & Computing, 43*, 548–551. doi:10.1007/BF02351026

Linkov, F., LaPorte, R., Padilla, N., & Shubnikov, E. (2010). Global networking of cancer and NCD professionals using internet technologies: The supercourse and mhealth applications. *Journal of Preventive Medicine and Public Health = Yebang Uihakhoe Chi, 43*(6), 472–478. Retrieved from http://www.ncbi.nlm.nih.gov/pubmed/21139407doi:10.3961/jpmph.2010.43.6.472

Linksys by Cisco. (2011). *Wireless-G broadband router WRT54GL*. Retrieved from http.//www.linksysbycisco.com/UK/en/products/WRT54GL.

Lipozencić, J., Celić, D., Strnad, M., Toncić, R. J., Pasić, A., Rados, J., & Znaor, A. (2010). Skin cancers in Croatia, 2003-2005: Epidemiological study. *Collegium Antropologicum, 34*, 865–869.

Lipton, R. (2004). *Information graphics and visual clues*. Gloucester, MA: Rockport Publishers.

Lipton, R. (2007). *The practical guide to information design*. Hoboken, NJ: Wiley.

Littlejohns, P., Wyatt, J. C., & Garvican, L. (2003). Evaluating computerised health information systems: Hard lessons still to be learnt. *British Medical Journal, 326*(7394), 860–863. doi:10.1136/bmj.326.7394.860

Liu, K., Liu, T., Shibata, K., & Inoue, Y. (2010). Visual estimation of lower limb motion using physical and virtual sensors. In *Proceedings of IEEE International Conference on Information and Automation (ICIA)*, (pp. 179 – 184). IEEE Press.

Liu, B.-C., Lin, K.-H., & Wu, J.-C. (2006). Analysis of hyperbolic and circular positioning algorithms using stationary signal strength difference measurements in wireless communications. *IEEE Transactions on Vehicular Technology*, *55*(2), 499–509. doi:10.1109/TVT.2005.863405

Li, X. (2006). RSS-based location estimation with unknown pathloss model. *IEEE Transactions on Wireless Communications*, *5*(12), 3626–3633. doi:10.1109/TWC.2006.256985

Lo, B. P. L., & Yang, G. Z. (2005). Key technical challenges and current implementations of body sensor networks. In *Proceedings of the 2nd International Workshop on Wearable and Implantable Body Sensor Networks*, (pp. 1-5). London, UK: IEEE.

Lober, W. B., Trigg, L. J., Karras, B. T., Bliss, D., Ciliberti, J., Stewart, L., & Duchin, J. S. (2003). Syndromic surveillance using automated collection of computerized discharge diagnoses. *Journal of Urban Health: Bulletin of the New York Academy of Medicine*, *80*(2), 97–106.

Lopez, D. M., & Blobel, B. (2009). A development framework for semantically interoperable health information systems. *International Journal of Medical Informatics*, *78*(2), 83–103. doi:10.1016/j.ijmedinf.2008.05.009

Lost it! (2011). *Website*. Retrieved February 22, 2011, from http://itunes.apple.com/us/app/lose-it/id297368629?mt=8#.

Lovelock, C. H. (1983). Classifying services to gain strategic marketing insights. *Journal of Marketing*, *47*(3), 9–20. doi:10.2307/1251193

Lovelock, C. H. (1996). *Service marketing* (3rd ed.). London, UK: Prentice Hall International.

Löwgren, J., & Stolterman, E. (2004). *Thoughtful interaction design: A design perspective on information technology*. Cambridge, MA: MIT Press.

Luff, P., & Heath, C. (1998). Mobility in collaboration. In *Proceedings of ACM 1998 Conference on Computer Supported Cooperative Work*. Seattle, WA: ACM Press.

Luinge, H. J., & Veltink, P. H. (2005). Measuring orientation of human body segments using miniature gyroscopes and accelerometers. *Medical & Biological Engineering & Computing*, *43*, 273–282. doi:10.1007/BF02345966

Luo, H., Liu, Y., & Das, S. K. (2006). Routing correlated data with fusion cost in wireless sensor networks. *IEEE Transactions on Mobile Computing*, *5*(11), 1620–1632. doi:10.1109/TMC.2006.171

Luo, H., Luo, J., Liu, Y., & Das, S. K. (2006). Adaptive data fusion for energy efficient routing in wireless sensor networks. *IEEE Transactions on Computers*, *55*(10), 1286–1299. doi:10.1109/TC.2006.157

Lupu, E., Dulay, N., Sloman, M., Sventek, J., Heeps, S., & Strowes, S. (2008). AMUSE: Autonomic management of ubiquitous e-health systems. *Concurrency and Computation*, *20*(3), 277–295. doi:10.1002/cpe.1194

Lyall, M. (2010). *Chronic diseases need attention of mHealth apps developers*. Retrieved February 14, 2011, from http://www.knowabouthealth.com/chronic-diseases-need-attention-of-mHealth-apps-developers/7339/.

Maharshi, A., Tong, L., & Swami, A. (2003). Cross-layer designs of multichannel reservation MAC under rayleigh fading. *IEEE Transactions on Signal Processing*, *51*(8), 2054–2067. doi:10.1109/TSP.2003.814465

Maibach, E., & Parrott, R. (1995). *Designing health messages: Approaches from communication theory and public health practice*. Thousand Oaks, CA: Sage Publications.

Malan, D., Fulford-Jones, T., Welsh, M., & Moulton, S. (2004). Codeblue: An ad hoc sensor network infrastructure for emergency medical care. In *Proceedings of the 1st International Workshop on Wearable and Implantable Body Sensor Networks*, (pp. 55-58). London, UK: IEEE.

Malecki, E. J., & Moriset, B. (2008). *The digital economy: Business organization, production processes, and regional developments*. Oxon, UK: Routledge.

Mallat, S. G. (1989). Theory for multiresolution signal decomposition: The wavelet representation. *IEEE Transactions on Pattern Analysis and Machine Intelligence*, *11*(7), 674–693. doi:10.1109/34.192463

Mallat, S., & Zhong, S. (1992). Characterization of signals from multiscale edges. *IEEE Transactions on Pattern Analysis and Machine Intelligence*, *14*(7), 710–732. doi:10.1109/34.142909

Malmivuo, J., & Plonsey, R. (1995). *Bioelectromagnetism.* New York, NY: Oxford University Press.

Mamlin, B. W., & Biondich, P. G. (2005). AMPATH medical record system (AMRS): Collaborating toward an EMR for developing countries. In *Proceedings of the AMIA Annual Symposium,* (pp. 490–494). AMIA.

Mamlin, B. W., Biondich, P. G., Wolfe, B. A., Fraser, H., Jazayeri, D., & Allen, C. ... Tierney, W. M. (2006). Cooking up an open source EMR for developing countries: OpenMRS - A recipe for successful collaboration. In *Proceedings of the AMIA Annual Symposium,* (pp. 529–533). AMIA.

Mandelli, A., & Parolini, C. (2003). Imprese e tecnologie digitali: La rete avanza. In Biffi, A., & Dematté, C. (Eds.), *L'araba Fenice: Economia Digitale Alla Prova Dei Fatti* (pp. 3–62). Milano, Italy: Etas.

Mandl, K. D., Overhage, J. M., Wagner, M. M., Lober, W. B., Sebastiani, P., & Mostashari, F. (2004). Implementing syndromic surveillance: A practical guide informed by the early experience. *Journal of the American Medical Informatics Association, 11*(2), 141–150. doi:10.1197/jamia.M1356

Manhattan Research. (2009). *Physician smart phone adoption rate to reach 81% in 2012.* Retrieved February 21, 2011, from http://www.manhattanresearch.com/newsroom/Press_Releases/physician-smartphones-2012.aspx.

Mansfield, P. (1977). Multi-planar image formation using NMR spin-echos. *Journal of Physics. C. Solid State Physics, 10,* 55–58. doi:10.1088/0022-3719/10/3/004

Manzoor, A., Truong, H. L., & Dustdar, S. (2008). On the evaluation of quality of context. In *Proceedings of the Third European Conference in Smart Sensing and Context,* (pp. 140 – 153). Zurich, Switzerland: IEEE.

Manzoor, A., Truong, H. L., & Dustdar, S. (2009). Quality aware context information aggregation system for pervasive environments. In *Proceedings of the International Conference on Advanced Information Networking and Applications Workshops,* (pp. 266 – 271). Bradford, UK: IEEE Press.

Manzoor, A., Truong, H. L., & Dustdar, S. (2009). Using quality of context to resolve conflicts in context-aware systems. In *Proceedings of QuaCon* (pp. 144–155). Springer. doi:10.1007/978-3-642-04559-2_13

Marmarelis, V. Z. (2004). *Nonlinear dynamic modeling of physiological systems.* New York, NY: John Wiley InterScience.

Mars, M., & Seebregts, C. (2008). *Country case study for ehealth South Africa.* Retrieved from http://www.ehealth-connection.org/content/country-case-studies.

Martinez-Ramirez, A., Lecumberri, P., Gomez, M., & Izquierdo, M. (2010). *Tri-axial inertial magnetic tracking in quiet standing analysis using wavelet transform.* Paper presented at the International Multi-Conference on Engineering and Technological Innovation, IMETI. Miami, FL.

Martins, H. M. G., Nightingale, P., & Jones, M. R. (2005). *Any time, any place? Temporal and spatial organisation of doctors' computer usage in a UK hospital department.* Paper presented at the Healthcare Computing Conference. Harrogate, UK.

Mason, M. (2011). *South Asians hit with heart attacks earlier than rest of world: Heart disease top killer.* Retrieved February 14, 2011, from http://www.google.com/hostednews/canadianpress/article/ALeqM5jR6gAxqnoC9T-KNq-Ck5XbOXbkeA?docId=5895164.

Massey, J. T., & Johns, R. J. (1981). A short history of the collaborative biomedical program. *Johns Hopkins APL Technical Digest, 2,* 141–142.

Masys, D. (1998). Advances in information technology: Implications for medical education. *The Western Journal of Medicine, 168*(5), 341–347.

Mathies, M., Coster, A., Lovell, N., & Celle, B. (2008). Accelerometry: Providing an integrated, practical method for long-term, ambulatory monitoring of human movement. *Journal Physiological Measurement, 25*(2).

Matthews, R., McDonald, N. J., Hervieux, P., Turner, P. J., & Steindorf, M. A. (2007). A wearable physiological sensor suite for unobtrusive monitoring of physiological and cognitive state. In *Proceedings of the International Conference of IEEE Engineering in Medicine and Biology Society,* (pp. 5276 – 5281). IEEE Press.

Mayagoitia, R. E., Nene, A. V., & Veltink, P. H. (2002). Accelerometer and rate gyroscope measurement of kinematics: An inexpensive alternative to optical motion analysis systems. *Journal of Biomechanics, 35,* 537–542. doi:10.1016/S0021-9290(01)00231-7

Mayer, R. E. (2001). *Multimedia learning.* Cambridge, UK: Cambridge University Press.

Mayer, R. E., & Moreno, R. (2002). Animation as an aid to multimedia learning. *Educational Psychology Review, 14*(1), 87–99. doi:10.1023/A:1013184611077

Mayer, R. E., & Moreno, R. (2003). Nine ways to reduce cognitive load in multimedia learning. *Educational Psychologist, 38*(1), 43–52. doi:10.1207/S15326985EP3801_6

Mazuelas, S., Bahillo, A., Lorenzo, R., Fernandez, P., Lago, F., & Garcia, E. (2009). Robust indoor positioning provided by real-time RSSI values in unmodified WLAN networks. *IEEE Journal of Selected Topics in Signal Processing, 3*(5), 821–831. doi:10.1109/JSTSP.2009.2029191

McCally, R. L. (2005). The master's degree program in applied biomedical engineering. *Johns Hopkins APL Technical Digest, 26*(3), 214–218.

McCann, D. G. C., & Cordi, H. P. (2011). Developing international standards for disaster preparedness and response: How do we get there? *World Medical & Health Policy, 3,* 5. Retrieved March 29, 2011, from http://www.psocommons.org/wmhp/vol3/iss1/art5.

McCann, J., Hurford, R., & Martin, A. (2005). *A design process for the development of innovative smart clothing that addresses end-user needs from technical, functional, aesthetic and cultural view points.* Paper presented at the Ninth IEEE International Symposium on Wearable Computers (ISWC 2005). Osaka, Japan.

McDonald, C., Huff, S., Mercer, K., Hernandez, J. A., & Vreeman, D. J. (Eds.). (2010). *Logical observation identifiers names and codes (LOINC®): Users' guide.* Indianapolis, IN: Regenstrief Institutes, Inc.

McGee, M. K. (2010). *Text messages boost patient outcomes.* Retrieved February 14, 2011, from http://www.informationweek.com/news/healthcare/mobile-wireless/showArticle.jhtml?articleID=227500893&subSection=News.

McMaster, O. S. C. A. R. (2011). *Web page.* Retrieved May 12, 2011, from http://en.wikipedia.org/wiki/OSCAR_McMaster.

MD National Council on Radiation Protection and Measurements. (1986). *Biological effects and exposure criteria for radio frequency electromagnetic fields. Report 86.* Washington, DC: MD National Council on Radiation Protection and Measurements.

Mechael, P., & Slonininsky, D. (Eds.). (2008). *Towards the development of an mhealth strategy: A literature review.* New York, NY: The World Health Organization. Retrieved from http://mobileactive.org/files/file_uploads/WHOHealthReviewUpdatedAug222008_TEXT.pdf.

MEDgle Inc. (2011). *The details.* Retrieved on June 15, 2011 from http://www.medgle.com/front.jsp?task=technology&section=details.

Medic, P. H. R. (2010). *Website.* Retrieved February 22, 2011, from http://itunes.apple.com/us/app/medic-phr/id336885531?mt=8.

Medical. (2011). *Web page.* Retrieved May 12, 2011 from http://medical.sourceforge.net.

MedMarket Diligence. (2002). *Report #S150.* Retrieved from http://mediligence.com/web-files/prod01.htm.

Medscape. (2010). *Website.* Retrieved February 9, 2011, from http://itunes.apple.com/us/app/medscape/id321367289?mt=8#.

Menz, H. B., Lord, S. R., & Fitzpatrick, R. C. (2003). Acceleration patterns of the head and pelvis when walking are associated with risk of falling in community-dwelling older people. *Journal of Gerontology, 58,* 446–452.

Merckel, C. (1972). Microwave and man - The direct and indirect hazards, and the precautions. *California Medicine, 117*(1), 20–24.

Microchip. (2004). *High precision temperature-to-voltage converter.* Technical Report. Retrieved from http://ww1.microchip.com.

Microsemi. (2005). *Ambient light detector, LX1972.* Technical Report. Retrieved from www.microsemi.com.

Microsoft Infopath. (2010). *Web page.* Retrieved December 14, 2010, from http://office.microsoft.com/en-us/infopath.

Miller, J., & Mukerji, J. (2003). *MDA guide version 1.0.1.* Tech. Rep. No. omg/2003-06-01. New York, NY: Object Management Group (OMG).

Miller, E. A., & Pole, A. (2010). Diagnosis blog: Checking up on health blogs in the blogosphere. *American Journal of Public Health*, *100*(8), 1514–1519. doi:10.2105/AJPH.2009.175125

Mišic, J., Shafi, S., & Mišic, V. B. (2006). Performance of a beacon enabled IEEE 802.15.4 cluster with downlink and uplink traffic. *IEEE Transactions on Parallel and Distributed Systems*, *17*, 361–376. doi:10.1109/TPDS.2006.54

Misra, R. (2007). *The significance of design: A multimodal analysis of government and non-government websites*. Unpublished Doctoral Dissertation. New York, NY: Columbia University.

Misra, R., & Wallace, B. C. (2011a). Improving the design of health information websites: A study of users' expectations. *Design Principles and Practices: An International Journal*, *5*. Retrieved from http://www.Design-Journal.com.

Misra, R., & Wallace, B. C. (2011b). Evaluating the design of two government and two non-government HIV/AIDS websites. *The International Journal of Health, Wellness and Society*, *1*. Retrieved from http://www.HealthandSocietyJournal.com/.

Mitseva, A., Kyriazakos, S., Litke, A., Papadakis, N., & Prasad, N. (2009). ISISEMD: Intelligent system for independent living and self-care of seniors with mild cognitive impairment or mild dementia. *The Journal on Information Technology in Healthcare*, *7*(6), 383–399.

MobiHealth Project. (2004). *Website*. Retrieved from http://www.mobihealth.org/.

Mokdad, A. H., Stroup, D. F., & Giles, W. H. (2003). Public health surveillance for behavioral risk factors in a changing environment recommendations from the behavioral risk factor surveillance team. *Recommendation and Reports*, *52*, 1-12. Retrieved from http://www.cdc.gov/mmwr/Preview/Mmwrhtml/rr5209a1.htm.

Mol, A., & Law, J. (1994). Regions, networks and fluids: Anaemia and social topology. *Social Studies of Science*, *24*, 641–671. doi:10.1177/030631279402400402

Moretti, F., & Witte, S. S. (2008). Using new media to improve learning: Multimedia connect for HIV/AIDS reduction and the triangle initiative. In Wallace, B. C. (Ed.), *Toward Equity in Health: A New Global Approach to Health Disparities* (pp. 277–296). New York, NY: Springer Publications.

Morgan, D. J., Day, H. R., Furuno, J. P., Young, A., Johnson, J. K., Bradham, D. D., & Perencevich, E. N. (2010). Improving efficiency in active surveillance for methicillin-resistant Staphylococcus aureus or vancomycin-resistant Enterococcus at hospital admission. *Infection Control and Hospital Epidemiology*, *31*, 1230–1235. doi:10.1086/657335

Moritz, W. E., & Huntsman, L. L. (1975). A collaborative approach to bioengineering education. *IEEE Transactions on Bio-Medical Engineering*, *22*, 124–129. doi:10.1109/TBME.1975.324431

Moruzzi, M. (2009). *E-health e fascicolo sanitario elettronico*. Milano, Italy: Il Sole 24 Ore.

Muhlsteff, J., & Such, O. (2004). Dry electrodes for monitoring of vital signs in functional textiles. In *Proceedings of the 26th Annual International Conference of the IEEE, Engineering in Medicine and Biology Society*, (pp. 2212 – 2215). San Francisco, CA: IEEE Press.

Müller, H., Gao, X. W., & Lin, C. (Eds.). (2006). Special issue. *Computerised Medical Imaging and Graphics*, *30*(6-7).

Müller, H., Gao, X. W., & Luo, S. (Eds.). (2008). *Computer Methods and Programs in Biomedicine*, *92*(3). doi:10.1016/j.cmpb.2008.07.004

Murota, T., Kato, A., & Okumura, T. (2010). Emergency management for information systems in public health: A case study of the 2009 pandemic-flu response in Japan. In *Proceedings of the Pervasive Computing and Communications Workshops (PERCOM Workshops), 8th IEEE International Conference*, (pp. 394 – 399). IEEE Press.

Murray, C. J. L., Lopez, A. D., & Wibulpolprasert, S. (2004). Monitoring global health: Time for new solutions. *British Medical Journal*, *329*, 1096–1100. doi:10.1136/bmj.329.7474.1096

Murray-Johnson, L., & Witte, K. (2003). Looking toward the future: Health message design strategies. In *Handbook of Health Communication* (pp. 473–495). Mahwah, NJ: Lawrence Erlbaum.

Murugappan, M., Rizon, M., Nagarajan, R., Yaacob, S., Hazry, D., & Zunaidi, I. (2008). Time-frequency analysis of EEG signals for human emotion detection. In *Proceedings of the 4th Kuala Lumpur International Conference on Biomedical Engineering*. Kuala Lampur, India: IEEE.

MyHeart Project. (2006). *Website*. Retrieved from http://www.hitech-projects.com/euprojects/myheart/.

Mylrea, K. C., & Siverston, S. E. (1975). Biomedical engineering in health care—Potential vs reality. *IEEE Transactions on Bio-Medical Engineering, 22*, 114–118. doi:10.1109/TBME.1975.324429

MySQL. (2010). *Web page*. Retrieved December 14, 2010, from http://www.mysql.com.

Nakahara, S., Saint, S., Sann, S., Ichikawa, M., Kimura, A., & Eng, L. (2010). Exploring referral systems for injured patients in low-income countries: A case study from Cambodia. *Health Policy and Planning, 25*(4), 319–327. doi:10.1093/heapol/czp063

Nannings, B., & Abu-Hanna, A. (2006). Characterizing decision support telemedicine systems. *Methods of Information in Medicine, 45*(5), 523–527.

Natesan, T. R. (2001). Web based multi-functional virtual instrument for telemedicine. *Medindia Networking for Health*. Retrieved from http://www.medindia.net/articles/webmedicine.htm

National Department of Health. (2003). *Strategic framework for the modernisation of tertiary hospital services*. Retrieved from http://www.doh.gov.za/mts/docs/framework.html.

National Department of Health. (2007). *The national strategic tramework for eHR implementation in South Africa*. Pretoria, South Africa: South African National Department of Health. Retrieved from http://www.pnc.gov.za/images/stories/focus_area/report/ehr_fm.pdf.

National Instruments. (2009). Working with LabVIEW filtering VIs and the LabVIEW. *Digital Filter Design Toolkit VIs*. Retrieved from www.ni.com.

National Radiological Protection Board. (1993). Board statement on restrictions on human exposure to static and time-varying electromagnetic fields. *Documents of the PRPB, 4*(5).

Neisse, R., Wegdam, M., & Van-Sinderen, M. (2008). Trustworthiness and quality of context information. In *Proceedings of the 9th International Conference for Young Computer Scientists, International Symposium on Trusted Computing*, (pp. 1925–1931). Zhang Jia Jie, China: IEEE.

NEMA. (2004). *Digital imaging and communications in medicine (DICOM)*. Fredericksburg, VA: NEMA.

Neuman, M. R. (2000). Biomedical sensors. In Bronzino, J. D. (Ed.), *The Biomedical Engineering Handbook* (2nd ed.). Boca Raton, FL: CRC Press LLC.

NeuroMind. (2010). *Website*. Retrieved February 22, 2011, from http://itunes.apple.com/us/app/neuromind/id353386909?mt=8#.

Neurosurgeon, D. (2011). *Blog*. Retrieved February 22, 2011, from http://blog.digitalneurosurgeon.com/?page_id=639.

Newhouse, V. L., Bell, D. S., & Tackel, I. S. (1989). The future of clinical engineering in the 1990s. *Journal of Clinical Engineering, 14*, 417.

Ng, N., Hakimi, M., Van Minh, H., Juvekar, S., Razzaque, A., & Ashraf, A. (2009). Prevalence of physical inactivity in nine rural indepth health and demographic surveillance systems in five Asian countries. *Global Health Action, 28*, 2.

NM-IBIS. (2011). *Evidence based public health practice*. Retrieved March 19, 2011, from: http://ibis.health.state.nm.us/resources/EvidenceBased.html.

Nobel Foundation. (2009). *The nobel prize in physics 2009*. Retrieved from http://nobelprize.org/nobel_prizes/physics/laureates/2009/index.html.

Nokes, L., Jennings, D., Flint, T., & Turton, B. (1995). *Introduction to medical electronics applications*. London, UK: Butterworth-Heinemann.

Nokia. (2011). *SAR information*. Retrieved from http://sar.nokia.com/sar/index.jsp.

Nongkynrih, B., Anand, K., Pandav, C. S., & Kapoor, S. K. (2010). Introducing regular behavioural surveillance into the health system in India: its feasibility and validity. *The National Medical Journal of India, 23*(1), 13–17.

Noor, A. M., Gikandi, P. W., Hay, S. I., Muga, R. O., & Snow, R. W. (2004). Creating spatially defined databases for equitable health service planning in low-income countries: The example of Kenya. *Acta Tropica, 91*, 239–251. doi:10.1016/j.actatropica.2004.05.003

Normann, R. (1984). *Service management strategy and leadership in service business*. Chichester, UK: John Wiley & Sons.

Northrop, R. B. (2003). *Signals and systems analysis in biomedical engineering*. Boca Raton, FL: CRC Press.

Nsubuga, P., White, M. E., Thacker, S. B., Anderson, M. A., Blount, S. B., & Broome, C. V. ... Trostle, M. (2006). Public health surveillance: A tool for targeting and monitoring intervention. In *Disease Control Priorities in Developing Countries* (2nd Ed), (pp. 997-1018). New York, NY: Oxford University Press.

Nsubuga, P., Nwanyanwu, O., Nkengasong, J. N., Mukanga, D., & Trostle, M. (2010). Strengthening public health surveillance and response using the health systems strengthening agenda in developing countries. *BMC Public Health*, *3*, 10.

Nursing. (2006). Replacing bar coding: Radio frequency identification. *Nursing, 36*(12), 30.

Nusca, A. (2009). *Smartphone vs. feature phone arms race heats up: Which did you buy?* Retrieved January 30, 2011, from http://www.zdnet.com/blog/gadgetreviews/smartphone-vs-feature-phone-arms-race-heats-up-which-did-you-buy/6836.

O'Connor, M. C. (2011a). Study determines optimized, RFID-enabled resupply system for nurse stations. *RFID Journal*. Retrieved July 1, 2011 from http://www.rfidjournal.com/article/view/8552.

O'Connor, M. C. (2011b). Saint Luke's hospital of Kansas City saves thousands with RFID. *RFID Journal*. Retrieved July 1, 2011 from http://www.rfidjournal.com/article/view/8560.

O'Donovan, K. J., Kamnik, R., O'Keeffe, D. T., & Lyons, G. M. (2007). An inertial and magnetic sensor based technique for joint angle measurement. *Journal of Biomechanics*, *40*, 2604–2611. doi:10.1016/j.jbiomech.2006.12.010

Oakes, J. B. (1975). Clinical engineering-The problems and promise. *Science*, *190*, 239–242.

Oakley, A. (2006). *Introduction to telemedicine* (2nd ed.). London, UK: RSM Books.

Odlum, M. (2010). *An exploratory analysis of factors associated with use and comprehension of the internet and a continuity of care document for persons living with HIV in New York City*. Unpublished Doctoral Dissertation. New York, NY: Columbia University.

OECD. (2010). *Improving health sector efficiency: The role of information and communication technologies*. Paris, France: OECD.

Oehler, R. L., Smith, K., & Toney, J. F. (2010). Infectious diseases resources for the iphone. *Clinical Infectious Diseases*, *50*(9), 1268–1274. doi:10.1086/651602

Ogirala, A., Murari, A., Hawrylak, P. J., & Mickle, M. H. (2011). Gen 2 timing analysis in state plane: Optimum parameter and command configuration for memory operations. *Journal of Computer Technology and Application*, *3*(3).

Oh, H., Rizo, C., Enkin, M., & Jadad, A. (2005). What is eHealth: A systematic review of published definitions. *Journal of Medical Internet Research*, *7*(1), e1. doi:10.2196/jmir.7.1.e1

Oliveira, M., Hairon, C., Andrade, O., Moura, R., Sicotte, C., & Denis, J.-L. ... Martin, H. (2010). A context-aware framework for health care governance decision-making systems: A model based on the Brazilian digital TV. In *Proceedings of the IEEE International Symposium on a World of Wireless, Mobile and Multimedia Networks*, (pp. 1 – 6). Montreal, Canada: IEEE Press.

Ono, N., Hayashi, Y., Kisuki, A., & Ikeda, Y. (1996). *Anechoic chamber and wave absorber patent*. US Patent no.5.510.792. Washington, DC: US Patent Office.

Open Healthcare. (2011). *Web page*. Retrieved May 12, 2011, from http://www.openhealth.org.

OpenEMR. (2011). *Web page*. Retrieved January 15, 2011, from http://www.oemr.org.

OpenMRS. (2010). *Web page*. Retrieved December 14, 2010, from http://www.openmrs.org.

OpenVista. (2011). *Web page*. Retrieved January 15, 2011, from http://worldvista.sourceforge.net/openvista/index.html.

Orava, M. (2002). Globalising medical services: Operational modes in the internationalization of medical service firms. *International Journal of Medical Marketing*, *2*(3), 232–240. doi:10.1057/palgrave.jmm.5040081

Oreilly, T. (2007). *What is web 2.0: Design patterns and business models for the next generation of software*. Retrieved from http://oreilly.com/web2/archive/what-is-web-20.html.

Orlikowski, W. J., & Yates, J. (2002). It's about time: Temporal structuring in organizations. *Organization Science, 13*(6), 684–700. doi:10.1287/orsc.13.6.684.501

Ortiz, A. P., Soto-Salgado, M., Suárez, E., Del Carmen Santos-Ortiz, M., Tortolero-Luna, G., & Pérez, C. M. (2011). Sexual behaviors among adults in Puerto Rico: A population-based study. *Journal of Sexual Medicine, 8*(9), 2439–2449. doi:10.1111/j.1743-6109.2011.02329.x

Orwat, C., Graefe, A., & Faulwasser, T. (2008). Towards pervasive computing in health care - A literature review. *BMC Medical Informatics and Decision Making, 8*(26).

Osman, M. A. R., Rahim, M. K. A., Azfar, M., Samsuri, N. A., Zubir, F., & Kamardin, K. (2011). Design, implementation and performance of ultra-wideband textile antenna. *Progress in Electromagnetic Research B, 27*, 307–325.

Osservatorio ICT in Sanità. (2008). *ICT e innovazione in sanità: Nuove sfide e opportunità per i CIO*. Milano, Italy: Politecnico di Milano, Dipartimento di Ingegneria gestionale.

Osservatorio ICT in Sanità. (2011). *ICT in sanità: L'innovazione in cerca di autore*. Milano, Italy: Politecnico di Milano, Dipartimento di Ingegneria gestionale.

Otal, B. (2010). *Optimization of wireless ambient and body sensor networks for medical applications.* PhD Dissertation. Catalunya, Spain: Universitat Politècnica de Catalunya (UPC).

Otal, B., & Habetha, J. (2005). *Power saving efficiency of a novel packet aggregation scheme for high-throughput WLAN stations at different data rates.* Paper presented at the IEEE Vehicular Technology Conference. Stockholm, Sweden.

Otal, B., Alonso, L., & Verikoukis, C. (2009). Highly reliable energy-saving MAC for wireless body sensor setworks in healthcare systems. *IEEE Journal on Selected Areas in Communications, 27*(4), 553–565. doi:10.1109/JSAC.2009.090516

Otal, B., Alonso, L., & Verikoukis, C. (2010). *Design and analysis of an energy saving distributed MAC mechanism for wireless body sensor networks.* EURASIP Journal on Wireless Communication and Networking.

Ottenbacher, J., Kirst, M., Jatoba, L., Großmann, U., & Stork, W. (2008). An approach to reliable motion artifact detection for mobile long-term ECG monitoring systems using dry electrodes. *Latin American Congress on Biomedical Engineering, 18*(3), 440 - 443.

Ouchi, K., Suzuki, T., & Doi, M. (2002). Lifeminder: A wearable healthcare support system using user's context. In *Proceedings of ICDCSW,* (pp. 791-792). ICDCSW.

Pagliari, C., Sloan, D., Gregor, P., Sullivan, F., Detmer, D., & Kahan, J. P. (2005). What is eHealth: A scoping exercise to map the field. *Journal of Medical Internet Research, 7*(1), e9. doi:10.2196/jmir.7.1.e9

Painter, C. C., & Shkel, A. M. (2001). Structural and thermal analysis of a MEMS angular gyroscope. In *Proceedings of Smart Structures and Materials 2001: Smart Electronics and MEMS,* (pp. 86-94). IEEE.

Palpanas, T., Papadopoulos, D., Kalogeraki, V., & Gunopulos, D. (2003). Distributed deviation detection in sensor networks. *SIGMOD Record, 32*(4). doi:10.1145/959060.959074

Pan, J., & Tompkins, W. J. (1985). A real-time QRS detection algorithm. *IEEE Transactions on Bio-Medical Engineering, 32*(3), 230–236. doi:10.1109/TBME.1985.325532

Pansiot, J., Stoyanov, D., Mcilwraith, D., et al. (2007). Ambient and wearable sensor fusion for activity recognition in healthcare monitoring systems. In *Proceedings of the Internatinal Workshop on Wearable and Implantable Body Sensor Networks,* (pp. 208-212). Berlin, Germany: Springer.

Pantelopoulos, A., & Borbakis, N. (2010a). A survey on wearable health care systems based on knitted integrated sensors. *IEEE Transactions on Systems, Man, and Cybernetics, 40*(1), 1–12. doi:10.1109/TSMCC.2009.2032660

Pantelopoulos, A., & Bourbakis, N. G. (2010b). A survey on wearable sensor-based systems for health monitoring and prognosis. *IEEE Transactions on Systems, Man and Cybernetics. Part C, Applications and Reviews, 40*, 1-12. doi:10.1109/TSMCC.2009.2032660

Paoletti, M., & Marchesi, C. (2006). Discovering dangerous patterns in long-term ambulatory ECG recordings using a fast QRS detection algorithm and explorative data analysis. *Computer Methods and Programs in Biomedicine, 82*(1), 20–30. doi:10.1016/j.cmpb.2006.01.005

Papanek, V. (1984). *Design for the real world: Human ecology and social change.* Chicago, IL: Academy Chicago Publishers.

Paradiso, R., Loriga, G., & Taccini, N. (2005). A wearable health care system based on knitted integrated sensors. *IEEE Transactions on Information Technology in Biomedicine, 9,* 337–344. doi:10.1109/TITB.2005.854512

Parazzini, M., Sibella, F., Paglialonga, A., & Ravazzani, P. (2010). Assessment of the exposure to WLAN frequencies of a head model with a cochlear implant. *Bioelectromagnetics, 31*(7), 546–555. doi:10.1002/bem.20601

Parker, G., Proudfoot, J., Hadzi, P. D., Manicavasagar, V., Adler, E., & Whitton, A. (2010). Community attitudes to the appropriation of mobile phones for monitoring and managing depression, anxiety, and stress. *Journal of Medical Internet Research, 12*(5).

Park, T. R., Kim, T. H., Choi, J. Y., Choi, S., & Kwon, W. H. (2005). Throughput and energy consumption analysis of IEEE 802.15.4 slotted CSMA/CA. *Electronics Letters, 41*(18), 1017–1019. doi:10.1049/el:20051662

Partners in Health. (2010). *Electronic medical records publications.* Retrieved December 14, 2010, from http://www.pih.org/pages/electronic-medical-records-publications.

Patel, A., & Schmidt, N. (2011). Application of structured document parsing to focused web crawling. *Computer Standards & Interfaces, 33*(3), 325–331. doi:10.1016/j.csi.2010.08.002

Patrick, K., Griswold, W., Raab, F., & Intille, S. (2008). Health and the mobile phone. *American Journal of Preventive Medicine, 35*(2), 177. doi:10.1016/j.amepre.2008.05.001

Pattem, S., Krishnamachari, B., & Govindan, R. (2004). The impact of spatial correlation on routing with compression in wireless sensor networks. In *Proceedings of the Third International Symposium on Information Processing in Sensor Networks,* (pp. 28-35). Berkeley, CA: ACM.

Peirce, L., & Bakke, E. (2010). *Healthcare perceptions and mobile phone use: A predictive model of text-based health communication.* Paper presented at the Annual Meeting of the International Communication Association. Suntec City, Singapore. Retrieved from http://www.allacademic.com/meta/p404783_index.

Perez-Rivera, B., & Langston-Davis, N. (2008). A model for comprehensive community-wide asthma education using partnerships and the public school curriculum. In Wallace, B. C. (Ed.), *Toward Equity in Health: A New Global Approach to Health Disparities* (pp. 529–545). New York, NY: Springer Publications.

Perry, M., O'Hara, K., Sellen, A., Brown, B., & Harper, R. (2001). Dealing with mobility: Understanding access anytime, anywhere. *ACM Transactions on Computer-Human Interaction, 8*(4), 323–347. doi:10.1145/504704.504707

Pessi, A. T., & Businger, S. (2009). Relationships among lightning, precipitation, and hydrometeor characteristics over the north Pacific ocean. *Journal of Applied Meteorology and Climatology, 48*(4), 833–848. doi:10.1175/2008JAMC1817.1

Peterson's. (2011). *Graduate programs in engineering and applied sciences* (46th ed.). Princeton, NJ: Peterson.

Peura, R. A., Boyd, J. R., Shahnarian, A., Driscoll, W. G., & Wheeler, H. B. (1975). Organization and function of a hospital biomedical engineering internship program. *IEEE Transactions on Bio-Medical Engineering, 22,* 134–140. doi:10.1109/TBME.1975.324433

Pine, J. (1993). Mass customizing products and services. *Planning Review, 22*(4), 7–55.

Pink, D. H. (2005). *A whole new mind: Moving from the information age to the conceptual age.* New York, NY: Riverhead Books.

Pires, A., & Miguel, R. (2009). Design de vestuário para a estimulação sensorial de crianças com atrasos ao nível do desenvolvimento psicomotor. In *Proceedings of Congresso E_design – Visões para o Ensino na Europa nos Novos Contextos Ambientais e Económicos, CPD – Centro Português de Design.* Lisbon, Portugal: IEEE.

Plux, S. A. (2011). *bioPlux research.* Retrieved 14 February 2011, from http://www.plux.info/biopluxresearch.

Polar Electro Oy. (2006). *RS100 training computer - running & multisport - get active - heart rate monitors - polar electro - global English.* Retrieved 7 April 2011, from http://www.polar.fi/en/products/get_active/running_multisport/RS100.

Poljicanin, T., Pavlić-Renar, I., & Metelko, Z. (2005). CroDiab net--Electronic diabetes registry. *Acta Medica Croatica, 59,* 185–189.

Poljicanin, T., Šekerija, M., & Metelko, Z. (2010). CroDiab web and improvement of diabetes care at the primary health care level. *Acta Medica Croatica, 64,* 349–354.

Pollard, J. K., Santarelli, C., Rohman, S., & Fry, M. E. (2002). Wireless and web-based medical monitoring in the home. *Medical Informatics and the Internet in Medicine, 27*(3), 219–227. doi:10.1080/1463923021000014130

Pollin, S., Ergen, M., Ergen, S., Bougard, B., Der Perre, L., & Moerman, I. (2008). Performance analysis of slotted carrier sense IEEE 802.15.4 medium access layer. *IEEE Transactions on Wireless Communications, 7*(9), 3359–3371. doi:10.1109/TWC.2008.060057

Porter, M. E. (2001). Strategy and the internet. *Harvard Business Review, 79*(2), 63–78.

Porter, M., & Millar, V. E. (1985). How information gives you competitive advantage. *Harvard Business Review, 63*(4), 149–160.

Prandelli, E., & Verona, G. (2011). *Vantaggio competitivo in rete: Dal Web 2.0 al cloud computing.* Milano, Italy: McGraw Hill.

Preuveneers, D., & Berbers, Y. (2008). Mobile phones assisting with health self-care: A diabetes case study. In *Proceedings of the 10th international Conference on Human Computer interaction with Mobile Devices and Services.* Amsterdam, The Netherlands: ACM.

Preuveneers, D., Berbers, Y., Shvaiko, P., Euzenat, J., & Léger, A. (2006). Quality extensions and uncertainty handling for context ontologies. In *Proceedings of C&O,* (pp. 62 – 64). C&O.

PricewaterhouseCoopers. (2007). *The economics of IT and hospital performance.* Retrieved July 14, 2011 from http://www.pwc.com/us/en/healthcare/publications/the-economics-of-it-and-hospital-performance.jhtml.

Prochaska, J. O. (2008). New paradigms for inclusive health care: Toward individual patient and population health. In Wallace, B. C. (Ed.), *Toward Equity in Health: A New Global Approach to Health Disparities* (pp. 61–78). New York, NY: Springer Publications.

Pubsearch. (2010). *Website.* Retrieved February 22, 2011, from http://itunes.apple.com/us/app/pubsearch/id287239420?mt=8#.

Pye, D. (1995). *The nature and aesthetics of design.* New York, NY: Cambium Press.

Qi, Y. (2003). *Wireless geolocation in a non-line-of-sight environment.* Ph.D. Dissertation. Princeton, NJ: Princeton University.

Qian, Y., Gao, X. W., Loomes, M., Comley, R., Barn, B., Hui, R., & Tian, Z. (2011). *Content-based retrieval of 3D medical images.* Paper presented at the Third International Conference on eHealth, Telemedicine, and Social Medicine, eTELEMED 2011. Guadeloupe, France.

RAFT. (2011). *Website.* Retrieved from http://raft.hcuge.ch.

Raghupathi, W., & Umar, A. (2008). Exploring a model-driven architecture (MDA) approach to health care information systems development. *International Journal of Medical Informatics, 77*(5), 305–414. doi:10.1016/j.ijmedinf.2007.04.009

Ragil, C. (Ed.). (2005). Striving for cableless monitoring. *Philips Medical Perspective Magazine, 8,* 24 - 25.

Rahman, Z. (2004). E-commerce solution for services. *European Business Review, 16*(6), 564–576. doi:10.1108/09555340410565396

Rakowitz, B. (2011). How (in-)complete are study reports? *Deutsche Medizinische Wochenschrift, 136*(15), 752.

Rashidi, H. H., & Buehler, L. K. (2000). *Bioinformatics basics: Applications in biological science and medicine.* Boca Raton, FL: CRC Press.

Ratner, B. D., Hoffman, A. S., Schoen, F. J., & Lemons, J. E. (2004). *Biomaterials science: An introduction to materials in medicine* (2nd ed.). San Diego, CA: Academic Press.

Ravenscroft, A. (2009). Social software, Web 2.0 and learning: Status and implications of an evolving paradigm. *Journal of Computer Assisted Learning, 25*(1), 1–5. doi:10.1111/j.1365-2729.2008.00308.x

Rayport, J. F., & Jaworski, B. J. (2001). *E-commerce.* New York, NY: McGraw Hill.

Razzaque, M. A., Dobson, S., & Nixon, P. (2005). *Categorization and modelling of quality in context information.* Paper presented at the Workshop on AI and Autonomic Communications. New York, NY.

Rehabilitation Engineering and Assistive Technology Society of North America (RESNA). (2011). *Website.* Retrieved from http://resna.org.

Repovs, G., & Baddeley, A. (2006). The multi-component model of working memory: Explorations in experimental cognitive psychology. *Neuroscience, 139*(1), 5–21. doi:10.1016/j.neuroscience.2005.12.061

Requena-Carrion, J., & Leder, R. S. (2009). The natural history of the engineering in medicine and biology society from a modern perspective. In *Proceedings of the IEEE Engineering in Medicine and Biology Society Conference 2009,* (pp. 1086-1088). IEEE Press.

Research2Guideance. (2010). *Mobile health market report 2010-2015.* Retrieved February 14, 2011, from http://www.research2guidance.com/shop/index.php/mHealth-report.

Revere, L., Black, K., & Zalila, F. (2010). RFIDs can improve the patient care supply chain. *Hospital Topics, 88*(1), 26–31. doi:10.1080/00185860903534315

Rhea, S. (2010). Going mobile: Wireless devices and technology bring surge in advanced applications for health monitoring and treatment, but legal and privacy issues remain. *Modern Healthcare, 40*(18), 28–30. Retrieved from http://www.ncbi.nlm.nih.gov/pubmed/20480559

Ricci, A., Facen, A., Grisanti, M., Boni, A., Munari, I. D., Ciampolini, P., & Morandi, C. (2010). Low-power transponders for RFID. In Yan, L., Zhang, Y., Yang, L. T., & Chen, J. (Eds.), *RFID and Sensor Networks: Architectures, Protocols, Security, and Integrations* (pp. 59–95). Boca Raton, FL: Auerbach Publications, Taylor & Francis Group.

Rifkin, J. (2000). *The age of access: The new culture of hypercapitalism, where all of life is a paid-for experience.* New York, NY: Tarcher/Putnam.

Rinderle-Ma, S., Reichert, M., & Jurisch, M. (2011). On utilizing web service equivalence for supporting the composition life cycle. *International Journal of Web Services Research, 8*(1), 41–67. doi:10.4018/jwsr.2011010103

RIS. (2011). *Website.* Retrieved from http://en.wikipedia.org/wiki/Radiology_information_system.

Roark, D. C., & Miguel, K. (2006). RFID: Bar coding's replacement? *Nursing Management, 37*(2), 28–31. doi:10.1097/00006247-200602000-00009

Rodrigues, S., Miguel, R., Lucas, J., Gaiolas, C., Araújo, P., & Reis, N. (2009). *Wearable technology - Development of polypyrrole textile electrodes for electromyography.* Paper presented at the BIODEVICES 2009 - International Conference on Biomedical Electronics and Devices. Porto, Portugal.

Rodrigues, S., Miguel, R., Reis, N., Araújo, P., & Lucas, J. (2008). *Wearable technology for muscle activity monitoring.* Paper presented at the CONTROLO 2008 - 8th Portuguese Conference on Automatic Control. Vila Real, Portugal.

Rodrigues, J. J. P. C., Pereira, O. R. E., & Neves, P. A. C. S. (2011). Biofeedback data visualization for body sensor networks. *Journal of Network and Computer Applications, 34*(1), 151–158. doi:10.1016/j.jnca.2010.08.005

Roine, R., Ohinmaa, A., & Hailey, D. (2001). Assessing telemedicine: A systematic review of the literature. *Canadian Medical Association Journal, 165*(6), 765–771.

Ruefli, T. W., Whinston, A., & Wiggins, R. R. (2001). The digital technological environment. In Wind, J., & Mahajan, V. (Eds.), *Digital Marketing* (pp. 26–58). New York, NY: John Wiley & Sons.

Rullani, E. (2001). New/net/knowledge economy: Le molte facce del postfordismo. *Economia e Politica Industriale, 110,* 6–31.

Sabinet. (2010). *Minister of health calls for national telemedicine strategy.* Retrieved November 19, 2010, from http://www.sabinetlaw.co.za/health/articles/minister-health-calls-national-telemedicine-strategy.

Sainz, B., de la Torre, I., Bermejo, P., García, E., Díaz, F. J., Díez, J. F., … de Castro, C. (2010). Evolución, beneficios y obstáculos en la implantación del historial clínico electrónico en el sistema sanitario. *Revista esalud. com, 6*(22).

Salah, A. A., Bicego, M., Akarun, L., Grosso, E., & Tistarelli, M. (2007). *Hidden Markov model-based face recognition using selective attention.* Paper presented at the Human Vision and Electronic Imaging XII. San Jose, CA.

Salomann, H., Kolbe, L., & Brenner, W. (2006). Self-services in customer relationships: Balancing high-tech and high-touch today and tomorrow. *E-Service Journal, 4*(2), 65–84. doi:10.2979/ESJ.2006.4.2.65

Saltzman, W. M. (2009). *Biomedical engineering.* Cambridge, UK: Cambridge University Press.

Samara, T. (2007). *Design elements: A graphic style manual: Understanding the rules and knowing when to break them.* Gloucester, MA: Rockport Publishers.

Samsung. (2011). *SAR information.* Retrieved from http://www.samsung.com/uk/support/sar/sarMain. do?prd_mdl_name=SCH-I510.

Sanders, D., Mukhi, S., Laskowski, M., Khan, M., Podaima, B. W., & McLeod, R. D. (2008). A network-enabled platform for reducing hospital emergency department waiting times using an RFID proximity location system. In *Proceedings of the International Conference on Systems Engineering (ICSENG 2008)*, (pp. 538-543). ICSENG.

Sarkar, U., Piette, J. D., Gonzales, R., Lessler, D., Chew, L. D., & Reilly, B. (2008). Preferences for self-management support: Findings from a survey of diabetes patients in safety-net health systems. *Patient Education and Counseling, 70*(1), 102–110. doi:10.1016/j.pec.2007.09.008

Sawhney, M., & Parikh, D. (2001). Where value lives in a networked world. *Harvard Business Review, 79*(1), 79–86.

Schmiedl, U. P., & Rowberg, A. H. (1990). Literature review: Picture archiving and communication systems. *Journal of Digital Imaging, 3*(3), 178–194. doi:10.1007/BF03167608

Schneck, D. J., & Bronzino, J. D. (2002). *Biomechanics: Principles and applications.* Boca Raton, FL: CRC Press. doi:10.1201/9781420040029

Schulz, S., Suntisrivaraporn, B., Baader, F., & Boeker, M. (2009). SNOMED reaching its adolescence: Ontologists' and logicians' health check. *International Journal of Medical Informatics, 78*(1), 86–94. doi:10.1016/j.ijmedinf.2008.06.004

Schumm, J., Axmann, S., Arnrich, B., & Tröster, G. (2010). Automatic signal appraisal for unobtrusive ECG measurements. *International Journal of Bioelectromagnetism, 12*(4), 158–164.

Schwan, H. P. (1984). The development of biomedical engineering: Historical comments and personal observations. *IEEE Transactions on Bio-Medical Engineering, 31*(12), 730–736. doi:10.1109/TBME.1984.325328

Schwartz, M. D. (1984). The emerging field of clinical engineering and its accomplishments. *IEEE Transactions on Bio-Medical Engineering, 31*(12), 743–748. doi:10.1109/TBME.1984.325233

Schwartz, M. D., & Long, F. M. (1975). A survey analysis of biomedical engineering education. *IEEE Transactions on Bio-Medical Engineering, 22*, 119–124. doi:10.1109/TBME.1975.324430

Scilingo, E. P., Gemignani, A., Paradiso, R., Taccini, N., Ghelarducci, B., & Rossi, D. D. (2005). Performance evaluation of sensing fabrics for monitoring physiological and biomechanical variables. *IEEE Transactions on Information Technology in Biomedicine, 9*(3), 345–352. doi:10.1109/TITB.2005.854506

Seebregts, C. J., Mamlin, B. W., Biondich, P. G., Fraser, H. S., Wolfe, B. A., & Jazayeri, D. (2009). The OpenMRS implementers network. *International Journal of Medical Informatics, 78*(11), 711–720. doi:10.1016/j.ijmedinf.2008.09.005

Semmlow, J. L. (2004). *Biosignal and medical image processing: MATLAB-based applications.* Boca Raton, FL: CRC Press Taylor & Francis.

Settle, D. (2010). Greater than the sum. *Global Health.* Retrieved from http://www.globalhealthmagazine.com/top_stories/greater_than_the_sum/.

Shapiro, C., & Varian, H. R. (1999). *Information rules: A strategic guide to the network economy.* Boston, MA: Harvard Business School Press.

Sharp. (2006). *GP2Y1010AU0F compact optical dust sensor*. Technical Report. Retrieved from www.sharp-world.com.

Shaw, M. (2001). Finding and using secondary data on the health and health care of populations. In Stevens, A., Fitzpatrick, R., Abrams, K., Brazier, J., & Lilford, R. (Eds.), *The Advanced Handbook of Methods in Evidence Based Healthcare* (pp. 164–189). London, UK: SAGE Publications.

Sheikh, K., Wegdam, M., & Van-Sinderen, M. (2007). Middleware support for quality of context in pervasive context-aware systems. In *Proceedings of the International Conference on Pervasive Computing and Communications Workshops*, (pp. 461–466). White Plains, NY: IEEE Press.

Sheikh, K., Wegdam, M., & Van-Sinderen, M. (2008). Quality-of-context and its use for protecting privacy in context aware systems. *Journal of Software*, *3*(1), 83–93.

Shekelle, P., & Goldzweig, C. L. (2009). *Costs and benefits of health information technology: An updated systematic review*. London, UK: The Health Foundation.

Shi, G., Zou, Y., Jin, Y., Cui, X., & Li, W. J. (2009). Towards HMM based human motion recognition using MEMS inertial sensors. In *Proceedings of the 2008 IEEE International Conference on Robotics and Biomimetics*. Bangkok, Thailand: IEEE Press.

Shortliffe, E. H., & Ciminio, J. J. (2006). *Biomedical informatics: Computer applications in health care and biomedicine*. New York, NY: Springer Verlag.

Shylie, M. (2009). Functional independence measure. *The Australian Journal of Physiotherapy*, *n.d.*, 55.

Shyu, M.-L., Chen, S.-C., & Luo, H. (2002). Optimal bandwidth allocation scheme with delay awareness in multimedia transmission. In *Proceedings of ICME*, *2002*, 37–540.

Siika, A. M., Rotich, J. K., Simiyu, C. J., Kigotho, E. M., Smith, F. E., & Sidle, J. E. (2005). An electronic medical record system for ambulatory care of HIV-infected patients in Kenya. *International Journal of Medical Informatics*, *74*(5), 345–355. doi:10.1016/j.ijmedinf.2005.03.002

Sixsmith, A., & Johnson, N. (2004). A smart sensor to detect the falls of the elderly. In *Proceedings of the IEEE Pervasive Computing*, (pp. 42–47). IEEE Press.

Slack, C. (2007). The robot surgeon. *Proto Magazine*. Retrieved June 17, 2011 from http://www.protomag.com/assets/the-robot-surgeon?page=1.

SmartCare. (2011). *Web page*. Retrieved May 12, 2011, from http://www.smartcare.org.zm.

Society for Biomaterials (SFB). (2011). *Website*. Retrieved from http://www.biomaterials.org/index.cfm.

Sood, S., Mbarika, V., Jugoo, S., Dookhy, R., Doarn, C. R., Prakash, N., & Merrell, R. C. (2007). What is telemedicine? A collection of 104 peer-reviewed perspectives and theoretical underpinnings. *Telemedicine Journal and e-Health*, *13*(5), 573–590. doi:10.1089/tmj.2006.0073

Spanjers, I. A. E., Wouters, P., van Gog, T., & van Merriënboer, J. J. G. (2011). An expertise reversal effect of segmentation in learning from animated worked-out examples. *Computers in Human Behavior*, *27*(1), 46–52. doi:10.1016/j.chb.2010.05.011

Spinelli, R. (2008). The digital economy: A conceptual framework for a new economic paradigm. *The Journal of Business*, *8*(1/2), 53–59.

SQL. (2010). *Web page*. Retrieved December 14, 2010, from http://www.sql.org.

St. Jude Children's Research Hospital. (2011). *How Cure4Kids can help*. Retrieved February 14, 2011, from https://www.cure4kids.org/ums/home/.

Stansfield, S. (2005). Structuring information and incentives to improve health. *Bulletin of the World Health Organization*, *83*, 562.

Stauch, G., Oberholzer, M., Kuakpaetoon, T., & Schattka, S. (2005). *Telepathology in developing countries in south east Asia: Results, limits, future Phnom Penh project*. Paper presented at the 3rd International Conference on Telemedicine & Multimedia Communication. Poland.

Stauffer, C., & Grimson, W. E. (2000). Learning patterns of activity using real time tracking. *IEEE Transactions on Pattern Analysis and Machine Intelligence*, *22*(8), 747–757. doi:10.1109/34.868677

Steadham, S. V. (1980). Learning to select a needs assessment strategy. *Training and Development Journal*, *34*(1), 56–61.

Steele, B. G., Holt, R. N. L., Belza, B., Ferris, S., Lakshminaryan, S., & Buchner, D. M. (2000). Quantitating physical activity in COPD using a triaxial accelerometer. *Chest, 117*, 1359–1367. doi:10.1378/chest.117.5.1359

Stevens, A., Fitzpatrick, R., Abrams, K., Brazier, J., & Lilford, R. (2001). Methods in evidence based healthcare and health technology assessment: An overview. In Stevens, A., Fitzpatrick, R., Abrams, K., Brazier, J., & Lilford, R. (Eds.), *The Advanced Handbook of Methods in Evidence Based Healthcare* (pp. 1–5). London, UK: SAGE Publications.

STMicroelectronics. (2009). *LPR530AP MEMS motion sensor: dual axis pitch and roll 300/s analog gyroscope.* Technical Report. Retrieved from www.nex-robotics.com.

Stonebraker, M., & Cetintemel, U. (2005). One size fits all: An idea whose time has come and gone. In *Proceedings of the 2005 International Conference on Data Engineering.* IEEE.

Store, A. (2011). *Website.* Retrieved February 22, 2011, from http://itunes.apple.com/us/genre/ios-medical/id6020?mt=8.

Stoto, M. A. (2008). Public health surveillance in the twenty-first century: Achieving population health goals while protecting individuals' privacy and confidentiality. *The Georgetown Law Journal, 96*, 703–719.

Strang, T., & Linnhoff-Popien, C. (2004). A context modeling survey. In *Proceedings of the Workshop on Advanced Context Modelling Reasoning and Management as part of UbiComp*, (pp. 33 – 40). Nottingham, UK: IEEE.

Strauss, A. L., Shizuko, F., Sucker, B., & Wiener, C. (1997). *Social organization of medical work.* New Brunswick, NJ: Transaction Publisher.

Strecher, V. J., Greenwood, T., Wang, C., & Dumont, D. (1999). Interactive multimedia and risk communication. *Journal of the National Cancer Institute. Monographs, 25*, 134–139.

Stroetmann, K. A., Jones, T., Dobrev, A., & Stroetmann, V. N. (2006). *eHealth is worth it: The economic benefits of implemented eHealth solutions at ten European sites.* Luxembourg: Commission of the European Communities.

Subramaniam, S., Palpanas, T., Papadopoulos, D., Kalogeraki, V., & Gunopulos, D. (2006). Online outlier detection in sensor data using non-parametric models. In *Proceedings of VLDB 2006.* VLDB.

Such, O., & Muehlsteff, J. (2006). The challenge of motion artifact suppression in wearable monitoring solutions. In *Proceedings of the 3rd IEEE/EMBS International Summer School on Medical Devices and Biosensors*, (pp. 49 – 52). Cambridge, MA: IEEE Press.

Sung-Eui, C. (2005). Developing new frameworks for operations strategy and service system design in electronic commerce. *International Journal of Service Industry Management, 16*(3), 294–314. doi:10.1108/09564230510601413

Swedberg, C. (2010a). RFID-based hand-hygiene system prevents health-care acquired infections. *RFID Journal.* Retrieved June 11, 2010, from http://www.rfidjournal.com/article/view/7660.

Swedberg, C. (2010b). Boeing, Fujitsu to offer airlines a holistic RFID solution. *RFID Journal.* Retrieved February 19, 2011, from http://www.rfidjournal.com/article/view/8099.

Swedberg, C. (2011a). Pittsburgh researchers develop implantable RFID for orthopedic device. *RFID Journal.* Retrieved June 20, 2011, from http://www.rfidjournal.com/article/view/8538.

Swedberg, C. (2011b). Wi-Fi system monitors health of cardiac patients. *RFID Journal.* Retrieved July 1, 2011, from http://www.rfidjournal.com/article/view/8535.

Sweller, J. (1994). Cognitive load theory, learning difficulty, and instructional design. *Learning and Instruction, 4*(4), 295–312. doi:10.1016/0959-4752(94)90003-5

Systems Architecture, N. E. D. S. S. (2001). *Centers for disease control and prevention.* Retrieved by January 15, 2011, from http://www.cdc.gov/nedss/BaseSystem/NEDSSsysarch2.0.pdf.

Szczepaniak, M. C. (2011). *Real-time outbreak and disease surveillance laboratory.* Retrieved January 11, 2011, from https://www.rods.pitt.edu/site/content/view/14/77/.

Szczepański, A., Saeed, H., & Ferscha, A. (2010). A new method for ECG signal feature extraction. In *Proceedings of the International Conference on Computer Vision and Graphics*, (pp. 334 – 341). IEEE.

Taflove, A. (1998). *Advances in computational electromagnetics: The finite difference time domain method.* London, UK: Artech House.

Takeda, R., Tadano, S., Natorigawa, A., Todoh, M., & Yoshinari, S. (2009). Gait posture estimation using wearable acceleration and gyro sensors. *Journal of Biomechanics*, *42*, 2486–2494. doi:10.1016/j.jbiomech.2009.07.016

Tan, X., Guo, X. M., Cheng, M., & Yan, Y. (2007). Wireless telemedicine physiological monitoring center based on virtual instruments. In *Proceedings of the Bioinformatics and Biomedical Engineering*, (pp. 1157 – 1160). Wuhan, China: IEEE Press.

Tan, C., & Wang, H. (2008). Body sensor network security: An identity-based cryptography approach. In *Proceedings of WiSec 2008*. WiSec.

Tang, S., Yang, J., & Wu, Z. (2007). A context quality model for ubiquitous applications. In *Proceedings of the IFIP International Conference on Network and Parallel Computing Workshops*, (pp. 282 – 287). IEEE Press.

Tao, Y., & Miao, J. (2002). The management and realizing of image data flow in PACS. *Chinese Journal of Radiology*, *36*(10), 171–173.

Tapscott, D. (2001). Rethinking strategy in a networked world. *Strategy + Business, 24*, 1-8.

Tatbul, N., Buller, M., Hoyt, R., et al. (2004). Confidence based data management for personal area sensor networks. In *Proceeedings of the 1st International Workshop on Data Management for Sensor Networks*. VLDB.

Tattersall, J. E. H., Scott, I. R., Wood, S. J., Nettell, J. J., Bevir, M. K., & Wang, Z. (2001). Effects of low intensity radiofrequency electromagnetic fields on electrical activity in rat hippocampal slices. *Brain Research*, *904*(1), 43–53. doi:10.1016/S0006-8993(01)02434-9

Taussig, K. S. (1997). Calvinism and chromosomes: Religion, the geographical imaginary, and medical genetics in the Netherlands. *Science as Culture*, *4*(29), 495–524. doi:10.1080/09505439709526483

Taylor, J., Dearnley, C., Laxton, J., Coates, C., Treasure-Jones, T., & Campbell, R. (2010). Developing a mobile learning solution for health and social care practice. *Distance Education*, *31*(2), 175–192. doi:10.1080/01587919.2010.503343

Taylor, P. (1998). A survey of research in telemedicine: Telemedicine services. *Journal of Telemedicine and Telecare*, *4*(2), 63–71. doi:10.1258/1357633981931948

Taylor, R., Bower, A., Girosi, F., Bigelow, J., Fonkych, K., & Hillestad, R. (2005). Promoting health information technology: Is there a case for more-aggressive government action? *Health Affairs*, *24*(5), 1234–1345. doi:10.1377/hlthaff.24.5.1234

Tech Briefs, N. A. S. A. (2011). *Electrocardiography (ECG) necklace.* Retrieved 13 June 2011, from http://www.techbriefs.com/component/content/article/10231.

Technology, H. M. (2010). Mobile on the rise. *ProQuest Medical Library*, *31*(3), 8.

Teece, D. J. (1986). Profiting from technological innovation: Implications for integration, collaboration, licensing and public policy. *Research Policy*, *15*(6), 285–305. doi:10.1016/0048-7333(86)90027-2

TeleMed. (1997). Proceedings of International Conference on Telemedicienne and Telecare (Telemed'96). *Journal of Telemedicine and Telecare*, *3*, 1–120.

TeleMed. (1998). Proceedings of international conference on telemedicienne and telecare (Telemed 1997). *Journal of Telemedicine and Telecare*, *4*, 1–112.

Telemedicine. (2005). *Website.* Retrieved from http://www.kpk.gov.pl/pliki/2493/Telemedicine_Conference%20in%20Poland.pdf.

Teutsch, S. M., & Churchill, R. E. (Eds.). (2000). *Principles and practice of public health surveillance.* New York, NY: Oxford University Press.

Thacker, S. B. (2003). *HIPAA privacy rule and public healthL Guidance from CDC and the U.S. Department of Health and Human Services.* Retrieved Mach 05, 2011, from http://www.cdc.gov/mmwr/preview/mmwrhtml/m2e411a1.htm.

Thacker, S. B., Stroup, D. F., & Dicker, R. C. (2003). Health data management for public health. In F. D. Scutchfield & C. W. KecK (Eds.), *Principles of Public Health Practices*, (p. 225). New York, NY: Thomson Delmar Learning.

The CTIA Wireless Association. (2010). *CTIA announces 2010 e-tech awards winners*. Retrieved February 16, 2011, from http://www.ctia.org/media/press/body.cfm/prid/1939.

The Economist. (2006). *The medical uses of mobile phones show they can be good for your health*. Retrieved January 30, 2011, from http://www.economist.com/node/5655105.

The Whitaker Foundation. (2011). *A history of biomedical engineering (May 2002)*. Retrieved from http://bmes.seas.wustl.edu/WhitakerArchives/glance/history.html.

Thiemjarus, S., Lo, B., & Yang, G. (2006). A spatio temporal architecture for context aware sensing. In *Proceedings of the International Workshop on Wearable and Implantable Body Sensor Networks (BSN)*, (pp. 1-4). Washington, DC: IEEE Press.

Thomas, D. R. E. (1978). Strategy is different in service businesses. *Harvard Business Review*, *56*(4), 158–165.

Thom, H. (1996). *Introduction to shortwave and microwave therapy*. Springfield, IL: Charles C. Thomas.

Thompkins, W. J. (1993). *Biomedical digital signal processing*. Englewood Cliffs, NJ: Prentice-Hall.

Tian, Z., Lu, W., Wang, T., Ma, B., Zhao, Q., & Zhang, G. (2008). Application of a robotic telemanipulation system in stereotactic surgery. *Stereotactic and Functional Neurosurgery*, *86*, 54–61. doi:10.1159/000110742

Tian, Z., Lu, W., Zhao, Q., Yu, X., Qi, S., & Wang, R. (2008a). From frame to frameless stereotactic operation—Clinical application of 2011 cases. *Lecture Notes in Computer Science*, *4987*, 18–24. doi:10.1007/978-3-540-79490-5_4

Tian, Z., Wang, T., Liu, Z., Zhao, Q., Du, J., & Liu, D. (1998). Robot assisted system in stereotactic neurosurgery. *Academic Journal of PLA Postgraduate Medicine School*, *1*, 4–5.

Ting, J. S. L., Tsang, A. H. C., Ip, A. W. H., & Ho, G. T. S. (2011). Professional practice and innovation: RF-MediSys: A radio frequency identification-based electronic medical record system for improving medical information accessibility and services at point of care. *Health Information Management Journal*, *40*(1), 25–32.

Ting, S. L., Kwok, S. K., Tsang, A. H. C., & Lee, W. B. (2011). Critical elements and lessons learnt from the implementation of an RFID-enabled healthcare management system in a medical organization. *Journal of Medical Systems*, *35*(4), 657–669. doi:10.1007/s10916-009-9403-5

Tinniswood, A. D., & Gandhi, O. P. (1998). Computations of SAR distributions for two anatomically based models of the human head using CAD files of commercial telephones and the parallelized FDTD code. *IEEE Transactions on Antennas and Propagation*, *46*, 829–833. doi:10.1109/8.686769

Tirtom, H., Mehmet, E., & Erkan, Z. E. (2008). Enhancement of time-frequency properties of ECG for detecting micropotentials by wavelet transform based method. *Expert Systems with Applications*, *34*(1), 746–753. doi:10.1016/j.eswa.2006.10.009

Tocci, R. (1988). *Digital system- Principles and applications* (4th ed.). Englewood Cliffs, CA: Prentice-Hall International.

Tolven Healthcare. (2011). *Web page*. Retrieved May 12, 2011, http://www.tolven.org.

Tomasi, E., Facchini, L. A., & Maia, M. F. (2004). Health information technology in primary health care in developing countries: A literature review. *Bulletin of the World Health Organization*, *82*(11), 867–874.

Tong, L., Zhao, Q., & Mergen, G. (2001). Multipacket reception in random access wireless networks: From signal processing to optimal medium access control. *IEEE Communications Magazine*, *39*(11), 108–112. doi:10.1109/35.965367

Torzyn, N. T., McKinney, W. D., Abbott, E. L. Jr, Cook, A. M., & Gillott, D. H. (1975). Biomedical engineering program to upgrade biomedical equipment technicians. *IEEE Transactions on Bio-Medical Engineering*, *22*, 145–147. doi:10.1109/TBME.1975.324435

Trindade, I. G., Pereira, M., Salvado, R., Lucas, J., Garcia, N. M., Silva, J. S., et al. (2010). *Intelligent clothing for health care*. Paper presented at the Symposium de Materiais e Processos Inovadores. Covilhã, Portugal.

Trindade, I., Lucas, J., Miguel, R., Alpuim, P., Carvalho, M., & Garcia, N. M. (2010). *Portable systems for health care*. Paper presented at the The IEEE 12th International Conference on e-Health Networking, Applications and Services (IEEE HealthCom 2010). Lyon, France.

Trusted Opensource Records for Care and Health. (2011). *Web page*. Retrieved May 12, 2011, from https://launchpad.net/trusted. XML. (2010). *Web page*. Retrieved December 14, 2010, from http://www.w3.org/XML.

Tsui, F. C., Espino, J. U., Wagner, M. M., Gesteland, P., Ivanov, O., & Olszewski, R. T. ... Moore, A. (2002). *Data, network, and application: Technical description of the Utah RODS winter olympic biosurveillance system*. Retrieved January 05, 2011, from http://rods.health.pitt.edu/LIBRARY/AMIA02-TsuiJue-Final.pdf.

Tuomainen, M., Mykkänen, J., Luostarinen, H., Pöyhölä, A., & Paakkanen, E. (2007). Model-centric approaches for the development of health information systems. *Studies in Health Technology and Informatics*, *129*(1), 28–32.

Turban, E., Aronson, J., & Liang, T. (2005). *Decision support systems and intelligent systems* (7th ed.). Upper Saddle River, NJ: Prentice Hall.

Turner, C., Bishay, H., Peng, B., & Merifield, A. (2006). The ALPHA project: An architecture for leveraging public health applications. *International Journal of Medical Informatics*, *75*(10-11), 741–754. doi:10.1016/j.ijmedinf.2005.10.006

Turner, L., & Mickle, M. H. (2007). Overview primer on near-field UHF versus near-field HF RFID tags. *International Journal of Radio Frequency Identification Technology and Applications*, *1*(3), 291–302. doi:10.1504/IJRFITA.2007.015852

U.S Census Bureau. (2011). *International database-World population summary*. Retrieved January 10, 2011, from http://www.census.gov/ipc/www/idb/worldpopinfo.php.

U.S. Department of Health and Human Services. (2011). *Health information privacy*. Retrieved March 13, 2011, from http://www.hhs.gov/ocr/privacy.

United Nations. (2008). *The millennium development goals report*. Retrieved from http://www.un.org/millenniumgoals/pdf/The%20Millennium%20Development%20Goals%20Report%202008.pdf.

Universal Doctor Speaker. (2010). *Website*. Retrieved February 22, 2011, from http://itunes.apple.com/us/app/universal-doctor-speaker-for/id364812043?mt=8.

University Health Network. (2011). *Patient education: Improving health through education*. Retrieved February 14, 2011, from http://www.uhn.ca/patients_&_visitors/health_info/topics/pen/index.asp.

Ursutiu, D., Cotfas, D. T., Ghercioiu, M., Samoila, C., Cotfas, P. A., & Auer, M. (2010). WEB instruments. In *Proceedings of the Education Engineering (EDUCON) – The Future of Global Learning Engineering Education*, (pp. 585 - 590). Madrid, Spain: IEEE Press.

Ursutiu, D. (2010). Wireless sensor networks and cloud instruments for web based measurements, guest editorial. *International Journal of Online Engineering*, *6*(4), 4–5.

US Centers for Disease Control and Prevention. (2004). *About chronic disease: Definition, overall burden, and cost effectiveness of prevention*. Washington, DC: National Center for Chronic Disease Prevention and Health Promotion. Retrieved June 27, 2011, from http://www.cdc.gov/chronicdisease/about/index.htm.

US Department of Health and Human Services. (1996). *Guide to clinical preventive services: Report o the U.S. preventive services task force* (2nd ed.). Washington, DC: US Preventive Services Task Force.

Valdani, E. (2000). I quattro fondamenti dell'economia digitale. *Economia & Management*, *3*, 51–67.

Valenzuela, R. A. (1993). A ray tracing approach to predicting indoor wireless transmission. In *Proceedings of the IEEE Vehicular Technology Conference*, (pp. 214 – 218). Secaucus, NJ: IEEE Press.

Values, S. A. R. (2011). *The complete SAR list for all phones (Europe)*. Retrieved from http://www.sarvalues.com/eu-complete.html.

Van Halteren, A., Bults, R., Wac, K., Konstantas, D., Widya, I., & Dokovsky, N. (2004). Mobile patient monitoring: The MobiHealth system. *The Journal on Information Technology in Healthcare*, *2*(5), 365–373.

Van, L. K., & Gellersen, H. W. (2004). A study in distributed wearable activity recognition. In *Proceedings of the 8th IEEE International Symposium on Wearable Computers (ISWC)*, (pp. 142-149). Washington, DC: IEEE Press.

Velikina, R., Dato, V., & Wagner, M. M. (2006). Governmental public health. In Wagner, M. M., Moore, A. W., & Aryel, R. M. (Eds.), *Handbook of Biossurveilance* (pp. 67–87). Burlington, MA: Elsevier Academic Press. doi:10.1016/B978-012369378-5/50007-7

Venkatasubramanian, K. K., & Gupta, S. K. S. (2010). Physiological value-based efficient usable security solutions for body sensor networks. *ACM Transactions on Sensor Networks*, 6(4), 1–36. doi:10.1145/1777406.1777410

Viana, W., Filho, J. B., Gensel, J., Villanova-Oliver, M., & Martin, H. (2008). PhotoMap: From location and time to context-aware photo annotations. *Journal of Location Based Services*, 2(1), 211–235. doi:10.1080/17489720802487956

Vicari, S. (2001a). Il management della virtualità. In Vicari, S. (Ed.), *Economia Della Virtualità* (pp. 5–59). Milano, Italy: Egea.

Vicari, S. (2001b). Dalla catena alla rete virtuale del valore. In Vicari, S. (Ed.), *Il Management Nell'era Della Connessione* (pp. 3–50). Milano, Italy: Egea.

Villalonga, C., Roggen, D., Lombriser, C., Zappi, P., & Tröster, G. (2009). Bringing quality of context into wearable human activity recognition systems quality of context. In *Proceedings of the First International Workshop on Quality of Context*, (pp. 164 – 173). Springer.

Vinjumur, J. K., Becker, E., Ferdous, S., Galatas, G., & Makedon, F. (2010). Web based medicine intake tracking application. In *Proceedings of the 3rd International Conference on Pervasive Technologies Related To Assistive Environments*. IEEE.

Vistumbler. (2011). *Website*. Retrieved from http://www.vistumbler.net/.

Vital Wave Consulting. (2009). *mHealth for development: The opportunity of mobile technology for healthcare in the developing world*. Washington, DC: UN Foundation-Vodafone Foundation Partnership. Retrieved form http://www.globalproblems-global-solutions-files.org/unf_website/assets/publications/technology/mHealth/ mHealth_for_Development_full.pdf.

Vogt, R. L., Larue, D., Klaucke, D. N., & Jillson, D. A. (1983). Comparison of an active and passive surveillance system of primary care providers for Hepatitis, Measles, Rubella, and Salmonellosis in Vermont. *American Journal of Public Health, 73*, 795–797. doi:10.2105/AJPH.73.7.795

Wagner, M. M., Moore, A. W., & Aryel, R. M. (Eds.). (2006). *Handbook of biosurveillance*. Burlington, MA: Elsevier Academic Press.

Wallace, B. C. (2005). *HIV/AIDS peer education training manual: Combining African healing wisdom and evidence-based behavior change strategies*. Philadelphia, PA: StarSpirit Press.

Wallace, B. C. (2008). Introduction: The forces driving and embodied within a new field of equity in health. In Wallace, B. C. (Ed.), *Toward Equity in Health: A New Global Approach to Health Disparities*. New York, NY: Springer Publications.

Walsham, G., & Sahay, S. (2006). Research on information systems in developing countries: Current landscape and future prospects. *Information Technology for Development*, 12(1), 7–24. doi:10.1002/itdj.20020

Wang, H., Choi, H., Agoulmine, N., Deen, M. J., & Hong, J. W. (2010). Information-based sensor tasking wireless body area networks in u-health systems. In *Proceedings of the 6th International Conference on Network and Service Management*, (pp. 517 – 522). Niagara Falls, Canada: IEEE Press.

Wang, X. (2004). Wide-band TD-CDMA MAC with minimum-power allocation and rate- and BER-scheduling for wireless multimedia networks. *IEEE/ACM Transactions on Networking*, 12(1), 103–116. doi:10.1109/TNET.2003.822663

Wang, Z. M., Pierson, R. Jr, & Heymsfield, S. B. (1992). The five-level model: A new approach to organizing body-composition research. *The American Journal of Clinical Nutrition, 56*, 19–25.

Wang, Z., & Gu, H. (2009). A review of TeleMedicine in China. *Journal of Telemedicine and Telecare, 15*, 23–27. doi:10.1258/jtt.2008.080508

Warakagoda, N. D., & Hogskole, N. T. (1996). *A hybrid ANN-HMM ASR system with NN based adaptive preprocessing*. Retrieved from http://jedlik.phy.bme.hu/~gerjanos/HMM/hoved.html.

Weaver, J. B., Mays, D., Weaver, S. S., Hopkins, G. L., Eroglu, D., & Bernhardt, J. M. (2010). Health information-seeking behaviors, health indicators, and health risks. *American Journal of Public Health, 100*(8), 1520–1525. doi:10.2105/AJPH.2009.180521

Webopedia. (2010). *Mobile phone*. Retrieved January 30, 2010, from http://www.webopedia.com/TERM/M/mobile_phone.html.

Webster, J. G., & Cook, A. M. (1979). *Clinical engineering: Principles and practices*. Tanglewood Cliffs, NJ: Prentice Hall.

Weed, H. R. (1975). Biomedical engineering— Practice or research? *IEEE Transactions on Bio-Medical Engineering, 22*, 110–113. doi:10.1109/TBME.1975.324428

Wennberg, D., , Bennett, G., O'Malley, S., Lang, L., & Marr, A., (2010). Randomized trial of a telephone care-management strategy. *The New England Journal of Medicine, 363*, 1245–1255. Retrieved from http://www.nejm.org/doi/full/10.1056/NEJMsa0902321doi:10.1056/NEJMsa0902321

Wessel, R. (2010). Airbus signs contract for high-memory RFID tags. *RFID Journal*. Retrieved February 19, 2011, from http://www.rfidjournal.com/article/view/7323.

Westbrook, J. I., Gosling, A. S., & Coiera, E. (2004). Do clinicians use online evidence to support patient care? A study of 55.000 clinicians. *Journal of the American Medical Informatics Association, 11*(2), 113–120. doi:10.1197/jamia.M1385

Whitney, L. (2011). *Report: Apple remains king of app-store market*. Retrieved February 16, 2011, from http://news.cnet.com/8301-13579_3-20032012-37.html.

Whitten, P., & Love, B. (2005). Patient and provider satisfaction with the use of telemedicine: Overview and rationale for cautious enthusiasm. *Journal of Postgraduate Medicine, 51*(4), 294–299.

WHO. (1990). Diabetes care and reasearch in Europe: The Saint Vincent declaration. *Diabetes Mellitus, 7*, 360.

WHO. (1999). *Recommended surveillance standards*. Retrieved February 05, 2011, from http://www.who.int/csr/resources/publications/surveillance/whocdscs-risr992.pdf.

WHO. (2001). *Protocol for the assessment of national communicable disease surveillance and response systems*. Retrieved February 05, 2011, from http://www.who.int/csr/resources/publications/surveillance/whocdscs-risr20012.pdf.

WHO. (2002). *Establishing a dialogue on risks from electromagnetic fields*. Retrieved from http://www.who.int/entity/peh-emf/publications/en/emf_final_300dpi_ALL.pdf.

WHO. (2006a). *eHealth tools and services: Needs of the member states*. Geneva, Switzerland: WHO.

WHO. (2006b). *Building foundations for eHealth: Progress of member states*. Geneva, Switzerland: WHO.

WHO. (2010a). *WHO endorses new rapid tuberculosis test: A major milestone for global TB diagnosis and care*. Retrieved March 29, 2011, from http://www.who.int/mediacentre/news/releases/2010/tb_test_20101208/en/.

WHO. (2010b). *Surveillance recommendations for member states in the post-pandemic period*. Retrieved March 20, 2011, from http://www.who.int/csr/resources/publications/swineflu/surveillance_post_pandemic_20100812/en/.

WHO. (2011a). *Health topics*. Retrieved March 20, 2011, from http://www.euro.who.int/en/what-we-do/health-topics.

WHO. (2011b). *Establishing a robust and sustainable human resources information systems in Kenya*. Retrieved from http://www.who.int/workforcealliance/forum/2011/hrhawardscs5/en/index.html.

WHO-CheSS. (2011). *Country health systems surveillance: Health statistics and health information systems*. Retrieved October 20, 2011, from http://www.who.int/healthinfo/country_monitoring_evaluation/en/index.html.

WHOSIS. (2011). *Statistical information system*. Retrieved February 11, 2011, from http://www.who.int/whosis/en/.

Wicks, A. M., Visich, J. K., & Li, S. (2006). Radio frequency identification applications in hospital environments. *Hospital Topics, 84*(3), 3–8. doi:10.3200/HTPS.84.3.3-9

Wiki. (2010). *Website.* Retrieved from http://en.wikipedia. org/wiki/Submarine_communications_cable.

Wiki-2. (2011). *Website.* Retrieved from http:// en.wikipedia.org/wiki.

Wiki-3. (2011). *Website.* Retrieved from http:// en.wikipedia.org/wiki/Telecommunications_indus-try_in_China.

Wiki-4. (2011). *Website.* Retrieved from http:// en.wikipedia.org/wiki/Integrated_Services_Digital_Net-work.

Wilkins, K., Nsubuga, P., Mendlein, J., Mercer, D., & Pappaioanou, M. (2008). The data for decision making project: Assessment of surveillance systems in developing countries to improve access to public health information. *The Journal of the Royal Institute of Public Health and Hygiene, 122,* 914–922.

Willemsen, A. T., van Alste, J. A., & Boom, H. B. (1990). Real-time gait assessment utilizing a new way of accelerometry. *Journal of Biomechanics, 23,* 859–863. doi:10.1016/0021-9290(90)90033-Y

Williamson, L., Stoops, N., & Heywood, A. (2001). Developing a district health information system in South Africa: A social process of technical solution? In Patel, V. L., Rogers, R., & Haux, R. (Eds.), *MEDINFO 2001* (pp. 773–777). Amsterdam, The Netherlands: IOS Press.

Williamson, R., & Andrews, B. J. (2001). Detecting absolute human knee angle and angular velocity using accelerometers and rate gyroscopes. *Medical & Biological Engineering & Computing, 39,* 294–302. doi:10.1007/BF02345283

Wilson, E. A. H., & Wolf, M. S. (2009). Working memory and the design of health materials: A cognitive factors perspective. *Patient Education and Counseling, 74*(3), 318–322. doi:10.1016/j.pec.2008.11.005

Winger, R., & Edelman, D. (1989). *The segment-of-one-marketing.* Boston, MA: The Boston Consulting Group.

Winslow, C. E. A. (1920). The untilled fields of public health. *Science, 51,* 23. doi:10.1126/science.51.1306.23

Winston, W., & Goldberg, J. (2004). *Operations research: Applications and algorithms.* Ottawa, Canada: Duxbury Press.

Wong, R. (2005). *Early CBRN attack detection by computerized record surveillance (ECADS) project: RODS user manual.* Retrieved February 05, 2011, from http://openrods.sourceforge.net/contrib/AMITA_RODS3_documentation.zip.

Woo, A., Madden, S., & Govindan, R. (2004). Networking support for query processing in sensor networks. *Communications of the ACM, 47*(6), 47–50. doi:10.1145/990680.990706

Woods, L. M., Coleman, M. P., Lawrence, G., Rashbass, J., Berrino, F., & Rachet, B. (2011). Evidence against the proposition that "UK cancer survival statistics are misleading": Simulation study with national cancer registry data. *British Medical Journal, 342,* 399. doi:10.1136/bmj.d3399

Wootton, R. (1998). Telemedicine in the national health service. *Journal of the Royal Society of Medicine, 91*(12), 614–621.

World Health Organization. (2003). *Unit costs for patient services.* Retrieved from http://www.who.int/choice/costs/unit_costs/en/index.html.

World Health Organization. (2011a). *Facing the facts: The impact of chronic disease in Canada.* Retrieved February 14, 2011, from http://www.who.int/chp/chronic_disease_report/media/CANADA.pdf.

World Health Organization. (2011b). *Preventing chronic diseases: A vital investment.* Retrieved February 14, 2011, from http://www.who.int/chp/chronic_disease_report/English%20compressed.ppt.

Wright, J., Williams, R., & Wilkinson, J. R. (1998). Health needs assessment: Development and importance of health needs assessment. *British Medical Journal, 316,* 1310–1313. doi:10.1136/bmj.316.7140.1310

Wu, G., Talwar, S., Johnsson, K., Himayat, N., & Johnson, K. D. (2011). M2M: From mobile to embedded internet. *IEEE Communications Magazine, 49*(4), 36–43. doi:10.1109/MCOM.2011.5741144

Wyatt, J. C. (1996). Commentary: Telemedicine trials—Clinical pull or technology push? *British Medical Journal, 313,* 1380. doi:10.1136/bmj.313.7069.1380

Xing, G., Tan, R., Liu, B., Wang, J., Jia, X., & Yi, C. (2009). Data fusion improves the coverage of wireless sensor networks. In *Proceedings of the International Conference on Mobile Computing and Networking*, (pp. 157-168). Beijing, China: IEEE.

Xiong, J., Seet, B.-C., & Symonds, J. (2009). Human activity inference for ubiquitous RFID-based applications. In *Proceedings of the 2009 Symposia and Workshops on Ubiquitous, Autonomic and Trusted Computing*, (pp. 304-309). IEEE.

Xu, W., & Campbell, G. (1992). A near perfect stable random access protocol for a broadcast channel. In *Proceedings of the IEEE International Conference Comunications (ICC)*, (pp. 370 – 374). Chicago, IL: IEEE Press.

Yang, C. C., & Hsu, Y. L. (2010). A review of accelerometry-based wearable motion detectors for physical activity monitoring sensors. *Sensors in Biomechanics and Biomedicine, 10*.

Yang, G.-Z. (Ed.). (2006). *Body sensor networks*. London, UK: Springer-Verlag. doi:10.1007/1-84628-484-8

Yu, Y., Krishnamachari, B., & Prasanna, V. K. (2004). Energy-latency tradeoffs for data gathering in wireless sensor networks. In *Proceedings of IEEE INFOCOM 2004 - Conference on Computer Communications - Twenty-Third Annual Joint Conference of the IEEE Computer and Communications Societies*, (pp. 244-255). Hong Kong, China: IEEE Press.

Yuen, W.-H., Lee, H., & Andersen, T. D. (2002). A simple and effective cross layer networking system for mobile ad hoc networks. In *Proceedings of PIMRC, 2002*, 1952–1956.

Yu, X., Liu, Z., Tian, Z., Li, S., Huang, H., Xiu, B., & Zhao, Q. (2000). Stereotactic biopsy for intracranial space-occupying lesions: Clinical analysis of 550 cases. *Stereotactic and Functional Neurosurgery, 75*, 103–208. doi:10.1159/000048390

Zadeh, L. A. (1965). Fuzzy sets. *Information and Control, 8*(3), 338–353. doi:10.1016/S0019-9958(65)90241-X

Zambuto, R. P. (2004). Clinical engineers in the 21st century. *IEEE Engineering in Medicine and Biology Magazine, 23*(3), 37–41. doi:10.1109/MEMB.2004.1317980

Zapartan, A. (2010). *Tag4 applet - The cloud instrument.* Unpublished Master's Thesis. Cluj-Napoca, Romania: Technical University of Cluj-Napoca. Retrieved from http://www.scribd.com/doc/46245362/Alin-Zapartan-Tag4Applet.

Zarcadoolas, C., Pleasant, A. F., & Greer, D. S. (2006). *Advancing health literacy: A framework for understanding and action.* San Francisco, CA: Josey-Bass.

Zeithaml, V. A., & Bitner, M. J. (2000). *Service marketing: Integrating customer focus across the firm.* New York, NY: McGraw Hill.

ZEPRS. (2011). *Web page.* Retrieved May 12, 2011, from http://www.ictedge.org/zeprs.

Zhang, H., & Shen, H. (2009). Balancing energy consumption to maximize network lifetime in data-gathering sensor networks. *IEEE Transactions on Parallel and Distributed Systems, 20*(10), 1526–1539. doi:10.1109/TPDS.2008.252

Zhao, J., Zhang, Z., Guo, H., Ren, L., & Chen, S. (2010). Development and recent achievements of telemedicine in China. *Telemedicine and e-Health, 16*(5), 634-638.

Zhao, J. A., Xu, Y. X., & Chen, J. (1998). The implementation of telemedicine network group. *China Hospital Management, 18*, 27–28.

Zhijiang, D., Zhiheng, J., & Minxiu, K. (2006). Virtual reality-based telesurgery via teleprogramming scheme combined with semi-autonomous control. In *Proceedings of the 27th Annual International Conference, Engineering in Medicine and Biology Society*, (pp. 2153-2156). Shanghai, China: IEEE.

Zhu, J. H., & Wang, W. (2005). Diffusion, use, and effect of the internet in China. *Communications of the ACM, 48*(4), 49–53. doi:10.1145/1053291.1053317

Zipson, L. (2010). Smartphone vulnerabilities. In *Network Security Pre-Press.* Oxford, UK: Mayfield Press.

About the Contributors

Joel J. P. C. Rodrigues (S'01 - M'06 - SM'06), is a Professor in the Department of Informatics of the University of Beira Interior, Covilhã, Portugal, and a Researcher at the *Instituto de Telecomunicações,* Associated Lab, Portugal. He received a five-year B.S. degree (licentiate) in Informatics Engineering from the University of Coimbra, Portugal, and the M.Sc. degree and Ph.D. degree in Informatics Engineering from the University of Beira Interior, Portugal. His main research interests include delay-tolerant networks, sensor networks, high-speed networks, e-Learning, e-Health, and mobile and ubiquitous computing. He is the leader of the NetGNA Research Group (http://netgna.it.ubi.pt) and the founder and leader of the IEEE ComSoc CSIM Special Interest Group on modeling and simulation tools (http://mst.it.ubi.pt). He is the Secretary of the IEEE ComSoc Technical Committee on eHealth and the Vice-Chair of the IEEE ComSoc Technical Committee on Communications Software. He has authored or coauthored over 170 technical papers in refereed international journals and conferences, book chapters, a book, and a patent. He is the editor-in-chief of the *International Journal on E-Health and Medical Communications*, the editor-in-chief of the *Recent Patent on Telecommunications Journal,* and also served several Special Issues as a Guest Editor (*IEEE Transactions on Multimedia, Elsevier Journal of Network and Computer Applications, IET Communications, Journal of Communications,* etc.). He has served as General Chair, Technical Program Committee Chair, and symposium Chair for many international conferences, including IEEE ICC/GLOBECOMs, CAMAD, MAN, ITST, ICNC, SoftCOM, among others. He participated in tens of international TPCs and several editorial review boards (including *IEEE Communications Magazine, International Journal of Communications Systems*, etc.). He is a licensed professional engineer (as a senior member), and he is member of ACM SIGCOMM, a member of the Internet Society, an IARIA fellow, and a senior member of the IEEE Computer Society, IEEE Communications Society, and IEEE Education Society.

Isabel de la Torre Díez was born in Zamora, Spain, in 1979. She received her M.S. and Ph.D. degrees in telecommunication engineering from the University of Valladolid, Spain, in 2003 and 2010, respectively. Currently, she is an Associate Professor in the Department of Signal Theory and Communications at the University of Valladolid. Her teaching and research interests include development of telemedicine applications, EHRs (Electronic Health Records), EHR standards, biosensors, e-learning, and e-commerce applications. She is author or co-author of nine papers in SCI journals, more than twenty papers in peer-reviewed conference proceedings, two books, and eleven international book chapters.

Beatriz Sainz de Abajo is a Telecommunications Researcher and teacher in the University of Valladolid (Spain). She has a PhD from the University of Cordoba, a Master's in Data Networks and Transportation and a Master's in Occupational Health and Safety. In recent years, she has published several books and book chapters related to access networks, broadband, and e-commerce. Other activities include research papers presented at international conferences and participation in research projects and publication of scientific papers in international journals. She has devoted all her professional life to the investigation of telecommunications regulation matters and to the teaching of novel telecommunications systems. Her fields of experience are Internet services for SMEs and telecommunications policy in the information society. Currently, her research interests include improving the QoS of e-commerce, e-marketing, e-learning, telemedicine, and also digital content both from the user's standpoint and from the competitive market vision and also contributing to the promotion of the entrepreneurial character of the University.

* * *

Nazim Agoulmine (Senior IEEE member) is a full Professor at the University of Evry and Head of LRSM Research Group in the IBISC Lab (France). He received his Engineer degree in 1988 from USTHB (Algeria) and his Master and PhD degrees in Computer Science, respectively, in 1989 and 1992, from the University of Paris XI (France). His research interests include wired/wireless network management/control, autonomic/sensor networks. He is an area editor of the Elsevier's *International Journal on Computer Networks* and a guest editor of *IEEE Communication Magazine, International Journal of Network and System Management,* etc. He has been TPC member (CNSM, IM, NOMS, LANOMS, etc.) and general of international conferences/workshops (IEEE/IM2011, IEEE/LANOMS2009, IEEE/BCN2009, etc). He is co-author of books in network architecture/management and on autonomic networks. He has participated as an expert to European projects RACE(Advance), ESPRIT(Pemmon), ACTS(ICM), IST(Flowthru), ITEA(Adanets), etc., and for research agencies ANR(France), NSERC, FCAR(Canada), HETAC(Ireland), NRK(South Korea).

Sarah Alofaysan is currently pursuing a Master's degree in Health Informatics from King Saud bin Abdulaziz University for Health Sciences in Saudi Arabia. She is concurrently working as a Program Analyst at the National Guard Health Affairs, the leading healthcare provider and healthcare research institute in the region. Her research interests span several fields including health and technology, data warehousing, mobile health, e-Health, data mining, and decision making. Mrs. Alofaysan started her career by earning a Bachelor degree in Information Technology form the College of Computer Sciences at King Saud University. She then worked as a Systems Developer at Ejada Systems, a leading IT services and solutions provider in the Middle East and North Africa. There she worked on the implementation of several governmental projects in transportation, healthcare, and banking sectors. Currently, Mrs. Alofaysan is working on the implementation of Enterprise Data Warehouse at the National Guard Health Affairs.

Luis Alonso obtained the PhD from UPC (Barcelona) in 2001 and got a permanent tenured position at the same University becoming an Associate Professor in 2006. He has been co-founder of the Wireless Communications and Technologies Research Group (WiComTec), to which currently belongs. His current research interests are within the field of medium access protocols, radio resource management, cross-layer optimization, cooperative transmissions, cognitive radio, and QoS features for all kind of wireless communications systems. He has been collaborating with some telecommunications companies working as a consultant for several research projects. He is currently the Project Coordinator of two research projects funded by the European Union, and he has been the coordinator of another three European Projects as well. He is currently the Scientist in Charge of a project that is being carried out in coordination with the Spanish Railway Infrastructure Administrator. He is author of thirty research papers in international journals and magazines, one book, six chapters of books, and more than ninety papers in international congresses and symposiums.

Adina Astilean, PhD, is Professor in the Automation Department at Technical University of Cluj-Napoca, Romania. Her research interests mainly include analysis and development of intelligent control systems, discrete event systems and data communication. She is the author or coauthor of more than 130 papers, published in various scientific journals, refereed conference proceedings and books. Adina Astilean was also member in many conference program committees and symposiums and reviewer in the fields of distributed systems, telemedicine, control engineering, and data communications. She coordinated and was involved in more than 20 national and international research projects. She supervised more than 30 master and PhD students.

Camelia Avram, PhD, is Assistant Professor at Technical University of Cluj-Napoca, Automation Department, Romania. Her research interests concentrate on: designing and implementing of real time applications, discrete event systems, and data communication. Her interests in She is author of 2 books and book chapters and more than 35 conference and journal publications. She also took part of 8 national and international research contracts.

Ahmad Azar has received the M.Sc. degree (2006) in System Dynamics and Ph.D degree (2009) in Adaptive Neuro-Fuzzy Systems from Faculty of Engineering, Cairo University (Egypt). He is currently Assistant Professor in the department of Electrical Communication and Electronics Systems Engineering, Modern Science and Arts University (MSA), Egypt. Dr. Ahmad Azar has worked in the areas of System Dynamics, Intelligent Control and Modelling in Biomedicine, and is the author of more than 35 papers in these subjects. He is an editor of two Books in the field of Fuzzy logic systems and biomedical Engineering. Dr. Ahmad Azar is the Editor in Chief of *International Journal of System Dynamics Applications (IJSDA)* as well as being the editor of a lot of international journals. His biography was selected to appear in the 27th Edition of *Who's Who in the World*, Marquis *Who's Who, USA*, 2010. His current research focuses on the soft computing techniques and intelligent control systems.

Agustín Llamas Ballestero was born in Zamora, Spain. He is a Telecommunications Researcher in the University of Valladolid (Spain). He has participated in an investigation projects in area of e-Health. In the last months, he has worked with Electronic Health Records (EHR). With respect to broadband networks and services, he collaborated with the university as administrator systems. The fields of his short experience are network management. Currently, he is working about technical characteristics of the EHR which have been studied theoretically. He received his degree in Technical Telecommunications Engineering (speciality: Telematics) in 2011 from the University of Valladolid.

Clara Benevolo holds a degree in Business and Economics from the University of Genoa (Italy). She is an Associate Professor in Management at the same institution. She teaches management, international management, and marketing e-business. Her research interests include service and tourism firms, global strategies, internationalization processes and entry modes to foreign markets, relationships between internationalization and adoption of ICT.

Elizabeth Borycki holds a PhD in Health Policy, Management, and Evaluation from the University of Toronto, Toronto, Canada. Elizabeth is an Assistant Professor at the School of Health Information Science at the University of Victoria, Victoria, British Columbia, Canada. Dr. Borycki's research interests include: clinical informatics, patient safety, human factors, educating health professionals about electronic health records, and health services research. Elizabeth has authored and co-authors numerous articles and book chapters examining the effects of health and clinical information systems upon health professional work processes and patient care outcomes. Elizabeth currently sits on the editorial board of *Computers in Biology and Medicine*. She has also edited a number of books in health informatics. She is currently Canada's Health Informatics Association (COACH) academic representative to the International Medical Informatics Association (IMIA) and represents North America as a Vice President on the Board of Directors of IMIA.

Diana Bri was born in Gandia, Valencia (Spain) on February 5, 1986. She received her B.Sc. in Telecommunications Engineering in 2007 at Universitat Politècnica de Valencia (UPV) and a Master's degree called "Master en Tecnologías, Sistemas y Redes de Comunicaciones" in 2011 at UPV. She is currently a Ph.D. student in the Department of Communications of the UPV. Currently, she works as researcher in the Research Institute for Integrated Management of Coastal Areas (IGIC). Until 2011, she had some scientific papers published in several international conferences, several educational papers and some chapters of book. Besides, she had several papers published in international journals (most of them with JCR). Ms. Bri has been technical committee member in several conferences.

Min Chen was an Assistant Professor in School of Computer Science and Engineering at Seoul National University (SNU). He was a Research Associate in Dept. of Computer Science at University of British Columbia (UBC) for half year. He has worked as a Post-Doctoral Fellow in Dept. of Electrical and Computer Engineering at UBC for three years since Mar. 2009. Before joining UBC, he was a Post-Doctoral Fellow at SNU for one and half years. He has published more than 90 technical papers. He is the sole author of a textbook, *OPNET Network Simulation* (Tsinghua Univ. Press, 2004). Dr. Chen received the Best Paper Runner-up Award from The Fifth International Conference on Heterogeneous Networking for Quality, Reliability, Security and Robustness (QShine) 2008. He serves as editor or associate editor for Wiley *International Journal of Security and Communication Networks, Journal of Internet Technology, KSII Transactions on Internet and Information Systems, IET Communications, International Journal of Sensor Networks (IJSNet)*. He is a managing editor for *International Journal of Autonomous and Adaptive Communications Systems*. He has worked as session chairs in several conferences, such as VTC'08, QShine'08, ICACT'09, Trientcom'09, and ICC'09. He is a TPC co-chair of BodyNets 2010. He is a symposia co-chair and workshop chair of CHINACOM 2010. He is the co-chair of MMASN-09, UBSN-10, and NCAS-11. He was the TPC chair of ASIT-09, ASIT-10, TPC co-chair of PCSI-09, PCSI-10, and UMES-11 publicity co-chair of PICom-09. He serves as the corresponding guest editors for several international journals, such as *ACM/Springer Mobile Networks and Applications (MONET), International Journal of Communications System (IJCS)*. He is an IEEE senior member.

Richard Comley has over 30 years experience in the areas of signal processing and algorithms. He received his PhD in 1978 from City University, London, for work on EEG signal processing and is currently the Associate Dean for Research in the School of Engineering and Information Sciences (EIS) at Middlesex University. Current interests include surveillance and navigation systems, brain-computer interfaces, and distributed architectures. In his role as Associate Dean for Research, he has responsibility for all research activities in the EIS School, which includes approx. £3.5m of project grants, £0.5m RAE funding, and approx 60 research students.

Liezl van Dyk is a Senior Lecturer in Industrial Engineering at Stellenbosch University, South Africa and holds post graduate qualifications in Industrial Engineering, Systems Engineering, and Teaching and Training Practice. She is heading the Health Systems Engineering research team at her department with a specific personal interest in Telemedicine. As such, she is a member of the organizing committee of the South African Telemedicine and eHealth conference (www.satelemedicine.co.za) as well as one of the facilitators of a post graduate certificate course in Telemedicine. She is also a member of the Biomedical Engineering Research Group (www.sun.ac.za/berg) at Stellenbosch University.

Marijan Erceg, MD, MSc in 1987 graduated Medicine, 1994 MSc degree at the University of Zagreb, School of Medicine, 2006 specialization of Epidemiology. Current position: Head of Department of Health Statistics and Medical Informatics in the Croatian National Public Health Institute. His Research interest includes Medical Informatics (data structure and organization, electronic health record, standardization in medical informatics) and Public Health (national public health information system, e-health principles, information based cardiovascular prevention, web technologies in health promotion). His Professional activities include membership in medical informatics and public health associations. Some of his recent projects include Development of National health indicators information system; Development of *Croatian Journal of Public Health.*

José Bringel Filho is a Postdoctoral Research Fellow at University of Evry Val d'Essonne (UEVE) and member of LRSM team (IBISC laboratory) led by Nazim Agoulmine. He received his B.S. degree in Computer Science from Federal University of Piauí (UFPI) in 2000 (Brazil), his M.S. degree in Computer Science from Federal University of Ceará (UFC – Great team) in 2004 (Brazil), and his Ph. D. degree in Computer Science from University of Grenoble (UJF – Steamer team) in 2010 (France). He was a NII Internship Student at National Institute of Informatics (Tokyo – Japan) in 2009 (March-July), working under the supervision of Prof. Ichiro Satoh. His research interests have included context-aware systems, quality, and privacy of context information, context-based access control models, semantic-based knowledge representation and reasoning applied to ubiquitous and pervasive systems.

Kristina Fišter, MD, PhD in 2001 graduated Medical school, 2007 MSc degree, and 2011 PhD, all at the University of Zagreb. Current position: Research Fellow at the University of Zagreb, School of Medicine, Andrija Štampar School of Public Health. Her research interests include epidemiology and public health (obesity; prevention of cardiovascular diseases and type 2 diabetes; women of childbearing age; mental and neurological public health; public health information systems; e-health; predictive systems); medical informatics (data structure and organization; electronic health record; standardization; data analysis and knowledge discovery; free-text analysis); the science of peer review. Her professional activities include membership in medical, obesity, medical informatics, and public health associations. Some of her recent projects include International Cooperative Action on Grid Computing and Biomedical Informatics between the EU, Latin America, the Western Balkans and North Africa, ACTION Grid - FP7; Regionalism of behavioral cardiovascular risks – model of intervention.

Silviu Folea, PhD, is Associate Professor at Technical University of Cluj-Napoca, Automation Department, Romania. His research interests include: embedded systems—hardware and software, reconfigurable systems, data acquisition, wireless networks and low power sensors. His software interests include LabVIEW graphical programming for Real Time, FPGA or PDA modules with courses taught at bachelor and master degree. Professor Folea has fifteen years of design experience in the embedded systems domain and in university teaching. He is the author of 6 books and book chapters and of more than 60 conference and journal publications, some indexed in international databases. Professor Folea took part in more than 25 research contracts. Some of the most important and interesting research contracts were carried out in collaboration with National Instruments Corporate USA. Two patents resulted from these research contracts in the USA. He worked for National Instruments Romania between the years 2005 and 2007.

Xiaohong Gao is a reader on imaging sciences at Middlesex University in London, UK. Her research interests span from computer vision on head motion detection, traffic sign recognition, and colour image retrieval to medical applications including telemedicine, medical informatics, and image processing. She has published widely on these fields and attracted many funding awards from both UK research councils (EPSRC, JISC, and the Royal Society) and European Commission (EC). Her latest EC funded FP7 project, WIDTH (2011-2014), is working on warehousing images in the digital hospital.

Miguel Garcia was born in Benissa, Alicante (Spain) on December 29, 1984. He received his M.Sc. in Telecommunications Engineering in 2007 at Universitat Politècnica de Valencia (UPV) and a Master's degree called "Master en Tecnologías, Sistemas y Redes de Comunicaciones" in 2008 at UPV. He is currently a Ph.D. student in the Department of Communications of the UPV. He has been a CCNA instructor since 2007. Currently, he works as researcher in Research Institute for Integrated Management of Coastal Areas (IGIC). Until 2011, he had more than 40 scientific papers published in several international conferences and more than 25 papers published in international journals (most of them with JCR). Mr. Garcia has been technical committee member in several conferences and journals. Miguel is associate editor of *International Journal Networks, Protocols and Algorithms* and *Advances in Network and Communications*. He is IEEE graduate student member.

Nuno M. Garcia is an Invited Professor at the University of Beira Interior, Covilhã, Portugal, and a Professor at the School of Communication, Arts and Information Technologies of the Lusophone University of Humanities and Technologies in Lisbon, Portugal. He holds a PhD degree from the University of Beira Interior, Covilhã, Portugal. He is currently coordinator of the Assisted Living Computing and Telecommunications Laboratory, a research group within the Institute of Telecommunications pole at the University of Beira Interior. His main interests include Next-Generation Networks, advanced algorithms for bio-signal processing, distributed and cooperative protocols. He is main author of several international and European patents. He is an ISOC member and a IEEE Member.

Hongwei Ge received B.S. and M.S. degrees in mathematics from Jilin University, China, and the Ph.D degree in Computer Application Technology from Jilin University, in 2006. He is currently a Vice Professor in the College of Electronic and Information Engineering, Dalian University of Technology, Dalian, China. His research interests are computational intelligence, optimization and modeling, system control, social network, and bioinformatics. He has published more than 40 papers in these areas. His research was featured in the *IEEE Transactions on Systems, Man, and Cybernetics*, the *Computers and Structures*, the *Nonlinear Analysis: Real World Applications*, the *Advances in Soft Computing,* and the *Nero-Computing*.

Antônio Tadeu A. Gomes is a Researcher at the National Laboratory for Scientific Computing (LNCC), Brazil. He is Head of the Mechanisms and Architectures for Tele-informatics Research Group (MARTIN), and the Executive Officer of the Brazilian National System for High-Performance Computing (SINAPAD). He received his Ph.D. in Computer Science from the Pontifical Catholic University of Rio de Janeiro (PUC-Rio), Brazil, in 2005. His research interests include quality of service, mobile computing, high-performance computing, and software architecture and modeling. He is a member of the Association for Computing Machinery (ACM) and the Brazilian Computer Society (SBC). He is recipient of the productivity research award PQ-2 from the Brazilian Research Council (CNPq).

John Hale is a Professor of Computer Science and Faculty Researcher in the Institute for Information Security at the University of Tulsa. He received his Bachelor of Science in 1990, Master of Science in 1992, and Doctorate degree in 1997, all in Computer Science from the University of Tulsa. Dr. Hale has overseen the development of the premier information assurance curriculum in the nation. In 2000, he earned a prestigious National Science Foundation CAREER award for his education and research initiatives at iSec. His research interests include cyber attack modeling, analysis and visualization, enterprise security management, secure operating systems, distributed system verification, and policy coordination.

Peter J. Hawrylak, is an Assistant Professor in the Electrical Engineering department at The University of Tulsa (TU), is vice-chair of the AIM RFID Experts Group (REG), and chair of the Healthcare Initiative (HCI) sub-group of the AIM REG. Dr. Hawrylak is a member of The University of Tulsa's Institute for Information Security (iSec), which is a NSA (U.S. National Security Agency) Center of Excellence. Peter has four (4) issued patents in the RFID space and numerous academic publications. Peter's research interests are in the areas embedded system security, RFID, embedded systems, and low power wireless systems. He is Associate Editor of the *International Journal of Radio Frequency Identification Technology and Applications (IJRFITA)* journal published by InterScience Publishers, which focuses on the application and development of RFID technology.

Mowafa Househ is an Assistant Professor and the Research Director at the College of Public Health and Health Informatics. Dr. Househ worked as a planning and research analyst with the Northern Health Authority and an instructor at the University of Northern British Columbia for over three years prior to coming to Saudi Arabia. One of Dr. Househ's main achievements is being the first researcher to introduce the Action Case research method to health informatics research. Dr. Househ's research interests cover a range of topics that include: mobile health, E-learning, collaborative technologies, knowledge, translation, action case, and mixed methods research.

Mihai Hulea, PhD, is Assistant Professor at Technical University of Cluj-Napoca, Automation Department, Romania. His research interests include: distributed control systems, real-time systems, and traffic control systems. His software interests include design and development of distributed applications based on J2EE and .NET platforms and also development applications for devices with limited resources. He is author of 3 books and book chapters and 25 conference and journal publications. He also took part of 6 national and international research contracts.

Davor Ivankovic, MD, DPH, PhD, 1969 graduated Medicine, 1972 DPH, 1976 MSc degree, and 1986 PhD degree at the University of Zagreb, School of Medicine, Specialist in Epidemiology 1989. Current position: professor of Medical statistics at the University of Zagreb, School of Medicine. Research interest: Medical Statistics (Research design and data analysis in biomedical research, statistical peer review) & Public health (methodology of Health Care Quality Assurance, Health measurement). Professional activities: membership in medical informatics, biometrics and public health associations. Recent projects: Regionalism of behavioral cardiovascular risks – model of intervention; Prediction models in medicine; How to measure Health?.

Débora Helena Job worked during three years as a network analyst at the Internet Data Center of Unisys Network in Brazil. Between 2008 and 2010, she pursued a M.Sc. degree in Computing and System Engineering in the Military Institute of Engineering (IME), Brazil. After obtaining the M.Sc. degree, between 2010 and 2011 she has held a position of research assistant at the National Laboratory for Scientific Computing (LNCC), Brazil, where this work has been developed. Currently, she is with Altran Brazil.

Josipa Kern, PhD in 1972 graduated Mathematics, 1981 MSc degree, and 1990 PhD at the University of Zagreb, Faculty of Science and Mathematics. Her current position is a professor of Medical informatics at the University of Zagreb, School of Medicine. Research interest: Medical Informatics (data structure and organization, electronic health record, standardization in medical informatics, data analysis and knowledge discovery, free-text analysis) and Public health (public health information system, e-health principles, information based cardiovascular prevention, predictive systems).Professional activities: membership in medical informatics and public health associations, president of national Technical Committee for standardization in medical informatics (HZN/TC215). Her recent projects include International Cooperative Action on Grid Computing and Biomedical Informatics between the EU, Latin America, the Western Balkans and North Africa (ACTION Grid - FP7; Regionalism of behavioral cardiovascular risks – model of intervention; Prediction models in medicine.

Andre Kushniruk is a Professor in the School of Health Information Science at the University of Victoria. Dr. Kushniruk conducts research in a number of areas including evaluation of the effects of technology, human-computer interaction in health care and other domains as well as cognitive science. His work is known internationally and he has published widely in the area of health informatics. He focuses on developing new methods for the evaluation of information technology and studying human-computer interaction in health care in studies of both technology designed for healthcare providers and patients. He has been a key researcher on a number of national and international collaborative projects. He holds undergraduate degrees in Psychology and Biology, as well as a M.Sc. in Computer Science from McMaster University and a Ph.D. in Cognitive Psychology from McGill University.

Kai Lin is an Assistant Professor at the School of Computer Science and Engineering, Dalian University of Technology. He received his B.S. degree in the School of Electronic and Information Engineering, Dalian University of Technology, Dalian, China in 2001, and obtained M.S. and PhD degree from the College of Information Science and Engineering, Northeastern University, Shen Yang, China in 2005 and 2008, respectively. His research interests include wireless networks, ubiquitous computing, and embedded technology.

Jaime Lloret received his M.Sc. in Physics in 1997, his M.Sc. in electronic Engineering in 2003 and his Ph.D. in telecommunication engineering (Dr. Ing.) in 2006. He is a Cisco Certified Network Professional Instructor. He worked as a network designer and as an administrator in several enterprises. He is currently Associate Professor in the Polytechnic University of Valencia and he is the research line coordinator of the "Communications and Remote Sensing" of the Integrated Management Coastal Research Institute. He is coordinating the "Active and Collaborative Techniques and use of Technologic Resources in the Education (EITACURTE)" Innovation Group. He is the director of the University Expert Certificate "Redes y Comunicaciones de Ordenadores" and of the University Expert Certificate "Tecnologías Web y Comercio Electrónico." He is currently the Cognitive Networks Technical Committee (IEEE Communications Society) Vice-chair for the Europe/Africa Region. He has 1 research book, and more than 155 research papers published in national and international conferences, international journals (most of them with Impact Factor in Journal Citation Report), and books. He has 11 educational books, and more than 55 papers published in international conferences, journals and books of education. He has been the co-editor of 15 conference proceedings and guest editor of several international books and journals. He is editor-in-chief of the international journal *Networks Protocols and Algorithms*, editor-in-chief of the international journal *Advances in Network and Communications*, IARIA Journals Board Chair (8 Journals) and he is associate editor of several international journals. He has been involved in more than 120 Program committees of international conferences and in several organization and steering committees until 2010. He has been the general chair of SENSORCOMM 2007, UBICOMM 2008, ICNS 2009, and ICWMC 2010 and co-chairman of ICAS 2009 and INTERNET 2010. He is the co-chairman of IEEE MASS 2011, SCPA 2011 and ICDS 2012, and chairman eKNOW 2012. He is IEEE Senior Member and IARIA Fellow Member.

Martin Loomes is Dean of Engineering and Information Sciences at Middlesex University. His research falls at the cusp between Computer Science, Mathematics and Psychology, with a particular focus on the ways theories are formulated, presented and used in complex tasks, particularly those with a safety-critical aspect. He has published widely in the area of image analysis applied to activities including medical imaging, handwriting analysis and face recognition. He has held grants from a wide variety of sources including the EPSRC, ESRC, European Commission and US Department of Homeland Security, with recent awards in the areas of image analysis and visual analytics (the use of visualisation to support the analysis of complex heterogeneous data sets).

José Mendes Lucas graduated in Textile Engineering by the University of Beira Interior (UBI) in 1981. In 1983 he concluded the Master of Science in Textile Science at Clemson University (USA). In 1987, he concluded the PhD degree in the same university in Textile and Polymer Science, field of Colour Science. He is a Researcher at Textile and Paper Research Unit of UBI. He is the author and co-author of several papers in textile physics and smart clothing areas. He is Associate Professor, the Director of PhD Program in Textile Engineering and Textile Area Coordinator of Textile and Paper Research Unit of UBI.

Henrique Martins is an Internal Medicine Specialist. He obtained his PhD degree from the Judge Business School, University of Cambridge with a thesis on "The use of Mobile ICT in Clinical Settings." He holds a Master in Management from the University of Cambridge and a Masters in HIV/AIDS from the University of Barcelona. He has several publications in the area of Mobile computing in healthcare and currently, he works as an Internist and CMIO—Chief Medical Information Officer at the Hospital Fernando Fonseca where he also coordinates the Center for Research and Creativity in Informatics (www.ci2.pt), where he supervises projects in mobile computing and intelligent systems. He teaches health management, leadership, and medical informatics in Portugal and abroad.

Rui Alberto Lopes Miguel is graduated in Textile Engineering by the University of Beira Interior (UBI). He started his professional activity in 1979 in the Wool Industry as production and quality control director. In 1987, he started his academic career at UBI in the field of Textile Engineering and Fashion Design. In 1992 he started the doctoral works at CSIC-Barcelona in the field of fabric mechanics and performance. In 2000, he presented the PhD thesis in Textile Engineering at UBI. He is researcher at Textile and Paper Research Unit of UBI. He is author and co-author of several papers in textile physics, smart clothing and fashion design areas. He is responsible of many studies and projects with the industry. He was a consultant of Portuguese Air Force. He is Associate Professor, the Director of Master Program in Branding and Fashion Design and the Head of the Textile Department of UBI.

Rupananda Misra has worked for over 13 years in Philadelphia, Pennsylvania in the United States as a Professor at The Art Institute of Philadelphia, and as an Adjunct Associate Professor at Drexel University—focusing on the teaching of interactive multimedia technologies. In addition, he serves as a member of the adjunct faculty teaching Health Communication courses at West Virginia University, Morgantown, West Virginia. His education and training for this work includes a Master's degree in Communications from Fort Hays State University, Hays, Kansas; and, a Doctoral degree in Education/ Communication from Columbia University, New York, New York. Dr. Misra completed a two-year post doctoral fellowship in Health Informatics at Columbia University, New York, New York.

Begonya Otal is a Postdoctoral Researcher at the Department of Neurosciences of the Institute of Biomedical Research August Pi Sunyer (IDIBAPS)—Hospital Clinic of Barcelona. She is currently working in a research project aiming to study functional connectivity networks in brain diseases using fMRI, network theory and computational modelling. In 2001, she obtained her M.Sc. degree in Tele-communications Engineering from the Polytechnic University of Catalonia (UPC), Barcelona. From 2001 to 2006, she worked as a Research Scientist for Philips Research Europe (Aachen, Germany) and was involved in a number of industrial and public-funded projects, and participated in standardization activities. She co-authored more than 20 invention disclosures from which 7 became patent application. From 2006 to 2009, she performed her Ph.D. in the Technology Center for Communications of Catalonia (CTTC), where she was awarded with a grant, and published several journal, conference papers and book chapters. Her research was mainly focused on the optimisation of wireless body sensor networks in the medical domain.

Mauricio Papa is an Associate Professor for the Department of Computer Science at The University of Tulsa. He also serves as Faculty Director of the Institute for Information Security, which supports a multi-disciplinary program of study and research tackling cyber security issues on a global scale. Dr. Papa received his Bachelor of Science in electrical engineering from Universidad Central de Venezuela in 1992 and his Master of Science in electrical engineering and Doctorate degree in Computer Science from TU in 1996 and 2001, respectively. His primary research area is critical infrastructure protection. Propelled by a world-class research program in SCADA network security, Dr. Papa and his team designed and constructed a novel process control network test bed to address cyber security needs for the critical infrastructure. He also conducts research in distributed systems, network security, cryptographic protocol verification, and intelligent control systems.

Tamara Poljičanin, MD, MSc, PhD in 1998 graduated Medicine at the University of Zagreb, School of Medicine. 2004 MSc degree earned at the Faculty of Science and Mathematics, and 2010 PhD at the School of Medicine, both at the University of Zagreb. Specialist in Epidemiology 2005. Current positions: Head of the Division of Epidemiology, Vuk Vrhovac University Clinic, Merkur Clinical Hospital, Zagreb; Project Manager, National Diabetes Registry. Her research interests include epidemiology (diabetes mellitus, registries, epidemiological methods), organization of health care (quality of care, quality management), data collection and analysis, modeling. Her professional activities include membership in epidemiological, public health, and diabetes associations. Some of her recent projects include EUBIROD – EUropean Best Information through Regional Outcomes in Diabetes supported by the European Commission; Frequency of Chronic Complications of Diabetes in the Republic of Croatia; Type 1 Diabetes Mortality in Zagreb – Trends; Prevalence and Risk Factors of Depression in Diabetic Patients.

Nakeisha Schimke is a Postdoctoral Researcher with the Institute of Bioinformatics and Computational Biology at The University of Tulsa (TU). Dr. Schimke's research interests include health information privacy and neuroinformatics.

Paula Sofia Sousa graduated in Biomedical Sciences (University of Beira Interior, Covilhã, Portugal) in 2008, and in 2010 she completed the Master's degree in Biomedical Sciences (University of Beira Interior, Covilhã, Portugal), in which she demonstrated a great interest in biomedical signal analysis and processing. Currently, she is involved in research activities in the Assisted Living Computing and Telecommunications Laboratory – AALab, a research group within the Network Group of Institute of Telecommunications at the University of Beira Interior, Covilhã, Portugal. Her research interests are based on health monitoring, including biomedical applications and instrumentation, and medical signal acquisition, analysis, and processing.

Slavica Sović, MD in 2001 graduated School of Medicine, PhD candidate at the University of Zagreb, School of Medicine. Her current position is a research fellow at the University of Zagreb, School of Medicine. Her research interests include medical informatics and public health. Her professional activities include membership in medical informatics and public health associations. She also had work on the project: How to Measure Health?

Riccardo Spinelli received his PhD in Service Management and Economics from the University of Genoa (Italy). He is an Assistant Professor in Management at the same institution. He teaches International Management and Marketing. His research interests include the foundations of the digital economy, the relationship between the development of e-business and the internationalization of firms, the application of ICT in SMEs and the management of SMEs.

Maria Jacoba (Miekie) Treurnicht is a young Industrial Engineer continuing her postgraduate studies at Stellenbosch University in South Africa. She is a senior research student in the Health Systems Engineering research group at Stellenbosch University and served in a variety of assistantship positions in research and teaching. During her studies, she was involved in a various consulting, system design and evaluation projects. She is a member of the Institute of Industrial Engineers (IIE), IIE Society of Health Systems, and the Operations Research Society of South Africa (ORSSA). Apart from winning departmental prizes at her university, she also won a student paper competition at the IIE Society of Health Systems (SHS) and American Society for Quality (ASQ) conference, held in Atlanta, Georgia, USA. As part of her personal aim to perform research that would make a difference in the developing world, she regularly presents at conferences in e-Health and Industrial Engineering.

Isabel G. Trindade graduated in Technological Physics from the University of Lisbon, Lisbon, Portugal, and received the Ph.D. degree in Electrical and Computer Engineering in 2000. During her Ph.D., she worked at the Data Storage Systems Center, Carnegie Mellon University, Pittsburgh USA. She worked three years with the industry in USA and England in the field of magnetic thin film devices. In 1995, she joined the Univertsity of Porto, where she was responsible for two projects funded by the Portuguese Ministry of Science and Technology; PTDC/CTM/66558/2006, "Strain Sensor Arrays for e-Textile and Health Care," and POCI/DG/CTM/63999/2006, "Micro-Devices and Nanostructures: Parametric Models, Prototype Fabrication and its Optimization." She is currently Research Assistant at Universidade da Beira Interior and UMTP, Covilhã, Portugal, working in the field of functional materials, sensors and actuators, and smart clothing. She also has interests in micro and nanotechnologies, and in technological basis entrepreneurship.

Carlos Turró received his M.Sc. Telecommunication Engineering in 1992 and his Ph.D. in Telecommunication Engineering (Dr. Ing.) in 2003. He works as network administrator and Head of Media Services at the Polytechnic University of Valencia. He has published more than 30 research papers in national and international conferences, international journals and books. He has also been reviewer for IEEE and IARIA journals. Currently his research interests deal with the delivery of media content on the Computer Network of the University and to the Internet and on the development of novel e-learning applications.

Christos Verikoukis got his Ph.D. from the Technical University of Catalonia in 2000. He is currently a Senior Researcher at CTTC and an Adjunct Professor at UB. His area of expertise is in the design of energy efficient layer 2 protocols and RRM algorithms, for short range wireless cooperative and network coded communications. Dr. Verikoukis has participated in and coordinated several national and European projects. He has published 35 journal papers and over 80 conference papers. He is also co-author in 2 books, 12 chapters in different books and in 2 patents. Dr. Verikoukis has participated more than 20 competitive projects (IST, ICT, CELTIC, MEDEA+, CATRENE, Marie-Curie, COST) while he has served as the Principal investigator in 3 national projects in Greece and Spain as well as the technical manager in 5 Marie-Curie and 2 Celtic projects. In addition Dr. Verikoukis has served as an external consultant to different companies (e.g., Lantiq S.A., VIDAVO S.A.) He has served as co-editor in 5 special issues while he has participated in the organization of several international conferences. He is also a regular reviewer in a number of international journals. He has appointed to serve as a reviewer in FP7 projects and as an evaluator in ARTEMIS-JU and in research funded programs in Greece and in Spain. He has supervised 10 Ph.D. students and 2 Post Docs researchers since 2004.

Emeritus Silvije Vuletić, MD, DPH, PhD in 1956 graduated Medicine, 1959 Diploma of Public Health, and 1965 PhD at the University of Zagreb, School of Medicine. Previous position: Professor of Medical Statistics. Current position: Professor Emeritus at the University of Zagreb. His research interests include Health survey and surveillance, qualitative and quantitative methods in public health, naturalistic inquiry, behavioral cardiovascular risk factors at the population level and intervention with aim to consolidate prevalence and incidence of such risks. His professional activities include membership in public health and medical informatics associations. Some of his recent projects include International Cooperative Action on Grid Computing and Biomedical Informatics between the EU, Latin America, the Western Balkans and North Africa (ACTION Grid - FP7); Regionalism of behavioral cardiovascular risks – model of intervention.

Barbara C. Wallace is a Clinical Psychologist, Professor of Health Education, Coordinator of the Program in Health Education, Director of the Research Group on Disparities in Health, and Director of Global HELP (Health Education and Leadership Program)—within the Department of Health and Behavior Studies, Teachers College, Columbia University. She has been honored for her outstanding and unusual contributions to psychology with the status of Fellow— within Divisions 50 (Addictive Behaviors) and 45 (Society for the Psychological Study of Ethnic Minority Issues) of the American Psychological Association. Among her 7 academic books, Dr. Wallace notes two relevant books, in particular: *HIV/AIDS Peer Education Training Manual: Combining African Healing Wisdom and Evidence-Based Behavior Change Strategies* (2005); and, *Toward Equity in Health: A New Global Approach to Health Disparities* (2008). She is also Editor-in-Chief of the online *Journal of Equity in Health*.

Artur Ziviani received the B.Sc. degree in Electronics Engineering in 1998 and the M.Sc. degree in Electrical Engineering (with emphasis in Computer Networking) in 1999, both from the Federal University of Rio de Janeiro (UFRJ), Brazil. In December 2003, he received the Ph.D. degree in Computer Science from the University Pierre et Marie Curie (Paris 6), Paris, France, where he has also been a lecturer during the 2003-2004 academic year. Since September 2004, he is with the National Laboratory for Scientific Computing (LNCC), located in Petrópolis, Brazil, where he heads with Antonio Tadeu Azevedo Gomes the MARTIN R&D group. From September 2008 to January 2009, he was a visiting researcher at the INRIA's ASAP and D-NET teams in France. His research interests include network measurements, mobile computing, complex networks, and computer-aided healthcare. He is recipient of the productivity research award PQ-1D from the Brazilian Research Council (CNPq). He is also a member of SBC (the Brazilian Computing Society) and a Senior Member of both IEEE and ACM.

Index

CPSIA information can be obtained at www.ICGtesting.com
Printed in the USA
BVOW042117020412

286316BV00015B/2/P